Voice Quality Measurement

Voice Quality Measurement

Editors

Raymond D. Kent, Ph.D.
Department of Communicative Disorders
University of Wisconsin, Madison
Madison, Wisconsin

Martin J. Ball, Ph.D.
University of Ulster at Jordanstown
Newtownabbey, North Ireland

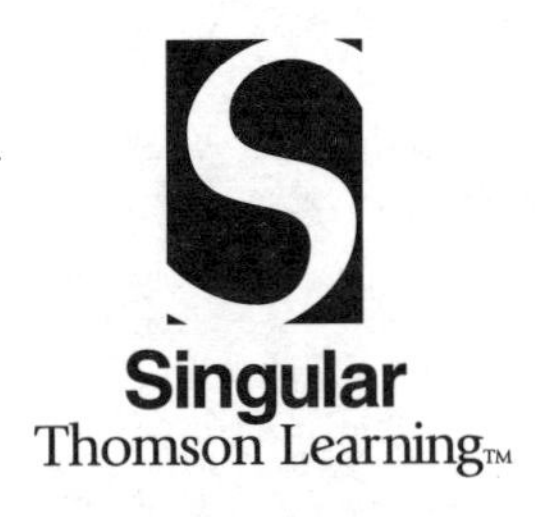

Singular
Thomson Learning™

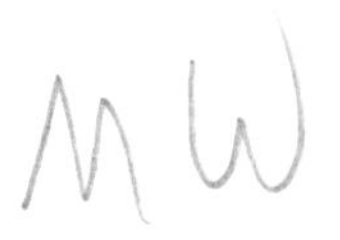

Singular Publishing Group
A Division of Thomson Learning
401 West "A" Street, Suite 325
San Diego, California 92101-7904

Singular Publishing Group publishes textbooks, clinical manuals, clinical reference books, journals, videos, and multimedia materials on speech-language pathology, audiology, otorhinolaryngology, special education, early childhood, aging, occupational therapy, physical therapy, rehabilitation, counseling, mental health, and voice. For your convenience, our entire catalog can be accessed on our website at **http://www.singpub.com.** Our mission to provide you with materials to meet the daily challenges of the ever-changing health care/educational environment will remain on course if we are in touch with you. In that spirit, we welcome your feedback on our products. Please telephone (**1-800-521-8545**), fax (**1-800-774-8398**), or e-mail (**singpub@singpub.com**) your comments and requests to us.

Typeset in 10/12 Palatino Light by D & G Limited, LLC
Printed in Canada by Transcontinental Printing

Library of Congress Cataloging-in-Publication Data

Voice quality measurement / edited by Raymond D. Kent, Martin J. Ball.
p. cm.
Includes bibliographical references and index.
ISBN 1-56593-991-3 (hbk. : alk. paper)
1. Voice disorders. 2. Voice—Physiological aspects. I. Kent, Raymond D. II. Ball, Martin J. (Martin John)
RF510.V67 1999
616.85'5—dc21

99-19664
CIP

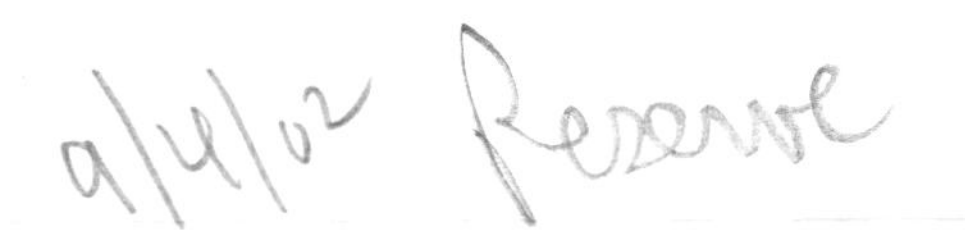

Contents

Preface

This book had its inspiration in the editors' belief that recent research on voice quality has reached a level that invites an integration and stock-taking. Voice quality is a concept that is at once widely recognized and very difficult to define in a way that is universally satisfactory. The term is used by many specialists for many different purposes. Voice quality can range from the ideal to the acceptable to the disordered, and numerous methods have been applied to its measurement.

Perceptual assessment of voice quality has a long history but also, we believe, a new horizon. For that reason, we invited contributors with expertise in this area to prepare chapters that present perspectives and ideas on how voice quality can be assessed perceptually. These eight chapters, which comprise Part I of the book, prove that perceptual assessment is not merely a historic legacy but, in fact, a progressive arena of theory and practice. The contributors point the way to greater validity and reliability in the perceptual definition of voice qualities. This progress is especially important to those who believe that voice quality is ultimately a perceptual phenomenon and that all attempts to study it must of necessity deal with perceptual judgments.

A variety of instrumental (acoustic and physiologic) methods also have been applied to the study of voice quality; and in this area, too, progress has been considerable. Part II contains six chapters pertaining to these methods. At the very least, instrumental procedures afford a degree of quantification and an essential replicability. Of the many different methods that have been proposed, several of the most productive ones are represented in Part II. The methods differ not only in kind but also in their refinements and accumulated database. We chose not to impose an artificial uniformity on these chapters but rather to give the experts the opportunity to present the methods as they thought best.

Part III considers voice states and disorders, that is, voice qualities associated with emotional states, development and aging, personality, and a number of vocal and related pathologies. These 10 chapters discuss phenomena that have come into relief largely through the application of methods such as those described in the first two parts of the book. These chapters are partly a chronicle of progress but also a compass that points to future work. They reflect how voice quality permeates a spectrum of issues in human communication.

Research moves forward on the wheels of technology, driven by the engine of scientific inquiry. This is true of voice quality, even though some might believe that voice quality is so subjective as to be nearly diaphanous. We think that the chapters in this book demonstrate convincingly that voice quality is the subject of earnest scientific study that has harnessed technology and empirical method to reach new depths of understanding.

We deeply appreciate the contributors' enthusiasm for our idea of bringing together in a single volume contemporary statements about voice quality. We feel that the chapters individually and collectively point to an important conclusion: Although voice quality measurement is a difficult task, it is an important objective in the laboratory, the clinic, and the studio, and recent advances carry exciting potential.

Contributors

Evelyn Abberton
Department of Phonetics and Linguistics
University College London
United Kingdom

Abeer A. Alwan
Associate Professor
Electrical Engineering Department
University of California, Los Angeles
Los Angeles, California

Martin J. Ball, Ph.D
University of Ulster at Jordanstown
Newtownabbey, Northern Ireland

Philbert T. Bangayan, M.S.
Research Scientist
Rockwell Science Center
Thousand Oaks, California

Diane M. Bless, Ph.D.
Professor
University of Wisconsin–Madison
Madison, Wisconsin

Eugene H. Buder, Ph.D.
School of Audiology and Speech-Language Pathology
Memphis Speech and Hearing Center
The University of Memphis
Memphis, Tennessee

Daniel E. Callan
Visiting Researcher
ATR Human Information Processing Laboratories
Kyoto, Japan

Michael P. Cannito, Ph.D.
Associate Professor
School of Audiology and Speech-Language Pathology
Memphis Speech and Hearing Center
The University of Memphis
Memphis, Tennessee

Nadine P. Connor, Ph.D.
Research Director
Division of Otolaryngology—Head and Neck Surgery
Department of Surgery
University of Wisconsin Hospital and Clinics
Madison, Wisconsin

Kim Corbin-Lewis, Ph.D.
Assistant Professor
Department of Communicative Disorders and Deaf Education
Utah State University
Logan, Utah

Bert Cranen
Department of Language and Speech
Nijmegen University
Nijmegen, The Netherlands

F. de Jong, M.D.
Department of Voice and Speech Pathology
University Hospital Nïmegen
Nïmegen, The Netherlands

Craig Dickson

Gerald J. Docherty, Ph.D.
Senior Lecturer
Department of Speech
University of Newcastle-Upon-Tyne
United Kingdom

John H. Esling
Associate Professor
Department of Linguistics
University of Victoria
Victoria, British Columbia, Canada

Charles N. Ford, M.D.
Professor and Chairman
Division of Otolaryngology—Head and Neck Surgery
University of Wisconsin Hospital and Clinics
Madison, Wisconsin

Adrian Fourcin
Professor
Department of Phonetics and Language
University College London
United Kingdom

Bruce R. Gerratt, Ph.D.
Division of Head and Neck Surgery
UCLA School of Medicine
Los Angeles, California

Robert E. Hillman, Ph.D.
Voice and Speech Laboratory
Massachusetts Eye and Ear Infirmary
& Harvard Medical School
Boston, Massachusetts

Minoru Hirano, M.D., Ph.D.
President
Kurume University
Kurume, Japan

Harry Hollien, Ph.D.
IASCP
University of Florida
Gainseville, Florida

Philip Hoole
Institut für Phonetik
Ludwig-Maximilians-Universität
Munich, Germany

Thomas S. Johnson, Ph.D.
Professor and Head
Department of Communicative Disorders and Deaf Education
Utah State University
Logan, Utah

Raymond D. Kent, Ph.D.
Department of Communicative Disorders
University of Wisconsin, Madison
Madison, Wiconsin

Shigeru Kiritani
Professor
Department of Cognitive and Speech Sciences
Faculty of Medicine
University of Tokyo
Tokyo, Japan

Gudrun Klasmeyer, Dipl.-ING
Technical University Berlin
Berlin, Germany

James B. Kobler, Ph.D.
H. P. Mosher Laryngological Research Laboratory
Massachusetts Eye and Ear Infirmary & Harvard Medical School
Boston, Massachusetts

Jody Kreiman, Ph.D.
Associate Professor
Division of Head and Neck Surgery
University of California, Los Angeles, School of Medicine
Los Angeles, California

John Laver
Professor of Phonetics
Institute for Advanced Studies in the Humanities
University of Edinburgh
Edinburgh, Scotland

Sue Ellen Linville, Ph.D.
Associate Professor
Marquette University
Milwaukee, Wisconsin

Christopher Long
Professor
Institute for Advanced Studies in the Humanities
University of Edinburgh
Edinburgh, Scotland

Anja Lowit-Leuschel, Ph.D.
University of Strathclyde
Department of Speech and Language Therapy
Glasgow, Scotland

Lesley Mathieson, F.R.C.S.L.T.
Visiting Lecturer in Voice Pathology
Department of Linguistic Science
The University of Reading
Reading, Berkshire
United Kingdom

Kazunori Mori, M.D.
Assistant Professor
Department of Otolaryngology—
Head and Neck Surgery
Kurume University
Kurume, Japan

Nelson Roy, Ph.D.
Assistant Professor
The University of Utah
Department of Communication
Disorders
Salt Lake City, Utah

Walter F. Sendlmeier
Professor
Institut fur Kommunikationswissenschaft
Technische Universität Berlin
Berlin, Germany

Stephen M. Tasko
Doctoral Student
University of Wisconsin–Madison
Madison, Wisconsin

Gayle E. Woodson, M.D., F.A.C.S.
Professor of Otolaryngology
University of Tennessee, Memphis
College of Medicine
Memphis, Tennessee

Wolfram Ziegler, Ph.D.
Clinical Neuropsychology Research Group
Department of Neuropsychology
City Hospital Bogenhausen
München, Germany

PART I

Perceptual Assessments

Some would argue that voice quality can be described and assessed only by auditory–perceptual means. It is only in this way, they might say, that voice quality exists at all. Attempts to reach objective measurement may destroy the very concept that is under study. Others would maintain that auditory–perceptual methods are indispensable as a reference for more objective procedures such as acoustic or physiologic analysis, but the instrumental methods can add to the understanding of the perceptual entities and scales. That is, even though instrumental methods may be more quantitative and "objective," they cannot stand alone—perceptual judgment is necessary for a voice quality to be identified. Perceptual and instrumental approaches are complementary, and the central task is to bring them into a unified picture. Still others might claim that auditory–perceptual methods are prone to various sources of error and, if these methods are used, steps should be taken to ensure the validity and reliability of the data obtained. There is a need for better methods and there is a reasonable likelihood that this need can be met. Perhaps a few would hold no hope whatever for auditory–perceptual judgments as a way of assessing voice quality. These individuals may emphasize the discrepancies among published studies and the looming problems of validity and interjudge agreement. Certainly, each of these opinions has been expressed formally or informally in the history of voice quality studies. The diversity of opinion reflects the theoretical and empirical challenge inherent to the study of voice quality.

A common feature to the chapters in Part I is that they offer improvements and sophistication in auditory–perceptual studies of voice quality. The procedures and recommendations vary greatly from chapter to chapter. Taken together, these chapters comprise a small book in themselves, a kind of collective expertise on how voice quality can be studied perceptually.

Lesley Mathieson's chapter opens the topic with a consideration of the continuum of voice qualities from normal to disordered. Such a continuum is explicitly or implicitly assumed in many studies of voice quality, and this chapter discusses the steps to defining such a continuum. One may ask if normal and disordered voice should be considered as variations along a single continuum or if they should be regarded as essentially different phenomena? The answer to this question is critical to a number of important issues, including the way in which normative data are used in the evaluation of voice quality disorder. Harry Hollien takes on the task of defining ideal voice quality. This issue is worthy in its own right to give a sense of what the ideal is, but it also serves to fix one end of the continuum of voice quality. Is there a single ideal voice quality, or are there several possible ideals? How can ideal voice quality be recognized? John Esling describes cross-linguistic aspects of voice. It is important to know in what way voice quality may be a universal property of voice versus a language-specific property. Cross-language variations are needed for a proper account of the role of voice quality in linguistics but also for an appreciation of how vocal pathologies may have both universal and language-specific aspects. John Laver analyzes the articulatory aspects of voice, demonstrating the potential variety of voice types. Laver's classification system is one of the richest and most detailed, affording a highly sensitive description of voice quality variations. Issues of transcription of voice quality are considered by Esling, Craig Dickson, and Martin Ball. Their chapter sets forth transcription tools and procedures by which quality variations can be coded. Dysprosody is the subject of the chapter by Anja Lowit-Leuschel and Gerry Docherty. Dysprosody, like prosody, has been variously defined in a large number of papers. Lowit-Leuschel and Docherty focus on variations in f_0 because these variations are most closely related to voice quality issues. Their chapter points the way to consistent definition and description of this important aspect of speech that is often interwoven with other aspects of voice quality. Jody Kreiman and Bruce Gerratt summarize several studies and report new data on the fundamental issue of the measurement of voice quality. Their review points up the difficulties that must be addressed if one is to use auditory perceptual methods to assess voice quality. They recommend that efforts be made to model individual differences in perception of voice quality. Finally, Daniel Callan, Ray Kent, Nelson Roy, and Stephen Tasko present a neural network approach in which acoustic and perceptual data are mutually considered in a Kohonen self-organizing map. This chapter shows how a two-layer network can be trained to reflect nonlinear regularities inherent in acoustic and perceptual data on voice quality.

In a sense, Part I is an introduction to the other two parts of the book because it identifies many of the critical issues involved in the measurement of voice quality and the relevance of these issues to theoretical and practical matters, such as delineating the types of voice quality in a language or determining clinical variants of voice quality

CHAPTER 1

Normal–Disordered Continuum

Lesley Mathieson

The human voice is the sound by which spoken language is transmitted. Not only does it make speech audible, but it can convey a wide range of information about the speaker's identity, physical health, emotional status, and personality. Most people give little thought to their voices unless they have vocal problems, and many have little awareness of this important component of self-image. The simplest definition of a normal human voice is that it is the acoustic product of a normal vocal tract that is functioning normally. Problems arise, of course, from the word *normal* within this definition. Every human voice is unique because of the various anatomical, physiological, psychological, cultural, sociolinguistic, and behavioral factors that contribute to the final product. These elements are not static, however, and in addition to variations in voices between individuals, the speaker's voice changes to varying degrees from day to day and throughout the lifespan. A propitious combination of factors can result in what might be regarded as a beautiful, or superior, voice but there is unlikely to be global agreement on a particular voice. A normal voice is generally unremarkable, with an abnormal voice ranging from the esthetically unpleasing to the functionally inefficient. Complete absence of phonation is the lowest point on the normal-disordered voice continuum, on which there are no clear boundaries.

A normal voice is audible in a wide range of acoustic settings, even with relatively high levels of ambient noise. It is appropriate for the gender and age of the speaker and is capable of fulfilling its paralinguistic and linguistic functions to the speaker's satisfaction. It should not deteriorate with use nor should there be any discomfort or pain associated with phonation. Each voice is primarily dependent on the anatomical structure of the vocal tract, which varies in dimensions and proportions from one individual to another and so provides the basis for a voice unique to each speaker. These anatomical features cannot be changed voluntarily and will always influence phonation, even when attempts are made to disguise them. Only disease or structural damage to the larynx and the related structures can alter this fundamental architecture. It has to be remembered, however, that age-related histological, skeletal, and physiological changes affecting the voice are taking place from birth onwards. Also contributing to vocal permanence are the voice settings resulting from the muscle tension adjustments acquired from one's cultural group. These are established during child-rearing and education and are subsequently reinforced and modified during an adult's social and professional life. They can affect habitual pitch, pitch range, loudness, vocal note quality, and nasal resonance. The vocal settings of particular groups can be imitated, but the original setting tends to reassert itself unless it is extinguished through retraining and practice.

1. VOCAL TRACT ANATOMY AND PHYSIOLOGY

The vocal tract is described in relation to the area between the vocal folds (the glottis) and the supra- and subglottic structures. The supraglottic tract extends from the laryngeal ventricles and false vocal folds, through the oropharynx to the oral and nasal cavities. The false vocal folds, or ventricular folds, are not involved in normal phonation but contribute to laryngeal valving for airway protection during swallowing. The pharynx, superior to the false vocal folds, is formed by the superior, middle, and inferior pharyngeal constrictor muscles. The relative degrees of constriction of these muscles affect the dimensions of the pharynx and the rigidity of the pharyngeal walls. These changes, in conjunction with changes in oral cavity dimensions, affect the formants of the fundamental vocal note. The subglottic tract includes the trachea, bronchi, and lungs. Changes in the supraglottic tract influence resonation of the vocal note, with air pressure changes effected by the subglottic tract. Whatever the acoustic, emotional, or linguistic subtleties of a voice, it is the macroscopic and microscopic biomechanics of the vocal tract structures that determine the sounds produced.

1.1. The Vocal Folds

The two vocal folds meet anteriorly to form the anterior commissure. Each vocal fold consists of the vocalis muscle, which is covered by four histologically different layers of mucosa: the epithelium and the three layers of the lamina propria. The superficial, gelatinous layer of the lamina propria is known as Reinke's space. The intermediate layer consists of elastic fibers and the deep layer is composed of collagen fibers. The vocalis muscle is referred to as the *body* of the vocal fold and the mucosa is the *cover*.

1.1.1. Fundamental Vocal Note Production

The fundamental vocal note is the product of pulmonic air passing between the adducted vocal folds causing them to open and close. This opening and closing constitutes one vibratory cycle during which subglottic pressure rises below the adducted folds until it overcomes the resistance and a puff of air is released. At the same time, the air pressure between the vocal folds drops (the Bernoulli effect) and the vocal folds are drawn together again with a further rise in subglottic air pressure. An undulating wave of movement of the vocal fold mucosa travels from the inferior to the superior surface of the vocal folds during each vibratory cycle. The inferior edges of the vocal folds adduct initially followed by complete adduction of the folds and then a gradual peeling apart, with the superior edges being the last to lose contact.

The *quality* of the fundamental vocal note depends on the competency of vocal fold adduction and the periodicity, amplitude, and symmetry of the mucosal waves. The vibratory characteristics of the vocal folds are, in turn, dictated by their viscosity, density, and elasticity, which derive from the degree of tension of the vocalis muscle and the histological structure of the lamina propria and epithelium. Research into vocal fold structure has identified that the layers of the lamina propria are morphologically distinct (Gray, Hirano, & Sato, 1993; Hirano, 1981) and therefore differ in their vibratory characteristics. More recent work has highlighted also the importance of the extracellular matrix to vocal fold mechanics (Hammond,

Zhou, Hammond, Pawlak, & Gray, 1997). All these features of vocal fold structure are potential variables in the production of a vocal note. For example, histological studies (Hirano & Sato, 1993) have demonstrated that the layers of the lamina propria are not fully defined until the midteens, while in later life the characteristics of these layers, particularly the elastic and collagen fibers, change significantly. These changes, in combination with age-related atrophic deterioration of the vocalis muscle, create a structure with markedly different vibratory characteristics throughout the lifespan that are reflected in the normal voice.

The vocal folds also determine the frequency, or pitch, of the vocal note according to their length, tension, and mass. Increases in vocal fold length and tension increase frequency, with increased mass reducing frequency. There are three distinct vocal fold vibratory patterns that relate to the three main vocal registers: vocal fry (or creak), modal, and falsetto. Vocal fry is characterized by a long closed phase in each vibratory cycle and occurs within the frequency range of 20–60 Hz. In the modal register, which is generally used for speech, the vocal folds make complete closure during the closed phase in a frequency range of 100–300 Hz. In falsetto, the vocal folds are thin, short, and tense, with vocal fold adduction incomplete.

2. ACOUSTIC FEATURES OF NORMAL PHONATION

The acoustic features of a voice can be described perceptually and analyzed instrumentally for certain parameters that reflect the structure and function of the larynx and the supra- and subglottic vocal tract (Kent & Read, 1992). These parameters relate to vocal note quality, habitual pitch, and pitch and loudness range and stability. The relative degree of hypo- or hypernasality can also be included. The parameters can be perceived and measured as separate entities but in reality they are interdependent. An acoustic profile of a voice can be compiled for these parameters and compared against normative data.

2.1. Fundamental Vocal Note Quality

The term fundamental note quality refers to the quality of the sound produced by the adducted vocal folds, themselves, during phonation. Normal voice consists of periodic waves and random noise. When voices are described in perceptual terms such as "breathy" and "rough," reference is being made to the relatively high noise component of the vocal note. A low signal-to-noise ratio indicates that the proportion of periodic waveforms (i.e., the signal) is being reduced by an increase in aperiodic waveforms (i.e., noise). An increase of noise in this ratio is typical of many pathological voices.

2.2. Vocal Pitch

Pitch is the perceived correlate of frequency. *Speaking fundamental frequency* (SF_0) is measured in hertz, or cycles per second, of vocal fold vibration. Extensive normative data have been collated by Baken (1987) that demonstrate the variations of mean SF_0 according to gender, age, and phonatory tasks performed. Average SF_0 for men is 128 Hz, for women 225 Hz, and for children 265 Hz. *Pitch perturbation* is cycle-to-cycle variation that is known as jitter. Jitter is frequently a feature of disordered voices, but is also present in voices that fall within normal limits, such as some normal elderly voices. The term *pitch range* refers to the entire range of frequencies that can be achieved by the voice. Maximum frequency range can extend from a lowest F_0 of 77 Hz to a highest F_0 of 567 Hz in a young man. The voices of women of a similar age can range from 134 Hz to 895 Hz.

2.3. Loudness

Loudness is the perceived correlate of intensity, or amplitude, with loudness range and stability capable of being measured. Shimmer is the term used to refer to *amplitude perturba-*

tion. An individual with normal vocal capabilities is able to phonate satisfactorily at the same low intensity in both speaking and singing. An individual with a normal voice can reach a *forte* intensity of 80 dB and a *fortissimo* of about 90 dB with the speaking voice (Haki, 1996). The shouting voice reaches an average of 100 dB, and this intensity can be matched in singing by the normal voice.

3. PHONATION IN DISCOURSE

Although anatomical features and musculoskeletal settings give rise to vocal permanence, paralinguistic features are the constantly changing aspects of vocal behavior that reflect emotion and help to convey a nonverbal message. A speaker unconsciously employs variations of pitch, loudness, and vocal quality to enhance or contradict the words being uttered. In this way, a listener can acquire some insight into the speaker's true feelings and the speaker is able to give indications of the emotions when it is difficult or socially inappropriate to make an overt statement. Paralinguistic features can also be consciously manipulated so the speaker can either convey an emotion that is not actually being felt or to influence a listener's behavior intentionally. The voice also has an important linguistic function in segmental and suprasegmental phonology. In its segmental role, it is an integral part of individual phonemes where the ability to coordinate phonation and articulation is essential for intelligibility. The suprasegmental features of speech that compose prosody are conveyed by vocal pitch and loudness in conjunction with segment duration and the use of pause.

Emotion produces vocal tract changes that, in turn, affect various vocal parameters. Scherer, (1995) in a paper on emotion and voice reported that frequency range has the most powerful effect on listener judgments of emotion. A narrow frequency range is perceived as sadness or neutrality, with a wide frequency range expressing high arousal, whether negative or positive.

4. THE SINGING VOICE

The singing voice occupies a special position in the normal-disordered voice continuum because the pitch and loudness range required is frequently more extensive than in speaking. In addition, different vocal behaviors are used that can highlight the onset of voice problems before they are apparent in the speaking voice. The physiological demands in operatic singing, for example, are greater than when speaking. To produce and sustain the vocal note at appropriate loudness levels, capacity and control of subglottic air has to be developed. Singers use significantly higher subglottic air pressures than nonsingers and, consequently, even minor respiratory deficiences can affect the professional voice user (Akerlund & Gramming, 1994; Carroll et al., 1996). It has also been observed that the closed quotient of the vocal fold vibratory cycle is longer in trained singers and this leads to the hypothesis that there might be greater stresses on the histological structure of the vocal fold mucosa for a singer (Howard, Lindsey, & Allen, 1990). Carroll et al. (1996) have suggested that because of the differences observed in trained singers from the generally used vocal parameter norms, separate normative data should be used for these vocal athletes.

4.1. Vibrato

Vibrato is a particular, normal vocal behavior that occurs in some singing that would be regarded as grossly abnormal in speech. It varies according to the type and culture of the singing: Western operatic singing achieves its warm, rich tone through a singer's use of vibrato. In physical terms, this consists of a fundamental frequency undulation at a rate of 5–7 Hz over a range of 1 semitone. This is the result of pulsating contractions of the cricothyroid muscle (Sundberg, 1995) in association with oscillations of the soft palate, the epiglottis, the lateral walls of the hypopharynx, and, in most singers, the inferior part of the oropharynx at some pitch and loudness levels. It is recognized as developing automatically in trained singers. (Sundberg suggests that the vibrato quality occurring in popular singing and in non-Western cultures appears to derive from subglottal pressure pulsations rather than the pulsations of the cricothyroid muscle.) Not only is there some vibrato rate variation between male and female operatic singers (with the average rate being slightly faster in females), but there is also some indication that the rate accelerates under emotional influences. Decrease in the vibrato rate tends to occur with aging and, when vibrato is excessively slow, it becomes an undesirable "wobble." Singers can have problems with vibrato when it varies from the standards of rate, frequency, and intensity called for in their singing style. Hyperfunctional laryngeal, thoracic, and abdominal musculature is usually involved. It is interesting to note that when the vocal characteristics of patients with pathological vocal tremor were compared with the vibrato features of opera singers in a study by Ramig and Shipp (1987), there were only minor differences. The rate was 6.8 Hz for vocal tremor patients and 5.5 Hz for the singers, with the regularity of the fundamental frequency variations in singers being somewhat greater.

4.2. Singing and Voice Disorder

The demands made by singing, particularly on professional singers, are more likely to result in vocal fold abnormalities than in average speakers. An untrained singer is also vulnerable when technique is poor. Even when there is no damage to the vocal fold mucosa, the superior vocal function required frequently leads a singer to perceive vocal problems when there is an inability to meet high standards. In these circumstances, there is no clinical voice disorder, but a demonstrable voice problem that can affect an individual's career and employment.

5. NORMAL–DISORDERED OVERLAP

5.1. Physiological Variants

Although it is possible for a relatively normal voice to be produced with minor abnormalities of the vocal tract, it is possible also for a wide range of vocal abnormality to be produced by an anatomically normal vocal tract with the potential for normal function. The point at which a voice is regarded as abnormal is inevitably ill-defined and, for that reason, the term normal-disordered voice continuum is more appropriate than using the terms normal or abnormal voice as discrete entities. An otherwise normal voice will be markedly different in various situations. The temporary changes that occur in extreme emotion, for example, might result in vocal features that could be judged as abnormal, if the voice sample were heard out of context. In grief, following prolonged sobbing, the nasal mucosa is swollen, resulting in hyponasal vocal resonance, with the speaking fundamental frequency lowered and the voice having a "wet" quality because of the additional secretions. A speaker who has been running and who is out of breath has a significantly reduced maximum phonation time so that phrase length is short. It is also difficult to increase vocal loudness in this situation, because the ability to increase subglottic air pressure is reduced by the constant need for rapid intakes of breath. The hyperfunctional "pressed" phonation required while carrying or pushing a heavy weight would be regarded as severely pathological if heard in isolation and resembles the phonation of certain neurological conditions, such as spasmodic dysphonia, causing hyperadduction of the vocal folds. These examples of "abnormal" voice are fleeting and reflect physiological conditions that interfere with phonation, with the voice subsequently returning to normal.

5.2. Individual Perception

The overlap between normal and abnormal voice and the criteria by which they are judged also vary from person to person. The professional singer, for example, might justifiably consider the inability to sing high notes that had been previously achieved as a voice problem. In contrast, other individuals might regard their voices as disordered only when marked changes severely reduce functional efficiency. Certain vocal features, such as creak, are regarded as normal when occurring intermittently or on falling intonation patterns. Excessive vocal creak, however, not only sounds abnormal but can result in damage to the vocal fold mucosa. In the early stages of an acquired voice disorder, the reduction in vocal capabilities might be apparent only in the upper part of the singing range initially, with speaking and shouting being within normal limits (Haki, 1996). As the condition deteriorates, singing, speaking, and shouting are all affected, either episodically or in a steadily declining pattern.

5.3. Vocal Fold Adduction

The overlap between the normal and the disordered is also observed in vocal fold behavior as well as in the sound of the voice. As the clinician frequently observes incomplete vocal fold adduction in dysphonic patients, it is easy to overlook that many speakers without voice problems have been shown to have glottic chinks and a degree of vocal bowing (Hirano & Bless, 1993). It is the degree of inadequacy of vocal fold adduction that is significant and, for the dysphonic individual, the extent to which it causes the voice to deviate from normal.

5.4. Sensory Changes

For the speaker, the initial indication of a problem is sometimes sensory rather than acoustic, with sensations ranging from increased phonatory effort through intermittent vocal tract discomfort to severe inflammatory or musculoskeletal pain. It has been found that individuals are generally reliable in distinguishing between the soreness arising from vocal fold inflammation and the aching resulting from musculoskeletal tension, even when they coexist (Mathieson, 1993). Such sensations usually result from hyperfunctional phonation. This might have a behavioral basis when the voice is being abused. It can also occur in cases of laryngeal abnormality when a speaker uses inappropriate compensatory strategies in an attempt to improve the voice.

6. CLINICAL VOICE DISORDERS

A disordered voice can be abnormal in one or more of its parameters, but the common feature of most dysphonias is a change in the quality of the fundamental vocal note, frequently referred to as hoarseness. In general, complaints about dysphonia concern hoarseness much more frequently than abnormal pitch or loudness (Dejonckere, 1995). On acoustic analysis, this is a reduction in the signal-to-noise ratio that is perceived, depending on the laryngeal biomechanics, as "breathiness" or "roughness" (Hirano, 1981). In these instances, the vocal folds have increased the quotient of aperiodic waveforms being produced with a consequent reduction in the periodic waveforms. This is perceived as a high noise component of the vocal note. Abnormalities of vocal tract structure and function cause changes in the signal-to-noise ratio because they give rise to abnormal patterns of adduction or vibration of the vocal folds or related vocal tract structures. "Breathiness" is caused by air leakage via the glottis, resulting in excessive high frequency noise because of inefficient vocal fold closure (Hirano, 1981). This can be from mass lesions, such as nodules, which physically obstruct complete adduction of the folds with a resulting glottic chink. Alternatively, neurological and nonorganic conditions can also result in glottic chinks of various configurations. The irregular glottal pulses caused by asymmetry in vocal fold mass or by atrophy of the vocalis muscle, result in "roughness" (Dejonckere, 1995). This irregularity is measured by jitter ratio, which is higher in pathological voices. In recent years, the complexities of the vibratory patterns occurring in rough voice have become the subject of nonlinear dynamic analysis, which, it is suggested, might explain various vocal irregularities (Baken, 1994; Herzel, Berry, Titze, & Saleh, 1994).

Vocal abnormality can be episodic in an individual who is able to produce normal voice at times, with episodes of dysphonia correlating with voice use or the stress of various life events. It has to be remembered, of course, that a structurally normal vocal tract is capable of producing a vocal note of abnormal quality, intentionally or unintentionally.

6.1 Incidence

The incidence of voice problems is difficult to ascertain. Statistics based on individuals who are seen by otolaryngologists will exclude those who do not regard their voices as sufficiently abnormal or functionally unsatisfactory to seek help. Enderby and Philipp (1986) suggested that in England the annual incidence of dysphonia could be 28 per 100,000 population. This estimate is probably low. A review of initial contacts of patients referred to the Speech and Language Therapy Department at Northwick Park and St Mark's Hospitals, London, England over a representative 6-month period produced an annual figure of 121 cases of dysphonia per 100,000 population (Mathieson, unpublished data 1997). This figure might be influenced by a number of factors, including the development of multidisciplinary voice clinics in the past 10 years, together with a greater public awareness of the importance of investigating the causes of vocal symptoms. Wilson (1979) thought that the incidence of voice disorders in children was between 5% and 6%. Boys tend to present with voice problems, usually those related to vocal abuse, more frequently than girls. In addition to a child's gender it seems that the social environment is also relevant. In a study of 362 children of 12–13 years, Multinovic (1994) found 3.92% of the children who lived in a rural setting had voice problems. In contrast, 43.67% of the urban group had similar difficulties. It is generally agreed, however, that more women than men have voice problems, but the reasons for this are speculative. Fritzell (1996) raises the possibility that women might have a greater need to speak than men, but also suggests that perhaps the female voice is less able to cope with the demands made on it. This latter hypothesis is also raised by Hammond et al. (1997) who quantified the hyaluronic acid composition of the lamina propria in men and women and concluded that the vocal folds of men and women were morphologically distinct. The greater thickness of the lamina propria in men appears to be due, in part, to the quantity of hyaluronic acid in the vocal fold structure, which acts as a shock absorber. The high incidence of vocal nodules in women and relatively few cases in men is possibly because of the higher fundamental frequency in women, which leads to greater impact stress.

The incidence of vocal pathology also correlates with lifestyle. Professional voice users such as singers, actors, and teachers, who all use their voices for longer periods in public settings than most people, are vulnerable, particularly if they have had no vocal training (Fritzell 1996). Voice problems are also more frequent in those who smoke and who drink large amounts of alcohol because of the resulting changes in the vocal fold mucosa resulting in increased mass.

6.2. Etiology

Clinical voice disorders can be congenital or acquired and have traditionally been classified as organic and nonorganic. This classification is unsatisfactory for clinicians, as it disregards the underlying etiology of the problem that must be understood and dealt with if the dysphonia is to be resolved. Vocal fold nodules, for example, are changes in the mucosa secondary to impact stress. Although they are an organic manifestation, they are secondary to hyperfunctional phonatory behavior. Subepithelial vocal fold cysts, on the other hand, tend to occur independently and not as the result of vocal abuse. Voice disorder resulting from vocal fold cysts, therefore, is primarily organic. Understanding the primary cause of a problem is fundamental to its successful resolution. Consequently, changing phonatory behavior is essential to resolving vocal fold nodules, with surgical aspiration of a vocal fold cyst the first course of action.

Voice disorders, therefore, fall broadly into the categories of behavioral (functional) and organic etiologies. Behavioral disorders range from muscular tension disorders, with or without mucosal changes such as nodules and polyps, to psychogenic causes of various types and severity. Organic etiologies can be divided into four subcategories: structural, neurogenic, endocrine, and laryngeal disease. Descriptions of these clinical voice disorders, and their evaluation and treatment, can be found in various texts. (Aronson, 1990; Boone & McFarlane, 1988; Colton & Casper, 1990; Dworkin & Meleca, 1996; Greene & Mathieson, 1989; Mathieson, 1997).

Although vocal acoustics provide some indication of laryngeal biomechanics, the underlying cause of vocal change must never be presumed, whatever the apparent precipitating factor. For example, although teachers often use their voices excessively in noisy conditions and can be more susceptible to voice disorders than others, laryngeal examination is essential to determine laryngeal status. All dysphonias that continue for 3 weeks or more in the absence of an upper respiratory tract infection must be investigated by a laryngologist to exclude or confirm malignancy and analyze laryngeal structure and function before further treatment is carried out. It is also significant when a voice falls within normal limits but has changed from what is normal for a particular speaker.

6.3. Hyperfunctional Voice Disorders

Voice disorders from excessive tension of the extrinsic and intrinsic laryngeal musculature, whether or not there are histological vocal fold changes, constitute the major proportion of the dysphonias presenting in routine ear, nose, and throat clinics and voice clinics. This hyperfunctional phonation occurs for a wide range of reasons, but in all speakers, the vocal folds are adducted with excessive effort so that there are high levels of impact stress on the vocal fold mucosa. These speakers often use hard glottal attack excessively and perform even nonphonatory tasks, such as throat clearing, with considerable force. Many such speakers are generally tense and tend to use excessive effort to undertake any task, including phonation. Others are generally noisy and speak loudly whatever the context or the environment, even if they are not unduly tense. They will speak against high levels of background noise and shout exuberantly at sports events and parties. When some speakers attempt to increase vocal loudness in the absence of a naturally well-produced voice, they encounter difficulties if they have to give presentations or project their voices to a group of listeners. Although muscle tension dysphonias are commonly associated with excessive vocal loudness, similar voice problems will occur if a speaker is using an unduly raised or lowered speaking fundamental frequency. Laryngeal examination in hyperfunctional dysphonia might reveal normal vocal folds, when the abnormal voice is intermittent, but vocal nodules, edema, polyps, and other vocal fold mucosa changes will be seen in more extreme cases of vocal fold abuse.

6.4. Psychogenic Voice Disorders

Psychogenic dysphonias occur as the result of abnormal function of an anatomically and neurologically normal vocal mechanism. The underlying psychological state of the patient is the primary cause of the problem, however, rather than more superficial misuse or abuse. Inevitably there is an overlap between many categories of voice disorder and they cannot be regarded as being mutually exclusive. The most dramatic manifestation of psychogenic voice disorder is the total voice loss of conversion symptom aphonia. The primary advantage of the unconsciously produced symptom is the inability to communicate effectively, with the secondary gain being the care and attention that the voice loss generates. Laryngoscopic examination classically reveals bowed vocal folds that remain firmly apart even when the speaker is apparently making every effort to phonate.

6.5. Gender-related Voice Problems

Normal vocal tract structure and potentially normal function are also underlying to mutational falsetto, or puberphonia, in which a postpubertal male continues to produce prepubertal voice. This is a condition that can usually be rectified rapidly with appropriate voice therapy.

The central point of the normal-disordered continuum might be identified as the transsexual speaker. Whether male or female, transsexuals have normal voices, which they regard as inappropriate because they desire characteristics, including the voice, of the opposite gender. Both the individual with mutational falsetto and the transsexual speaker vividly demonstrate that an abnormal voice cannot be evaluated by acoustic analysis, instrumental or perceptual, in isolation. The voice is an important part of a speaker's self-image and it will be regarded as abnormal if it does not accord with either the image presented to the public or to the speaker's internal image.

6.6. Alaryngeal Voice

Although laryngeal voice is our preoccupation in this text, for the sake of completeness, it should be mentioned that at the end of the normal-disordered voice continuum there is alaryngeal voice, which demonstrates that a similar acoustic signal can be generated outside the vocal tract. Following laryngectomy, pseudovoice or esophageal voice can be produced at the site of the pharyngoesophageal segment (P-E segment) with either pulmonic or injected air. When efficient, it is similar to vocal fold voice perceptually and acoustic analysis confirms similar parameter measures (Williams & Watson, 1987). Laryngectomees are the prime example of the importance of having a voice that is regarded as normal for both the practicalities of communication and for conveying an appropriate self-image.

7. IMPAIRMENT, DISABILITY, AND HANDICAP

Voice disorders have social, lifestyle, and employment consequences, and the effects of dysphonia can be classified according to the World Health Organization *International Classification of Impairments, Disabilities and Handicaps* (WHO, 1980). This classification is used as a conceptual framework to describe the consequences of a disease or disorder. An *impairment* represents dysfunction of abnormal structures, with *disability* referring to changes in behavior and performance as a result of the impairment. When these impairments or disabilities place the individual at a disadvantage to others, this is referred to as *handicap.*

In their study of of 133 patients who completed open-ended questionnaires Scott, Robinson, Wilson, and Mackenzie (1997) found that the total number of problems associated with having a voice disorder was listed as 467. Of these, 60% were classified as impairments, 26% as disabilities, and 14% were handicap related. The majority of impairments were concerned with altered voice and throat symptoms with symptoms, such as a lump in the throat, choking, and dizziness being in the minority. Lack of vocal clarity and the inability to increase vocal loudness against background noise or when talking to a group constituted most of the disability category. Singing difficulty was noted by more than a quarter of the subjects. The 31 respondents who reported handicaps cited employment-related difficulties as a result of their voice disorders, as well as the effects on family and friends. Psychological and emotional issues also fell into this category. As Scott et al. pointed out, despite extensive literature and research into a wide range of aspects of voice disorders, this was the first study to categorize patients' self-reported problems related to dysphonia. Clinicians' awareness of the impairment, disability, and handicap issues in this field should facilitate the development of problem-specific strategies in treating voice disorders.

REFERENCES

Akerlund, L., & Gramming, P. (1994). Average loudness level, mean fundamental frequency and subglottal pressure: Comparison between female singers and nonsingers. *Journal of Voice, 8*(3), 263–270.

Aronson, A. E. (1990). *Clinical voice disorders: An interdisciplinary approach* (3rd ed.). New York: Thieme Stratton, Inc.

Baken, R. (1987). *Clinical measurement of speech and voice.* London: Taylor and Francis.

Baken, R. (1994). The aged voice: A new hypothesis. *Voice, 3*(2), 57–73.

Boone, D., & McFarlane, S. C. (1988). *The voice and voice therapy* (4th ed.). Englewood Cliffs, NJ: Prentice-Hall.

Carroll, L. M., Sataloff, R. T., Heuer, R. J., Spiegel, J. R., Radionoff, S. L., & Cohn, J. R. (1996). Respiratory and glottal efficiency measures in normal classically trained singers. *Journal of Voice, 10*(2), 139–145.

Colton, R. H., & Casper J. K. (1990). *Understanding voice problems: A physiologic perspective for diagnosis and treatment.* Baltimore: Williams and Wilkins.

Dejonckere, P. H. (1995) Principal components in voice pathology. *Voice, 4*(2), 96–105.

Dworkin, J. P., & Meleca R. J. (1996) *Vocal pathologies.* San Diego: Singular Publishing Group, Inc.

Enderby, P., & Philipp, R. (1986). Speech and language handicap: Towards knowing the size of the problem. *British Journal of Disorders of Communication, 21,* 151–165.

Fritzell, B. (1996). Voice disorders and occupations. *Logopedics Phoniatrics Vocology, 21*(1), 7–12.

Gray, S. D., Hirano, M., & Sato, K. (1993). Molecular and cellular structure of vocal fold tissue. In I. R. Titze (Ed.), *Vocal fold physiology* (pp. 1–35). San Diego: Singular Publishing Group, Inc.

Greene, M. C. L., & Mathieson, L. (1989). *The voice and its disorders.* (5th ed.). London: Whurr.

Haki, T. (1996). Comparative speaking, shouting and singing voice range profile measurements: Physiological and pathological aspects. *Logopedics Phoniatrics Vocology, 21*(3/4), 123–129.

Hammond, T. H., Zhou, R., Hammond, E. H., Pawlak, A., & Gray, S. D. (1997). The intermediate layer: A morphologic study of the elastin and hyaluronic acid constituents of normal human vocal folds. *Journal of Voice, 11*(1), 59–66.

Herzel, H., Berry D., Titze, I. R., & Saleh, M. (1994). Analysis of vocal disorders with methods from nonlinear dynamics. *Journal of Speech and Hearing Research, 37*(5), 1008–1019.

Hirano, M. (1981). *Clinical examination of voice.* Vienna: Springer Verlag.

Hirano, M., & Bless, D. (1993). *Videostroboscopic examination of the larynx.* San Diego: Singular Publishing Group, Inc.

Hirano, M., & Sato, K. (1993). *Histological color atlas of the human larynx.* San Diego: Singular Publishing Group, Inc.

Howard, D. M., Lindsey, G. A., & Allen, B. (1990). Toward the quantification of vocal efficiency. *Journal of Voice, 4,* 205–212.

Kent, R., & Read, C. (1992). *The acoustic analysis of speech.* San Diego: Singular Publishing Group, Inc.

Mathieson, L. (1993). Vocal tract discomfort in hyperfunctional dysphonia. *Voice, 2*(1), 40–48.

Mathieson, L. (1997). Voice disorders following road traffic accidents (editorial review). *Journal of Laryngology and Otology, 111,* 903–906.

Morrison, M., & Rammage, L. (1994). *The management of voice disorders.* London: Chapman and Hall Medical.

Multinovic, Z. (1994). Social environment and incidence of voice disturbances in children. *Folia Phoniatrica 46*(3), 135–138.

Ramig, L., & Shipp, T. (1987). Comparative measures of vocal tremor and vocal vibrato. *Journal of Voice, 1*(1), 162–167.

Scherer, K. R. (1995). Expression of emotion in voice and music. *Journal of Voice, 9* (3), 235–248.

Scott, S., Robinson, K., Wilson, J. A., & Mackenzie, K. (1997). Patient-reported problems associated with dysphonia. *Clinical Otolaryngology, 22,* 37–40.

Sundberg, J. (1995). Acoustic and psychoacoustic aspects of vocal vibrato. In P. H. Dejonckere, M. Hirano, & J. Sundberg., (Eds.), *Vibrato* (pp. 35–62). San Diego: Singular Publishing Group, Inc.

World Health Organization. (1980). International Classification of Impairments, Disabilities and Handicaps.

Williams, S. E., & Watson, J. B. (1987). Speaking proficiency variations according to method of alaryngeal voicing. *Laryngoscope, 97*(6), 737–739.

Wilson, K. (1979). *Voice problems of children* (2nd ed.). Baltimore: Williams and Wilkins.

CHAPTER 2

The Concept of Ideal Voice Quality

Harry Hollien

It is a little difficult to separate voice quality from voice; so too is it somewhat of a problem to separate "ideal" voice quality from "ideal" speech. Indeed, these entities trade on each other and, if narrowly defined, any one of them will be quite restrictive. When blurred together, they can be said to have provided a base for the numerous pedagogues who have had "ideal" as their ideal. As a group, they extend back to ancient Greek and Roman times. Unfortunately, their goals have not led to much success in practice. After all, if you were to argue that ideal voice quality (or the ideal voice or ideal speech) could not exist as a single entity, you would be on pretty firm ground. What would be "ideal" in one situation, might not be suitable for a second. As an example, consider opera singers. The kind of energy and pacing they produce when singing on the stage would knock your socks off if they attempted to communicate with you in that same fashion in, say, an elevator. And how about that low, vibrant, throbbing voice a man might employ when courting his intended? It might be "ideal" in that situation; but how about its applicability to a business conference? Indeed, there probably are dozens (maybe hundreds) of different voice qualities that could be classed as "ideal"; that is, if you take into account the circumstances under which they were produced.

1. "IDEAL" HAS A LONG, LONG HISTORY

Just as with the "ideal speaker" or "natural pitch level," the concept of ideal voice quality probably developed several millennia ago. To establish a really good appreciation of this abstraction, it probably would be necessary to study the relevant writings and opinions of pedegogues from as far back as the Greek, Roman, and Renaissance periods. On the other hand, there is little argument but that the thinking and approaches professed in those bygone days were both contradictory and crude; most deserved only to be discarded.

Yet the concept of "ideal" is a hardy one; it continues up to the present. Well, at least it did until not so long ago. Included among its proponents have been public speaking teachers, elocutionists, speech pathologists, and, even, phoneticians. Indeed, books on public speaking published during the middle of the 20th century pretty much set the tone. For example, in 1940 Hoffman wrote that he agreed with Quintilian and quoted him as having said that a "good speaker must be a good man." Later Hoffman carries this thought on into a "quality of voice" discussion. Of course, currently anyway, the omission of women from this definition would create a firestorm, but, perhaps more important, it must be conceded that at least some of the most mesmerizing orators in history hardly can be thought of as "good men." In any event, the cited example neatly illustrates the struggles engaged in by many authors in order to establish "ideal" status for a communicative act. Some of them (see Rasmussen, 1949) even recommend working toward these goals without defining them. In any case, most of these attempts fail and for good reason.

1.1. Other Examples

All types of communication specialists can be observed seeking the "ideal." To illustrate: It is not all that difficult to accept as meritorious the "imagery" procedures used by singing teachers. For example, a few have been observed attempting to cultivate an ideal quality by instructing their pupils to "sing through the top of your head." In all fairness, this approach, although not anatomically possible, can be effective when employed by a talented teacher who knows exactly what quality she wants to hear; it only becomes garbled when she attempts to write down what she meant by the instruction. Thus even though legitimate, this technique and related ones demonstrate that vocal music specialists have developed a complex structure of many "ideal" voice qualities (Hollien, 1993). Still not convinced? Consider singer Patti LuPone's performance in *Evita*. On first hearing her, I personally remember thinking that "here is a voice with hormones." On the other hand, would that same voice quality also be appropriate for *La Bohème's* Mimi?

But, back to public speaking teachers. They appear to have continued many of the ancient ideas about the "ideal" into the middle 1900s. Note, for example, the writings of Craig (1938) who disdained any approach to effective speech that was not "scientific." Her studies, she wrote, led her to the conclusion that the only possible basis for good speech is one where "you speak six inches in front of your lips." Yet other examples could be provided; ones where subjective attempts were made to define such entities as "good," "superior," or "ideal" voice quality, voice, speech, speaking ability, and/or singing skill. With little positive data to support them, these attempts tended to prove less than adequate. On the other hand, two (different) groups of professionals would appear to be in a better position to address this issue than those just considered. They are the speech pathologists and the phoneticians (phoneticians are sometimes referred to as speech or voice scientists).

1.2. The Speech Pathologists

Very few of these specialists appear willing to *define* ideal voice quality. Most of them address the problem by listing characteristics that should *not* be heard in the voice of a speaker. Nonetheless, early attempts at scaling these features have been noted (Stinchfield, 1928) and the "listing" approach is fairly widespread. For example, Anderson (1942) indicated that the superior voice should exhibit (paraphrased): (1) adequate intensity, (2) a clear, pure tone (see also Millar, 1993 for a discussion of clarity), (3) pleasing/effective fundamental frequency, (4) an ease and flexibility, (5) vibrant quality, (6) clearness and ease in diction, and so on. Some of his definitions appear associated with general speaking ability; only one directly addresses voice quality and, even in that instance, additional definitions appear necessary.

Most modern speech pathologists are silent on the issue or, again, list the "should nots." Still others (see especially Baken, 1987 or Kent, Kent, & Rosenbek, 1987) provide listings of the normal (or expected) levels and ranges of the constituent elements within voice or speech. Some of the other current authors, such as Wilson (1987), also attempt to describe the normal (not ideal) voice; he says it exhibits (paraphrased): (1) pleasing voice quality, (2) proper balance between nasal and oral resonance, (3) appropriate loudness, (4) modal fundamental frequency suitable for age/size/sex, and (5) appropriate inflections in fundamental frequency and vocal intensity. Still not at a desirable level but, as with Anderson, this approach begins to provide structural boundaries of at least some usefulness. Moreover, an organization of this type, coupled with data provided by researchers such as Kent et al. (1987) and the instrumental means to make advances (see Baken, 1987), should permit systematic, if modest, progress.

Other authors (Gelfer, 1996; Stemple, 1984) include esthetics in their discussions. However, when discussing voice (on the basis of its laryngeal quality, intensity, fundamental frequency, nasality, and variability constituents), Gelfer indicates that it is more important to define it on the basis of suitability, properness, and appropriateness than on superiority. Indeed, she probably is correct in suggesting that esthetics are more within the province of other professionals (such as singing teachers or drama coaches)—ones who attempt to upgrade the quality of voice from normal to good, superior, or ideal (see also Glasgow, 1961).

To summarize: It appears that no viable definitions or foci about "ideal" quality have emerged from the efforts of speech pathologists as a group.

1.3. The Phoneticians

Phoneticians—or speech scientists or voice scientists—have provided at least a little information about the issue under discussion. Some of the earliest phoneticians of merit (Bell, 1907; Scripture, 1902; Sweet, 1906) appeared to have flirted with the idea but not to have addressed it functionally.

1.3.1. Early Research on the Issue

It was during the middle years of the 20th century that a number of phonetic scientists seriously addressed the problem (see for example, Black, 1942; Cowan, 1936; Lewis & Tiffin, 1934; Lynch, 1934; Murray & Tiffin, 1934; Pronovost, 1943; Snidecor, 1952; Talley, 1937); they actually attempted to provide data on the "ideal" voice. Of course, these investigators quickly realized that because of differing demands, environments, and situations, the concept of "ideal" itself might be too difficult to tackle. That is, they judged that there was little merit in attempting to define the "ideal" either logically or on the basis of research results, as there simply had been too much clutter in earlier attempts to do so and appropriate data did not exist. Moreover, they recognized that the effects of environment, situation, mood, or emotional states had too much of an impact on voice to permit them to construct any but the most tentative hypotheses about the issue. Rather, these investigators approached the problem by studying speakers they identified as trained or superior; these were individuals who might approximate "the ideal." To permit better interpretation, they sometimes (but not always) contrasted the performance of their subjects to those (1) provided by untrained individuals or (2) perceived as exhibiting inferior voice/speech characteristics. Nearly all of the cited researchers focused on speaking fundamental frequency (SFF, F_0); others included intensity and/or prosody, and a few attempted direct analysis of "quality." Incomplete, of course, but their efforts led to a tentative structure about the attributes of a good voice. For example, Lynch (1934) found that her "trained" subjects (actors, theater faculty, etc.) exhibited a higher mean fundamental frequency than did her inexperienced talkers; they (the "trained" speakers) also exhibited greater SFF range and variability—as well as a generally slower speaking rate. What she did not do is determine if her experienced subjects actually were perceived as being superior to the control subjects; she just assumed that they were.

In a sense, Pronovost (1943) confirmed the Lynch evaluations, finding that his superior speakers had a rather high SFF. However, as he did not employ controls of any kind, his data also are of but limited usefulness. Cowan (1936) also added a modest new element to the effort. He did not employ controls either but did add intensity and certain prosodic features to his other suprasegmental analyses. As it can be assumed that professional actors from the New York stage probably speak in a manner superior to members of the general public, Cowan's data (when compared to those on average subjects) probably can be used to suggest that superior voices show a somewhat higher SFF, a higher intensity, a somewhat slower rate, and, especially, more variability than do ordinary speakers.

Lewis and Tiffin (1934) and Murray and Tiffin (1934) also attempted to upgrade what was known about "superior" voices. In the initial study, a small number of subjects (N = 6) were sorted on the basis of perceived "effectiveness" of voice and speech; in the second, a large number (N = 122) were perceptually divided into good and poor groups, with a third cohort (N = 22) selected from a "trained" population. These investigators then analyzed the speech and voice of the individuals and/or groups who had been placed in the different categories. As it turns out, their data (plus those from others in the listed group) tended to further confirm the previously cited relationships.

The sum total of these studies would suggest that good or superior (if not "ideal") speakers can be expected to exhibit somewhat higher SFF than do average talkers. They also can be expected to speak slower and, overall anyway, a little louder. Finally, they can be said to exhibit a somewhat more complex spectra (quality) than average speakers and one with reasonably good "consistency." Perhaps most important, nearly all investigators report that the better voices showed greater-to-much-greater variability in speaking fundamental frequency and intensity.

1.3.2. More Modern Approaches

Other than that to follow, little research on "ideal voice quality" has been or is being (currently) carried out. Again, organization of what is known about normal (rather than ideal) voice is the primary focus here. One of the leaders in this area is Laver (1980, 1993) who, of course, structures the normal voice on the basis of the available data on relevant features (see also Laver & Hanson, 1981). He provides lists (see especially, Laver, Wirz, MacKenzie, & Hiller, 1985), but then draws on the research to validate these features. However, even when he is working within the area of phonetics, Laver most often contrasts his normal descriptions to those for pathological voices rather than superior ones. However, he also presents an extensive and insightful review of phonatory features such as register (modal, creak, falsetto), as well as voice type (modal, whisper, breathiness, harsh), and these contrasts are quite useful. Nevertheless, Laver's focus is on the basic, functional description of voice rather on the higher "quality" levels of this behavior.

But, do any of these relationships lead us any closer to an understanding or even a basic definition of ideal voice quality? Probably not. What they may provide is a structure which permits some research on *good* voice/speech production.

2. A PERSPECTIVE

In all fairness, it must be obvious by now that the concept of "ideal voice quality" cannot be established on any basis close to universal. There simply are no characteristics that will always separate ideal voice from average voice—and do so in the many, many situations in which it is relevant to the process. Admittedly, there are speakers who are considered by many to exhibit superb voice quality. The American actor Henry Fonda was one such individual. Saying this, however, it must be conceded that his voice could not be considered ideal for all situations and there probably are people who would not class his voice as ideal in the first place.

Thus, it would seem that the goals of this chapter should not be overly ambitious—that is, to aspire to provide a full definition and description of "ideal voice quality." Rather and as with other chapters in this book, there should be a stretching of the concept's borders. On the other hand, the adopted focus should be one that extends beyond a limited description of *normal* voice and speech. Those operations also constitute boundaries established around what is both average and appropriate. Although it is a little difficult to organize them (Michel, 1985), at least some data for this purpose appear to be available. Accordingly, what will be attempted here is to build on materials (as well as on the relationships reported above) in an effort to expand the available structure from the "normal" *toward* the "ideal." In other words, questions can be asked about the constituent attributes of good or superior voice and speech. To address even these modest goals, it is necessary to limit the discussion even further. For one thing, defining what may be good in all situations and environments still cannot be attempted. Singing and dramatic portrayals, for example, have to be omitted, as do other specific and special phonatory productions. The focus then is on the definition/description of good voice (if not superior or exceptional) under general speaking conditions. Perhaps the term "preferred" (by the listener, that is) leads to a better definition here. A final limitation: The term "voice quality" is expanded a little to mean good voice or speech.

3. A RELEVANT STUDY

The next phase of our search for the "good voice" will build on what was previously gleaned from the data reported by the investigators already cited. To do so, however, it also is necessary to consider current research. The first set of relationships are drawn from an existing research program—one where some (but not all) of the substudies already have been published (Hollien, Gelfer, & Carlson, 1991; Hollien & Hollien, 1987). The thrust in this case was organized somewhat differently than those cited previously. In this instance, the speakers were required to rigorously control their speech, that is, their speaking fundamental frequency (SFF) and vocal intensity (VI). In certain of the several procedures employed, groups of auditors were permitted to rank the talkers' level of vocal excellence on the basis of a 5-point scale (1 = very much liked; 5 = very much disliked). Exacting controls of the talkers' productions were established and only those individuals who could meet rigid performance criteria were accepted as subjects. Specifically, each speaker had to produce a standard passage read orally (Fairbanks, 1960) at the controlled frequency and intensity levels found in Table 2–1. Even though an intensity effect was found in one instance (see table footnote), subjects were able to stay within the frequency-intensity ranges for the entire reading of the passage; indeed, no samples could have been used unless the subject met the appropriate SFF-VI criteria. The accuracy of these controls was verified by sound level meter readings and FFI-8 frequency analysis (Hollien, 1990).

In all, 80 subjects (half each, males and females) served as talkers; thus, there were 10 samples in each of the eight cells, with the sexes equally represented. Listeners were 80 different individuals selected primarily on the basis of age, educational/socioeconomic status, good health, and normal hearing ability (tested); they were divided into four cohorts, with 10 males and 10 females in each. To be specific, these listener groups consisted of (20 each): (1) young adults (age range: 20–30 years), (2) adults (30–40 years), (3) older adults (60–70 years), and (4) the elderly (80–86 years).

As may be seen from Tables 2–2 and 2–3, which present the *combined* mean scores for all four listener groups, the mid-intensity and low frequency conditions were pretty much dominant. As can be seen from consideration of Table 2–2, the most compelling relationship is that of intensity (mid-intensity to be specific), the second major effect is for low speak-

Table 2–1. The speaking fundamental frequency and intensity categories* for the 80 talkers.

Parameter	Condition		
	Low	***Medium***	***High***
Frequency (Hz)			
Male	95–115	120–135	140–165
Female	165–190	190–215	220-255
Intensity (dB)			
Male	60–65	70–75	80–85
Female	60–65	70–75	80–85

*The low-SFF, high-VI condition could not be included, as only three subjects (of the 10 needed) could perform the task. For a discussion of this problem, see Coleman, Mabis, and Hinson, 1977.

ing fundamental frequency. The primary domination of the mid-intensity plus low-SFF parameters may best be seen by observing the combined scores found on Table 2–3. The data for the low-SFF/low-VI cell show that listeners have a secondary preference for speakers who exhibit these features. Please note also that, although not shown, the absolute values found in these tables are truncated somewhat because of the different rating levels found among the four listener groups. However, even there, it was observed that mid-VI was almost always picked first and low-SFF second. Conversely, it also may be seen (Table 2–3) that auditors did not like speech at high intensities and high frequencies; indeed the high VI-SFF combination was always scored worst.

4. ADDITIONAL DATA

At first glance, these results do not appear to square very well with those drawn from the earlier research. However, these seeming differences may result, at least partly, from variation in the task-related environment. In the present case, the speakers met rigorous phonatory criteria; they were not preselected as trained or superior. Moreover, they represented reasonably large populations and the equipment was of modern laboratory quality. Although these "preference" type studies appear appropriate and stable, any conceptual advance will require that these data be synthesized with those from the previous studies—and new data added. Moreover, it would appear that the factors permitting assessment and identification of the quality under study must be considered one at a time. The order for these discussions is speaking fundamental frequency, vocal intensity, prosody, and voice quality.

4.1. Speaking Fundamental Frequency (SFF or F_0)

A great deal of research has been carried out on SFF (see summaries by Hollien, Hollien & DeJong, 1997; Pegoraro Krook, 1988). In virtually all instances, the foci have been on normal phonation as a function of age, sex, race, or some behavioral factor (singing, smoking, etc.). A summary of the expected SFF means, as a function of age and sex, is found in Figure 2–1. This figure, although based on the best information available, only provides estimates for normal speaking individuals. Thus, although it contains baseline material permitting contrasts from the normal to the superior voice, it does not also provide good predictions for any "special" or exceptional populations.

4.1.1. Mean F_0 Data

A seeming contradiction appears to exist if the materials considered up to this juncture are

Table 2–2. Mean preference scores for 80 listeners (combined from four age groups) when judging samples that were produced at combinations of low, middle, and high SFF and vocal intensity (excepting Low-SFF/High-VI). The smaller the value the more favorable the preference. Ranks are in parentheses.

Speaking Condition	*Frequency*	*Intensity*	*Combined*
Low	2.76 (1)	2.90 (2)	2.83 (1)
Middle	3.14 (2)	2.68 (1)	2.91 (2)
High	3.24 (3)	3.94 (3)	3.59 (3)

Table 2–3. Mean preference scores for the 80 listeners when responding to the low-to-high frequency and intensity combinations. Lower scores carry a higher acceptance. Ranks are in parentheses.

	Intensity		
Frequency	*Low*	*Medium*	*High*
Low	2.83 (2)	2.72 (1)	—*
Medium	3.02 (5)	2.91 (3)	3.54
(7)			
High	3.07 (6)	2.96 (4)	3.59
(8)			

*It proved impossible to obtain enough low-SFF/High-VI talkers to include data in that cell.

contrasted with each other and then to Figure 2–1. What can be seen is that the SFF levels for the early research cited (i.e., Black, 1942; Cowan, 1936; Lynch, 1934; Pronovost, 1943; etc.) would fall above the Figure 2–1 means and those from the preferences study (Hollien & Hollien, 1987; Hollien et al., 1991) would be at or below them. The answer to this apparent lack of agreement actually seems clearcut. All of the individuals identified in the earlier studies as having "trained" or "superior" voices were actors (some were actually among the leading actors of that period) and their presentations were either of dramatic material or bordering on it. Little wonder that their SFF was higher than that for adequate, average, or normal speakers. Further validation of this relationship is provided by (1) assessment of their level of vocal intensity (higher than average) and (2) the Brown, Morris, Hollien, and Howell (1991) study (even older professional actors and actresses tended to exhibit higher than average F_0). Finally (as a student at the University of Iowa), I personally heard several of the cited recordings . There is but little question that the professionals were producing fairly loud "stage speech" when they served as subjects in these investigations. In short, it appears fair to say that some of the findings from the earlier studies resulted from the "situation" encountered rather than the natural attributes of the subjects. Hence, the available data (plus observation by practitioners) suggest that good speech/voice quality is associated with lower-than-average (not higher) speaking fundamental frequency.

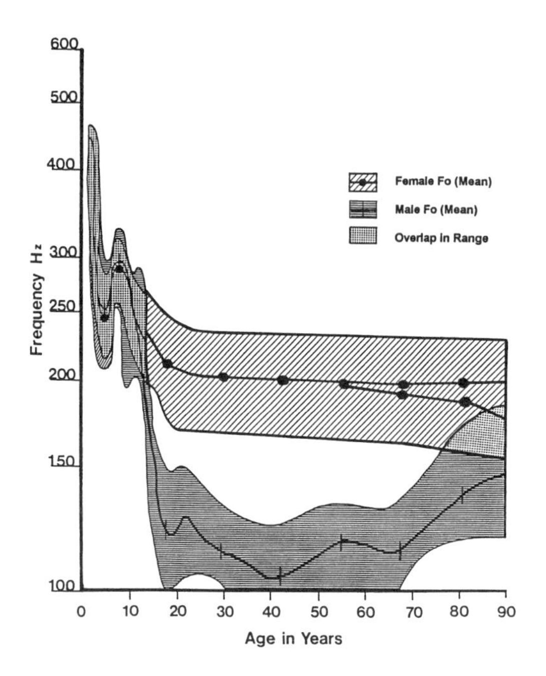

Figure 2–1. Graphic portrayal of generalized data for male/female speaking fundamental frequency levels as a function of age. The data are plotted in Hertz; variation around the means is indicated by the hatched areas. Note, there is now some question as to whether female SFF level remains constant or is lowered in older women.

4.1.2. SFF Variability

One nearly universal research finding is that there is a substantial correlation between good voice quality and high SFF variability. Practitioners appear to agree. In any event, all data generated to date support the idea that good speech and voice is associated with a higher than average F_0 variability. Terms such as flexible, dynamic, and supple are often applied to such variation.

4.2. Mean Vocal Intensity

In a sense, this characteristic relates fundamentally to mean SFF, for again a contradiction appears to exist. That is, the actors studied in the earlier investigations exhibited higher than average mean vocal intensity, whereas the preferred speakers in the later research spoke at levels that were the same or softer than most average or normal talkers. In this instance also, the relationship appears to relate to the nature of the speaker and the type of performance given (that is, the actors spoke louder). Hence, it may be deduced that, here too, good or superior quality can be associated with softer vocal intensities.

4.2.1. Vocal Intensity Variability

As with SFF, the relationship between increased intensity variation and better speech/voice quality appears to be nearly universal. Just about all of the research findings, plus many stated opinions, appear to support the postulate that one of the salient features of good quality is greater (but not extremely greater) variability in vocal intensity usage.

4.3. Prosody

Speech rate is a rather complex entity and how this prosodic feature operates to affect voice/speech *quality* is not very well understood. For example, Feldstein and Bond (1981) and Bond, Feldstein, and Simpson (1988) have reported that this speaking attribute is itself influenced by SFF and VI. Nevertheless, virtually all research has demonstrated that slower than average speaking rates (but not abnormally slow ones) can be associated with the perception of good speech. But, do these relationships also correlate with good voice quality? Probably not completely—especially if voice quality is defined in its narrowest sense. However, the suggestions by Feldstein and Bond are such that this factor could lead to judgments of better quality, at least, if the judgments are associated primarily with speaking as opposed to singing. This relationship is supported by (unpublished) data resulting from the preference studies described above (Hollien et al., 1991; Hollien & Hollien, 1987). In those instances, talkers judged as exhibiting the most pleasing speech/voice spoke at a measurably slower rate (if not a statistically significant one) than did those individuals whose speech was judged less pleasant. In short, if prosodic features can be associated with good or superior quality, a somewhat slower than normal speaking rate would appear to correlate positively with it.

4.4. Quality

This speaking attribute is, at once, the most central of all the factors and the most difficult to address (see also Michel, 1985). At its core is, of course, wave composition as measured by frequency spectra. The problem, however, lies not so much in just the manipulation of the partials (harmonic and otherwise) that make up this entity. Rather, the approach employed should involve both acoustic and perceptual research (see for example, Novak & Vokral, 1995; Zuckerman & Miyake, 1993). Unfortunately, however, such efforts appear lacking. To illustrate the needed perceptual approaches: Large numbers of speakers should be rated by large numbers of auditors in a variety of situations and by rigorous scaling (or related) procedures. Given those kinds of data, it might be possible to provide at least tentative (and, hopefully, testable) descriptions of good, superior, or ideal voice quality. Research of this type simply has not been carried out. Hence, although opinions abound, data are in very short supply. Worse yet, even those research materials that are available are quite limited in scope.

One area in which preference testing has been carried out is in the rather restricted domain of vowel quality. For example, when Fairbanks and Grubb (1961) attempted to specify the formants/allophones for the vowels of American English, they generated three types of samples: (1) approved, (2) most intelligible (identified), and (3) preferred. As it turns out, there appeared to be no discernible differences when the preferred vowels were contrasted to the other two sets nor when all three were compared to the patterns reported by Peterson and Barney (1952) or Wakita (1977). Nonetheless, the excellence of vowel quality should correlate (at least to some extent) with voice quality. Certainly, efforts should be made not just to ensure vowel accuracy, but also to upgrade their basic quality (Skinner, 1980).

But what of overall voice quality percepts? By and large they appear to be related to contrasts involving (1) voice degradation (Anders, Hollien, Hurme, Sonninen & Wendler, 1988; Baken, 1987; Gelfer, 1996; Hollien & Martin 1996; Sataloff, Bough, & Spiegal, 1994; Stemple, 1984; Wilson, 1987), (2) efforts to improve this characteristic (see, for example Theiler and Lippman, 1995), (3) the nature of specific elements within the general rubric of the factor (Schoenhardt & Hollien, 1982), or (4) how different classes of auditors make their judgments (Anders et al., 1988; Hollien & Hollien, 1987). Worse yet, the judgments, even when appropriate, are confounded because they are only a part of the overall matrix: one that consists of a number of attributes (Black, 1942; Cowan, 1936; Hollien et al., 1991; Hollien & Hollien, 1987). Accordingly, there is little here that can be done other than to rely on the subjective descriptions of practitioners who argue that good voice quality should be "pleasing" or "vibrant" or "full and deep" or "complex but consistent" or involving a "nasal-oral balance." Actually, their descriptions make a good deal of sense. Unfortunately, they lack the precision that would provide a basis for useful operational definitions. Indeed, there is no question but that they are quite difficult to define (Tveteras, 1992) or even transcribe (Ball, Code, Rahilly, & Hazlett, 1994).

5. CONCLUSIONS

It should be reiterated that the concept of "ideal voice quality" or even voice quality in general is an important one. Moreover, it is of *substantial* consequence to those of us (phoneticians, speech pathologists, speech teachers, drama coaches, and singing teachers) who deal with the concept on a daily basis. It also interfaces with many other factors. Two examples are: voice quality has an impact on social skills (Boice & Monti, 1982) and also is of influence when attempts are made to develop adequate speech synthesis systems (Paris, Gilson, Thomas, & Silver, 1995).

Yet, it also must be remembered that voice quality determinations are made on a level that can be more complex than that of basic speech perception; processes that are difficult in-and-of-themselves (Allen, 1994; Kingston & Diehl, 1994; Watson & Foyle, 1985). Worse yet, patterns can be established by auditors that limit judgmental class; in turn, these occurrences can serve to distort the ultimate classes (see modeling by Nearey, 1997). Thus, the question must be asked if any kind of relvant modeling can be carried out, especially as there are but few data and the processes involved tend to degrade the possibility of developing adequate structure. Actually the answer can be couched (at least tentatively) in the affirmative.

Reasonable estimates of the phonatory and prosodic features thought associated with good, or superior, voice quality can be found in Figure 2–2. Specifically, good (if not ideal) speech-voice quality can be said to exhibit the following characteristics.

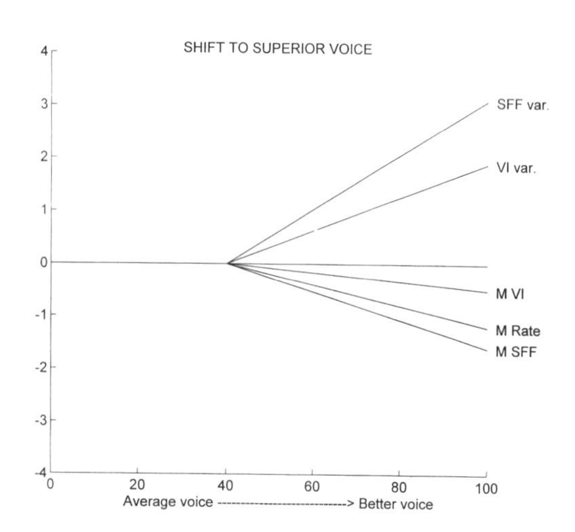

Figure 2–2. A model suggesting how various phonatory and prosodic features shift as human voices are upgraded from average to superior. The values portrayed are not calculated but rather included to suggest function. M-SFF = mean speaking fundamental frequency, SFF var. = speaking fundamental frequency variability, M VI = mean vocal intensity, VI var. = vocal intensity variability, and M Rate = mean speaking rate. Quality could not be portrayed.

1. The speakers will phonate at lower-than-average fundamental frequencies,
2. Superior voices will tend to be associated with average to softer than average vocal intensity,
3. Extensive variability will occur for both fundamental frequency and vocal intensities,
4. Speakers will speak at rates that are somewhat slower than average,
5. Although speaker's voice quality relationships are not shown in Figure 2–2, these will exhibit a well organized spectrum. That is, each voice will be broad band and not exhibit noise (such as breathiness, harshness, etc). As with all the other features, voice quality will be appropriate for the situation.

Is there any chance that the needs of the many professionals who would profit by identifications of "ideal voice quality" can ever be met? Only if the entire effort is structured to take into account the specific situation within which the speech-voice utterances are produced can the answer be "yes."

REFERENCES

Allen, J. (1994). How do humans process and recognize speech? *IEEE Transactions Speech, Audio Processing, 2,* 567–577.

Anders, L., Hollien, H., Hurme, P., Sonninen, A., & Wendler, J. (1988). Perception of hoarseness by several classes of listeners. *Folia Phoniatrica, 40,* 91–100.

Anderson, V. (1942). *Training the speaking voice.* New York: Oxford University Press.

Baken, R. (1987). *Clinical measurement of speech and voice*. Boston: College-Hill Press.
Ball, M. J., Code, C., Rahilly, J., & Hazlett, D. (1994). Non-segmental aspects of disordered speech: Developments in transcription. *Clinical Linguistics and Phonetics, 8,* 67–83.
Bell, A. G. (1907). *The mechanism of speech*. New York: Funk and Wagnalls.
Black, J. W. (1942). A study of voice merit. *Quarterly Journal of Speech, 28,* 67–74.
Boice, R., & Monti, P. (1982). Specification of nonverbal behaviors for clinical assessment. *Journal of Nonverbal Behavior, 7,* 79–94.
Bond, R. N., Feldstein, S., & Simpson, A. (1988). Relative and absolute judgements of speech rate from marked and content-standard stimuli. *Human Communication Research, 14,* 548–568.
Brown, W. S., Jr., Morris, R., Hollien H., & Howell, E. (1991). Speaking fundamental frequency characteristics as a function of age and professional singing. *Journal of Voice, 5,* 310–315.
Coleman, R. F., Mabis, J. H., & Hinson, J. (1977). Fundamental frequency-sound pressure level profiles of adult male and female voices. *Journal of Speech and Hearing Research, 20,* 197–204.
Cowan, M. (1936, December). Pitch and intensity characteristics of stage speech. *Archives of Speech,* Suppl., pp. 1–92.
Craig, A. E. (1938). *The junior speech arts*. New York: Macmillan and Co.
Fairbanks, G. (1960). *Voice and articulation drillbook*. New York: Harper Rowe.
Fairbanks, G., & Grubb, P. (1961). A psychophysical investigation of vowels. *Journal of Speech and Hearing Research, 4,* 203–219.
Feldstein, S., & Bond, R. N. (1981). Perception of speech rate as a function of vocal intensity and frequency. *Language and Speech, 24,* 387–394.
Glasgow, G. M. (1961). The effects of manner of speech on appreciation of spoken literature. *Journal of Educational Psychology, 52,* 322–329.
Gelfer, M. P. (1996). *Survey of communication disorders*. New York: McGraw-Hill Co.
Hoffman, W. G. (1940). *Public speaking today*. New York: McGraw-Hill Co.
Hollien, H. (1990). *The acoustics of crime*. New York: Plenum.
Hollien, H. (1993). That golden voice—Talent or training? *Journal of Voice, 7,* 195–205.
Hollien, H., Gelfer, M. P., & Carlson, T. (1991). Listening preferences for voice types. *Journal of Communication Disorders, 24,* 157–151.
Hollien, H., & Hollien, P. A. (1987). Listening preferences of the elderly. In R. Weiss & J-P. Köster (Eds.), *Festschrift Wängler* (pp. 121–140). Hamburg: Buske.
Hollien, H., Hollien, P. A., & DeJong, G. (1997). Effects of three parameters on speaking fundamental frequency. *Journal of the Acoustical Society of America, 102,* 2984–2992.
Hollien, H., & Martin, C. A. (1996). Conducting research on the effects of intoxication on speech. *Forensic Linguistics, 3,* 107–127.
Kent, R. D., Kent, J. F., & Rosenbek, J. C. (1987). Maximum performance tests of speech production. *Journal of Speech and Hearing Disorders, 52,* 367–387.
Kingston, J., & Diehl, R. (1994). Phonetic knowledge. *Language, 70,* 419–454.
Laver, J. (1980). *The phonetic description of voice quality*. Cambridge, UK: Cambridge University Press.
Laver, J. (1993). *Principles of phonetics*. Cambridge, UK: Cambridge University Press.
Laver, J., & Hanson, R. (1981). Describing the normal voice. In J. Darby (Ed.), *Speech evaluation in psychiatry*. New York: Grune and Stratton.
Laver, J., Wirz, S., MacKenzie, J., & Hiller, S. (1985). Vocal profile analysis in the description of voice quality. In V. Lawrence (Ed.), *Transactions, 14th Symposium, Care of the Professional Voice* (pp. 184–192). New York: The Voice Foundation.
Lewis, D., & Tiffin, J. (1934). A psychological study of individual differences in speaking ability. *Archives of Speech, 1,* 41–60.
Lynch, G. E. (1934). A phonophotographic study of trained and untrained voices reading factual and dramatic material. *Archives of Speech, 1,* 9–25.
Michel, J. (1985). The elusive nature of voice quality. In V. Lawrence (Ed.), *Transactions of the 14th Symposium: Care of the Professional Voice* (pp. 178–183). New York: The Voice Foundation.
Millar, S. (1993). In pursuit of clarity. *Language and Communication, 13,* 287–303.
Murray, E., & Tiffin, J. (1934). An analysis of some basic aspects of effective speech. *Archives of Speech, 1,* 61–83.
Nearey, T. M. (1997). Speech perception as pattern recognition. *Journal of the Acoustical Society of America, 101,* 3241–3254.
Novak, A., & Vokral, J. (1995). Acoustic parameters for the evaluation of voice for future voice professionals. *Folia Phoniaticia, 47,* 279–285.
Paris, C., Gilson, R., Thomas, M., & Silver, N. (1995). Effect of synthetic voice intelligibility on speech comprehension. *Human Factors, 37,* 335–340.

Pegoraro Krook, M. (1988). Speaking fundamental frequency characteristics of normal Swedish subjects obtained by glottal frequency analysis. *Folia Phoniaticia, 40,* 82–90.

Peterson, G., & Barney, H. L. (1952). Control methods used in the study of vowels. *Journal of the Acoustical Society of America, 24,* 175–184.

Pronovost, W. (1943). Experimental study of habitual and natural pitch levels of superior speakers. *Speech Monographs, 9,* 111–123.

Rasmussen, C. (1949). *Speech methods in the elementary schools.* New York: The Ronald Press.

Sataloff, R. T., Bough, I., Jr., & Spiegel, J. (1994). Arytenoid dislocation: Diagnosis and treatment. *Laryngoscope, 104,* 1353–1361.

Schoenhardt, C., & Hollien, H. (1982). A perceptual study of registration in female singers. *The NATS Bulletin, 39,* 22–28.

Scripture, E. W. (1902). *Elements of experimental phonetics.* New York: Scribner.

Skinner, E. (1980). *Good speech for the American actor* (cassette recording by E. Skinner & T. Monich; booklet by E. Skinner). New York: Drama Book Specialists.

Snidecor, J. S. (1952). The pitch and durational characteristics of superior female speakers, during oral reading. *Journal of Speech and Hearing Disorders, 16,* 44–52.

Stemple, J. (1984). *Clinical voice pathology.* Columbus, OH: Charles E. Merrill.

Stinchfield, S. M. (1928). *Speech pathology.* Boston: Expression Co.

Sweet, H. (1906). *A primer of phonetics* (3rd ed.). Oxford, UK: Clarendon Press.

Talley, C. H. (1937). A comparison of conversational and audience speech. *Archives of Speech, 2,* 28–40.

Theiler, A. M., & Lippman, L. G. (1995). Effects of mental practice and modeling on guitar and vocal performance. *Journal of General Psychology, 122,* 329–343.

Tveteras, G. (1992). Perceptual analysis of voice quality. *Scandinavian Journal of Logopedics and Phoniatrics,* 145–149.

Wakita, H. (1977). Normalization of vowels by vocal tract length and its application to vowel identification. *Transactions, Acoustics, Speech and Signal Processing,* ASSP-25, 183.192.

Watson, C. J., & Foyle, D. (1985). Central factors on the discrimination and identification of complex sounds. *Journal of the Acoustical Society of America, 78,* 375–379.

Wilson, D. (1987). *Voice problems in children* (3rd ed.). Baltimore: Williams and Wilkins.

Zuckerman, M., & Miyake, K. (1993). The attractive voice; what makes it so? *Journal of Nonverbal Behavior, 17,* 119–135.

CHAPTER 3

Crosslinguistic Aspects of Voice Quality

John H. Esling

1. THE SOCIAL CONTEXT OF VOICE QUALITY

There are a number of precedents in the description of the phonetic systems of languages of the world for positing that voice quality has a socially acquired and, therefore, a socially descriptive component. In fact, modern phonetics was founded on this principle. Sweet used the term *organic basis* in the sense of the long-term quality that distinguishes one language from another: "Every language has certain general tendencies which control its organic movements and positions, constituting its organic basis or basis of articulation" (1906, p. 74). Sweet's description is not meant to imply an anatomical distinction between speakers of different languages, but rather a different pattern of physiological behavior, for example, that the articulators have been "trained" to operate in different ways, depending on the phonetic constituents of the language that has been learned. Sapir, describing numerous phonological systems, provides an insightful perspective on patterning of sounds: "We are often under the impression that we are original or otherwise aberrant when, as a matter of fact, we are merely repeating a social pattern with the very slightest accent of individuality" (1927 in Laver & Hutcheson 1972, p. 72).

The challenge outlined by Sapir is to develop a methodology to inform which elements of voice quality are socially normative and which are relatively idiosyncratic. "There is always something about the voice that must be ascribed to the social background. . . . In spite of the personal and relatively fixed character of the voice, we make voluntary adjustments in the larynx that bring about significant modifications in the voice. Therefore, in deducing fundamental traits of personality from the voice we must try to disentangle the social element from the purely personal one" (Sapir 1927, in Laver & Hutcheson 1972, p. 73).

Sweet (1906, p. 74) commented generally on the typical postures or "neutral positions" that characterize several European languages. It should be pointed out that these characterizations are primarily auditory—that is, that the identification of long-term settings is based initially on the identification of qualities that are heard and placed within a systematic model of auditory categories. Thus, the "voluntary long-term muscular settings of the larynx and vocal tract" referred to by Laver (1970, p. 525) have auditory realizations that, given phonetic training in identifying the productions of a normal vocal tract, can be taken as indicative of those physiological adjustments.

Honikman (1964) made a number of auditory judgments of voice quality settings in European and Asian languages. The judgments are classified articulatorily, and the implication is that language learners can improve their auditory perception and their productive abilities by altering key postural parameters of their articulators. The term *articulatory setting* adopted by Honikman (1964) of the London school of Daniel Jones conveys the notion clearly that articulatory postures and patterns are "set" differently according to the sound system being acquired—that the "switches" for a number of articulatory parameters may be set differently depending on the language being learned. Catford (1964) outlines the "non-phonological function" of phonation "as a characteristic of the speaker as an individual, or of the language or dialect which the speaker is using: in this function, phonatory features may be indicative of the speaker's sex, age, health, social class, place of origin, etc." (p. 35). This is the sense in which Abercrombie uses the term "indexical" with reference to voice quality features (1967, pp. 5–9).

Abercrombie is explicit in dividing the aural medium into three strands, of which voice quality is the longest term and therefore the least likely to carry linguistic meaning while still likely to carry indexical significance (1967, pp. 89–95). Some of these indices are idiosyncratic, but a large proportion consist of regional indicators and social markers. The term *voice quality* refers to those features of speech present more or less all the time that a person is speaking—the background characteristics perceived as the most constant or persistent over time (see Esling, 1994). The notion of quasipermanence is enunciated quite clearly by Abercrombie (1967), who argues that although articulators do not remain in a permanent posture (otherwise segmental changes could not occur), our perception of articulator movement tends to fix them in space relative to each other. This implies that their average location over time can be calculated, either in terms of frequency of deviation from that average locus, the magnitude of that deviation, or the duration of one posture relative to others. It is also the hierarchical relationship between articulators that defines the prominence of one average location relative to another. Laver (1980, pp. 4–5) describes this as a figure-to-ground relationship of segmental fluctuations to voice quality.

Laver (1968) argues convincingly that social information, in addition to other traits, is likely to be conveyed at the long-term voice quality level of accent and cites ample evidence of voice quality settings that are associated with particular linguistic groups (Laver, 1980, pp. 4–7). In fact, it is not so much language that is the defining domain of voice quality variation, but rather social/regional affiliation that is the focus of production of voice quality; and code switching within a given sociolinguistic group may involve voice quality alterations. In the "matched-guise" tests of Lambert, Hodgson, Gardner, and Fillenbaum (1960), fluent bilinguals from Quebec produced phonetically comparable utterances in English and in French for rating by listeners. Listeners' assessments of the bilinguals on a number of social and psychological categories differed, even for the same speaker, according to what language was being spoken (see also Preston, 1989, pp. 50–51). Some of these holistic perceptual judgments could have been based on segmental or on intonational factors as well as on voice quality characteristics, but the matched-guise control assures that they were not based on individual features specific to the speaker. In a review of accommodation theory ("the general adjustment of a speaker's speech style in reaction to an interlocutor's speech style") in multiple language acquisition, Beebe and Zuengler (1983, p. 201) point out that it is not only the language code that can alter in social discourse, but also details of phonetic production. This is the level of "social intent"—the level above that of individual variation in speaker recognition—referred to by Nolan (1983, pp. 63–69).

Such observations prompt Laver (1980, pp. 2–3) to describe voice quality as social semiotic. The premise might be that if voice quality can be used paralinguistically to signal changes in affect, then voice quality can be used prototypically to reflect social identities at the level of linguistic groups. Preston (1992) reports a number of accent alterations in a sociolinguistic task in which White Americans were asked to "talk Black" and Blacks were asked to "talk White." Many of the features of Whites imitating Blacks were morphological or phonological; "much of the phonological imitation, however, took place at a non-segmental level" (p. 334). Changes to pitch, rate, and vocal quality included "slow speech, falsetto voice, deep voice, raspy voice, nasalization, and rapid speech" (pp. 334–335). It is likely that rate changes primarily influence the continuant/noncontinuant manner of articulation of consonants, although pitch could play a major role affecting the impression of the shape and size of the vocal tract, especially of the pharynx. "Deep voice" could be a result of creaky phonation or of a lowered larynx posture and "raspy voice" points either to harshness and/or to constrictive effects of the pharyngeal sphincter (see Esling, 1996). If pharyngealization occurred in the imitations together with high pitch (viz. falsetto), then it is possible that some of the imitations used raised larynx voice.[1]

Also using imitative methodology, Zuengler (1988) offers an insight into the most salient features that listeners perceive in a second language with which they are familiar. Results suggest that native speakers are not generally aware of what it is in another language that makes its accent different, aside from a few salient phonological features that stand out as stereotypical. Individual speakers differ widely in their phonetic awareness, which is in any case usually not explicit. The main features altered implicitly by native Spanish speakers mimicking an American accent in Spanish were consonants and "a large majority produced the American English retroflex [ɹ]" in place of the Spanish [r] (p. 41). It could be that those instances of [ɹ] represent a tendency toward a generally more retracted tongue tip position in the Hispanic imitation of an American accent, but this was not clear from the study. In the context of speaker recognition (Nolan, 1983), these alterations parallel the effect of self-presentation—that is, how speakers relate to a given sociolinguistic image and how they adopt a particular manner of speaking depending on interlocutor and other surrounding conditions.

Esling (1978a, 1978b) found that the auditory qualities judged to occur in the voices of one social class of speakers differ from the qualities judged to occur in another social class—even within the same city. "Certain of the features which comprise particular voice types observed in the Edinburgh linguistic community are socially stratified in their distribution, with certain features predominant in certain groups" (Esling, 1978a, p. 18). Standard Edinburgh English is judged to have an extremely creaky, moderately close jaw and slightly nasal voice; whereas broad Edinburgh dialect is judged to have an extremely harsh, moderately protruded jaw voice with laminal

[1]Raised larynx voice is a term chiefly employed in the UK for a distinct voice quality more often distinguished in higher pitched voices. Articulatory correlates are nearest to raising the larynx from neutral position, entailing tongue root retraction with implied aryepiglottic or laryngeal sphincter engagement.

articulation of the tongue and a pharyngeal quality that was defined only imprecisely at the time. The voice quality labels that were used included faucalized, pharyngealized, raised larynx, and tense voice (Esling, 1978a). The quality of broad Scots being described was presumably the same quality identified by Sweet (1906, p. 73) as "the pig's whistle"—presumably a narrowing just above the glottis related to ventricular closure—also cited by Abercrombie (1991). An impressionistically similar label used by Bell (1916, p. 19), albeit in reference to deaf speech, is "the cry of a peacock." There is little question that dialects of Scots are distinguished regionally by differences in voice quality. Catford has remarked on the differences in phonation between the Glasgow, Edinburgh, and North East regions, including the aforementioned "tense" component.

> Anterior, hard, voice is characteristic of many North German speakers. In Britain some degree of "anteriorness" is very common in the dialects of North East Scotland, especially Aberdeenshire and Banff, as opposed to the very lax, full-glottal, voice commonly heard in Central Scotland. (Catford, 1977, p. 103)

Only recently have experimental studies afforded some insight into the nature of these adjustments at the back of the vocal tract and how they are related. The quality referred to as "anterior" is most probably a function of the laryngeal sphincter (see Esling, 1996), closely related to raised larynx voice (see Laver, 1980).

The qualities raised larynx voice and lowered larynx voice,[2] and pharyngealized voice and faucalized voice, were examined in detail by Esling, Heap, Snell, and Dickson (1994). By controlling pitch and comparing postproduction auditory qualities of isolated vowels, raised larynx voice and pharyngealized voice were found to be related—occurring complementarily, so that productions of vowels with either pharyngealized voice or raised larynx voice quality were perceived as pharyngealized voice at low pitch but as raised larynx voice at higher pitch. Similarly, productions of vowels with either lowered larynx voice or faucalized voice quality were perceived to be lowered larynx voice at low pitch but faucalized voice at higher pitch. Thus, the larynx height descriptors are shown to be pitch dependent, with a connection drawn between raising the larynx and pharyngeal constriction.

Laryngoscopic experimentation reveals pharyngeal articulations to be primarily a function of the aryepiglottic sphincter mechanism, and that the articulatory posture for pharyngealized voice is indeed the same configuration required to produce what is identified at higher pitch as raised larynx voice (Esling, 1996). The qualities of lowered larynx voice and faucalized voice, on the other hand, involve a vertical expansion of the pharyngeal space. This implies that the "tense" quality identified in the broad Edinburgh dialect sample in 1978 was either faucalized or raised larynx but not both and, in either case, was predominantly high pitched. Incidences of lowered larynx voice are articulatorily consistent with judgments of faucalized voice, but represent a lower level of pitch of the individual speaker's voice. It is likely, in retrospect, that the Scots dialect voices reflected a vertically expanded pharynx, produced with either higher pitch or, in some cases, low pitch, and that a degree of pharyngeal constriction was occasionally present—being interpreted at high pitch as intermittent raised larynx voice.

When contemplating distinctions that differentiate social groups, it must also be remembered that gender and age cut across group lines. Pitch differences, which average higher for females than for males, exert considerable influence on the perceptual quality ascribed to any voice. The mechanics of voicing (vocal fold vibration) can also be shown to dif-

[2]Lowered larynx voice is a term mostly used in the UK, a distinct quality identified primarily in lower pitched voices. Its articulatory correlates are a lowering of the larynx from neutral position, resulting in an "expanded" pharynx.

fer systematically for females, with a generally smoother vibratory pattern and less variability over time (Monsen & Engebretson, 1977). Females have been shown to produce breathier voice than males in some samples (of English) or to be perceived as breathier (Henton & Bladon, 1985; Klatt & Klatt, 1990). Furthermore, the aging process has an effect on the production and perception of the voice within and across social group lines. Some of the changes that occur with aging are physiological (see Hollien, 1987), but others may be the result of accommodating to an elder style of discourse.

2. VOICE QUALITY INDICES

Abercrombie (1967) mentions two specific voice quality indices: "nasal twang," apparently a reference to some southern U.S.A. accents (p. 30) and its opposite, denasal (largely through velarization) or "adenoidal" quality that Abercrombie associates with the accent of Liverpool (p. 95). The one defining feature of Received Pronunciation (RP), Abercrombie writes, is its "extensive" use of creaky voice (1991, p. 48), implying more than just a phrase-final incidence. Catford (1977) also comments that creaky voice occurs "with low pitch in certain types of British English" (p. 101), and he cites the social incidence of voice qualities that depend on the position of the larynx such as "anterior voice" in many Scots dialects. The same quality, "sometimes approaching strangulation" and "combined with high key" was noted by Sweet (1906, p. 73) as characteristic of some Scottish and Saxon German pronunciations. Using Laver's terminology, this quality can be described as a function of the laryngeal sphincter—the posture for pharyngealized or raised larynx voice, with raised pitch (see Esling 1996). Furthermore, Catford implies that certain types of British speech such as RP are distinctive in voice quality from other varieties because of "stretches of utterances" that are characterized by low-pitched creakiness (p. 100). Sweet was very clear that "controllable organic positions" over the long term "may—and often do—characterize the speech of whole communities" (1906, p. 73). Also in the Scottish phonetic tradition, A. G. Bell (1916) described some hearing-impaired speech as having been acquired in a way that apparently used the pharyngeal mechanism rather than the glottal mechanism for controlling pitch. Although described impressionistically, his observation is important in signaling that habitually maintained postures of certain articulators are responsible for qualities that distinguish one voice from another—a result of the process of the acquisition of accent.

Labov's earliest research suggests the importance of describing articulatory setting and its social distribution. To consolidate a number of related phonological variables, Labov drew attention to the level of voice quality setting and its economy of explanation. In his study of Martha's Vineyard, Massachusetts, Labov wrote that

> there are no less than 14 phonological variables which follow the general rule that the higher or more constricted variants are characteristic of the up-island "native" speakers, while the lower, more open variants are characteristic of down-island speakers under mainland influence. We can reasonably assume that this "close-mouthed" articulatory style is the object of social affect. It may well be that social evaluation interacts with linguistic structures at this point, through the constriction of several dimensions of phonological space. Particular linguistic variables would then be variously affected by the overall tendency towards a favored articulatory posture, under the influence of the social forces we have been studying. (1972, p. 40)

Trudgill (1974) devised a set of rules to describe Norwich English in which generalizations at the level of voice quality contribute to the economy of explanation of lower-level phonological processes. Working-class Norwich speech is described as creaky, higher in pitch, louder, and more fronted than middle-class Norwich speech, with greater tongue lowering, larynx raising, and nasality. These latter features suggest the possibility of a raised setting of the pharynx (slight pharyngealization) that would contrast with a lowered-larynx, lengthened-pharynx setting.

Laver and Trudgill (1979) offer explicit suggestions as to the types of features that act as markers of linguistic group membership and that can presumably be used to alter images in sociolinguistic switching circumstances. Among them are nasality in Received Pronunciation in Britain and also in many Australian (see Pittam, 1987b) and American accents, and velarization in Liverpool or Birmingham, for example. Although social class may be marked by a preference for particular settings, these preferences also depend on regional standards of accent. For instance, although a nasal setting carries high social prestige when associated with certain accents (RP or Standard Edinburgh English), it stands out as an undesirable feature to many listeners when associated with other accents (see Pittam, 1994). Laver and Trudgill also cite the paralinguistic function of long-term settings: harsh phonation with raised pitch and loudness for anger in English or a "smiling" spread lip setting to signal cheerfulness or even derision, depending on the dynamic features (of intonation, for example) that accompany it. Velarization is reported to be used as a marker of a threatening tone of voice in Bangkok Thai (Harris, 1987; Laver, 1994). Although the emotive indices of voice quality have been studied in detail (summarized in Pittam, 1994), it is important for the purposes of the analysis of voice quality in accent to differentiate physiologically induced changes in the voice from the relatively more voluntary paralinguistic modifications to an underlying setting or complex of settings that mark a speaker's social roles and, indeed, self-concept.

The long-term state of the lips is compared crosslinguistically by Honikman (1964), who notes that French involves considerable mobility and rounding, and English remains rather neutral, with Russian maintaining a horizontally spread posture and only infrequent rounding. She also notes that the jaw remains close and moves comparatively little in British English, although in French the jaw lowers more often. Accents of India are described as having a minimally contracted labial setting with the jaw held loosely open. As for lingual settings, English is characterized as primarily apical (tongue tip articulation) and alveolar, with French characterized as laminal (tongue blade articulation) and dental. By contrast, Turkish and Iranian (Farsi) are described as dental but also apical, implying a different auditory effect, as the tongue occupies a different space in the front of the oral cavity. In Russian, the prevalence of palatalized sounds is noted, implying a habitually high and spread posture of the tongue body for ease of articulation. The tendency of Russian speech to have a high back, velarized overlay is noted by Harris (1987). An important aspect of Honikman's pedagogical and observational methodology—training second-language speakers and teachers to modify parameters of setting selectively—is the notion of muscular development, where facial, mandibular, and lingual muscles can be seen to adopt a familiar setting from constant use. This is presumably a function of the reflex system of muscular toning. The relaxed state of many facial articulators in the pronunciation of English is contrasted with the more strongly contracted state of the lips and cheeks in the pronunciation of French, as an example.

Esling and Wong (1983) have described a set of parameters that can be taken to characterize a general variety of American English. They suggest that ease of articulation can be defined in terms of the settings of the various articulators relative to the predominant places of articulation of most consonantal and vocalic segments. This implies that a shorter distance between the central "hub" of most articulations and any given articulation defines the ease of achieving that articulation. This principle also implies that shifting pronunciation from one language to another may be accomplished most efficiently by moving habitual articulatory postures for speech to a location closer to the average position of segmental articulations of the target language. A further corollary implication that can also be explored is that instances of language change are accomplished by slightly altering articulatory posture, which in turn produces minute, subphonemic changes in the phonetic quality of certain susceptible segments. Such speculation merits a new systematic approach to the perceptual testing of phonetic production in psycholinguistics.

3. TECHNIQUES OF ANALYSIS OF SOCIAL MARKERS IN VOICE QUALITY

Elaborate acoustic studies have been carried out to isolate long-term changes that occur when bilinguals switch languages. Comparing long-term average spectral (LTAS) characteristics of native-language texts and an English text read by Arabic, French, and Cantonese speakers showed a high probability of differentiating the three language groups across both sets of texts (Esling, 1983). This suggests that the phonetic features of the three language samples contrast in long-term (recurring) acoustic information independently of text.

An initial methodology for voice quality analysis developed by Esling and Dickson (1985) resulted in an interesting comparison of four dialect samples of English against a set of phonetically performed model voices. Each of the four dialects correlated with a different set of phonetic models. Standard Edinburgh English correlated with nasal voice and palatalized voice, with broad Edinburgh dialect correlated with lowered larynx voice and close jaw voice (and also palatalized and faucalized voice). Urban Black Houston, Texas, speech correlated with velarized voice, raised larynx voice, and faucalized voice (and also laryngopharyngealized voice), although urban working-class Vancouver, B.C., speech correlated with laryngopharyngealized voice, uvularized voice, dentalized voice, retroflex articulation, and close rounded voice (along with faucalized voice). The acoustic correlation for Standard Edinburgh English fits with earlier auditorily based judgments of nasality and lingual fronting (Esling, 1978a, 1978b). The acoustic correlation for broad Edinburgh dialect is less obvious, but the subsequent discovery of a relationship between lowered larynx voice and faucalized voice (Esling et al., 1994) may explain why lowered larynx voice was identified as the principal acoustic feature, with faucalized voice being noticed in the auditory analysis. Close jaw quality (as well as palatalized quality) may be accounted for by the auditory judgments of protruded jaw, tongue blade articulation, and palatoalveolarized voice. Velarization was predicted auditorily in the Houston sample, and the matching of the raised larynx model with the Houston voices and of the laryngopharyngealized model with the Vancouver working-class voices may relate to the extreme lingual retraction required for both of those settings (Esling et al., 1994). The correlation of close rounding with the Vancouver voices may also be due to the similarity of its acoustic characteristics with extreme tongue backing. In any case, the parallel between matching by acoustic model and auditorily based judgments of quality remained ill defined in the early studies.

In an LTAS evaluation of French and Dutch bilinguals in Belgium, Harmegnies and Landercy (1985) found that "changing languages introduces more variability than changing texts (within a given language)" and, as variability between individual speakers is even greater, "the language spoken introduces some specific variability which probably arises from some language features" (p. 72). They mention the possibility that the presence of nasal vowels in French may account for the spectral differences observed between French and Dutch. They also note that as the subjects of the study are bilingual, the differences observed between the spectra of the two languages are probably less than would be expected in a general monolingual population. Harmegnies and Landercy (1986) reiterate that when a bilingual Belgian produces a phonetically balanced utterance in each language, the change in language introduces a systematic shift in LTAS.

The acoustic and statistical techniques developed in Harmegnies (1988) were used by Esling, Harmegnies, and Delplancq (1991) to analyze the long-term spectra of social groups in the Survey of Vancouver English. Based on the analysis of an identical reading passage from 192 subjects in the survey, spectra across age groups are weakly but positively differentiated, suggesting that speakers in the same age group share some long-term speech features, at least in oral reading style. Spectra across socioeconomic status (SES) groups are more strongly differentiated, suggesting that certain long-term speech features are shared by members of one SES group but differ from the features used in the speech of other groups. Whether these features are directly related to sustained articulatory postures, to common patterns of articulatory movement between postures, or to related phenomena such as pitch differences is difficult to establish precisely. What is clear is that for a relatively uniform variety of English (compared to British English, for example), socially differentiated levels of the Vancouver anglophone community exhibit distinct long-term traits in their speech that can be used to identify and distinguish them from one another.

Elaborate acoustic studies have been carried out to identify the features that change when such shifts occur. Harmegnies, Esling, and Delplancq (1989) identify and rank groups of settings that deliver similar spectral results. Although not all deliberate changes to voice quality exert a major influence on the LTAS, changes in laryngeal setting produce the greatest differences from the neutral setting. This agrees with Nolan's (1983) conclusions. Of the supralaryngeal settings, only raised larynx voice was observed to have an effect equal in significance to adjustments in laryngeal setting. Harmegnies, Delplancq, Esling, and Bruyninckx (1994) hierarchically summarize the acoustic effects that several phonetically controlled setting changes produce, both in English and French, and highlight which of those features produce the greatest effects. Phonatory features are again found to produce a larger effect than supralaryngeal features, but the effect of raised larynx is nearly as great as of phonation type. This result confirms the finding of Pittam (1987a) that creaky voice, breathy voice, and whispery voice yield significant differences in LTAS, but that nasal voice is not significantly differentiated using LTAS. These findings may account for some of the difficulties encountered in trying to isolate long-term supralaryngeal features and relate them to vowel shifts in Vancouver English in Esling (1987, 1991) and in Esling and Warkentyne (1993).

A description of Danish articulatory setting by Collins and Mees (1995) links pharyngeal and laryngeal phenomena. In characterizing Danish as both palatalized and laryngopharyngealized, part of the tongue is assumed to be raised, with the tongue root adopting a retracted posture. This action of pharyngealization, related to a closing off of the larynx as implied by using "laryngo," is accompanied by a quality of "tight" phonation akin to Catford's category of "anterior voice" (1977, p. 418). The recurring effect of the *stød* quality in Danish reinforces the interpretation that the larynx is "shutting down" beginning with the glottal vocal folds, ventricular folds, and finally the aryepiglottic folds at the most extreme degree of laryngopharyngealization. This movement can be regarded as the same physiological gesture responsible for pharyngeal and pharyngealized consonants in Semitic languages—as a sequence for laryngeal protective closure (see Esling, 1996). The interesting difference is that the Danish articulatory setting involves larynx lowering (instead of raising, which would be expected for full protective closure) that affords expanded chamber resonance above the sphinctered epilarynx during the radical retraction of the tongue. The setting of Danish is an illustration of the close relationship between long-term posture and the segmental incidence of articulatory features.

Harmegnies and Landercy (1994) argue that speakers' phonetic ability to modify minute details of articulatory production over the long term has been demonstrated in the research literature, but that the degree of change in articulatory posture that is perceptually significant to the hearer has not been demonstrated. As already pointed out by Laver and Trudgill (1979), listeners are adept at judging the physical characteristics of a speaker (including age) from the voice alone, at least for a linguistic community with which they are familiar. A relevant test of the theory of voice quality would be to measure how well listeners can judge physical characteristics of speakers from linguistic communities with which they are not familiar, the hypothesis being that many of these extralinguistic indexical features belong to the sustained, nonvarying, long-term component of accent, and that they are, like the more rapidly fluctuating components of accent, acquired in the context of a particular language group and social surrounding. Impressions of a speaker's sex are also fairly accurate based on vocal clues (Laver & Trudgill, 1979, pp. 11–12), but with some reported intentional deviation from the expected average, so that it is logical to predict that other social norms of group affiliation are also reflected in vocal clues at the long-term level.

In a comprehensive evaluation of voice quality in Catalan/Spanish bilinguals, not only was variability within the language group found to be less than between languages, but variability was also lower in general in the bilinguals' nondominant language (Bruyninckx, Harmegnies, Llisterri, & Poch-Olivé, 1994). This suggests a split between two codes, marked by a systematic shift in long-term accent features, where the second language exhibits tighter consistency than the first. Such a finding corresponds well with the restricted variability that has been observed to characterize second-language learners' segmental phonological systems and prosodic/ intonational patterns (Tarone, 1978).

4. SUMMARY

The systematic application of experimental techniques to the acoustic characteristics of speakers' voices in a series of studies on bilingual language production leads researchers such as Harmegnies and his colleagues to conclude that the significant variability of LTAS between languages "is properly to be found in voice quality shifts due to variation in the dominant features of articulatory behaviors" (Bruyninckx et al., 1994, p. 29).

The application of sociolinguistic and dialect survey techniques indicates further that long-term features of accent are not only language specific, but that they also vary according to the socioeconomic status of the speaker within the linguistic community. Regional variation in voice quality has been explored by Foldvik in Norway (1981) and by Elert and Hammarberg in Sweden (1991). Significant findings in the extensive Swedish survey include the identification of pitch parameters and creaky phonation, as well as of raised larynx quality as SES markers. It is these qualities of the pharynx and larynx that LTAS analyses indicate have the most critical acoustic effect on voice quality and which auditory analyses associate with the activity of laryngeal protective closure.

A relatively unexplored and interesting area of long-term quality is the effect of different degrees of sustained pharyngeal constriction on glottal phonation. An exploration of this relationship would help to clarify the role of raised larynx voice quality as a significant feature in altering the acoustic spectrum in the same way that phonatory settings alter the spectrum. Pharyngeal constriction can also involve pharyngeal trilling. The phenomenon of pharyngeal trilling is described as a periodic vibration of the aryepiglottic folds that is slower than the vibratory cycle of the vocal folds, but faster than trilling by other articulators in the mouth (Esling, 1996). Larynx raising, as found in pharyngealization, and larynx lowering, as accompanying breathy voicing, appear to have an influence on overall voice quality that is nearly as significant as the effect of glottal phonation type and pitch (Harmegnies et al., 1989). In fact, pharyngeal adjustments, pitch, and phonation share an interdependent relationship that may determine the major part of how voice quality is perceived.

REFERENCES

Abercrombie, D. (1967). *Elements of general phonetics*. Edinburgh: Edinburgh University Press.

Abercrombie, D. (1991). *Fifty years in phonetics*. Edinburgh: Edinburgh University Press.

Beebe, L. M., & Zuengler, J. (1983). Accommodation theory: An explanation for style shifting in second language dialects. In N. Wolfson & E. Judd (Eds.), *Sociolinguistics and language acquisition* (pp. 195–213). Rowley, MA: Newbury House.

Bell, A. G. (1916). *The mechanism of speech* (8th ed.). New York: Funk & Wagnalls Co.

Bruyninckx, M., Harmegnies, B., Llisterri, J., & Poch-Olivé, D. (1994). Language-induced voice quality variability in bilinguals. *Journal of Phonetics, 22*, 19–31.

Catford, J. C. (1964). Phonation types. In D. Abercrombie, D. B. Fry, P. A. D. MacCarthy, N. C. Scott, & J. L. M. Trim (Eds.), *In honour of Daniel Jones: Papers contributed on the occasion of his eightieth birthday 12 September 1961* (pp. 26–37). London: Longmans, Green & Co.

Catford, J. C. (1977). *Fundamental problems in phonetics*. Edinburgh: Edinburgh University Press; Bloomington: Indiana University Press.

Collins, B., & Mees, I. M. (1995). Approaches to articulatory setting in foreign-language teaching. In J. Windsor Lewis (Ed.), *Studies in general and English phonetics: Essays in honour of Prof. J.D. O'Connor* (pp. 415–424). London: Routledge.

Elert, C-C., & Hammarberg, B. (1991). Regional voice quality variation in Sweden. *Actes du XIIème Congrès International des Sciences Phonétiques* (Vol. 4, pp. 418–420). Aix-en-Provence: Université de Provence.

Esling, J. H. (1978a). The identification of features of voice quality in social groups. *Journal of the International Phonetic Association, 8*, 18–23.

Esling, J. H. (1978b). *Voice quality in Edinburgh: A sociolinguistic and phonetic study*. Unpublished doctoral dissertation, University of Edinburgh.

Esling, J. H. (1983). Quantitative analysis of acoustic correlates of supralaryngeal voice quality features in the long-time spectrum. In A. Cohen & M. van den Broecke (Eds.), *Abstracts of the Xth International Congress of Phonetic Sciences* (p. 363). Dordrecht: Foris.

Esling, J. H. (1987). Vowel shift and long-term average spectra in the Survey of Vancouver English. *Proceedings of the XIth International Congress of Phonetic Sciences* (Vol. 4, pp. 243–246). Tallinn: Academy of Sciences of the Estonian SSR.

Esling, J. H. (1991). Sociophonetic variation in Vancouver. In J. Cheshire (Ed.), *English around the world: Sociolinguistic perspectives* (pp. 123–133). Cambridge, UK: Cambridge University Press.

Esling, J. H. (1994). Voice quality. In R. E. Asher & J. M.Y. Simpson (Eds.), *The encyclopedia of language and linguistics* (pp. 4950–4953). Oxford, UK: Pergamon Press.

Esling, J. H. (1996). Pharyngeal consonants and the aryepiglottic sphincter. *Journal of the International Phonetic Association, 26*, 65–88.

Esling, J. H., & Dickson, B. C. (1985). Acoustical procedures for articulatory setting analysis in accent. In H. J. Warkentyne (Ed.), *Papers from the Fifth International Conference on Methods in Dialectology* (pp. 155–170). Victoria, BC: University of Victoria.

Esling, J. H., Harmegnies, B., & Delplancq, V. (1991). Social distribution of long-term average spectral characteristics in Vancouver English. *Actes du XIIème Congrès International des Sciences Phonétiques* (Vol. 2, pp. 182–185). Aix-en-Provence: Université de Provence.

Esling, J. H., Heap, L. M., Snell, R. C., & Dickson, B. C. (1994). Analysis of pitch dependence of pharyngeal, faucal, and larynx-height voice quality settings. *ICSLP 94* (pp. 1475–1478). Yokohama: Acoustical Society of Japan.

Esling, J. H., & Warkentyne, H. J. (1993). Retracting of /æ/ in Vancouver English. In S. Clarke (Ed.), *Focus on Canada* (pp. 229–246). Amsterdam/Philadelphia: John Benjamins.

Esling, J. H., & Wong, R. F. (1983). Voice quality settings and the teaching of pronunciation. *TESOL Quarterly, 17*, 89–95.

Foldvik, A. K. (1981). Voice quality in Norwegian dialects. In T. Fretheim (Ed.), *Nordic prosody II* (pp. 228–232). Trondheim, Norway: Tapir.

Harmegnies, B. (1988). *Contribution à la caractérisation de la qualité vocale*. Unpublished doctoral dissertation, Université de l'Etat à Mons, Belgium.

Harmegnies, B., Delplancq, V., Esling, J., & Bruyninckx, M. (1994). Effets sur le signal vocal de changements délibérés de qualité globale en anglais et français. *Revue de Phonétique Appliquée, 111*, 139-153.

Harmegnies, B., Esling, J. H., & Delplancq, V. (1989). Quantitative study of the effects of setting changes on the LTAS. In J. P. Tubach & J. J. Mariani (Eds.), *European conference on speech communication and technology* (Vol. 2, pp. 139–142). Edinburgh: CEP Consultants.

Harmegnies, B., & Landercy, A. (1985). Language features in the long-term average spectrum. *Revue de Phonétique Appliquée, 73–74-75*, 69–79.

Harmegnies, B., & Landercy, A. (1986). Comparison of spectral similarity indices for speaker recognition. *Proceedings of the 12th International Congress on Acoustics, 1*, A1–A4, Toronto.

Harmegnies, B., & Landercy, A. (1994). Effets sur la qualité vocale de modifications délibérées d'éléments de la sphère audio-phonatoire. *Revue de Phonétique Appliquée, 111*, 123–137.

Harris, J. G. (1987). *Linguistic phonetic notes (1969-1979)*. Bangkok: Chulalongkorn University.

Henton, C. G., & Bladon, R. A. (1985). Breathiness in normal female speech: Inefficiency versus desirability. *Language and Communication, 5*, 221–227.

Hollien, H. (1987). "Old voices": What do we really know about them? *Journal of Voice, 1*, 2–17.

Honikman, B. (1964). Articulatory settings. In D. Abercrombie, D. B. Fry, P. A. D. MacCarthy, N. C. Scott, & J. L. M. Trim (Eds.), *In honour of Daniel Jones: Papers contributed on the occasion of his eightieth birthday 12 September 1961* (pp. 73–84). London: Longmans, Green & Co.

Klatt, D. H., & Klatt, L. C. (1990). Analysis, synthesis, and perception of voice quality variations among female and male talkers. *Journal of the Acoustical Society of America, 87*, 820–857.

Labov, W. (1972). *Sociolinguistic patterns*. Philadelphia: University of Pennsylvania Press.

Lambert, W. E., Hodgson, R. C., Gardner, R. C., & Fillenbaum, S. (1960). Evaluational reactions to spoken languages. *Journal of Abnormal Social Psychology, 60*, 44–51.

Laver, J. (1968). Voice quality and indexical information. *British Journal of Disorders of Communication, 3*, 43–54.

Laver, J. (1970). The synthesis of components in voice quality. *Proceedings of the Sixth International Congress of Phonetic Sciences, Prague, 1967* (pp. 523–525). Prague: Academia.

Laver, J. (1980). *The phonetic description of voice quality*. Cambridge, UK: Cambridge University Press.

Laver, J. (1994). *Principles of phonetics*. Cambridge, UK: Cambridge University Press.

Laver, J., & Hutcheson, S. (Eds.). (1972). *Communication in face to face interaction*. Harmondsworth, UK: Penguin Books.

Laver, J., & Trudgill, P. (1979). Phonetic and linguistic markers in speech. In K. R. Scherer & H. Giles (Eds.), *Social markers in speech* (pp. 1–32). Cambridge, UK: Cambridge University Press; Paris: Editions de la Maison des Sciences de l'Homme.

Monsen, R. B., & Engebretson, A. M. (1977). Study of variations in the male and female glottal wave. *Journal of the Acoustical Society of America, 62*, 981–991.

Nolan, F. (1983). *The phonetic bases of speaker recognition*. Cambridge, UK: Cambridge University Press.

Pittam, J. (1987a). Discrimination of five voice qualities and prediction to perceptual rating. *Phonetica, 44*, 38–49.

Pittam, J. (1987b). Listeners' evaluations of voice quality in Australian English speakers. *Language and Speech, 30*, 99–113.

Pittam, J. (1994). *Voice in social interaction: An interdisciplinary approach*. Thousand Oaks, CA: Sage Publications.

Preston, D. R. (1989). *Sociolinguistics and second language acquisition*. Oxford, UK: Basil Blackwell.

Preston, D. R. (1992). Talking black and talking white: A study in variety imitation. In J. H. Hall, N. Doane, & D. Ringler (Eds.), *Old English and new: Studies in language and linguistics in honor of Frederic G. Cassidy* (pp. 327–355). New York: Garland Publishing.

Sapir, E. (1927). Speech as a personality trait. *American Journal of Sociology, 32*, 892–905.

Sweet, H. (1906). *A primer of phonetics* (3rd ed. revised). Oxford, UK: Clarendon Press.

Tarone, E. E. (1978). The phonology of interlanguage. In J. C. Richards (Ed.), *Understanding second and foreign language learning: Issues and approaches* (pp. 15–33). Rowley, MA: Newbury House.

Trudgill, P. (1974). *The social differentiation of English in Norwich*. Cambridge, UK: Cambridge University Press.

Zuengler, J. (1988). Identity markers and L2 pronunciation. *Studies in Second Language Acquisition, 10*, 33–49.

CHAPTER 4

Phonetic Evaluation of Voice Quality

John Laver

Analyzing the quality of speakers' voices and understanding the underlying physiological actions has captured the interest of scholars from classical times onwards (Laver 1978, 1981). But the scientific study of the voice and its quality has only comparatively recently attracted the detailed attention of more modern subjects concerned with speech. Phonetics has been one of these subjects, together with speech science and speech pathology (Abercrombie, 1967; Baer, Sasaki, & Harris, 1987; Bless & Abbs, 1983; Catford, 1964; Fujimura, 1988; Gauffin & Hammarberg, 1991; Greene & Mathieson, 1989; Hirano, 1981; Hollien, 1974; Laver, 1968, 1980, 1991a, 1994; Luchsinger & Arnold, 1965; Nolan, 1983; Pittam, 1994; Stevens & Hirano 1981; Sweet, 1877; Titze & Scherer, 1983). This chapter offers a perspective on the evaluation of voice quality from the descriptive viewpoint of a phonetician.

1. ORGANIC AND PHONETIC ASPECTS OF VOICE QUALITY

The characteristic sound of a speaker's voice arises from the interaction of two different types of factors, *organic* and *phonetic* (Abercrombie, 1967; Laver, 1980). Organic factors are structural, with phonetic factors dealing with neuromuscular patterns of voluntary control. Organic factors derive from biologically determined architectural and mechanical aspects of the speech apparatus, with phonetic factors being the result of socially and idiosyncratically learned muscular habits acquired over the lifetime of a speaker.

Organic design is reflected in the geometry, dimensions, and mass of the vocal apparatus (Abercrombie, 1967; Laver, 1991b). Major elements are the overall length of the vocal tract; the residual shape and volume of the three cavities that make up the tract—the mouth, the pharynx, and the nasal cavity; the size, mass, and shape of the upper and lower jaws; the size and distribution of the teeth; the volume of the tongue; the structural and mechanical make-up of the larynx; and the volume and power of the respiratory system. The variation of voice quality arising from interpersonal details of the vocal architecture of different speakers is at least as marked as the variation of their facial appearance.

Organic factors include both healthy and pathological elements (Mackenzie Beck, 1988, 1997). They are subject to genetic and environmental variation, trauma, and disease. These influences therefore include slow life cycle structural and mechanical changes of growth in youth and atrophy in old age and more rapidly occurring, ephemeral conditions such as tonsillitis, a cold, laryngitis, or hormonal effects of the menstrual cycle. Longer term pathological conditions affecting the characteristic quality of the voice can include tumors of the tongue, pharynx, or larynx that distort their normal physiological function in speech (Mackenzie Beck, Wrench, Jackson, Soutar, Robertson, & Laver, 1998) or edema due to thyroid pathology or polyps or nodules on the vocal folds (Mackenzie Beck, Laver, & Hiller, 1991). Equally, the trauma of surgery or accident can have long-term structural and mechanical effects.

Organic and phonetic factors necessarily interact in the perceptual outcome of every detail of the production of speech—in the phonatory activities of the larynx and the articulatory activities of the organs of the supralaryngeal vocal tract, alike. This is true of all aspects of speech, whether the focus of attention is on short-lived segments or syllables or on events of longer duration such as whole utterances or on the quasi-permanent, characteristic quality of a speaker's habitual voice. This chapter addresses the last of these aspects of speech, the quality of a speaker's habitual voice.

Some phoneticians use the term "voice quality" to refer, implicitly or explicitly, to the perceptual quality arising from the phonatory activities of the larynx alone. Others use "voice quality" for the perceptual quality arising from the combination of laryngeal and supralaryngeal activities together. In this chapter, I will take the latter approach. Specifically, the premise is that the interaction of organic and phonetic factors, operating in both phonation and articulation, generates a relatively consistent perceptual quality heard as running through the momentary variations of the consonants, vowels, and syllables of spoken utterances. It is this long-running, speaker-characterizing, general perceptual quality that is here called *voice quality* (Laver, 1980, 1991b, 1994; Laver & Hanson, 1981); and I distinguish between *articulatory aspects of voice quality* and *phonatory aspects of voice quality* as two major strands together making up the overall composite quality of the voice. Implicit in this approach is the view that the voice can be analyzed as the product of auditorily separable components.

Against the background that both articulatory and phonatory aspects of voice quality are necessarily a blend of organic and phonetic factors, this chapter concentrates on the phonetic analysis of articulatory and phonatory actions that contribute to a speaker's habitual voice quality. Readers with an interest in specifically organic factors of voice quality are recommended to read Mackenzie Beck's comprehensive overview chapter (1997).

2. THE CONCEPT OF SETTINGS IN THE PHONETIC ANALYSIS OF VOICE QUALITY

A key concept in the phonetic analysis of voice quality is that of a *setting* (Abercrombie, 1967; Esling, 1978, 1994; Honikman, 1964; Laver, 1968, 1975, 1979, 1980, 1991a, 1991b, 1994; Nolan, 1983; Pittam, 1994). Honikman (1964) originally presented the idea of a setting in the context of teaching the pronunciation of a foreign language and particularly sought to relate the performance of individual articulations to common aspects:

> Articulatory setting does not imply simply the particular articulations of the individual

> speech sounds of a language, but is rather the nexus of these isolated facts and their assemblage, based on their common, rather than their distinguishing, components. The isolated articulations are mutually related parts of the whole utterance; they are clues, as it were, to the articulatory plan of the whole; the conception of articulatory setting seeks to incorporate the clues or to see them as incorporated in the whole. Thus an articulatory setting is the gross oral posture and mechanics, both external and internal, requisite as a framework for the comfortable, economic and fluent merging and integrating of the isolated sounds into that harmonious, cognizable whole which constitutes the established pronunciation of a language. (p. 73)

Abercrombie (1967) does not use the word "setting"as such, although he acknowledges Honikman's original conception. He also distinguishes between organic and phonetic aspects of voice quality in terms relating to the possibility of control:

> The components of voice quality are of two different kinds, those which are outside the speaker's control, and those which are within it. The latter components can therefore be acquired, by learning from other people, while the former can not . . . [The latter components] originate in various muscular tensions which are maintained by the speaker the whole time he is talking, and which keep certain of the organs of speech adjusted in a way which is not their relaxed position of rest. These adjustments give a kind of general "set" or configuration of the vocal tract, which inevitably affects the quality of sound which issues from it. (Though acquired by learning, the habit of such muscular tensions can, once acquired, be so deeply rooted as to seem as much an unalterable part of a person as his anatomical characteristics.) (pp. 92–93)

Abercrombie's position is that a setting is most easily thought of as a common constraining tendency on the production of individual segments, biasing the detailed performance of segments toward a particular posture of the vocal tract or favoring a given mode of vibration of the vocal folds. An alternative approach is that a setting is best regarded as an emergent property of segmental performance. The first view is that settings are superimposed on the flow of segments, with the second that a setting is abstracted from the flow of segments as a second-order analysis. But, of course, both segments and settings are analytic abstractions from the same observed stream of speech performance, merely calculated on different time bases. Segments are short-lived, with settings being long term, but both are merely different facets of the same phenomena.

In a strict theoretical approach, segments and settings would be of equal analytically complementary status; neither one nor the other would be subordinate. The concepts of both segments and settings are useful and their interrelationship is interesting. The notion of the segment as an entity has stood the test of time as a convenient fiction in the analysis of speech (Laver, 1994), and the related and complementary concept of the setting may also prove to be of value, having many applications. This metatheoretical debate does not need to be resolved here, however. In this chapter, for convenience, an articulatory setting is represented in terms of a configuration of the vocal apparatus, sometimes as if constraining segmental performance and sometimes as if emerging from it.

If characteristic articulatory positions for every type of segment were plotted, weighted for their typical frequency of occurrence in the habitual speech of a given speaker speaking in a neutral tone of voice, then the result would be a particular long-term-average configuration of the vocal tract. This configuration would represent the common articulatory tendency underlying (or arising from) the momentary actions of segmental performance, and it is this common configuration, with its auditory consequences, that is being referred to in this chapter as a setting. At the phonatory level, the pictorial concept of"configuration" is not quite so cogent. But the idea of a setting of the phonatory mechanism is closely similar to that of an articulatory setting, in that both concern the setting up of the structural mechanism for speech to favor a particular mode of detailed articulatory or phonatory action.

A simple example of an articulatory setting is a speaker who maintains a lip-rounded position (a *labialized setting*) as a habitual tendency during speech. Occasional segments will have phonological requirements for a spread lip position or for closed lips that override or preempt the tendency to maintain a rounded-lip position. But for all segments where the phonological requirement is neutral, the constraints of the habitual setting apply and contribute to the speaker-characterizing voice quality.

A comparable example of an articulatory setting involving a constriction at a particular part of the vocal tract is that of a *velarized setting,* where a tendency to keep the body of the tongue in a raised and backed position audibly colors all except velar segments.

A phonatory example is a speaker who maintains a *whispery phonation type* throughout all voiced segments in speech as a habitual, speaker-characterizing tendency.

3. SEGMENTAL SUSCEPTIBILITY TO THE EFFECT OF A SETTING

The relationship between segmental performance and the constraining effect of a given setting cannot be properly understood without an understanding of the concept of *segmental susceptibility* (Laver, 1979). Mention has already been made of phonological requirements that override the biasing effect of a setting on the performance of a segment. An articulatory example here is a nasal setting. Nasality as a component of voice quality is redundant during the production of a segment that is already phonologically nasal. Conversely, nasality as a voice quality setting does not normally make segments whose phonological status is obligatorily oral, such as oral stops and fricatives, into phonetically nasal segments. But all segments where nasality is not inherently present or absent for reasons of phonological distinctiveness, for example vowels in English, may normally be susceptible to the nasalizing effects of a nasal setting.

The susceptibility of segments to the biasing effect of given settings is therefore governed by the phonetic issue of whether their production relies on the same articulatory system or not and whether phonological constraints make the operation of the setting redundant or preempt it. The appropriateness of equating a setting with a long-term-average articulatory posture therefore has to be conditioned by the susceptibility relationships between the setting and the segments involved. The relevant long-term average can only be suitably applied to the set of susceptible segments. All calculations of a long-term average (whether of articulatory position, auditory impression, or acoustic spectrum) based on all segments, susceptible and nonsusceptible alike, will give obvious inaccuracies.

4. THE NEUTRAL REFERENCE SETTING

It is helpful to define individual settings in relation to a *neutral reference setting.* The neutral setting is solely a convenient theoretical construct and carries no implication of normality, nor of identifying a representative rest position of the vocal organs. Laver and Hanson (1981) offer a detailed acoustic characterisation of neutral settings at both the articulatory and phonatory levels, as would be produced by an adult male speaker of average supralaryngeal and laryngeal anatomy.

For *articulatory settings,* the neutral reference setting is one where the vocal tract is in a long-term average posture where:

> the vocal tract is as nearly as anatomy allows in a posture giving equal cross-section to the vocal tract along its full length;
>
> the tongue is in a regularly curved convex shape;
>
> the velum is in a position of closure with the back wall of the pharynx, except for phonemically nasal segments;
>
> the lower jaw is held slightly open; the lips are held slightly open, without rounding or spreading. (Laver, 1994, pp. 402–403)

More specifically, the conditions that must apply are:

> the length of the vocal tract must not be muscularly distorted,
>
> the vocal tract must not be muscularly distorted at any point, by the action of the lips, the jaw, the tongue or the pharynx. (Laver, 1994, p. 404)

In this neutral configuration, the vowel that would be produced is schwa, the central unrounded [ə].

Any individual setting can then be evaluated as a violation of at least one of these conditions to some particular degree. Almost nobody's habitual voice quality seems to be characterized by full conformity to all of the neutral supralaryngeal factors in the description presented. In any individual speaker, there may be a tendency toward a particular constriction being maintained at some point along the length of the tract; the lips might be rounded, spread, or protruded; the larynx may be held lower or higher in the throat than a neutral position requires; the velum may open for a greater number of segments than phonological requirements justify; the jaw could be held in a slightly more open position; or the tongue tip may be held curved slightly upwards; or the body of the tongue may constrict the velar region, or the root of the tongue may be retracted towards the pharynx, and so on—or any physiologically compatible combination of any of these and to different degrees of local constriction from neutral to extreme. Laver (1980, 1994) offers an extensive description of such supralaryngeal settings.

For *phonatory settings*, the neutral reference setting is one where"voicing must show modal phonation; the average muscular tension throughout the vocal apparatus must be moderate; the prosodic features of pitch and loudness must be set at moderate values for mean, range and variability" (Laver, 1994, p. 403).

Modal phonation is as defined by Hollien (1972, 1974). More generally, the neutral phonatory setting is one where:

> only the true vocal folds must be in vibration;
>
> the vibration of the true vocal folds must be regularly periodic, without audible roughness arising from dysperiodicity;
>
> the vibration of the folds must be efficient in air use, without audible friction;
>
> the degree of muscle tension in all phonatory muscle systems must be moderate. (Laver, 1994, p. 404)

Very few adults speak with a fully neutral type of phonation. Variation of the conditions just described leads to the phonatory setting being labeled as *harsh* (dysperiodicity, with frequency jitter or intensity shimmer); or *creaky* (low-frequency, irregular pulses); or *whispery* (with audible friction caused by air leaking through a slightly open glottis); or *breathy* (with lax muscular tension of all the phonatory muscle systems leading to much greater air wastage than in the case of whispery voice); or *falsetto* (high pitch range, with increased longitudinal muscular tension of the vocal folds and thin fold-edges)—or several types of combinations of these modes of phonation (such as *whispery voice, whispery creaky voice,* etc.), within certain limitations on physiological or acoustic compatibility. Whisperiness and creakiness are perhaps the most common of all these variations from neutral, modal phonation.

Laver (1980, 1994) offers a detailed account of the physiological and acoustic characteristics of these phonatory settings (as does Catford 1964, although he does not use the term phonatory settings, preferring phonation types). Laver, Hiller, Mackenzie, and Rooney, (1986) and Laver, Hiller, and Mackenzie Beck (1992) give accounts of acoustic investigations into some of these phonation types, exploring the possibility of automatic, computer-based acoustic screening for laryngeal pathology.

5. SCALAR DEGREES OF SETTINGS

The discussion of segmental susceptibility to the biasing effects of a setting so far apply to speech that can be regarded as *normal,* in that the requirements of phonology are respected in the combined acoustic product. When a setting is applied more pervasively to otherwise nonsusceptible segments, so that in the case of an extreme nasal setting the segments that in other speakers are normally oral fricatives are made into nasal fricatives, then this can be regarded as an instance of *disordered* speech. The alternative terms abnormal or pathological are so heavily loaded with assumptions that they are perhaps better avoided (see also the chapter in this volume on the normal-disordered voice continuum by Lesley Mathieson).

Because of its violation of normal phonological expectations and because of the excessive attenuation of the acoustic power of the susceptible segments affected, an extreme degree of nasality causes significant problems of intelligibility and merits the attention of speech therapy. This may offer a reasonable defense of the use of the term "disordered" in this context. As a rule of thumb, therefore, the boundary between normal and disordered degrees of a setting can be set at the point where the degree of the setting gives cause to consider the voice a potential case for rehabilitative treatment, under-defined though the social or clinical criteria may be in this discussion.

Some settings (in a given language) are by their phonetic nature phonologically irrelevant. Examples include habitually whispery voice, where the speaker-characterizing fact that instances of phonetic voicing exhibit simultaneous glottal friction is no obstacle to the maintenance of the phonologically crucial voiced/voiceless distinction. In such cases, the differentiation of normal from disordered voice quality relies on the audible balance of periodic vibration of the vocal folds versus aperiodic glottal friction. When the periodic vibration dominates the audible impression, the voice can be said to be relatively normal; when the aperiodic component of whisperiness dominates (which is much more rarely encountered), then the voice can be regarded as relatively disordered.

The perceptible differences of degrees of a setting can extend from neutral to nonneutral, where a range of both normal and disordered possibilities are included within the continuum of the nonneutral range. If six scalar degrees of nonneutral settings are proposed beyond neutral, then scalar degrees 1 to 3 can be regarded as covering the range of settings displayed in normal voices. Scalar degree 1 shows a just noticeable divergence from the neutral specification, scalar degree 2 a slight amount, and scalar degree 3 a moderate amount. Thereafter, scalar degrees 4, 5, and 6 represent notable, severe, and extreme amounts, respectively. By definition, scalar degrees 1 to 3 represent degrees of a setting that one would expect to find in the normal population and scalar degrees 4 to 6 almost exclusively in the population of speakers with voice and speech disorders (or perhaps in momentary, paralinguistic extremes of emotional expression).

One example of specific criteria for some of the different scalar degrees is the case of degrees of lip rounding in a labialized setting. Scalar degrees 1 to 3 show open rounding and 4 to 6 close rounding. Within these bands, scalar degree 3 shows an average lip position corresponding to the rounding in the vowel [ɔ], the position for 4 is as for the vowel [o], and for 6 is as for [u]. It may be important to note that lip rounding as a setting takes account only of the two-dimensional shape of the lip opening, from side to side. The analysis of whether the lips are simultaneously protruded is handled separately as a setting of longitudinal extension of the vocal tract by the lips, discussed next.

It may be helpful now to return to the evaluation of nasality as a component of voice quality, for another example of specific criteria for different scalar degrees. We have seen that a neutral degree would show nasality only on phonemically nasal segments. As making certain anticipatory adjustments to oncoming segments is necessary to maintain fluent connected speech, a neutral degree of nasality would also include a small amount of allophonic nasalization of vowels preceding nasal consonants. But this anticipatory allophonic accommodation would be limited to the minimum duration consistent with maintaining fluent pronunciation. Allophonic nasalization in English slightly exceeds this physiological minimum, and so the voice quality associated with the typical pronunciation of all accents of English would have to be judged as showing nasality at scalar degree 1 at least.

For scalar degree 2 of nasality, open vowels before nasal consonants show nasalization throughout their medial phase (Laver, 1994), rather than only during the transition toward the following nasal consonants. By scalar degree 3, the medial phases of both open and close vowels are audibly nasalized. The threshold to a degree of nasality that may be regarded as a mild disorder of speech comes at scalar degree 4, where semi-vowels [w] and [j], and [r] and [l] become nasalized. Scalar degree 5 shows nasality on voiced fricative consonants, and the extreme nasality of scalar degree 6 is manifested by audible nasality throughout all segments in speech except oral stops. For nasality to go beyond this to the point of ubiquity in speech, not only destroys much of intelligible communication, it takes voice quality beyond the reach of a descriptive system designed for general applicability into organic cases of cleft or paralyzed palates with continuous audible nasal escape.

6. MEASURING VOICE QUALITY AS A COMPOSITE PROFILE OF MULTIPLE SETTINGS

Settings can be systematically grouped in relation to the functional subsystem of the vocal apparatus involved. At the highest level of classification, we have seen that it is convenient to distinguish between articulatory settings and phonatory settings, depending on whether the articulatory function of the supralaryngeal vocal tract or the phonational function of the larynx is involved. At the same level of analysis, one might usefully add classes of settings that affect the range of articulatory action, or factors of general muscular tension.

Within each of the above classes it is possible to distinguish a variety of subclasses and individual settings. Thus within the overall class of articulatory settings, three general categories of settings are those that affect the longitudinal axis of the vocal tract, the cross-sectional characteristics, or the velopharyngeal system, respectively. Each of these can be subdivided. Within the longitudinal category, for example, two subgroups of individual settings can be identified: those that change the vertical position of the larynx versus those that affect the contribution of the lips to the overall length of the vocal tract.

Any voice can be analyzed as a composite profile of settings, assessed in terms of whether each individual category of setting displays a neutral or a nonneutral degree and, if nonneutral, the applicable scalar degree. Laver, Wirz, Mackenzie, and Hiller (1985), Laver, Wirz, Mackenzie, and Hiller (1991) and Mackenzie Beck (1988) report the outcomes of a 6-year, collaborative project by a team of phoneticians, speech therapists, and speech scientists to develop a scheme of Vocal Profile Analysis (VPA) on this basis. The work was funded by the British government's Medical Research Council. Readers interested in the applications of the VPA system to the analysis of voices in speech therapy and speech pathology, sociolinguistics, and paralinguistic research are referred to those publications. The following comments are confined to illustrations of the general approach of the VPA project as one example of methods for the evaluation of voice quality.

Figure 4–1 and Figure 4–2 have been developed from the original work of the VPA project and exemplify parts of a possible protocol for a written record of perceptual judgments of an individual speaker's voice. Figure 4–1 shows a protocol for the assessment of supralaryngeal settings and Figure 4–2 a protocol for phonatory settings.

Repeated listenings to 45-second recorded samples of continuous speech are necessary to reach an overall impression of the profile of a speaker's characteristic long-term-average settings in all the categories of an overall VPA protocol. With suitable perceptual training, supported by practical materials and illustrative tapes identifying labeled examples of the individual scalar degrees of each type of

Category	Setting	Scalar Degrees						
		neutral	1	2	3	4	5	6
Longitudinal	Laryngeal							
	raised larynx							
	lowered larynx							
	Labial							
Cross Sectional	labiodentalization							
	labial protrusion							
	Labial							
	lip-rounded							
	lip-spread							
	Mandibular							
	close jaw							
	open jaw							
	Lingual Tip/Blade							
	advanced tip/blade							
	retracted tip/blade							
	Lingual Body							
	advanced body							
	retracted body							
	raised body							
	lowered body							
	Lingual Root							
	constricted pharynx							
	expanded pharynx							
Velopharyngeal	Velic Coupling							
	nasal							
	denasal							

Figure 4–1. A perceptual protocol for analyzing supralaryngeal settings in voice quality.

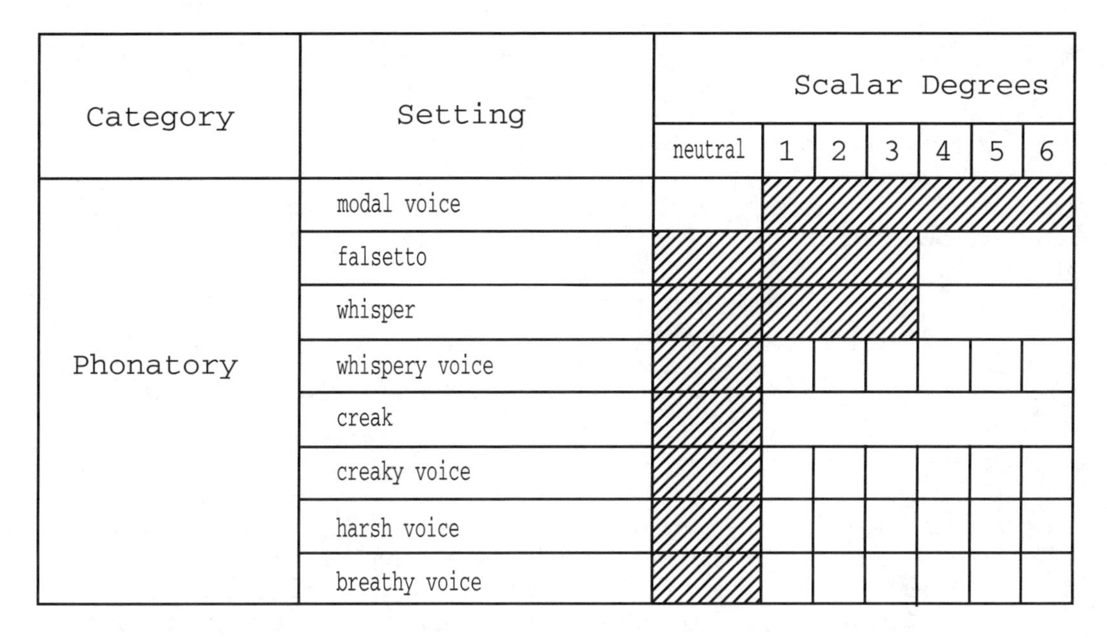

Category	Setting	Scalar Degrees						
		neutral	1	2	3	4	5	6
Phonatory	modal voice							
	falsetto							
	whisper							
	whispery voice							
	creak							
	creaky voice							
	harsh voice							
	breathy voice							

Figure 4–2. A perceptual protocol for analyzing phonatory settings in voice quality.

setting (both normal and disordered), therapists and others on VPA courses have reached good consistency of performance. The reliability of trained judges has been assessed in groups in Edinburgh, London, Vancouver, and Madison, WI, and performance between and within judges to within one scalar degree typically runs at about 75% and to within two scalar degrees at over 90%.

The process of completing a protocol such as the one illustrated in Figures 4–1 and 4–2 is that the analyst, preferably listening to a good quality tape recording of continuous speech or the reading of a standard passage, evaluates each category of setting separately. Taking the supralaryngeal settings from Figure 4–1, examples that potentially can distort the longitudinal axis of the vocal tract, the first judgment to make is whether the particular speaker uses a neutral setting in this regard, or not. If neutral, that box is ticked. If nonneutral, a decision is required between raised versus lowered larynx and a scalar degree allocated in the light of the instruction and demonstrations given during the training of the person doing the rating.

In a few categories in Figures 4–1 and 4–2, the number of scalar degrees is reduced from 6 to 1 or 2. In the case of settings of the root of the tongue, subtly increasing degrees of pharyngeal constriction or expansion are hard to discern perceptually, so the analytic nonneutral possibilities for pharyngeal constriction are reduced to a decision between constriction within a normal range versus constriction of an excessive, disordered degree. Denasal settings are given the same consideration.

In the case of phonatory settings, both falsetto and whisper (as the sole phonation present) are assumed to be evidence of a disorder that might merit therapeutic attention. A decision on falsetto phonation is treated only as a yes/no question. Logically, falsetto is either present or absent and does not vary in degree. A similar position applies to the whisper type of phonation (as distinct from whispery voice): Ticking the whisper category indicates the presence of whisper as the sole phonation being used. If whisper modulates another mode of phonation with simultaneous periodic vibration of the vocal folds, where the vibrating folds fail fully to close off the glottal space at their maximum approximation, then this is identified by ticking the whispery voice box. The creak type of phonation (vocal fry or glottal fry in North American terminology) versus creaky voice is treated under the same convention, although creak alone is not defined here as disordered.

Compound phonation types such as whispery creaky voice can be annotated by ticking the boxes for whispery voice and creaky voice in appropriate scalar degrees reflecting the judgment about relative balance of the whisperiness and creakiness components. Correspondingly, for harsh whispery voice, the boxes for harsh voice and whispery voice should be ticked; for whispery falsetto, the boxes for whispery voice and falsetto should be ticked; and for creaky falsetto, the boxes for creaky voice and falsetto should be ticked.

Breathy voice does not enjoy such versatility. It cannot combine with any other mode of phonation, because of the laxness of all the contributory muscle systems allowing the vocal folds to "flap in the breeze," as it were, in a very inefficient use of the air supply. It can, however, be assessed as having different scalar degrees. In an extreme (scalar degree 6) version exhibiting very strong signs of speech disorder, breathy voice allows only very short utterances, at very low intensity. In a slight to moderate version (scalar degree 2 or 3), breathy voice is used paralinguistically in English to signal intimacy, with whispery voice at the same degrees conventionally signaling confidentiality.

It is sometimes the case in phonatory settings that laryngeal vibration switches audibly from moment to moment between two modes, although often with one mode perceptually dominating. An example would be a voice that mixed predominantly whispery voice with momentary bursts of creakiness. This is dealt with by annotating the relevant scalar degree box with "i" for "intermittent." If whispery voice persists throughout, with creakiness being momentarily added from time to time, the whispery voice box can be ticked, with creaky voice being annotated with an "i"; but if whispery voice alternates with creaky voice, then both whispery voice and creaky voice can be annotated with an "i." The same treatment would be applied to a voice that alternated between falsetto and another phonation type.

Once all settings have been analyzed, the protocol is suitable for use as a permanent record in the speaker's file, and is available for quantified comparison against later performance, perhaps after therapy or other treatment where relevant.

7. ORGANIC AND PHONETIC EQUIVALENCES IN VOICE QUALITY

Finally, we return to the distinction between organic and phonetic aspects of voice quality. The same perceptual effect in two speakers can sometimes have a phonetic cause in one case but an organic cause in the other. An articulatory example is a case where one speaker has adopted as a habitual phonetic style of speaking a *labiodentalized setting*, in which the lower lip tends to be held close to or touching the upper teeth. Another speaker may have an undershot lower jaw, so that there is an anatomically induced, organic labiodental approximation of the lower lip and the upper teeth. Both the phonetic and the organic causes produce a constriction of the vocal tract at the labiodental place of articulation, with audible labiodentality affecting susceptible segments.

A similar example would be where one speaker phonetically adopted a *palatalized setting* where the body of the tongue tended to be held high and fronted in the mouth, where another speaker (say one with Down syndrome) showed organic underdevelopment of the mid-face but with relatively normal development of the lower jaw and tongue (Mackenzie Beck, 1988). Both the phonetic and the organic causes would produce a constriction of the vocal tract at the palatal region, with similar audible effects on susceptible segments.

A phonatory example is one where a speaker characteristically uses a whispery voice setting, where it is a matter of phonetic habit that the vocal folds fail to close completely during phonation, with continuous leakage of air through the glottis during voicing resulting in audible friction. Another speaker may produce a very similar phonatory quality of whispery voice, but where the reason for the audible friction is not phonetic habit but an organic semiparalysis of one vocal fold such that the speaker cannot achieve complete closure of the glottis during phonation. Many similar examples could be offered from both articulation and phonation.

The articulatory examples can be thought to show *configurational equivalence* between the phonetic and the organic situations. The phonatory examples show *phonatory equivalence* between the phonetic and organic cases. The equivalence of phonetic and organic aspects of voice quality in this illustration have profound implications for general phonetic theory. In order for general phonetic theory to work at all, phoneticians accept the generalizing assumption that virtually all speakers can be analyzed as if they were performing their articulatory and phonatory actions on an idealized, standard vocal apparatus. In effect, general phonetic theory so far has formally ignored interspeaker differences at the organic level, and has treated the perceptual quality of what is heard as fully explainable by appeal to the notion of phonetic quality alone (Laver, 1994). It is plain that the concept of phonetic quality, and that of voice quality, cannot be fully understood without an adequate understanding of the nature of organic factors in speech in general, and in voice quality in particular.

REFERENCES

Abercrombie, D. (1967). *Elements of general phonetics.* Edinburgh, Scotland: Edinburgh University Press.

Baer, T., Sasaki, K., & Harris, K. (Eds.). (1987). *Laryngeal function in phonation and respiration.* San Diego, CA: College-Hill Press.

Bless, D., & Abbs, J. H. (Eds.). (1983). *Vocal fold physiology: Contemporary research and clinical issues.* San Diego, CA: College-Hill Press.

Catford, J. C. (1964). Phonation types. In D. Abercrombie, D. B. Fry, P. A. D. MacCarthy, N. C. Scott, & J. L. M. Trim (Eds.), *In honour of Daniel Jones* (pp. 26–37). London: Longmans, Green.

Esling, J. (1978). *Voice quality in Edinburgh: A sociolinguistic and phonetic study.* Doctoral dissertation, University of Edinburgh, Scotland.

Esling, J. (1994). Voice quality. In R. E. Asher & J. M. Y. Simpson (Eds.), *The encyclopedia of language and linguistics* (pp. 4950–4953). Oxford, UK: Pergamon Press.

Fujimura, O. (Ed.). (1988). *Vocal fold physiology: Voice production, mechanisms and functions.* New York: Raven Press.

Gauffin, J., & Hammarberg, B. (Eds.). (1991). *Vocal fold physiology: Acoustic, perceptual, and physiological aspects of voice mechanisms.* San Diego, CA: Singular Publishing Group.

Greene, M. C. L., & Mathieson, L. (1989). *The voice and its disorders* (5th ed.). London: Whurr.

Hirano, M. (1981) *Clinical examination of voice.* New York: Springer-Verlag.

Hollien, H. (1972). Three major vocal registers: A proposal. In *Proceedings of the Seventh International Congress of Phonetic Sciences* (Montreal) (pp. 320–331).

Hollien, H. (1974). On vocal registers. *Journal of Phonetics, 2,* 125–143.

Honikman, B. (1964). Articulatory settings. In D. Abercrombie, D. B. Fry, P. A. D. MacCarthy, N. C. Scott, & J. L. M. Trim (Eds.), *In honour of Daniel Jones* (pp. 73–84). London: Longmans, Green.

Laver, J. (1968). Voice quality and indexical information. *British Journal of Disorders of Communication, 3,* 43–54.

Laver, J. (1975). *Individual features in voice quality.* Unpublished doctoral dissertation, University of Edinburgh, Scotland.

Laver, J. (1978). The concept of articulatory settings: An historical survey. *Historiographia Linguistica, 5,* 1–14.

Laver, J. (1979). The description of voice quality in general phonetic theory. *Edinburgh University Department of Linguistics Work in Progress, 12,* 30–52 (reprinted in J. Laver [1991b] *The Gift of Speech: Papers in the Analysis of Speech and Voice* [pp. 184–208.] Edinburgh University Press).

Laver, J. (1980). *The phonetic description of voice quality.* Cambridge, UK: Cambridge University Press.

Laver, J. (1981). The analysis of vocal quality: From the classical period to the twentieth century. In R. E. Asher & E. J. A. Henderson (Eds.), *Towards a history of phonetics* (pp. 79–99). Edinburgh, Scotland: Edinburgh University Press.

Laver, J. (1991a). *The gift of speech: Papers in the analysis of speech and voice.* Edinburgh,

Scotland: Edinburgh University Press. (Issued in paperback 1996, as *The Gift of Speech: Readings in the Analysis of Speech and Voice*.)

Laver, J. (1991b). Voice quality. In W. Bright (Ed.), *Oxford international encyclopedia of linguistics* (Vol. 4, pp. 231–232). London: Oxford University Press.

Laver, J. (1994). *Principles of phonetics*. London: Cambridge Textbooks in Linguistics Series, Cambridge University Press.

Laver, J., & Hanson, R. J. (1981). Describing the normal voice. In J. Darby (Ed.), *Speech evaluation in psychiatry* (pp. 57–78). New York: Grune and Stratton.

Laver, J., Hiller, S. M., & Mackenzie Beck, J. (1992). Acoustic waveform perturbations and voice disorders. *Journal of Voice, 6*, 115–126.

Laver, J., Hiller, S. M., Mackenzie, J., & Rooney, E. (1986). An acoustic screening system for the detection of laryngeal pathology. *Journal of Phonetics, 14*, 517–524.

Laver, J., Wirz, S., Mackenzie, J., & Hiller, S. M. (1985). Vocal profile analysis in the description of voice quality. In V. Lawrence (Ed.), *Transactions of the 14th Symposium on the Care of the Professional Voice* (pp. 184–192). New York: The Voice Foundation.

Laver, J., Wirz, S., Mackenzie, J., & Hiller, S. M. (1991). A perceptual protocol for the analysis of vocal profiles. In J. Laver (Ed.), *The gift of speech: Readings in the analysis of speech and voice* (pp. 265–280). Edinburgh, Scotland: Edinburgh University Press.

Luchsinger, R., & Arnold, G. E. (1965). *Voice, speech, language: Clinical communicology—Its physiology and pathology*. Belmont CA: Wadsworth.

Mackenzie Beck, J. (1988). *Organic variation and voice quality*. Unpublished doctoral dissertation, University of Edinburgh, Scotland.

Mackenzie Beck, J. (1997). Organic variation of the vocal apparatus. In W. J. Hardcastle & J. Laver (Eds.), *The handbook of phonetic sciences* (pp. 256–297). Oxford/Cambridge, MA: Blackwell.

Mackenzie Beck, J., Laver, J., & Hiller, S.M. (1991). Structural pathologies of the vocal folds. In J. Laver (Ed.), *The gift of speech: Readings in the analysis of speech and voice* (pp. 281–318). Edinburgh, Scotland: Edinburgh University Press.

Mackenzie Beck, J., Wrench, A., Jackson, M., Soutar, D., Robertson, A. G., & Laver, J. (1997). Surgical mapping and phonetic analysis in intra-oral cancer. In W. Zeigler & K. Deger (Eds.), *Clinical phonetics and linguistics* (pp. 485–496). London: Whurr.

Nolan, F. (1983) *The phonetic bases of speaker recognition*. Cambridge: Cambridge University Press.

Pittam, J. (1994). *Voice in social interaction: An interdisciplinary approach*. Thousand Oaks, CA: Sage.

Stevens, K. N., & Hirano, M. (Eds.). (1981). *Vocal fold physiology*. Tokyo: University of Tokyo Press.

Sweet, H. (1877). *A handbook of phonetics*. Oxford: Clarendon Press.

Titze, I. R., & Scherer, R. C. (Eds.). (1983). *Vocal fold physiology: Biomechanics, acoustics, and phonatory control*. Denver, CO: The Denver Center for the Performing Arts.

CHAPTER

5

The Transcription of Voice Quality[1]

Martin J. Ball, John Esling, and Craig Dickson

Although the history of interest in voice quality dates back at least as far as Henry Sweet (e.g., 1890), there was for many years little agreement on how to classify voice quality or how to transcribe it as part of a phonetic transcription. Indeed, there is not even agreement on precisely what the term covers, in that it is often restricted to aspects of voice quality derived from vocal fold activity, rather than the fuller meaning that encompasses features derived from supralaryngeal settings of the articulators. Authors such as Nolan (1983) have used the phrase *long-term quality* as an alternative; however, in this chapter we retain the traditional term, but with a wide application to account for voice quality derived from airflow features, vocal fold activity, and supralaryngeal activity.

1. DESCRIBING VOICE QUALITY

Impressionistic descriptive labels for voice quality have been in use for a long time and include such terms as "light" and "guttural" for normal speakers and "hoarse" and "strangled" for those with voice disorders. As Laver (1980) points out, these terms are holistic, in that they encompass the range of phonatory and articulatory settings that have been used to produce a particular voice quality, but they are also imprecise, in that no particular settings are described that combine to give a particular voice type.

Interestingly, work within voice disorders has often favored the retention of impressionistic labels, whereas work within phonetics has tended to avoid them. To move beyond these

[1]An earlier version of this chapter appeared in the *Journal of the International Phonetic Association.* It is reproduced here with permission.

labels, an attempt was made some years ago to see whether a set of 15 disordered "cardinal voice qualities" could be established for speech and language pathologists in much the same form as the cardinal vowel system (Winter & Martin, 1981). It was hoped that these cardinal vowel qualities could be learned simply as numbers (rather than as names such as "husky" etc.), and then a disordered voice could be described in terms of which cardinal voice quality it was nearest to. However, although some of these voice types did seem to be easy to learn for some of the subjects in the study, the authors admit that, overall, the results were disappointing.

Interest in voice quality among phoneticians has grown over the last 20 years or so. Work by Laver (1975) and Esling (1978), for example, paved the way for Laver's subsequent major publications (1979, 1980). These, together with Catford's (1977) classification of phonatory types, provide phoneticians with a widely accepted taxonomy of phonatory and articulatory settings that can be used to describe voice quality (see Esling, 1994).

However, one must be aware of what is meant by some of the voice quality terms used. With phonation types, the use of a term such as whisper, for example, does not imply normally that every single segment is uttered using the whisper phonation type. Normally, this would be understood to mean that expected voiced sounds were made with whisper, but that expected voiceless sounds were still voiceless. In this way, the phonological contrast between voiced and voiceless sounds is maintained. The same would apply for most of the phonatory voice quality types described in this chapter.

With voice quality types dependent on supralaryngeal settings, again we will not imply necessarily that all segments are uttered with the setting type specified. For example, nasalized voice does not mean that all sounds are uttered with a lowered velum; rather the term suggests a perceptually greater use than normal of nasal and nasalized articulations. However, a heavily nasalized voice quality may well be derived from virtually total use of a lowered velum, and this can be marked by use of symbols marking degree of a particular quality (described later). Another example would be that given in Laver (1980) of velarization, where he notes that this setting is likely to shift the articulatory location of any given segment toward the velar location or to add a secondary velar articulation to the primary. He also points out that different sounds will be differently susceptible to this process, and so any particular setting will only have an intermittent effect throughout an utterance.

Indeed, for a variety of reasons, voice qualities may be intermittent in another sense, in that they only occur within certain frequency ranges (e.g., creak), or for paralinguistic reasons (e.g., whisper to mark confidentiality), or for sociolinguistic reasons (e.g., switching into or out of a particular articulatory setting associated with a regional accent).

2. TRANSCRIBING VOICE QUALITY

There has until recently been no widely recognized symbol system for the transcription of voice quality. This is partly because many phoneticians would regard voice quality as extralinguistic in most instances (see Laver, 1980) and partly due to the difficulty of arranging segmental and suprasegmental symbolization together. Laver's (1980) study of voice quality did provide a large set of symbols for many of the voice qualities he described. He also suggested a way of setting a voice quality symbol to one side of the normal segmental transcription. It was not altogether clear how, for example, one might notate a change from one voice quality to another within an utterance—which might be useful for transcribing both normal and disordered speakers. Also, some of the types described lacked a symbol (e.g., faucalized voice), and others used symbols since superseded in the IPA by new forms (e.g., palatalized, tip, and blade articulations) or ambiguous symbols (e.g., the plus and double plus for palatoalveolar and alveolar, respectively).

Looking at the most recent revisions of the IPA (1989, 1993), it is found that diacritics are available for a small range of phonation types. These include voiceless and voiced, breathy voice, and creaky voice. Other common types, such as whisper, are not found. These diacritics are, however, suitable only for marking single segments. In other words, the voiceless diacritic can be used to mark, for example, a voiceless sonorant where a specific symbol is not provided; the voiced diacritic can be used to show a voiced fortis sound; and the breathy and creaky voice symbols can mark individual segments with these phonation types used contrastively in certain languages. Clearly, these diacritics are not even adequate to cover the range of voice types dependent on phonation, and, even if more were available, it would hardly be practicable to place such diacritics on every symbol within a transcription.

An important development occurred with the setting up at the 1989 Kiel Convention of the IPA of a subgroup to examine the transcription of disordered speech and voice quality. This subgroup produced a report recommending a set of symbols and diacritics called the "Extensions to the IPA," now commonly referred to as extIPA. This set of symbols is described in some detail in Duckworth, Allen, Hardcastle, and Ball (1990) and exemplified in Ball (1991) and Ball, Code, Rahilly, and Hazlett (1994). The current extIPA chart is available in ICPLA Executive Committee (1994). The extIPA symbols cover a variety of suprasegmental features, such as pausing, tempo, and loudness, as well as voice quality. For all these aspects of connected speech, Laver's notion of transcription was adapted through the adoption of the labeled brace. This enables a suprasegmental symbol to be separated from the main segmental transcription, and also allows for such features to be turned on and off during a transcription. The convention is: at the appropriate point within a transcription, a brace is used coupled with a suprasegmental symbol; the suprasegmental feature is then read as applying to the following string of segmental symbols until a further labeled brace marks the end of its domain of operation. We can illustrate this with the symbol for quiet speech: *p* (for *piano*): ['ðɪs ɪz 'nɔ˞məl 'spitʃ {*p* 'ðɪs ɪz 'kwaɪət 'spitʃ *p*}].

When it came to voice quality, the extIPA subgroup decided on a minimalist approach. As one of the main audiences for the extIPA symbols was expected to be speech and language pathologists, it was felt that what was necessary was a basic set of labels for the commonly occurring pathological voice types. To this end, the following range of phonation types was recognized: breathy/whispery, whisper, creak (and presumably creaky voice), ventricular and harsh, and falsetto. Apart from being limited, some of these are also ambiguous, in that the symbol for creak actually suggests creaky voice, and that no distinction is made between harsh voice made with the normal vocal folds and ventricular voice (and presumably diplophonia: double voice).

ExtIPA also recognized the need to transcribe voice qualities dependent on supralaryngeal articulatory settings. However, it notes only that the normal IPA diacritics can be used in conjunction with the V symbol for voice, and that new diacritics such as [ᶹ] can be adopted to mark labiodentalized voice. It does not enter the debate, however, of how to mark settings such as alveolarized or palatoalveolarized or faucalized, for which no IPA or extIPA diacritics existed. It became clear that those specializing in the investigation of voice quality required a more comprehensive set of transcription conventions than were available in extIPA.

3. THE VoQS SYSTEM

The VoQS system is a set of voice quality symbols devised to provide as full a coverage as possible, and derived with some addition and changes from the labels proposed by Laver (1980), but using the transcription convention for suprasegmentals introduced in the extIPA developments.

3.1. Airstream Types

As this system has been drawn up for use with both normal and disordered voice, we find that the symbols are divided into three main groups, as opposed to the typical two. In studies of normal voice, there are the categories of phonation and supralaryngeal setting, as noted previously; however, voice quality in disordered speech may be affected by the use of artificial and, therefore, nonnormal initiation and phonation. On the VoQS chart (see Figure 5–1), this category is given the overall heading of "airstream types" and covers esophageal (oesophageal) speech, tracheoesophageal speech, electrolarynx speech, and pulmonic ingressive speech.[2]

Of these, the last can be found in certain circumstances with normal speakers (for example, with alternative egressive and ingressive speech in counting), but is also encountered in certain speech disorders (see a description of its use with disfluent speech in Ball et al., 1994). The extIPA symbol for ingressive has been used here, but within the labeled brace format, as opposed to being added to a single symbol.

The other three symbols in this group are all used with mechanisms adopted by speakers who can no longer use the normal pulmonic egressive airstream with laryngeal phonation due, normally, to laryngectomy. It may well be argued that phonetic transcription is rarely undertaken with such speakers and so specific symbols are unnecessary. But, as was shown by Hewlett and Cohen (1993), it is possible to examine features of articulation in esophageal speech, and in such circumstances the VoQS symbol is a useful addition to the clinical phonetician's repertoire. Further, these particular symbols may well be useful as a shorthand method of specifying what alternative initiation/phonation mechanisms are being used by laryngectomy patients.

As with the extIPA symbols, an attempt has been made in devising these symbols to bring some kind of iconicity to their design. Whereas the Œ symbol of esophageal speech is only a visual reminder of the o-e digraph of the British spelling, the Ю is an attempt to represent the dual nature of this airstream/phonation combination. Esophageal speech involves the use of a moving column of air from the esophagus, which causes a vibration at the sphincteric pharyngoesophageal junction (acting as a pseudoglottis). The resultant airstream is then modified by the supraglottal articulators and resonators in the normal way. Lung air is not available for speech, as following the removal of the larynx, the trachea ends in a stoma in the throat. A variety of air-intake techniques are used by esophageal speakers and are described in, for example, Edels (1983). Voice quality in esophageal speech clearly differs from that in pulmonic speech; one major difference lies in the amount of air available. With esophageal speech, it has been shown (see Edels, 1983) that the reservoir is, in fact, the upper portion of the esophagus, holding about 15 ml of air for each air-charge, approximately 100 times less than that used in normal phonation. Apart from the shorter breath units, the use of the pseudoglottis at the pharyngoesophageal junction instead of the normal glottis results in a voice quality normally deemed unnatural.

In tracheoesophageal speech, the surgery leaves a slightly different result than that noted for esophageal speakers. Here, although the trachea still terminates with a stoma in the throat, a puncture is made between the trachea and the esophagus just at the level of the tracheal opening. The intention is that lung air can still be used for speech by redirecting exhaled air from the trachea, through the tracheoesophageal puncture and into the esophagus, from where it flows into the pharynx and upper vocal tract (see Perry, 1983). To produce a more

[2] **Ball (in press) suggests that various oralic airstreams used to produce percussive sounds can be symbolized by linking a glottal stop to the relevant place diacritic (i.e., bilabial, dental, or tongue blade). Ball (1998) suggests % as a symbol for a buccal airstream mechanism; but these are not included in the VoQS system.**

VoQS: Voice Quality Symbols

AIRSTREAM TYPES

Œ	oesophageal speech	И	electrolarynx speech
Ю	tracheo-oesophageal speech	↓	pulmonic ingressive speech

PHONATION TYPES

V	modal voice	F	falsetto
W	whisper	C	creak
Ṿ	whispery voice (murmur)	V̰	creaky voice
V̤	breathy voice	C̣	whispery creak
V!	harsh voice	V!!	ventricular phonation
V̬!!	diplophonia	Ṿ!!	whispery ventricular phon.
V̟	anterior or pressed phonation	W̠	posterior whisper

SUPRALARYNGEAL SETTINGS

L̝	raised larynx	L̞	lowered larynx
Vꟹ	labialized voice (open round)	Vʷ	labialized voice (close round)
V͍	spread-lip voice	Vᶹ	labio-dentalized voice
V̺	linguo-apicalized voice	V̻	linguo-laminalized voice
V˞	retroflex voice	V̪	dentalized voice
V͇	alveolarized voice	V͇ʲ	palatoalveolarized voice
Vʲ	palatalized voice	Vˠ	velarized voice
Vʶ	uvularized voice	Vˤ	pharyngealized voice
V̰ˤ	laryngo-pharyngealized voice	Vᴴ	faucalized voice
Ṽ	nasalized voice	V͊	denasalized voice
J̞	open jaw voice	J̝	close jaw voice
J͔	right offset jaw voice	J͕	left offset jaw voice
J̟	protruded jaw voice	Θ	protruded tongue voice

USE OF LABELED BRACES & NUMERALS TO MARK STRETCHES OF SPEECH AND DEGREES AND COMBINATIONS OF VOICE QUALITY

['ðɪs ɪz 'nɔ˞məl 'vɔɪs {3V! 'ðɪs ɪz 'veɹi 'hɑ˞ʃ 'vɔɪs 3V!} 'ðɪs ɪz 'nɔ˞məl 'vɔɪs wʌns 'mɔ˞ {L̞1V! 'ðɪs ɪz 'les 'hɑ˞ʃ 'vɔɪs wɪð 'loʊəd 'læɹɪŋks 1V!L̞}]

Figure 5–1. The VoQS Chart.

natural type of voice, artificial valves of different types may be fitted into the puncture, but the vibration for voice still occurs at the pharyngoesophageal junction. Although it is possible to use normal pulmonic egressive airflow with this voice type, thus increasing the length of the breath units, the voice quality is still markedly different from that of normal speech, nevertheless generally deemed more acceptable than that of simple esophageal speech.

Finally, in this group there is a symbol representing electrolarynx speech. This has been designed to represent a stylized version of the electric flash motif often found to warn of the presence of electricity. Electrolarynges are of various kinds, but all operate to produce an alternative noise source to the vibrating vocal folds. Most kinds can be turned on and off to mimic the difference between voiced and voiceless sounds, but users differ as to how well they manage to control this distinction (see Hewlett & Cohen, 1993). Clearly, if a transcription of an electrolarynx user is undertaken, the И symbol is to be read as meaning that an electrolarynx was in use as the noise source, but not that it was in use for all segments. Details of the accuracy of the voicing distinction can be marked through the choice of symbols, or through the use of the detailed phonation diacritics available in the extIPA set.

With this group of symbols we have attempted to provide a means of transcribing the major nonnormal initiation and phonation types. It is, however, not a comprehensive listing. There are various other, less usual airstream types that can be encountered in the clinic. These range from, for example, parabuccal voice formed in the mouth (see Luchsinger & Arnold, 1965) to neoglottal voice (see, for example, Ainsworth & Singh, 1990, 1992; Singh, 1993a, 1993b), in which surgery refashions the remnants of the larynx into a structure that can operate as a valve to act as a noise source for speech (though a tracheostoma valve may also need to be inserted). These initiation and phonation types are still, however, comparatively uncommon and so do not warrant an extension of the VoQS symbols at this moment.

3.2. Phonation Types

The next main grouping of symbols represents different phonation types, and is based closely on the Laver (1980) symbols. The four main phonation types—modal voice, falsetto, whisper, and creak—retain their single capital letter symbols: V, F, W, C. (Voiceless phonation is not symbolized, for in normal phonatory usage, voiced and voiceless phonation are mixed in an utterance, and the voiceless segments are symbolized through the use of segmental symbols. Even in other phonation types, the usual patterns are for the voiceless segements to remain as voiceless, with the normally voiced segments transferred to whisper, etc.) Combinatory phonation types are symbolized by the use of one of the four capital letters together with a relevant diacritic (some from the IPA list, others as proposed by Laver). On the chart in Figure 5–1, examples are given of whispery voice (or murmur), creaky voice, and breathy voice (these defined according to Catford, 1977). These use the modal voice symbol with added subscripts. Unfortunately, the terms breathy voice and whispery voice have not always been used consistently. We follow Catford's definitions, but it is clear that the subscript double dot ordained by the IPA to mark breathy voice, should be applied to what Catford terms whispery voice. The VoQS chart uses the single dot whisper diacritic beneath V for whispery voice, and the double dot for breathy voice. A possible solution to this discrepancy would be to denote whispery voice by the double dot diacritic, with breathy voice transcribed by V^h. However, until the IPA itself changes its terminology, we recommend retention of the original VoQS symbols.

Whispery creak is marked through adding the whisper diacritic to the creak symbol, with other examples not on the chart easily constructed to show the compound phonation types listed in Laver (1980), such as whispery creaky falsetto and whispery creaky voice (WF̰ and WV̰).

We depart from Laver (1980) in our symbols for harsh voice and ventricular phonation, in that we allow for discrimination between harshness with and without added ventricular phonation and for ventricular phonation without simultaneous vocal fold vibration. For harshness without ventricular involvement we use Laver's original symbol of the capital V plus exclamation mark. To show ventricular phonation alone we use the V plus two exclamation marks. This will not be confused with a scalar notation, as degree of harshness is shown by the use of numerals (see later). To transcribe diplophonia or double voice (that is the simultaneous use of ventricular and normal phonation) we add the IPA voice diacritic to the ventricular symbol. As also seen on the chart, other varieties of ventricular phonation can also be shown through the addition of different diacritics.

Following Catford (1977), we recognize that anterior and posterior location may need to be marked. Anterior vocal fold phonation has been termed "tight" voice and "pressed" phonation and involves the holding together of the arytenoid cartilages such that only the ligamental part of the glottis participates in phonation. Catford also notes that the usual variety of intercartilaginous whisper is made at the arytenoidal end of the glottis and so can be marked as posterior. We use the advanced and retracted diacritics with the relevant phonation symbol to show this distinction: V̟, W̠.

3.3. Supralaryngeal Settings

The VoQS system provides symbolization for some 26 different supralaryngeal settings that can affect voice quality. As noted, the use of a specific supralaryngeal setting label, such as palatalization, for example, does not imply that the speaker converts all other target articulations to the palatal place, nor that all possible articulations are made with secondary palatalization. It is to be read as denoting that a substantial amount of palatalization is used by the speaker—differences in degree are shown through the scalar notation described later.

The symbols in this section are derived from Laver's (1980) set, with some changes and additions. Most of these changes involve use of IPA diacritics changed or added since the 1989 revision, but also the use of IPA and extIPA diacritics instead of forms adopted by Laver. An example of the latter can be seen with the raised and lowered larynx symbols, which use capital L plus the raised and lowered diacritics of the IPA. The 1989 IPA change to superscript diacritics to mark secondary articulations can be seen in the symbols for labialized and labiodentalized voice, and for all secondary articulations from palatalized back. VoQS also provides a method of distinguishing between close and open rounded labialized voice. Clearly, these diacritics can also be used with single segments, if need be.

New IPA diacritics allow new distinctions to be made, so VoQS has symbols for linguoapicalized and linguolaminarized voice quality, as well as using older diacritics to mark dentalized and retroflex. New extIPA diacritics allow the marking of spread-lip shape and alveolarized (for other uses of the latter see Bernhardt & Ball, 1993). The alveolar diacritic is also used in conjunction with the palatalization superscript to mark palatoalveolarized voice. This diacritic has been designed as an equivalent to the dental diacritic: If the dental one is intended to represent a tooth, then the alveolar one is intended to represent the upper and lower edges of the alveolar ridge.

Palatalized, velarized, uvularized, and pharyngealized voice all use the new IPA convention for superscript diacritics (uvularized is not specified in either the 1989 or 1993 IPA chart, but is readily derived through analogy with the others). Laryngopharyngealized voice uses the basic pharyngealized symbol together with the IPA diacritic for retracted tongue root. This was felt to be a somewhat better choice than the simple retraction sign used by Laver. The next voice type is faucalized voice. This is described in Laver's (1980) account in some detail, although no separate symbol is provided for a voice quality marked by constriction of the faucal pillars (though it is noted that such constriction is often common in nasalized voice quality). The symbol adopted in VoQS is a superscript double-barred capital H. There are three reasons why this symbol was chosen: first, the use of capital letters in phonetic symbolization is normally restricted to posterior areas of the vocal tract; second, h-like symbols are generally associated with glottal and pharyngeal regions; and, finally, the symbol has a degree of iconicity, in that it can be seen as two uprights (for the pillars) being constricted by the double bar.

Nasalized and denasalized voice use the nasal and denasal diacritics from the IPA and extIPA, respectively. By analogy, one could also imagine the use of the extIPA diacritic for audible nasal escape being used to characterize the voice quality of a speaker with gross velopharyngeal inadequacy.

The final set of symbols are for use with mandible settings and atypical lingual settings. Laver's (1980) symbol set provided symbols for close, open, and protruded jaw positions, and these have been retained, except that IPA raised and lowered diacritics have been used with the capital J symbol for close and open jaw, respectively. To these have been added two further jaw symbols for right and left offset jaw voice. These diacritics might also be useful when applied to, for example, bilabial consonants to mark speakers who use laterally differentiated mouth shape (Sara Howard, personal communication). We also include a symbol for protruded tongue voice. Some disordered speakers adopt an articulatory setting characterized by long-term excessive protrusion of the tongue (see Bernhardt & Ball, 1993), sometimes to such an extent that the blade is visible. While extIPA does provide diacritics to mark interdental articulation, these would not normally characterize such excessive protrusion. Therefore, for VoQS we have adopted the theta used for the dental fricative, but in capital form. The use of this symbol would be read to mean that some amount of tongue tip protrusion was present throughout the utterance being transcribed: the degree could be shown through scalar marking described below.

3.4. Scalar Markings

Many of the voice quality types listed above can be described in scalar terms: that is to say in terms of what degree of the quality is present. For example, we can distinguish between slight, moderate and excessive nasality; between very harsh and less harsh voice; between greater or lesser tongue tip protrusion. Laver (1980) recognized this, and proposed that a three-term scale could be used, equivalent to the adjectives "slightly," "moderately," and "extremely." This three-term scale is marked through the use of the numerals 1–3, where the absence of a numeral is interpreted as either "moderate" degree or as degree being irrelevant. In the VoQS system, the numeral is placed before the appropriate voice quality symbol.

3.5. The Use of VoQS Symbols

We noted earlier that the VoQS system is designed to be used with the conventions for marking suprasegmentals found in the extIPA principles (see Duckworth et al., 1990): that is to say the use of labeled braces within a segmental transcription. There are, however, a couple of other points that need to be clarified: First, how do we show combinations of various voice quality types and how to we show intermittent voice quality?

With many of the combined phonation types—as we have discussed—it is possible to use several diacritics on a single symbol. However, with other combinations the result may well be illegible: To adapt Laver's (1980) example, velarized nasal whispery creaky voice would be shown as Ṿ̰̃ˠ. To avoid such clumsy symbolizations, separate voice quality symbols can be shown for such combinations: Vˠ Ṽ Ṿ V̰. Alternatively, a mixture of combined and separate symbols could be utilized, although the danger with this approach is that it might suggest that some of the features are more interconnected than others. This can be addressed if only phonatory or supralryngeal aspects of voice quality are combined together on one symbol. Clearly, a separate symbol policy is needed if one wishes to add a scalar numeral to any of the individual components of a particular voice quality combination.

Both in normal and disordered speakers, one may wish to mark in a transcription that a specific voice quality has been changed in degree or type during an utterance. For example, a harsh voice quality may become more or less harsh or falsetto may be turned on or off at particular moments. Using labeled braces makes it straightforward to deal with these alterations in voice quality. A labeled brace can be inserted at any point in a segmental transcription and so can mark changes in degree or the start point or end point of a particular voice quality. The final section on the VoQS chart (Figure 5–1) illustrates this usage.

4. CONCLUSION

We believe that the recent developments in the transcription of suprasegmental features in both normal and disordered speech require a comprehensive and principled method for the marking of long-term voice quality. The current IPA and extIPA provisions are not sufficient for this task, and we submit that the VoQS system goes a long way to meet this aim. We await with interest more feedback from practitioners, as the system can clearly evolve to meet their needs.

REFERENCES

Ainsworth, W. A., & Singh, W. (1990). Analysis of fundamental frequency and temporal characteristics of neoglottal, oesophageal and normal speech. *Proceedings of the International Acoustics Association, 12*(10), 25–32.

Ainsworth, W. A., & Singh, W. (1992). Perceptual comparison of neoglottal, oesophageal and normal speakers. *Folia Phoniatrica, 44,* 297–307.

Ball, M. J. (1991). Recent developments in the transcription of nonnormal speech. *Journal of Communication Disorders, 24,* 59–78.

Ball, M. J. (in press). On percussives. *Journal of the International Phonetic Foundation.*

Ball, M. J. (1998b). The phonetics of *Rubus idaeus. The Phonetician, 76,* 3.

Ball, M. J., Code, C., Rahilly, J., & Hazlett, D. (1994). Non-segmental aspects of disordered speech: Developments in transcription, *Clinical Linguistics and Phonetics, 8,* 67–83.

Bernhardt, B., & Ball, M. J. (1993). Characteristics of atypical speech currently not included in the extensions to the IPA. *Journal of the International Phonetic Association, 23,* 35–38.

Catford, J. C. (1977). *Fundamental problems in phonetics.* Edinburgh: Edinburgh University Press.

Duckworth, M., Allen, G., Hardcastle, W., & Ball, M. J. (1990). Extensions to the International Phonetic Alphabet for the transcription of atypical speech. *Clinical Linguistics and Phonetics, 4,* 273–280.

Edels, Y. (1983). Pseudo-voice: Its theory and practice. In Y. Edels (Ed.), *Laryngectomy: Diagnosis to rehabilitation* (pp. 107–141). London: Croom Helm.

Esling, J. H. (1978). *Voice quality in Edinburgh: A sociolinguistic and phonetic study.* Unpublished doctoral dissertation, University of Edinburgh.

Esling, J. H. (1994). Voice quality. In R. Asher & J. Simpson (Eds.), *The encyclopedia of language and linguistics* (pp. 4950–4953). Oxford: Pergamon Press.

Hewlett, N., & Cohen, W. (1993). *Voicing distinctions in electrolarynx speech.* Paper presented at the Third Congress of the International Clinical Phonetics and Linguistics Association, Helsinki.

ICPLA Executive Committee. (1994). The extIPA chart. *Journal of the International Phonetic Association, 24,* 95–98.

IPA. (1989). Report on the 1989 Kiel Convention. *Journal of the International Phonetic Association, 19,* 67–80.

IPA. (1993). Council actions on the revisions of the IPA. *Journal of the International Phonetic Association, 23,* 32–34.

Laver, J. (1975). *Individual features in voice quality.* Unpublished doctoral dissertation, University of Edinburgh, Scotland.

Laver, J. (1979). *Voice quality: A classified bibliography.* Amsterdam: John Benjamins.

Laver, J. (1980). *The phonetic description of voice quality.* Cambridge: Cambridge University Press.

Luchsinger, R., & Arnold, G. D. (1965). *Voice-speech-language: Its physiology and pathology* (G. E. Arnold & E. R. Finkbeiner, Trans.) Belmont, CA: Wadsworth.

Nolan, F. (1983). *The phonetic bases of speaker recognition.* Cambridge: Cambridge University Press.

Perry, A. (1983). The speech therapist's role in surgical and prosthetic approaches to speech rehabilitation, with particular reference to the Blom-Singer and Panjé techniques. In Y. Edels (Ed.), *Laryngectomy: Diagnosis to rehabilitation* (pp. 271–288). London: Croom Helm.

Singh, W. (1993a). Fistula speech. In W. Singh & D. Soutar (Eds.), *Functional surgery of the larynx and pharynx* (pp. 171–203). Oxford: Butterworth Heinemann.

Singh, W. (1993b). Parsimonious laryngectomee. In W. Singh & D. Soutar (Eds.), *Functional surgery of the larynx and pharynx* (pp. 116–146). Oxford: Butterworth Heinemann.

Sweet, H. (1890). *A primer of phonetics*. Oxford: Clarendon Press.

Winter, H., & Martin, S. (1981). The classification of deviant voice quality through auditory memory training. *British Journal of Disorders of Communication, 16*, 204–210.

CHAPTER 6

Dysprosody

Anja Lowit-Leuschel and Gerry Docherty

The term *dysprosody* covers a range of suprasegmental aspects of speech production, some of which fall outside the domain of a volume focusing on voice quality (e.g., speech rhythm, prosodic modulation of segmental realization (see Couper-Kuhlen [1986] or Nooteboom [1997] for overviews of prosodic aspects of speech). This chapter provides an evaluative overview of the assessment of that aspect of prosody that is most closely associated with the phonatory mechanism and thereby with other aspects of voice quality: namely, F_0 variation and intonation. We begin by considering the range of etiologies of impaired F_0 modulation and its associated functions. We focus, in particular, on dysarthria, as it is in motor speech disorders that prosodic impairment seems to be most consistently a critical feature. Following a discussion of some of the methodological difficulties associated with assessment of functional aspects of F_0 modulation, we survey the auditory procedures that have been proposed to assist in this task. Readers are referred to chapters in Part II of this volume for details of relevant instrumental techniques. Our review leads to the conclusion that there is still a considerable amount of work required before clinicians can call on diagnostically valuable probes in this area that have good reliability, validity, and sensitivity.

1. THE CAUSES OF DYSPROSODY

1.1. Diverse Causal Factors

A multitude of speech and language disorders have been shown to cause prosodic disturbances: fluent and nonfluent aphasia, foreign accent syndrome, right hemisphere damage, apraxia of speech, dysarthria, stuttering, voice disorders, hearing impairment, learning difficulties, autism, developmental speech and language disorders, and specific language impairment (SLI) (Hargrove & McGarr, 1994; Wells, Peppé, & Vance, 1995). Table 6–1 gives a selection of research reports that have indicated prosodic problems for the listed disorders. Some of these references have been taken from Wells et al. (1995), as well as from review articles on prosodic disturbance by Ackermann, Hertrich, and Ziegler (1993) and Weismer and Martin (1992). References to studies of dysprosody in dysarthria are not included in Table 6–1, as the prosodic problems associated with this disorder are described in more detail later.

Despite the great variety of etiologies related to prosodic problems, these problems do not typically play a central role in the majority of the disorders listed in Table 6–1, with other factors, such as language difficulties, typically being more noticeable.

However, the same cannot be said of dysarthria. Dysprosody, particularly in relation to F_0 modulation and voice quality, is evident in each of the six types of dysarthria identified by Darley, Aronson, and Brown (1975), frequently being one of the prominent symptoms of the disorder. The following section provides a brief summary of the pitch and voice characteristics identified in the flaccid, spastic, ataxic, hypokinetic, hyperkinetic, and mixed dysarthrias.

1.2. A Closer Look at Dysarthria

1.2.1. Flaccid Dysarthria

Flaccid dysarthria has not been the subject of a great deal of research from the point of view of prosodic characteristics. Darley et al.'s (1975) work is probably still the most extensive study that has been carried out. They report a high incidence of breathy voice characteristics, followed closely by "monopitch" (the term used by Darley et al. to refer to a reduction in the modulation of F_0 during speech production, in many cases to the extent that there is no modulation). Harsh voice quality was not a common symptom of their speakers.

Table 6–1. References to prosodic impairment associated with a diversity of etiologies.

Disorder	***References***
Aphasia	Benson & Geschwind, 1985; Berthier et al., 1991; Blumstein et al., 1987; Bryan, 1994; Cancelliere & Kertesz, 1990; Cooper et al., 1984; Coppens & Robey, 1992; Danly & Shapiro, 1982; Darby, 1993; Emmorey, 1987; Goodglass & Kaplan, 1972; Graff-Radford et al., 1986; Gurd et al., 1988; Lecours & Rouillon, 1976; Moen, 1990; Pitchford et al., 1997; Ryalls, 1982; Van Lancker & Sidtis, 1992
Right hemisphere	Behrens, 1987; Bryan, 1994; Colsher et al., 1987; Dordain et al., 1971, House et al., 1987; Ross & Mesulam, 1979; Ross et al., 1988; Shairo & anly, 1985; Tucker et al., 1977; Van Lancker & Sidtis, 1992; Weintraub et al., 1981
Speech apraxia	Kent & Rosenbek 1982, 1983; Square-Storer et al., 1988
Stuttering	Bergmann, 1986; Grube & Smith, 1989; Hall & Yairi, 1992; Harrington, 1986; Jäncke et al., 1996; Packman et al., 1996; Wingate, 1985
Hearing impairment	Friedman, 1985; Lane & Webster, 1991; Maassen & Povel, 1985; Parker & Rose, 1990; Rahilly, 1992
Learning difficulties	Heselwood et al., 1995; Jackson et al., 1997; Shriberg & Widder, 1990
Autism	Baltaxe, 1981; Baltaxe & Simmons, 1985; Erwin et al., 1991; Local & Wootton, 1995; Murayama et al., 1991; Rutter & Schopler, 1987
Developmental speech and language disorder	Hargrove & Sheran, 1989; Ruscello et al., 1991; Shriberg et al., 1986; Shriberg & Kwiatkowski, 1994; St. Louis et al., 1992; Wells & Local, 1993

1.2.2. Spastic Dysarthria

Similarly, not many researchers have focused on the pitch and voice characteristics of spastic dysarthric speakers, although Darley et al. (1975) observed a variety of pitch problems, such as monopitch, relatively low mean F_0 level, pitch breaks, as well as speakers with harsh, strained-strangled, or breathy voices.

1.2.3. Ataxic Dysarthria

The cerebellar or ataxic disorders have received more attention. Darley et al. (1975) report that their speakers exhibited a harsh voice quality and monopitch. Similar findings are reported by Amarenco, Chevrie-Muller, Roullet, and Bousser (1991), who observed a decrease in F_0 modulation. However, Hertrich and Ackermann (1993b) could find no evidence of reduced F_0 variation in their subjects with Friedreich ataxia. In addition to Darley et al.'s (1975) finding of harsh voice quality, Ackermann and Ziegler (1991) observed weak and breathy voices in their subjects, and Ackemann and Ziegler (1992) report the presence of a strident voice quality. A further observation concerning voice quality was the presence of voice tremor or increased jitter (Ackermann & Ziegler, 1991, 1992, 1994), which was thought to be related to postural tremor (Ackermann & Ziegler, 1991). Finally, Ackermann and Ziegler (1991, 1994) report increases in mean F_0 level. Ackermann and Ziegler (1994) hypothesize that this might stem from the increased vocal effort made by their speakers.

1.2.4. Hypokinetic Dysarthria

The disorder most commonly associated with prosodic problems is Parkinson disease, which is classified as resulting in hypokinetic dysarthria by Darley et al. (1975). They indicate monopitch as the primary symptom of this disorder, followed by harsh or breathy voice and a lowering in mean F_0 level. Subsequent studies have produced inconsistent findings in relation to lowering of mean F_0, as some researchers report having replicated Darley et al.'s (1975) results (Hertrich & Ackermann 1993a[1]), while others have found no abnormalities (Metter & Hanson, 1986; Zwirner, Murry, & Woodson, 1991), or have described increases in mean F_0 level (Canter, 1961; Illes, Metter, Hanson, & Iritani, 1988; Lowit-Leuschel, 1997; Ludlow & Bassich, 1983, 1984). The findings in respect of monopitch are more homogeneous and most researchers have indicated reductions in the modulation of F_0 (Ackermann & Ziegler, 1989; Canter, 1961; Kent ,1991; Logemann, Fisher, Boshes, & Blonsky, 1978; Ludlow & Bassich, 1983, 1984; Metter & Hanson, 1986; Uziel, Bohe, Cadilhac, & Passouant, 1975; Zwirner et al., 1991). In addition to the above reported symptoms, Chenery, Murdoch, and Ingram (1988) observed a hoarse, strained-strangled voice quality in their speakers, as well as periods of intermittent breathiness.

Another dysfunction involving the basal ganglia, thalamic infarction, has also received some attention. Ackermann, Ziegler, and Petersen (1993) report alterations in pitch level, monotonous speech, and hoarse or rough voice quality as their own as well as other researchers' findings.

1.2.5. Hyperkinetic Dysarthria

Further types of dysarthria identified by Darley et al. (1975) are hyperkinetic (chorea) and slow hyperkinetic dysarthria (athetosis, dyskinesia, dystonia). Again, Darley et al.'s (1975) work is the principal source of information about prosodic aspects of these disorders. According to their findings, chorea is associated with monopitch and harsh voice quality, although strained-strangled voice can occur in a few cases. Regarding the slow hyperkinesias, harsh, strained-strangled voice quality and monopitch were the most prominent pitch or voice problems and some subjects exhibited "voice stoppages."

[1]In relation to their male subjects.

1.2.6. Mixed Dysarthria

The final type of dysarthria to be discussed is mixed dysarthria, which results from disorders with multiple lesions in the nervous system. Darley et al. (1975) discuss amyotrophic lateral sclerosis (ALS), pseudobulbar palsy (PBP), bulbar palsy (BUL), multiple sclerosis (MS), and Wilson disease.

According to Darley et al. (1975), ALS speakers mainly present with harsh voice quality and monopitch. Low mean F_0 levels, strained-strangled voice, and breathy voice qualities were some of the more infrequent findings. The presence of low F_0 levels was confirmed by Caruso and Burton (1987). Strand, Buder, Yorkston, & Ramig's (1994) review of the disorder additionally reports the findings of a "wet hoarse" voice, tremor, and F_0 fluctuations. They also report findings of low mean F_0, vocal instability and increased shimmer and jitter from other studies which used acoustic analysis (Kent et al., 1992; Kent et al., 1991; Ramig, Scherer, Klasner, Titze, & Horii, 1990). Their own study does not add any new characteristics to the listed findings, but indicates that subjects can exhibit a variety of symptom patterns. The finding of variability was reproduced by Lowit-Leuschel (1997), who observed F_0 levels above, within, and below the normal range for her subjects. In contrast to Darley et al.'s (1975) findings, the subjects of this study showed no signs of reduced F_0 modulation.

PBP and BUL result in prosodic features similar to those of ALS (Darley et al., 1975), although BUL speakers do not exhibit low mean F_0 and strained-strangled voice characteristics. Darley et al.'s (1975) MS speakers, on the other hand, differed slightly from the other speakers with mixed dysarthria, and showed harsh or breathy voice, reduced F_0 control, and inappropriate F_0 levels. These results were confirmed by Fitzgerald, Chenery, and Murdoch (1987), who, in addition, observed monopitch in their speakers. In contrast, Lowit-Leuschel (1997) found a high degree of variation in the extent of F_0 modulation and mean F_0 level, with subjects performing within as well as above or below the normal range for these parameters. Finally, Wilson disease has again not received much attention in the research literature. Darley et al. (1975) report the presence of monopitch, low mean F_0, and harsh or strained voice quality. These results were largely supported in a subsequent study by Liao, Wang, Kwan, Kong, and Wu (1991).

1.3. Summary

In summary, aspects of prosody have been implicated across a wide variety of different types of communication impairment. The evidence in the literature suggests that the dysarthrias are notable by the fact that in many cases the prosodic characteristics are primary symptoms of the disorder. Most of the dysarthrias are associated with changes in aspects of performance related to F_0 and vocal quality, with the most common symptoms being alterations in the overall mean F_0 level, a reduction in the modulation of F_0, and breathy, harsh, or hoarse voice quality. It is not surprising then to find that a good deal of the work that has been carried out on the assessment of impaired prosody has arisen from investigators in this particular area. The key features of this work are next reviewed, following a brief excursus into some key background issues that need to be borne in mind when planning an assessment of F_0 variation in speech.

2. METHODOLOGICAL AND CONCEPTUAL ISSUES

Space restrictions permit no more than a brief overview of the methodological and conceptual issues surrounding the understanding of F_0 variation in speech. Readers are referred to Cruttenden (1997) and Ladd (1996) for fully detailed accounts of these. For the present purposes we highlight what we see as some of the key issues that need to be considered in carrying out an assessment of impaired F_0 variation.

2.1. Intonational "Meaning"

Functional speech assessment typically involves measuring performance against a normal baseline and computing some form of distance measure. For segmental assessment, the baseline is the "correct" production of the target corpus by a matched normal speaker or group of speakers. For analysis of the linguistic (and, in some cases, the paralinguistic) functions associated with F_0 variation (i.e., intonation) it is considerably harder to define the baseline for comparison. Compared to segmental analysis (where, for example, there would be an expectation that a visual stimulus showing a four-legged feline would consistently elicit the sequence [kat] from normal English speakers) the relationship between the phonetic form taken by a F_0 contour and the "meaning" that it conveys is much harder to define. It is possible to identify a number of facets of this complex relationship: (a) functional interpretation of F_0 movement is extremely context-sensitive, that is, the same contour may not carry the same shade of meaning across two different contexts; (b) it may be difficult to state exactly what a particular pragmatic function is, even if native speakers are in agreement about appropriacy (this may be because the functions of intonation are often emotional or affective and therefore difficult to state in concrete, consistent fashion); (c) intonation has a multiplicity of functions (syntactic, pragmatic, paralinguistic, social) with some of these being achieved simultaneously, that is, the functions are overlaid on one another, which makes it difficult to assess them independently; (d) linguistic use of F_0 variation is subject to considerable variation, both crossaccentually and sociolinguistically, and, at least for English, there are very few accounts of this variation, which means that for a very large number of speakers there is simply no existing account of normal patterns of intonation; (e) although it is possible to get native speaker judgments of appropriacy, listeners often report *degrees* of appropriacy, correlating with the likelihood or otherwise of the particular interpretation of the context—this underlies the point made in (a) that the functional interpretation of a particular pitch contour is hugely context-sensitive.

2.2. Analysis Framework

A second issue fundamental to assessment of intonation is related to the analysis framework that is chosen. In analyzing intonation, the investigator has to take a step back from the raw data (i.e., F_0 traces plotted on a hertz scale through time) due to the difficulties of interspeaker variation. To investigate the linguistic use of F_0 variation, it is important to be able to normalize across speakers with different mean speaking F_0 and F_0 range, with the result that subsequent analysis is based on some form of abstraction away from the physical level. This, in itself, is not too different from the situation that applies to segmental speech assessment (a segmental transcription normalizes across speakers and is a considerable abstraction away from actual speech production), but it is fair to say that in the field of intonation there is considerably greater controversy about the nature of the abstract representation and the various proposals are substantially different. Ladd (1996) points out that for most of the second half of this century, a basic distinction could be drawn between analyses that treated intonation contours as a sequence of level tones and others that interpreted them as being composed of sequences of pitch movements (e.g., fall, rise, or rise-fall). More recently, linguists specializing in intonational phonology have tended to converge toward what Ladd refers to as an autosegmental-metrical analysis framework (largely based on the seminal work of Liberman, 1975, and Pierrehumbert, 1980). Currently, the most popular version of this analytic framework is the so-called ToBI system (Beckman & Ayers, 1994) designed for transcribing the intonational characteristics of large speech corpora. Readers are referred to Cruttenden (1997) for an excellent overview and a balanced evaluation of these developments. It is notable that virtually none of these recent developments in intonational analysis have had any significant impact in the clinical arena, and it is fair to say that there is a considerable gap between current thinking in intonational phonology and the functional assessment of F_0 variation built in to existing clinical assessment procedures.

2.3. On the Interpretation of Impaired F_0 Variation

As with investigations of segmental impairment, difficulties arise in attempting to relate a particular pattern of impaired F_0 variation to a particular locus of breakdown within the speech processing chain. Although it is quite clear that any given F_0 contour is a function of both a linguistic plan and the execution of that plan by the vocal apparatus, it is not absolutely straightforward to dissociate these different aspects with confidence, which leads to difficulty in deciding whether an impairment should be attributed to difficulty at a lower or higher level of the processing chain (similar difficulties arise when investigating an individual's receptive abilities vis-à-vis prosody). A further ambiguity in interpretation can be attributed to the fact that the physiological basis of F_0 variation and intonation (i.e., the phonatory mechanism) is driven by the output from the respiratory system as well as by the tension and configuration of the laryngeal musculature. What this means is that any impairment to F_0 variation/intonation cannot automatically be attributed to a difficulty in laryngeal articulation, and it is necessary to devise probes that tap selectively into other potential contributing factors, including respiratory abilities, aspects of utterance planning, and even a speaker's ability to monitor pragmatic context, all of which could well be a factor in impaired patterns of intonation.

Taken together, the stated points suggest that functional assessment of F_0 variation is not without a number of significant challenges. However, bearing in mind the prevalence with which F_0 variation is implicated in communication impairment and its potential for contributing to degradation of speech intelligibility, it is not an area that can be ignored. In the following section we review a number of clinical assessment protocols that attempt to characterize this aspect of speech production. As explained earlier, our focus is on those protocols that rely primarily on auditory analysis by a clinician; readers are referred to Part II of this volume for details of instrumental assessment of F_0.

3. HOW CAN PITCH BE ASSESSED PERCEPTUALLY?

A variety of assessment protocols have been designed in order to assess F_0 variation and/or intonation. These assessments vary in their overall purpose, ranging from assessments of dysarthria to those of voice or even specifically for prosody (but not linked to a particular category of impairment). This section reviews several assessment procedures in the light of how F_0 or intonation are assessed (Sections 3.1–3.3) and how reliable, valid, and sensitive these methods are (Section 3.4). The assessment protocols discussed are three dysarthria tests, the Frenchay Dysarthria Assessment (Enderby, 1983), the Robertson Dysarthria Profile (Robertson, 1982), and the Motor Speech Examination (Darley et al., 1975); two "prosodic profiles," Crystal's (1982) Profile of Prosody (PROP) and Hargrove and McGarr's (1994) Prosody Teaching Model Checklist (PTMC); and voice evaluations by Wilson (1979), Boone (1983), and Wirz and Mackenzie-Beck (1995).

3.1. Dysarthria Tests

The Robertson Dysarthria Profile (Robertson, 1982) and the Frenchay Dysarthria Assessment (Enderby, 1983) are very similar in their analysis of F_0 variation and intonation. Some of the assessment is carried out on nonspeech tasks, where the patient's ability to vary F_0 is investigated by asking the individual to perform pitch glides (Robertson, 1982) or sing a scale (Enderby, 1983). The Frenchay Dysarthria Assessment (Enderby, 1983) furthermore proposes to evaluate a patient's phonation, loudness and F_0 variation in connected speech. The Robertson Dysarthria Profile (Robertson, 1982) suggests a slightly more detailed investigation of connected speech and looks at the appropriacy of intonation and stress patterns in reading, conversation, and contrastive stress drills. Both assessments are based on purely perceptual analyses and use a 5-point scale to score a patient's performance.

Darley et al.'s (1975) Motor Speech Examination generally adheres to the same pattern of investigation. F_0 is assessed in one nonspeech task, where the patient is asked to produce a prolonged [a]-vowel to judge the F_0 level and voice quality, as well as loudness and breath support. As opposed to the previous two tests, F_0 variation is not assessed in nonspeech tasks; instead, the assessment of this parameter is carried out in more detailed fashion in contextual speech. The data are collected in reading and spontaneous speech, and a patient's performance is then evaluated against a checklist based on the dimensions or speech characteristics identified in Darley et al.'s (1969a, 1969b) original study. The dimensions relating to F_0 are abnormal mean F_0 level, sudden, uncontrolled variations in F_0, and monopitch. In addition, the clinician is asked to listen for abnormal voice qualities such as harshness, hoarseness, breathiness, or strained-strangled voice. The assessment is again carried out by perceptual means, however, Darley et al. (1975) do not specify how the severity should be scored.

As can be seen from the description of the three dysarthria tests, the main focus of the analysis lies on the evaluation of mean F_0 level and variability, on the basis of either speech or nonspeech tasks. Only the Robertson Dysarthria Profile (Robertson, 1982) includes an assessment of intonation and this is restricted to the judgment of appropriacy. Darley et al.'s (1975) protocol provides the most detailed information for clinicians about what features of F_0 should be attended to and could be affected. This feature was most probably included to aid clinicians in identifying F_0 problems, however, it could also have the opposite effect and adversely influence the analysis by restricting the scope of investigation. Although Darley et al. (1975) indicate that their dimensions should be "borne in mind" (p. 95) during the analysis rather than adhered to strictly, some clinicians might be inclined to only listen out for the characteristics suggested by Darley et al. (1975), instead of approaching the data with an open mind. Disturbances not mentioned in the test's checklist might thus not be detected.

3.2. Prosodic Profiles

Two profiles that seek to give a broader assessment of prosody are discussed in this section, Crystal's PROP (1982) and Hargrove and McGarr's (1994) PTMC.

PROP is purely concerned with the functional aspect of F_0 variation, that is, intonation. Crystal (1982) adopted Halliday's (e.g., 1970) approach to the description of prosody and investigates three dimensions thought to characterize the linguistic use of F_0 variation, tonality (the way in which intonational contours are arrayed over stretches of speech and, in particular, the relationship between this and the syntactic structure of a phrase), tonicity (the use of F_0 variation to impart different degrees of prominence to components of a phrase), and tone (an analysis of the finite set of linguistically significant F_0 contours). The analysis is carried out perceptually and is scored descriptively; for example, the clinician is asked to note down all tones produced by a client. Although Crystal (1982) provides some guidelines for normal production, a client's performance is not scored on a scale comparable to the previously discussed tests. Instead, it is assumed that certain patterns or deficits might become apparent from the descriptive analysis. Although this scoring method ensures that clinicians approach the data with an open mind and score a client's performance in great detail, the lack of quantification could cause problems when attempts are made to compare clients with one other or the same client over time. This is particularly the case if spontaneous speech is used (as advised by Crystal, [1982]), as intonation patterns and tones vary considerably from utterance to utterance. An increase in number of observations of rising tones, for example, could arise from an improvement in a client's ability to produce the tone type, or simply because the second speech sample includes more structures requiring the particular tone.

The most comprehensive prosodic profile currently available is Hargrove and McGarr's (1994) PTMC. In contrast to Crystal (1982), the dynamic properties of both F_0 variation and intonation are investigated. The assessment is carried out on a sample of spontaneous speech. The features investigated with regard to F_0 are mean F_0 level, extent of F_0 modulation, "direction" (which refers to the types of pitch movement produced by a speaker), and F_0 range. Intonation is analyzed by looking at aspects of the internal structure of intonation contours, such as pitch of the first "full" syllable in a phrase (the "onset"), the tone assigned to the most prominent word within a phrase (the "nucleus"), and the pitch movement observed in phrase-final position (the "terminal contour"). An account is also given of aspects of the use of F_0 variation across utterances, including "pitch agreement" (the relationship between the F_0 level at the end of one utterance and the onset of the following utterance) and "cohesive devices" (the extent to which F_0 variation is used by speakers as a marker of the cohesiveness of a stretch of speech consisting of a number of utterances). Perceptual analysis can probably not be much more detailed; however, the value of the profile is seriously diminished by the scoring system, which, for all of the measures mentioned, consists simply of the labels "appropriate," "inappropriate," and "not judged." This limits the potential for making fine-grained judgments of differences in performance across and within speakers.

3.3. Voice Profiles

Tests designed for the assessment of disordered voice focus on a wide range of parameters, some of which can be unrelated to actual voice production, such as environmental factors, personality, or stress. A relatively large number of protocols have been published, all slightly varying in their focus. A common factor, however, is that most of them include an assessment of F_0 variation. This generally consists of an investigation of the overall mean F_0 level and a measure of F_0 variation or range (e.g., Boone, 1983; Wilson, 1979; Wirz & Mackenzie Beck, 1995). In this, these protocols do not differ significantly from the dysarthria tests previously described. Most assessments are carried out perceptually, although some researchers such as Boone (1983) suggest that parameters such as F_0 should be measured instrumentally. The perceptual assessments all use rating scales to score a speaker's performance, which are again comparable to the dysarthria assessments.

3.4. Discussion

As can be seen from the previous section, a variety of assessment procedures are available to investigate phonetic characteristics of F_0 variation (e.g., mean F_0 and F_0 dynamics). Despite the varying foci of these protocols, the tasks and measurement techniques do not differ hugely from each other. A smaller number of broader prosodic profiles investigate the linguistic use of F_0, either exclusively (Crystal, 1982) or in addition to its phonetic properties (Hargrove & McGarr, 1994).

Thus, existing assessments differ in the extent to which F_0 performance is investigated; only at the phonetic level (e.g., F_0 range and dynamics) or at the linguistic-functional level as well. In the field of dysarthria, there has been an argument in favor of the latter (e.g., Brewster, 1989; Lowit-Leuschel, 1997), mainly because phonetic and linguistic aspects of F_0 variation can either be affected independently or can be interrelated, a factor that can influence the diagnosis and have repercussions on the choice of therapy approach. In other disorders with a potential prosodic component, such as voice disorders, this argument might be less strong. However, as there is a complex mapping between the phonetic and linguistic aspects of prosody, it is likely that clients with similar phonetic profiles can show differences in the use of the linguistic parameters, and it therefore seems to be important to investigate both aspects of F_0 in any type of disorder. One could therefore argue that, with the exception of the profiles by Crystal (1982) and Hargrove and McGarr (1994), most tests that include an analysis of F_0 appear to lack in investigative detail by not assessing its linguistic functions.

A further issue that could be perceived as a limitation of all of the mentioned tests is the use of perceptual analysis techniques. Perceptual analysis has long been criticized for its high degree of subjectivity, its relatively low inter- and intrarater reliability, its questionable validity, and its reduction in sensitivity of measurement (Kent, 1994; Lowit-Leuschel, 1997). Subjectivity of measurement often arises from poorly defined terminology and the lack of widely accepted and available norms.

Descriptions of voice quality, such as hoarseness or harshness, have often been shown to be interpreted differently by experimenters (de Bodt, Wuyts, Van de Heyning, & Croux, 1997). Darley et al.'s (1975) dimension of "bizarreness of speech" has received similar criticism (Kent, 1994). In addition, certain parameters, such as habitual pitch, can differ across languages and even regional accents (Wirz & Mackenzie Beck, 1995), and clients might be described as having abnormalities when judged against the norms of the experimenter's accent. Subjective measurements can also affect the overall diagnosis, as demonstrated by Zyski and Weisiger (1987). They asked a number of listeners to reclassify Darley et al.'s (1975) original data and found considerable variations in diagnosis when a large number of speech dimensions were used by the listeners to make this diagnosis. Finally, subjectivity of measurement and judgment can lead to poor inter- and intrarater reliability. Sheard, Adams, and Davis (1991) and Kent (1994) have alerted to the low reliability of perceptual dysarthria tests such as Darley et al.'s (1975), and De Bodt et al. (1997) found similar results for a perceptual voice assessment (GRBAS, Hirano, 1981).

Validity is another important aspect of assessments that can be problematic for perceptual protocols. Research into the perception of rate in Parkinson disease has indicated that the evaluation can be influenced by prosodic factors such as voice quality (Weismer, 1984), pitch and loudness variation (den Os, 1985), or segmental features such as articulatory undershoot (Kent & Rosenbek, 1982; Ziegler, Hartmann, & von Cramon, 1988). As most aspects of prosody are interrelated during speech production, it is highly likely that the perception of pitch performance can also be affected by factors other than pitch, which, in turn, can affect the validity of the perceptual measure.

In view of these limitations of perceptual measurements, many researchers have turned to an instrumental analysis of voice and prosody. However, others are not satisfied that this move is an actual improvement. Wirz and Mackenzie Beck (1995), for example, state that "whilst these [physiological and acoustic techniques—AL/GD] have undoubtedly added greatly to our knowledge and have enabled more accurate and objective measurements of many aspects of vocal performance, it is unlikely that they will ever obviate the need for systematic perceptual assessment of voice quality" (p. 39). Their argument is based on the high costs of equipment, the discomfort and anxiety caused by invasive techniques, and more fundamentally, the fact that voice production is a result of a multitude of interrelated physiological processes, the dynamics of which cannot be captured with one measurement technique at a particular point in time. In addition, other researchers have argued that perceptual techniques have greater "face validity" (Wertz & Rosenbek, 1992) or "content validity" (Ludlow & Bassich, 1983), as it is ultimately the perceptual impression of the speaker that determines if a problem is present and to what degree.

In view of the multitude of arguments both for and against perceptual and instrumental measurement techniques, the most favorable solution seems to be a combination of both. This idea has recently been taken on in the field of dysarthria assessments (Lowit Leuschel, 1997; Robin, Klouda, & Hug, 1991). The literature on voice disorders does not yet seem to have produced an assessment that specifically advocates a combined analysis of each parameter, although "mixed" protocols are available (e.g., Boone, 1983). It might therefore be useful to take a perceptual voice assessment such as GRBAS (Hirano, 1981) or the Vocal Profile Analysis (Wirz & Mackenzie Beck, 1995) and supplement the perceptual evaluations by instrumental measures, such as advocated by Titze (1994) where possible.

4. SUMMARY

In this chapter, we have focused on the assessment of that aspect of dysprosody that is most closely linked to voice production, that is, F_0 variation. We have pointed out that impaired prosody is a feature of many types of communication impairment, but that it is a particularly common feature in the dysarthrias. Work in this area has identified impaired patterns of F_0 variation as being a key component of speech that sounds "dysprosodic." It was suggested that assessment of the functional aspects of F_0 variation are hindered by the complexity and relative opacity of the relationship between the phonetic features of F_0 and its corresponding functions, and that this contrasts sharply with the situation that applies to assessment of segmental aspects of speech production. We reviewed a selection of existing auditory procedures for the assessment of impaired F_0 variation. Generally these have focused primarily on the phonetic aspects of F_0 variation as opposed to its functional implications, and they are subject to a number of problems associated with auditory analysis, which detracts to some extent from their reliability, validity and sensitivity. Assessment of prosodic aspects of speech production, and particularly of impaired F_0 variation is an area that is clearly in need of much further work (particularly when compared to the amount of attention that has been paid to segmental aspects of speech production). We suggest that one fruitful line of investigation might be to look at how auditory and instrumental analyses can be used in complementary fashion to enhance assessment and subsequent clinical intervention in this area.

REFERENCES

Ackermann, H., Hertrich, I., & Ziegler, W. (1993). Prosodische Störungen bei neurologischen Erkrankungen—eine Literaturübersicht. *Fortschritte der Neurologie—Psychiatrie, 7,* 241–253.

Ackermann, H., & Ziegler, W. (1989). Die Dysarthrophonie des Parkinson Syndroms. *Fortschritte der Neurologie—Psychiatrie, 57,* 149–160.

Ackermann, H., & Ziegler, W. (1991). Cerebellar voice tremor: An acoustic analysis. *Journal of Neurology, Neurosurgery and Psychiatry, 54,* 74–76.

Ackermann, H., & Ziegler, W. (1992). Die zerebellare Dysarthrie—eine Literaturübersicht. *Fortschritte der Neurologie—Psychiatrie, 60,* 28–40.

Ackermann, H., Ziegler, W., & Petersen, D. (1993). Dysarthria in bilateral thalamic infarction. A case-study. *Journal of Neurology, 240*(6), 357–362.

Ackermann, H., & Ziegler, W. (1994). Acoustic analysis of vocal instability in cerebellar dysfunctions. *Annals of Otology, Rhinology and Laryngology, 103,* 98–104.

Amarenco, P., Chevrie-Muller, C., Roullet, E., & Bousser, M -G. (1991). Paravermal infarct and isolated cerebellar dysarthria. *Annals of Neurology, 30,* 211–213.

Baltaxe, C. A. M. (1981). Acoustic characteristics of prosody in autism. In P. Mittler (Ed.), *Frontiers of knowledge in mental retardation. Vol. 1: Social, educational, and behavioural aspects* (pp. 223–233). Baltimore: University Park Press.

Baltaxe, C. A. M., & Simmons, J. (1985). Prosodic development in normal and autistic children. In E. Schopler & G. Mesibov (Eds.), *Communication problems in autism* (pp. 95–126). New York: Plenum.

Beckman, M., & Ayers, G. (1994). *Guidelines for ToBi labelling.* Version 2.0. Columbus: Ohio State University, Department of Linguistics.

Behrens, S. J. (1987). The role of the right hemisphere in the production of linguistic prosody: An acoustic investigation. In J. H. Ryalls (Ed.), *Phonetic approaches to speech production in aphasia and related disorders* (pp. 81–92). Boston: College-Hill Press.

Benson, D. F., & Geschwind, N. (1985). Aphasia and related disorders: A clinical approach. In M. M. Mesulam (Ed.), *Principles of behavioural neurology* (pp. 193–238). Philadelphia: Davis.

Bergmann, G. (1986). Studies in stuttering as a prosodic disturbance. *Journal of Speech and Hearing Research, 29,* 290–300.

Berthier, M. L., Ruiz, A., Massone, M. I., Starkstein, S. E., & Leiguarda, R. C. (1991). Foreign accent syndrome: Behavioural and anatomical findings in

recovered and non-recovered patients. *Aphasiology, 5,* 129–147.
Blumstein, S. E., Alexander, M. P., Ryalls, J. H., Katz, W., & Dworetzky, B. (1987). On the nature of the foreign accent syndrome: A case study. *Brain and Language, 31,* 215–244.
Boone, D. (1983). *The voice and voice therapy*. Englewood Cliffs, NJ: Prentice-Hall.
Brewster, K. (1989). Assessment of prosody. In K. Grundy (Ed.), *Linguistics in clinical practice* (pp. 168–185). London: Taylor & Francis.
Bryan, K. (1994). *The right-hemisphere language battery* (2nd ed.). London: Whurr.
Cancelliere, A. E. B., & Kertesz, A. (1990). Lesion localization in acquired deficits of emotional expression and comprehension. *Brain and Cognition, 13,* 133–147.
Canter, G. J. (1961). *An investigation of speech characteristics of a group of patients with Parkinson's disease*. Unpublished doctoral dissertation, Northwestern University, Evanston, IL.
Caruso, A. J., & Burton, E. K. (1987). Temporal acoustic measures of dysarthria associated with amyotrophic lateral sclerosis. *Journal of Speech and Hearing Research, 30,* 80–87.
Chenery, H. J., Murdoch, B. E., & Ingram, J. C. L. (1988). Studies in Parkinson's disease: Perceptual speech analysis. *Australian Journal of Communication Disorders, 16,* 17–29.
Colsher, P. L., Cooper, W. E., & Graff-Radford, N. (1987). Intonational variability in the speech of right hemisphere damaged patients. *Brain and Language, 32,* 379–383.
Cooper, W. E., Soares, C., Nicol, J., Michelow, D., & Goloskie, S. (1984). Clausal intonation after unilateral brain damage. *Language and Speech, 27,* 17–24.
Coppens, P., & Robey, R. R. (1992). Crossed aphasia—New perspectives. *Aphasiology, 6,* 585–596.
Couper-Kuhlen, E. (1986). *An introduction to English prosody*. London: Edward Arnold.
Cruttenden, A. (1997). *Intonation* (2nd ed.). Cambridge, UK: Cambridge University Press
Crystal, D. (1982). *Profiling linguistic disability*. London: Edward Arnold.
Danly, M., & Shapiro, B. (1982). Speech prosody in Broca's aphasia. *Brain and Language, 16,* 171–190.
Darby, D. G. (1993). Sensory aprosodia—A clinical clue to lesions of the inferior division of the right middle cerebral artery? *Neurology, 43,* 567–572.
Darley, F. L., Aronson, A. E., & Brown, J. R. (1969a). Clusters of deviant speech dimensions in the dysarthrias. *Journal of Speech and Hearing Research, 12,* 462–496.
Darley, F. L., Aronson, A. E., & Brown, J. R. (1969b). Differential diagnostic patterns of dysarthria. *Journal of Speech and Hearing Research, 12,* 246–269.
Darley, F. L., Aronson, A. E., & Brown, J. R. (1975). *Motor speech disorders*. Philadelphia: W.B. Saunders Company.
de Bodt, M. S., Wuyts, F. L., Van de Heyning, P. H., & Croux, C. (1997). Test-retest study of the GRBAS scale: Influence of experience and professional background on perceptual rating of voice quality. *Journal of Voice, 11,* 74–80.
Dordain, M., Degos, J. D., & Dordain, G. (1971). Troubles de la voix dans les hemiplegies gauches. *Revue Laryngologica, Otolaryngologica et Rhinologica, 92,* 178–188.
Emmorey, K. D. (1987). The neurological substrates for prosodic aspects of speech. *Brain and Language, 30,* 305–320.
Enderby, P. M. (1983). *Frenchay Dysarthria Assessment*. San Diego: College-Hill Press.
Erwin, R., van Lancker, D., Guthrie, D., Schwafel, J., Tanguay, P., & Buchwald, J. S. (1991). P3 responses to prosodic stimuli in adult autistic subjects. *Electroencephalography and Clinical Neurophysiology, 80,* 561–571.
Fitzgerald, F., Chenery, H. J., & Murdoch, B. E. (1987). Speech and language disorders in multiple sclerosis. *Australian Journal of Human Communication Disorders, 15,* 15–36.
Friedman, M. (1985). Remediation of intonation contours of hearing-impaired students. *Journal of Communication Disorders, 18,* 259–272.
Goodglass, H., & Kaplan, E. (1972). *The assessment of aphasia and related disorders*. Philadelphia: Lea and Febiger.
Graff-Radford, N. R., Cooper, W. E., Colsher, P. L., & Damasio, A. R. (1986). An unlearned foreign "accent" in a patient with aphasia. *Brain and Language, 28,* 86–94.
Grube, M. M., & Smith, D. S. (1989). Paralinguistic intonation-rhythm intervention with a developmental stutterer. *Journal of Fluency Disorders, 14,* 185–208.
Gurd, J. M., Bessel, N. J., Bladon, R. A. W., & Bamford, J. M. (1988). A case study of foreign accent syndrome, with follow-up clinical, neuropsychological and phonetic descriptions. *Neuropsychologia, 26,* 237–251.
Hall, K. D., & Yairi. E. (1992). Fundamental frequency, jitter, and shimmer in preschoolers who stutter. *Journal of Speech and Hearing Research, 35,* 1002–1008.

Halliday, M. (1970. *A course in spoken English: Intonation*. Oxford, UK: Oxford University Press.
Hargrove, P. M., & McGarr, N. S. (1994). *Prosody management of communication disorders*. London: Whurr.
Hargrove, P. M., & Sheran, C. (1989). The use of stress by language-impaired children. *Journal of Communication Disorders, 22*, 361–373.
Harrington, J. (1986). Stuttering, delayed auditory feedback, and linguistic rhythm. *Journal of Speech and Hearing Research, 31*, 36–47.
Hertrich, I., & Ackermann, H. (1993a). Acoustic analysis of speech prosody in Huntington's and Parkinson's disease—A preliminary report. *Clinical Linguistics and Phonetics, 7*, 285–297.
Hertrich, I., & Ackermann, H. (1993b). Dysarthria in Friedreich's ataxia: Syllable intensity and fundamental frequency patterns. *Clinical Linguistics and Phonetics, 7*, 177–190.
Heselwood, B., Bray, M., & Crookston, I. (1995). Juncture, rhythm and planning in the speech of an adult with Down's syndrome. *Clinical Linguistics and Phonetics, 9*, 121–137.
Hirano, M. (1981). *Clinical examination of voice*. New York: Springer.
House, A., Rowe, D., & Standen, P. J. (1987). Affective prosody in the reading voice of stroke patients. *Journal of Neurology, Neurosurgery and Psychiatry, 50*, 910–912.
Illes, J., Metter, E. J., Hanson, W. R., & Iritani, S. (1988). Language production in Parkinson's disease: Acoustic and linguistic considerations. *Brain and Language, 33*, 146–160.
Jackson, S. A., Treharne, D. A., & Boucher, J. (1997). Rhythm and language in children with moderate learning difficulties. *European Journal of Disorders of Communication, 32*, 99–108.
Jäncke, L., Bauer, A., & Kalveram, K. T. (1996). Duration of phonation under changing stress conditions in stuttering and non-stuttering adults. *Clinical Linguistics and Phonetics, 10*, 225–234.
Kent, J. F., Kent, R. D., Rosenbek, J. C., Weismer, G., Martin, R. E., Sufit, R. L., & Brooks, B. R. (1992). Quantitative description of the dysarthria in women with amyotrophic lateral sclerosis. *Journal of Speech and Hearing Research, 35*, 723–733.
Kent, R. D. (1991). The acoustic and physiologic characteristics of neurologically impaired speech movements. In W. J. Hardcastle & A. Marchal (Eds.), *Speech production and speech modelling* (pp. 365–402). London: Kluwer Academic Publishers.
Kent, R. D. (1994). The clinical science of motor speech disorders: A personal assessment. In J. A. Till, K. M. Yorkston, & D. R. Beukelman (Eds.), *Motor speech disorders: Advances in assessment and treatment* (pp. 3–18). London: Paul H. Brooks Publishing Company.
Kent, R. D., & Rosenbek, J. C. (1982). Prosodic disturbance and neurologic lesion. *Brain and Language, 15*, 259–291.
Kent, R. D., & Rosenbek, J. C. (1983). Acoustic patterns of apraxia of speech. *Journal of Speech and Hearing Research, 26*, 231–249.
Kent, R. D., Sufit, R., Rosenbek, J. C., Kent, J. F., Weismer, G., Martin, R. E., & Brooks, B. R. (1991). Speech deterioration in amyotrophic lateral sclerosis: A case study. *Journal of Speech and Hearing Research, 34*, 1269–1275.
Ladd, H., & Webster, J. W. (1991). Speech deterioration in postlingually deafened adults. *Journal of the Acoustical Society of America, 89*, 859–866.
Lane, H., & Webster, J. W. (1991). Speech deterioration in postlingually deafened adults. *Journal of the Acoustical Society of America, 89*, 859–866.
Lecours, A. R., & Rouillon, F. (1976). Neurolinguistic analysis of jargonaphsia and jargonagraphia. In H. Whitaker & H. A. Whitaker (Eds.), *Studies in neurolinguistics*. (Vol. 2, pp. 95–144). London: Academic Press.
Liao, K. K., Wang, S. J., Kwan, S. Y., Kong, K. W., & Wu, Z. A. (1991). Tongue diskinesia as an early manifestation of Wilson disease. *Brain and Development, 13*, 451–453.
Liberman, M. (1975). *The intonational system of English*. Doctoral dissertation, Massachusetts Institute of Technology (published 1978 by the Indiana University Linguistics Club).
Local, J., & Wootton, A. (1995). Interactional and phonetic aspects of immediate echolalia in autism: A case study. *Clinical Linguistics and Phonetics, 9*, 155–184.
Logemann, J. A., Fisher, H. B., Boshes, B., & Blonsky, E. R. (1978). Frequency and cooccurrence of vocal tract dysfunction in the speech of a large sample of Parkinsonian patients. *Journal of Speech and Hearing Disorders, 43*, 47–57.
Lowit-Leuschel, A. (1997). *Prosodic impairment in dysarthria: An acoustic phonetic study*. Unpublished doctoral dissertation, University of Newcastle upon Tyne.
Ludlow, C. L., & Bassich, C. J. (1983). The result of acoustic and perceptual assessment of two types of dysarthria. In W. R. Berry (Ed.), *Clinical dysarthria* (pp. 121–154). San Diego: College-Hill Press.
Ludlow, C. L., & Bassich, C. J. (1984). Relationships between perceptual ratings and acoustic mea-

sures of hypokinetic speech. In M. R. McNeil, J. C. Rosenbek, & A. E. Aronson (Eds.), *The dysarthrias: Physiology, acoustics, perception, management* (pp. 163–196). San Diego: College-Hill Press.

Maassen, B., & Povel, D. J. (1985). The effect of segmental and suprasegmental corrections on the intelligibility of deaf speech. *Journal of the Acoustical Society of America, 78,* 877–886.

Metter, E. J., & Hanson, W. R. (1986). Clinical and acoustical variability in hypokinetic dysarthria. *Journal of Communication Disorders, 19,* 347–366.

Moen, I. (1990). A case of"foreign-accent syndrome." *Clinical Linguistics and Phonetics, 4,* 295–302.

Murayama, K., Greenwood, R. S., Rao, K. W., & Aylsworth, A. S. (1991). Neurological aspects of del(1q) syndrome. *American Journal of Medical Genetics, 40,* 488–492.

Nooteboom, S. (1997) The prosody of speech: melody and rhythm. In W. Hardcastle, & J. Laver (Eds.), *The handbook of phonetic sciences* (pp. 640–673). Oxford, UK: Blackwell.

Packman, A., Onslow, M., Richard, F., & Van Doorn, J. (1996). Syllabic stress and variability: A model of stuttering. *Clinical Linguistics and Phonetics, 10,* 235–263.

Parker, A., & Rose, H. (1990). Deaf children's phonological development. In P. Grunwell (Ed.), *Developmental speech disorders* (pp. 83–108). Edinburgh, UK: Churchill Livingstone.

Pierrehumbert, J. (1980). *The phonology and phonetics of English intonation.* Doctoral dissertation, Massachusetts Institute of Technology (published 1980 by the Indiana University Linguistics Club).

Pitchford, N. J., Funnell, E., Ellis, A. W., Green, S. H., & Chapman, S. (1997). Recovery of spoken language processing in a 6-year-old child following a left hemisphere stroke: A longitudinal study. *Aphasiology, 11,* 83–102.

Rahilly, J. (1991). *Intonation patterns in normal hearing and postlingually deafened adults in Belfast.* Unpublished doctoral dissertation, Queen's University of Belfast, Great Britain.

Ramig, L., Scherer, R., Klasner, E., Titze, I. R., & Horii, Y. (1990). Acoustic analysis of voice in amyotrophic lateral sclerosis: A longitudinal case study. *Journal of Speech and Hearing Disorders, 55,* 2–14.

Robertson, S. J. (1982). *Dysarthria profile.* London: Winslow Press.

Robin, D. A., Klouda, G. V., & Hug, L. N. (1991). Neurogenic disorders of prosody. In D. Vogel, & M. P. Cannito (Eds.), *Treating disordered speech motor control: For clinicians by clinicians* (pp. 241–271). Austin, TX: Pro-Ed.

Ross, E. D., & Mesulam, M. M. (1979). Dominant language functions of the right hemisphere? *Journal of Experimental Psychology, 102,* 508–511.

Ross, E. D., Edmondson, J. A., Seibert, G. B., & Homan, R. W. (1988). Acoustic analysis of affective prosody during right-sided Wada Test: A within-subject verification of the right hemisphere's role in language. *Brain and Language, 33,* 128–145.

Ruscello, D. M., St. Louis, K. O., & Mason, N. (1991). School-aged children with phonological disorders: Coexistence with other speech/language disorders. *Journal of Speech and Hearing Research, 34,* 236–242.

Rutter, M., & Schopler, E. (1987). Autism and pervasive developmental disorders: Concepts and diagnostic issues. *Journal of Autism and Developmental Disorders, 17,* 159–186.

Ryalls, J. H. (1982). Intonation in Broca's aphasia. *Neuropsychologia, 20,* 355–360.

Shapiro, B. E., & Danly, M. (1985). The role of the right hemisphere in the control of speech prosody in propositional and affective contexts. *Brain and Language, 25,* 19–36.

Sheard, C., Adams, R. D., & Davis, J. (1991). Reliability and agreement of ratings of ataxic dysarthric speech samples with varying intelligibility. *Journal of Speech and Hearing Research, 34,* 285–293.

Shriberg, L. D., & Kwiatkowski, J. (1994). Developmental phonological disorders. I: A clinical profile. *Journal of Speech and Hearing Research, 37,* 1100–1126.

Shriberg, L. D., Kwiatkowski, J., Best, S., Hengst, J., & Terselic-Weber, B. (1986). Characteristics of children with phonological disorders of unknown origin. *Journal of Speech and Hearing Disorders, 51,* 140–161.

Shriberg, L. D., & Widder, C. J. (1990). Speech and prosody characteristics of adults with mental retardation. *Journal of Speech and Hearing Research, 33,* 627–653.

Square-Storer, P., Darley, F. L., & Sommers, R. (1988). Nonspeech and speech processing skills in patients with aphasia and apraxia of speech. *Brain and Language, 33,* 65–85.

St. Louis, K. O., Hansen, G. G. R., Buch, J. L., & Oliver, T. L. (1992). Voice deviations and coexisting communication disorders. *Language, Speech, and Hearing Services in Schools, 23,* 82–87.

Strand, E. A., Buder, E. H., Yorkston, K. M., & Ramig, O. L. (1994). Differential phonatory characteristics of four women with amyotrophic lateral sclerosis. *Journal of Voice, 8,* 327–339.

Titze, I. R. (1994). Towards standards in acoustic analysis of voice. *Journal of Voice, 8,* 1–7.

Tucker, D. M., Watson, R. T., & Heilman, K. M. (1977). Discrimination and evocation of affectively intoned speech in patients with right parietal disease. *Neurology, 27*, 947–950.

Uziel, A., Bohe, M., Cadilhac, J., & Passouant, P. (1975). Les troubles de la voix et de la parole dans les syndromes parkinsoniens. *Folia Phoniatrica, 27*, 166–176.

Van Lancker, D., & Sidtis, J. J. (1992). The identification of affective-prosodic stimuli by left- and right-hemisphere-damaged subjects: All errors are not created equal. *Journal of Speech and Hearing Research, 35*, 963–970.

Weintraub, S., Mesulam, M. M., & Kramer, L. (1981). Disturbances in prosody: A right-hemisphere contribution to language. *Archives of Neurology, 38*, 742–744.

Weismer, G. (1984). Articulatory characteristics of Parkinsonian dysarthria: Segmental and phrase-level timing, spirantization, and glottal-subglottal coordination. In M. R. McNeil, J. C. Rosenbek, & A. E. Aronson (Eds.), *The dysarthrias: Physiology, acoustics, perception, management* (pp. 101–130). San Diego: College-Hill Press.

Weismer, G., & Martin, R. E. (1992). Acoustic and perceptual approaches to the study of intelligibility. In R. D. Kent (Ed.), *Intelligibility in speech disorders: Theory, measurement and management* (pp. 67–118). Amsterdam: John Benjamins.

Wells, B., & Local, J. (1993). The sense of an ending: A case of prosodic delay. *Clinical Linguistics and Phonetics, 7*, 59–73.

Wells, B., Peppé, S., & Vance, M. (1995). Linguistic assessment of prosody. In K. Grundy (Ed.), *Linguistics in clinical practice* (pp. 234–266). London: Whurr.

Wertz, R. T., & Rosenbek, J. C. (1992). Where the ear fits: A perceptual evaluation of motor speech disorders. *Seminars in Speech and Language, 13*, 39–54.

Wilson, D. K. (1979). *Voice problems of children* (2nd ed.). Baltimore: Williams and Wilkins.

Wingate, M. (1985). Stuttering as a prosodic disorder. In R. Curlee & W. Perkins (Eds.), *Nature and treatment of stuttering* (pp. 215–235). London: Taylor & Francis.

Wirz, S., & Mackenzie Beck, J. (1995). Assessment of voice quality: The vocal profile analysis scheme. In S. Wirz (Ed.), *Perceptual approaches to communication disorders*. London: Whurr.

Ziegler, W., Hartmann, E., & von Cramon, D. (1988). Word identification testing in the diagnostic evaluation of dysarthric speech. *Clinical Linguistic and Phonetics, 2*, 291–308.

Zwirner, P., Murry, T., & Woodson, GE. (1991). Phonatory function of neurologically impaired patients. *Journal of Communication Disorders, 24*, 287–300.

Zyski, B. J., & Weisiger, B. E. (1987). Identification of dysarthria types based on perceptual analysis. *Journal of Communication Disorders, 20*, 367–378

CHAPTER 7

Measuring Vocal Quality[1]

Jody Kreiman and Bruce Gerratt

Measurement validity—the extent to which a scale or instrument measures what it is intended to measure—is a central concern in the development and evaluation of any measurement system. Measures that are weakly or variably related to a concept are not useful indices of that concept (e.g., Carmines & Zeller, 1979; Crocker & Algina, 1986; Kerlinger, 1973). This chapter examines the validity of traditional scales such as breathiness, roughness, hoarseness, or harshness as measures of vocal quality. Although a few authors have expressed doubt about the validity of such scales (Jensen, 1965; Perkins, 1971), issues of the validity of perceptual measures are typically neglected in studies of voice, which more commonly focus on rater reliability (see Kreiman, Gerratt, Kempster, Erman, & Berke, 1993, for review).

The validity of traditional rating scales for vocal quality is important in part because perceptual ratings are often used clinically to evaluate vocal disorders (Gerratt, Till, Rosenbek, Wertz, & Boysen, 1991). Perceptual ratings are also used to validate acoustic and other instrumental, or "objective," measures of voice (e.g., de Krom, 1995; Fritzell, Hammarberg, Gauffin, Karlsson, & Sundberg, 1986; Hillenbrand, Cleveland, & Erickson, 1994; Martin, Fitch, & Wolfe, 1995; Sodersten, Hertegard, & Hammarberg, 1995). Vocal quality is an interaction between an acoustic voice signal and a listener; the acoustic signal itself does not possess quality, it evokes it in the listener. For this reason, acoustic measures are meaningful primarily to the extent that they correspond to what listeners hear (Gerratt & Kreiman, 1995; Kreiman & Gerratt, 1996).

Finally, scale validity is important because measurement protocols imply a model of the construct being measured. Therefore, studies of the validity of rating protocols for voice also

[1]**Adapted from Kreiman, J., & Gerratt, B.R., "Validity of rating scale measures of voice quality,"** ***Journal of the Acoustical Society of America,*** **104(3), September, 1998, pp. 1598–1608.**

serve to test the adequacy of the implied model of vocal quality. Because vocal quality is a perceptual response to an acoustic signal, rating protocols for vocal quality comprise a set of claims about both signals and listeners. When vocal quality is measured by means of ratings on scales for particular aspects of quality, this implies that the overall impression a listener receives from a voice can be decomposed into several perceptually distinct aspects corresponding to various terms such as breathiness and roughness. It is assumed that individual listeners can focus their attention on these different aspects of the stimuli and can make the judgments required. Finally and crucially, it is assumed that characteristics of the measurement tool remain constant across listeners and voices, so that different listeners use the scales in the same way and measurements of different voices can be meaningfully compared. This implies that quality is fairly constant across listeners, so that voice quality may be treated as an attribute of the voice signal itself, rather than as the product of a listener's perception. That is, traditional protocols for assessing voice quality necessarily treat individual differences in perception as noise and do not model them explicitly. Because voice signals provide listeners with large amounts of information (for example, about the identity and physical, mental, and emotional state of a speaker; see Kreiman, 1997, for review), such claims about the perceptual process have interest beyond their clinical applications, and the validity or invalidity of voice assessment protocols has important implications for models of auditory pattern recognition and perception of complex signals, in general.

1. DEFINING AND MEASURING OVERALL VOCAL QUALITY

Attempts at validating voice quality scales presuppose that vocal quality is definable. How do we define vocal quality or specific vocal qualities? In other words, what are descriptive ratings of pathologic voice intended to measure?

Traditionally, the overall quality (or timbre) of a sound has been defined as "that attribute of auditory sensation in terms of which a listener can judge that two sounds similarly presented and having the same loudness and pitch are dissimilar" (ANSI Standard S1.1.12.9, p. 45, 1960; cf. Helmholtz, 1885). Several complications ensue from this definition that make the study of quality more difficult than the study of pitch and loudness. As everything that is not pitch or loudness, quality includes the perceptual effects of the spectral envelope and its changes in time, periodic fluctuations of amplitude or fundamental frequency, and any noise component in the signal (Plomp, 1976) and thus is inherently multidimensional (unlike pitch and loudness, which have single acoustic correlates). Given this multidimensionality, the perceptual importance of different aspects of the voice may depend on context or attention (Gerratt, Kreiman, Antonanzas-Barroso, & Berke, 1993; Kreiman, Gerratt, Precoda, & Berke, 1992), so psychophysical functions relating acoustics to perception may be complex and difficult to derive. According to the ANSI standard definition, quality is a perceptual response in a particular task (determining that two sounds are dissimilar), and it is unclear how this definition might generalize to common, seemingly related tasks like identification or evaluation of single stimuli. Finally, recent evidence suggests that quality may not be independent of frequency and amplitude (Krumhansl & Iverson, 1992; Melara & Marks, 1990), again suggesting that straightforward specification of univariate relations between an acoustic signal and its perceived quality may not be possible.

Given these difficulties, most authors avoid studying quality as a whole, preferring instead to focus on single dimensions or specific aspects of quality (for example, breathiness, harshness, or strain).[2] One way to motivate

[2] This strategy applies in other areas also. For example, Pavlovic, Rossi, and Espesser (1990) argued that the term "quality" is ambiguous when applied to synthetic speech, and instead studied the acceptability, intelligibility, and naturalness of different tokens.

scales for specific aspects of quality is with reference to overall quality: Individual scales or sets of scales may be valid to the extent that as a group they measure overall quality. This approach is related to content validation, which assesses the extent to which test items adequately sample the content of the concept or domain being measured (e.g., Kerlinger, 1973). In this case, overall quality is the domain of content that a set of scales for individual qualities is intended to measure.

A few studies (Kempster, Kistler, & Hillenbrand, 1991; Kreiman & Gerratt, 1996; Kreiman, Gerratt, & Berke, 1994; Kreiman, Gerratt, & Precoda, 1990; Kreiman et al., 1992; Murry, Singh, & Sargent, 1977) have used multidimensional scaling (MDS) to determine how scales for particular qualities relate to overall pathologic vocal quality and to specify sets of scales that are necessary and sufficient to measure overall quality adequately. In MDS, the relationship between quality and the dimensions that result from scaling is straightforward, because listeners assess vocal quality directly by judging the similarity of pairs of voices. The adequacy of the scaling solution as a model of overall quality is estimated by R^2, the amount of variance in similarity ratings accounted for by the scaling solution.

Unfortunately, MDS studies of pathologic voice have not supported the validity of traditional rating scales as measures of overall vocal quality. Relationships that have emerged between scaling dimensions and traditional quality scales have been neither consistent nor straightforward. None of the traditional qualities has emerged consistently as a perceptual dimension in all these studies, and many dimensions have emerged that do not correspond to traditional qualities (for example, dimensions correlated with F_0 or formant frequencies, or dimensions interpreted as weighted sums of assorted acoustic variables (e.g., Kreiman et al., 1992; Matsumoto, Hiki, Sone, & Nimura, 1973; Murry & Singh, 1980). Derived dimensions that are correlated with ratings of particular qualities often account for very small amounts of variance in the underlying ratings of overall quality; for example, a breathiness dimension reported by Murry and Singh (1980) accounted for only 8% of the variance in the underlying similarity judgments. Correlations between ratings of particular qualities and the derived dimensions are often rather small (e.g.,"hoarseness" ratings in Murry and Singh [1980] accounted for only 25% of the variance on the dimension); and more than one quality may be associated with a single perceptual dimension (e.g., Kreiman et al., 1994). Scaling solutions have sometimes accounted for less than half of the variance in the underlying similarity judgments (Kreiman & Gerratt, 1996; Murry & Singh, 1980; Murry et al., 1977), suggesting that small sets of dimensions/features may not adequately model listener perceptions of overall quality. Finally, a recent study (Kreiman & Gerratt, 1996) suggested that traditional continuous scales may not be appropriate for describing overall quality. In that study, voices did not disperse in a perceptual space along continuous scale-like linear dimensions, but instead clustered together in groups that lacked subjective unifying percepts. Taken together, these studies provide little support for the validity of traditional scales as measures of overall vocal quality and suggest that it may be difficult, if not impossible, to devise standard scalar rating protocols to measure overall quality.

2. DEFINING PARTICULAR VOCAL QUALITIES

The use of MDS methodology implies the search for a model of overall vocal quality. For clinical purposes, however, it may not be necessary to model overall quality in detail. Instead, it may be adequate to focus quality assessment on a limited number of clinically significant perceptual dimensions, while neglecting other irrelevant aspects of vocal quality. If this is so, results of MDS studies are not necessarily useful for identifying or specifying the important dimensions, because the relationship between traditional rating scales and overall quality is not necessarily straightforward or even particularly interesting.

In this case, motivating and defining individual scales remain critical aspects of scale development, to specify what is being measured, to justify why those aspects of voice (and not others) are of interest, and to clarify the relationship among different scales. Few studies have investigated these issues. Individual scales are typically validated by appeals to intuition, consensual validity, face validity (Allen & Yen, 1979; Silverman, 1977), or by reference to their association with purported acoustic, aerodynamic, and/or physiological correlates. However, because appeals to face validity do not involve empirical examination of evidence or reference to theory, they are of little use in the assessment of measurement systems. Scale proliferation has occurred and is a well-documented problem in voice quality research. Previous reviews (e.g., Pannbacker, 1984; Perkins, 1971; Sonninen, 1970) have reported as many as 67 terms for vocal quality in the literature. This situation has not improved substantially in recent years: Gelfer (1988) lists 57 terms for voice quality, de Krom (1989) lists 28, and Titze (1995) lists 21 (cf. Ethington & Punch, 1994, who list 124 terms for musical timbre).

Issues of scale definition have also been neglected. Table 7–1 lists Fairbanks' (1940) definitions for breathiness, harshness, and hoarseness, along with composite contemporary definitions for the same qualities. (Complete sample definitions are given in Appendix 7–1.) Definitions have changed very little in the last 60 years, with perceptual scales for vocal qualities typically defined in terms of their hypothetical acoustic, physiologic, or aerodynamic correlates.

Such definitions present several problems. First, it is circular to define particular vocal qualities in terms of their purported acoustic, aerodynamic, and/or physiological correlates and then to validate acoustic, aerodynamic, and physiological measurements by their correlation with perceptual measures. Such practices resemble criterion validation, which assesses the strength of association between a measure and some theoretically important form of behavior external to the instrument (e.g., Kerlinger, 1973). In voice research, however, the critical step of validating the perceptual measure independently from the criterion has been omitted.

Second, the definitions in Table 7–1 assert correspondences between perceptual and objective measures that do not withstand empirical scrutiny. For example, these definitions indicate that roughness/harshness should correspond to aperiodicity or noise. Many studies have examined the relationship between measures of acoustic perturbation, spectral noise, and roughness, with variable results (Table 7–2). For example, correlations between the harmonics to noise ratio and roughness have ranged from –.28 to –.85; and correlations between various jitter measures and roughness have ranged from –.01 to +.69. A similar pattern emerges for breathiness, which by definition (Table 7–1) should correspond to presence of a glottal gap, turbulence noise, and weakness or lack of loudness (presumably by analogy to whisper). Reported associations between glottal gap size and rated breathiness have been moderate at best. The study usually cited in support of such a correspondence (Fritzell et al., 1986) based its conclusions on observations of only 8 patients. The authors reported a correlation of .70 between glottal insufficiency and breathiness, but this correlation reflects the influence of outliers in the data. When these are eliminated from the analysis, the correlation between gap and breathiness decreases to .57. Rammage, Peppard, and Bless (1992) reported similar correlations of .52–.61 between breathiness and glottal gap size. Other studies indicate that voices with a glottal gap may lack significant breathiness (e.g., Sodersten & Lindestad, 1990; Sodersten et al., 1995). Correlations between rated breathiness and aerodynamic measures have ranged from low ($r = .48$; Murry et al., 1977) to nonsignificant (Rammage et al., 1992); and correlations between breathiness and spectral noise measures also vary substantially (Table 7–3).

Several explanations are possible when consistent correlations between perceptual and instrumental measures do not emerge as predicted (Cronbach & Meehl, 1955). First, the

Table 7–1. Definitions for some pathologic vocal qualities.

Quality	*Definition*
breathiness	"Breathy quality results when the vocal cords fail to approximate completely as they vibrate, and a steady stream of air rushes audibly through the glottis and resonance cavities . . . Weakness of voice and breathiness are closely related, for it is impossible to produce extremely loud tones with breathy quality" (Fairbanks, 1940, pp. 209–210).
	Impression of turbulence noise and audible escape of air through the glottis due to insufficient closure; vocal folds are vibrating, but somewhat abducted (de Krom, 1995; Hammarberg & Gauffin, 1995; Sodersten & Lindestad, 1990).
harshness/ roughness	"Harsh quality is characterized by a noisy, rasping, unmusical tone" (Fairbanks, 1940, p. 213).
	A psycho-acoustic impression of aperiodic noise, presumably related to some kind of irregular vocal fold vibrations (Askenfelt & Hammarberg, 1986; Hirano, 1981; Martin et al., 1995).
hoarseness	"Hoarseness is the typical voice quality of the individual who has acute or chronic laryngeal infection or irritation . . . From both acoustical and causal points of view hoarseness combines the features of breathiness and harshness" (Fairbanks, 1940, p. 216).
	A combination of rough and breathy—that is, irregular vocal fold vibrations along with additive noise; wet or unpleasant sounding (Anders et al., 1988; Bassich & Ludlow, 1986; Martin et al., 1995).

problem may lie with the instrumental measure. For example, something may be wrong with the theoretical framework used to generate the predicted relationship, so that the perceptual measure is valid, but the objective measure is actually unrelated to it. Studies that seek new correlates for traditional qualities apparently assume that this is the case. This assumption has probably contributed to proliferation of measures associated with a particular quality, as investigators (assuming that the quality is valid) propose new measures when old ones are not supported empirically (e.g., Fukazawa, El-Assuooty, & Honjo, 1988; Hillenbrand et al., 1994; Michaelis, Gramss, & Strube, 1997; Mori, Blaugrund, & Yu, 1994; Wagner, 1995). It is also possible that the theoretical predictions are appropriate, but a problem exists with the procedure used to make the objective measurement. In voice research, this possibility has led to sequential refinements and adjustments to objective measures. For example, at least 10 measures of frequency perturbation have been proposed (e.g., Deal & Emanuel, 1978; Hecker & Kreul, 1971; Hollien, Michel, & Doherty, 1973; Lieberman, 1961; Takahashi & Koike, 1975) (see Baken, 1987, for review), and many more papers have described effects of recording and signal processing techniques on measured perturbation (e.g., Bielamowicz, Kreiman, Gerratt, Dauer, & Berke, 1996; Deem, Manning, Knack, & Matesich, 1989; Doherty & Shipp, 1988; Horiguchi, Haji, Baer, & Gould, 1987; Karnell, 1991; Perry, Ingrisano, & Scott, 1996; Titze, Horii, & Scherer, 1987; Titze & Winholtz, 1993; Vieira, McInnes, & Jack, 1997) (see Titze, 1995, for review), possibly because investigators assume that refinement of an algorithm will reveal an existing valid association between acoustic signal perturbation and voice quality scales such as roughness.

Table 7–2. Univariate correlations between rated roughness or harshness and selected acoustic measures.*

Acoustic Measure	***Correlation with Rated Roughness/Harshness***
H1–H2	–.42 (Kreiman et al., 1990)
	.18 (de Krom, 1994)
Harmonics to noise ratio	–.40 (Kreiman et al., 1990)
	–.28 —.59 (de Krom, 1994)
	–.85 (Martin et al., 1995)
Amplitude perturbation quotient	.67 (Hirano et al., 1988)
Mean shimmer	.66 (Martin et al., 1995)
Percent shimmer	.32 (Heiberger & Horii, 1982)
Amplitude variability index	.48 –.75 (Deal & Emanuel, 1978)
Normalized noise energy	.78 (Hirano et al., 1988)
Pitch perturbation quotient	.31 (Prosek et al., 1987)
	.65 (Hirano et al., 1988)
Percent jitter	–.01 (Heiberger & Horii, 1982)
	.57 (Kreiman et al., 1990)
Period variability index	.03 –.69 (Deal & Emanuel, 1978)

**Note:* Correlation values are Pearson's *r*. Please see individual studies for details of the acoustical measures and statistical techniques applied.

A third explanation for failures to find expected correlations between objective and perceptual measures of voice is that something is wrong with the techniques used to estimate the association between objective and perceptual measures. For example, results may reflect statistical or experimental artifacts, technical problems with a study, or sampling limitations. In this case, a true association between the acoustic and perceptual measures exists in theory, but estimates of it vary due to the particular population of speakers or signals chosen, the size of the sample, repeated sampling from the population, or random error. This possibility may explain the prevalence of repeated studies of the same measures and qualities in the literature (e.g., Dejonckere & Lebacq, 1996; de Krom, 1995; Fukazawa et al., 1988; Hanson, 1995; Shoji, Regenbogen, Yu, & Blaugrund, 1992; Wagner, 1995; McAllister, Sederholm, Ternstrom, & Sundberg, 1996).

Finally, failures to find expected correlations among objective and perceptual measures may indicate that something is wrong with the perceptual measures. A quality may be valid, but our perceptual measurement techniques inappropriate; alternatively, the quality may lack construct validity. The first possibility has generated papers evaluating different types of rating instruments (e.g., Gerratt et al., 1993; Toner & Emanuel, 1989). The second has motivated a variety of MDS studies, as discussed, along with a few papers evaluating scale validity. For example, Moody, Montague, and Bradley (1979) assessed the validity of the Wilson Voice Profile Analysis (VPA) system (Wilson, 1977) by comparing ratings of a set of children's voices with a set of ratings gathered in another study with a

Table 7–3. Univariate correlations between rated breathiness and selected acoustic measures.*

Acoustic Measure	*Correlation with Rated Breathiness*
H1–H2	.40 (de Krom, 1994)
First harmonic amplitude	.66 (Hillenbrand et al., 1994)
Spectral slope	.59 (Hammarberg et al., 1980)
	–.67 (Klich, 1982)
Spectral slope of residue signal	.59 (Prosek et al., 1987)
Breathiness index	.62 (Hillenbrand & Houde, 1996)
Harmonics to noise ratio	.26 (Kreiman et al., 1990)
	–.46 — –.69 (de Krom, 1994)
	–.25 (Martin et al., 1995)
Normalized noise energy	.73 (Hirano et al., 1988)
Vocal noise	.84 (Feijoo & Hernandez, 1990)
Aspiration noise	.14 –.72 (Klatt & Klatt, 1990)
Amplitude perturbation quotient	.60 (Prosek et al., 1987)
	.91 (Feijoo &Hernandez, 1990)
Mean shimmer	.07 (Kreiman et al., 1990)
	.42 (Martin et al., 1995)
Shimmer factor	.34 (Arends et al., 1990)
Pitch amplitude	–.75 (Prosek et al., 1987)
Pitch perturbation quotient	.38 (Prosek et al., 1987)
	.67 (Hirano et al., 1988)
Percent jitter	.55 (Eskenazi et al., 1990)
	.003 (Martin et al., 1995)
CPP-S	–.96 (Hillenbrand & Houde, 1996)
RPK	–.84 (Hillenbrand & Houde, 1996)
SPL	–.75 (Klich, 1982)

**Note:* Correlation values are Pearson's *r*. Please see individual studies for details of the acoustical measures and statistical techniques applied.

different perceptual instrument. Because ratings from the two studies were similar and both sets distinguished normal from clinical subjects, the authors argued that the validity of the VPA was "at least indirectly established" (p. 232). In another attempt at indirect scale validation, de Krom (1989) argued that the GRBAS rating protocol (Hirano, 1981) "is both well defined and sufficient to classify the variety of pathological voices" (p. 59), because the traditional definitions and proposed objective correlates of the different scales indicate that they are intended to measure different aspects of voice.

Other authors have used a "consensus model" (Sonninen & Hurme, 1992) to establish the validity of a rating instrument. For example, Hammarberg and Gauffin (1995) describe a process by which clinicians, through extensive discussion, agreed on a set of parameters to be measured and on definitions for those parameters. Similarly, Stewart et al. (1997) conducted a series of perceptual evaluations, successively incorporating suggestions of experienced clinicians to develop an instrument for rating the severity of symptoms of adductory spasmodic dysphonia. The instrument was considered valid when raters agreed that the scales were relevant and when interrater reliability for each scale (measured by intraclass correlations) exceeded .4. Note that consensual validation closely resembles face validation: A protocol is valid when raters declare it to be so, without respect to factors external to the agreement process. Raters' beliefs about the importance of different aspects of vocal quality may be shaped by many factors, including tradition, habit, peer beliefs, and particular clinical practice patterns. Thus consensual validation may lead to clinical acceptance of a protocol without knowledge of rater agreement or consideration of the adequacy of the set of scales as a de facto model of vocal quality. It is not a substitute for construct validation, through which concepts are validated by testing theoretically predicted relationships with external variables (Kerlinger, 1973).

Unfortunately, it is impossible to determine which explanation applies for failures to find consistent correlations between perceptual and objective measures of vocal quality. Ideally, comprehensive theoretical models of voice production, acoustics, and perception should generate predictions about which aspects of the acoustic signal are perceptually important. However, traditionally qualities are defined in terms of instrumental measures and instrumental measures are validated by their relationship to the same qualities. This circularity makes it impossible to interpret findings as evidence for or against the validity of the objective or perceptual measures. Experimental studies (in contrast to associative studies like those reviewed) could be used to address these concerns, but are uncommon in this research area. A few authors (e.g., Coleman & Wendahl, 1967; Heiberger & Horii, 1982; Hillenbrand, 1988; Wendahl, 1963, 1966a, 1966b; Yanagihara, 1967) have used speech synthesis to systematically examine the relationship between acoustic parameters and perceived vocal quality, but such studies have been few in number and limited in scope (see Hillenbrand, 1988, for review).

3. FACTOR ANALYSIS APPROACHES TO DERIVING SCALES FOR VOCAL QUALITY

A final difficulty with existing definitions for specific vocal qualities is that they do not appear to be specific enough to distinguish among related qualities (as they must to establish construct validity, which entails specifying both what a construct is and what it is not; Kerlinger, 1973). For example, both breathiness and roughness are associated by definition with noise, and several studies have reported that breathiness and roughness are correlated (Dejonckere, Obbens, de Moor, & Wieneke, 1993; Kreiman et al., 1994; Sederholm, McAllister, Sundberg, & Dalkvist, 1993; Takahashi & Koike, 1975). The two qualities have also been repeatedly associated with the same or similar acoustic measures (Tables 7–2 and 7–3); for example, significant correlations between the pitch perturbation quotient and the amplitude perturbation quotient and both breathiness and roughness have been reported (e.g., Feijoo & Hernandez, 1990; Hirano et al., 1988). These findings again suggest that these qualities cannot be separated in practice.[3]

[3]Breathiness and roughness have been used as examples here because fairly stable consensual definitions have emerged in the literature for these qualities, and because a large literature exists examining objective correlates of these qualities. However, a similar argument can be made for other vocal qualities. For example, hoarseness has been both positively and negatively associated with glottal flow levels, the harmonics-to-noise ratio, the relative intensity of the first harmonic, the

Some authors have attempted to address the problem of overlap and redundancy in the meanings of traditional quality scales through the use of factor analysis (FA) (e.g., Hammarberg, Fritzell, Gauffin, Sundberg, & Wedin, 1980; Isshiki, Okamura, Tanabe, & Morimoto, 1969; Isshiki & Takeuchi, 1970; Nieboer, De Graaf, & Schutte, 1988; Sederholm et al., 1993; Takahashi & Koike, 1975). In FA, a large set of rating scales is reduced to a small set of orthogonal factors that capture as much of the variance in the original scales as possible. FA is often used during test development to verify that the scales on a test instrument are clearly related to the theoretical dimensions of the construct being measured (for example, different dimensions of personality). Because output factors are orthogonal, FA potentially eliminates concerns about redundancies or overlap among the underlying scales. Further, in contrast to MDS, the relationship between the output factors and traditional labels for voice quality is straightforward in FA, because the factors are defined in terms of the scales. This relationship can be quantified by the extent to which each original rating scale loads on the output factors. However, results of FA studies may vary substantially, depending on the sample of voices and on the scales the author selects to study.

Two general approaches to FA have been used in voice quality research. In the first (Holmgren, 1967; Isshiki & Takeuchi, 1970; Nieboer et al., 1988; Takahashi & Koike, 1975), voices are rated on a relatively small set of semantic differential scales that have been selected to reflect an underlying set of factors. Because no standard factors have been established for voice quality, these studies have generally adopted factors (e.g., potency, evaluation, activity) and scales (e.g., sweet/sour, strong/weak, hot/cold; Osgood, Suci, & Tannenbaum, 1957) that are theoretically related, but not obviously applicable to voice quality. (An exception is Nieboer et al. [1988], who used voice-related scales and factors derived by Fagel, van Herpt, & Boves [1983].) Alternatively, investigators have asked listeners to rate voices on large sets of traditional voice quality scales that were not derived a priori from a set of hypothetical superordinate factors (Fagel et al., 1983; Hammarberg et al., 1980; Sederholm et al., 1993; Voiers, 1964). Rather than assuming an underlying set of factors for voice quality, these studies oversampled the semantic space for voices, in an attempt to ensure that all possible perceptual factors were represented.

Not surprisingly, findings have varied considerably across studies. For example, Isshiki and Takeuchi (1970) found factors they labeled rough, breathy, asthenic, and degree of hoarseness; Takahashi and Koike (1975) reported factors interpreted as pitch, loudness, and "evaluation of voice quality"; Nieboer et al. (1988) identified tempo, quality, and pitch factors; and factors labeled unstable/steady, breathy/overtight, hyper/hypofunctional, coarse/light, head/chest register emerged from the study by Hammarberg et al. (1980). Idiosyncrasies in labeling may obscure further differences between studies. For example, Isshiki's "breathiness" factor loaded highly on the scales dry, hard, excited, pointed, cold, choked, rough, cloudy, sharp, poor, and bad, with that in Hammarberg et al. (1980) corresponding to the scales breathy, wheezing, lack of timbre, moments of aphonia, husky, and not creaky. Restricted populations of speakers (Fagel et al., 1983; Holmgren, 1967; Nieboer et al., 1988; Voiers, 1964) and small sets of voices (for example, 16 in Isshiki and Takeuchi [1970], 24 [9 of whom were normal] in Takahashi and Koike [1975] and 17 in Hammarberg et al. [1980]) limit the extent to which results can be generalized to the full spectrum of vocal qualities. Finally, rating scales may load on more than one factor, leading to complicated relationships among factors; and several authors have questioned whether scales derived from FA truly measure independent aspects of voice

magnitude of a cepstral peak, jitter, breathiness, and roughness (Dejonckere & Lebacq, 1996; Hiraoka, Kitazoe, Ueta, Tanaka, & Tanabe, 1984; Wagner, 1995; Yumoto, Gould, & Baer, 1982; Yumoto, Sasaki, & Okamura, 1984).

quality (Dejonckere et al., 1993; Kreiman et al., 1994; Takahashi & Koike, 1975). Thus, FA has done little to clarify the issues of which scales for pathologic vocal quality are independent and valid.

4. RELIABILITY AS A TOOL FOR ASSESSING VALIDITY

As this review indicates, the literature on pathologic voice quality does not provide convincing or consistent evidence for the validity or invalidity of traditional scales for vocal quality. Although the validity of traditional scales for voice quality has never been formally established, there is little evidence that such scales are invalid, largely because of lack of research. However, because the validity of perceptual measures depends on characteristics of both listeners and stimuli, validity is partially determined by reliability. That is, because quality is a function of both listeners and stimuli, an unreliable test cannot be a valid measure of quality, because it does not model listener behavior accurately (e.g., Cone, 1977; Suen & Ary, 1989; Ventry & Schiavetti, 1980; Young & Downs, 1968). Thus, evidence about patterns of agreement and disagreement among listeners in their use of quality scales can provide evidence for or against the validity of the scales. If listeners cannot agree when making the required judgments, the critical assumption of listener equivalence is violated, and the validity of traditional protocols for quality assessment is not supported.

In the study reported later, we combined traditional approaches to reliability with new analyses designed to examine patterns of agreement and disagreement among listeners that bear on issues of measurement validity. Conventional statistical analyses of reliability do not provide enough information to answer questions about scale validity. Such analyses produce a single number representing the overall reliability of a set of ratings across all the voices and listeners in a study. This conventional approach derives from the literature on psychological test construction (Allen & Yen, 1979; Crocker & Algina, 1986), with listeners substituted for test items and voices substituted for examinees or subjects. Errors are assumed to be random in this model, so averaging together scores from a large number of raters will give the best estimate of the "true" score for a voice on a scale and the mean rating approaches the true score as the number of raters increases. Thus, reliability in classic theory is a function of both the average interrater correlation and the number of raters in a study.

In this traditional framework, reliability implies that another sample of listeners would produce the same mean ratings for the same test voices, but does not necessarily inform us of how the subjects would agree in their ratings of a new set of voices. Conventional reliability statistics are not informative about many other important aspects of listener performance. For example, they cannot indicate agreement for specific voice samples (Young & Downs, 1968), and they cannot capture information about systematic variations in reliability or agreement across raters or parts of the rating scale. Patterns of agreement and disagreement between listeners may provide evidence about the perceptual processes that underlie judgments of vocal quality. Such evidence may be helpful in establishing the validity of different scales for vocal quality and may help determine why measurement protocols may fail. Finally, because the validity of measurement systems ultimately depends on the success of the underlying perceptual model, such detailed knowledge about listener agreement may guide the design of future protocols for quality assessment.

5. METHOD

To determine if patterns of rater agreement support rating scale validity, we reevaluated existing data from experiments using unidimensional scales for different traditional vocal qualities or ratings of the similarity of pairs of voices. Data were drawn from four previously published studies (Kreiman & Gerratt, 1996; Kreiman et al., 1994; Kreiman et al., 1993;

Rabinov et al., 1995) and one unpublished study (Chhetri, 1997). Two of these studies (Kreiman et al., 1993; Rabinov et al., 1995) were specifically concerned with issues of rating reliability. Listeners in these studies judged the roughness of samples of pathologic voices and recorded their responses on equal-appearing interval (EAI) or visual analog (VA) scales.

Three other studies (Chhetri, 1997; Kreiman & Gerratt, 1996; Kreiman et al., 1994) used EAI scales to address more general issues of the perception of pathologic voice quality. Two groups of raters participated in the studies reported in Kreiman et al. (1994). The first group judged the similarity of pairs of voices with respect to breathiness or roughness. The second directly rated the breathiness or roughness of the individual voices. Raters in Kreiman and Gerratt (1996) judged the overall similarity of pairs of voices. Raters in Chhetri (1997) rated the severity of vocal pathology for samples of voices gathered pre- and postoperatively. Further details are given in Table 7–4.

For our current purposes, we calculated several traditional measures of overall intra- and interrater reliability and agreement for each data set. For each voice in the data sets, we also examined an additional measure, the empirical likelihood that two raters would agree in their ratings of a specific voice. These finer-grained analyses assessed how likely it was that individual raters would agree with one another for specific voice stimuli, rather than how well the population of raters agreed on average or how well the averaged data estimated the "true mean rating." This approach also allowed us to capture detailed information about variations in agreement across voices and parts of the rating scale. Similar analyses of intrarater agreement were undertaken, comparing the first and second rating of a voice by a single listener, to determine whether individuals were more self-consistent for some voices than for others.

To simplify comparisons among studies using VA and EAI scales, differences between pairs of ratings on the VA scale were converted from mm to "scale value equivalents." For example, a 100-mm VA scale was divided into 7 intervals of 14.3 mm each, analogous to a 7-point EAI scale. Pairs of ratings within 7.2 mm of each other were considered to agree exactly; ratings that differed by 21.5 mm (7.2 + 14.3) were considered to be within 1 scale value of each other and so on. For the 75-mm VA scale, a scale interval was defined as 10.7 mm. Thus, ratings differing by 5.4 mm or less were considered to agree exactly, and ratings differing by 16.1 mm or less were considered within 1 scale value of each other. Differences in mm and in scale value equivalents were highly correlated (data from Kreiman et al., 1993: $r = .98$; data from Rabinov et al., 1995: $r = .98$).

6. RESULTS

6.1. Intrarater Agreement: How Self-Consistent Were Listeners?

Traditional analyses of intrarater agreement examine overall levels of listener self-consistency, summed across voices. In contrast, Table 7–5 shows the likelihood that a given voice would be re-rated consistently, calculated across listeners. Numbers in this table represent the likelihood that a single rerating of a single voice would agree with the first rating by some amount (for example, exactly or within 1 scale value).

Listeners produced the same value when rerating a stimulus for 32%–50% of trials, depending on the study. Pooled across studies, a second rating agreed exactly with the first for 38.6% of repeated trials, and 76.8% of repeated ratings agreed with the first within 1 scale value. In comparison, across studies traditional test-retest agreement (calculated across voices for each listener, and then averaged across listeners) ranged from 72.5%–92.0% of ratings within ± 1 scale value.

Figure 7–1 shows how test-retest agreement varied across listeners and voices for EAI ratings of roughness (Figure 7–1A; Kreiman et al., 1993), VA ratings of roughness (Figure 7–1B; Rabinov et al., 1995), and ratings of overall similarity of pairs of voices (Figure 7–1C; Kreiman & Gerratt, 1996). In this figure, each point represents a single stimulus presented to

Table 7–4. Characteristics of the data sets.*

Study	***Raters***	***Speakers***	***Scale(s)***	***Rating Task***
Kreiman et al. (1993)	30 expert**	30 (22 disordered, 8 normal)	7 pt EAI 100 mm VA	Judgments of roughness Judgments of roughness
Kreiman et al. (1994)	5 expert	18 disordered	7 pt EAI	Paired comparison: Dissimilarity of pairs of voices with respect to breathiness
			7 pt EAI	Paired comparison: Dissimilarity of pairs of voices with respect to roughness
	8 expert	18 disordered	7 pt EAI	Judgments of breathiness
		18 disordered	7 pt EAI	Judgments of roughness
Rabinov et al. (1995)	10 expert	50 disordered	75 mm VA	Judgments of roughness
Kreiman & Gerratt (1996)	8 expert	80 disordered (Males)	7 pt EAI	Paired comparison: Overall dissimilarity of pairs of voices
		80 disordered (Females)	7 pt EAI	Paired comparison: Overall dissimilarity of pairs of voices
Chhetri (1997)	9 expert	32 disordered (pre/postoperative)	7 pt EAI	Judgments of severity of pathology

*EAI = equal-appearing interval scale; VA = visual analog scale.
**Data from experiments 1 and 2 have been combined.

a single rater; the difference between the first and second rating that voice received from that rater is plotted against the mean of that individual's two ratings for that voice. Because agreement is plotted against the mean rating for a given voice, the probability of agreement must be high when mean ratings are near scale endpoints. However, agreement in the midrange of a scale may be high (if a listener consistently rates voices as moderately pathologic) or low (if a listener responds with a large scale value on one occasion and a small value on another occasion).

As Figure 7–1 shows, for all three tasks individual listeners were often self-consistent in their use of these rating scales. In particular, individual listeners appeared to maintain stable standards for the midrange of a scale, so that many voices received ratings of 3, 4, or 5 both times they were rated.

Figure 7–2 summarizes the data from Figures 7–1A and 7–1B (Kreiman et al., 1993; Rabinov et al., 1995) by showing the overall probability of test-retest agreement (within 1 scale value) for individual voices. Levels of self-consistency for individual stimuli were quite high overall, with most values above .8. This suggests that individual listeners are able to make reasonably consistent judgments of traditional vocal qualities.

Table 7–5. Likelihood that a single rerating of a single voice would differ from the first rating by a given amount.*

Study/Scale	*N***	*Exact Agreement*	*Ratings Differ by 1 Scale Value*	*Ratings Differ by 2 Scale Values*	*Ratings Differ by 3 or More Scale Values*
Kreiman et al. (1993) (EAI/Roughness)	900	44.9%	38.6%	12.0%	4.6%
Kreiman et al. (1993) (VA/Roughness)	900	48.8%	33.6%	11.8%	5.9%
Kreiman et al. (1994) (EAI/Roughness)	144	38.9%	43.8%	11.1%	6.3%
Kreiman et al. (1994) (EAI/Breathiness)	144	47.2%	38.2%	11.1%	3.5%
Kreiman et al. (1994) (Dissimilarity/Roughness)	765	36.5%	36.9%	15.3%	11.4%
Kreiman et al. (1994) (Dissimilarity/Breathiness)	765	32.0%	40.5%	16.3%	11.1%
Rabinov et al. (1995) (VA/Roughness)	500	44.2%	35.4%	13.8%	6.6%
Kreiman & Gerratt (1996) (Dissimilarity/Male voices)	5056	36.6%	38.1%	16.4%	9.0%
Kreiman & Gerratt (1996) (Dissimilarity/Female voices)	5056	38.4%	38.9%	15.7%	7.0%
Chhetri (1997) (EAI/Severity)	66	50.0%	42.4%	6.1%	1.5%
Pooled data	14,296	38.6%	38.2%	15.3%	7.8%

*EAI = equal-appearing interval scale; VA = visual analog scale.

***N* = (# listeners) * (# repeated trials/listener). Differences between VA ratings were converted to scale value equivalents, as described in the text.

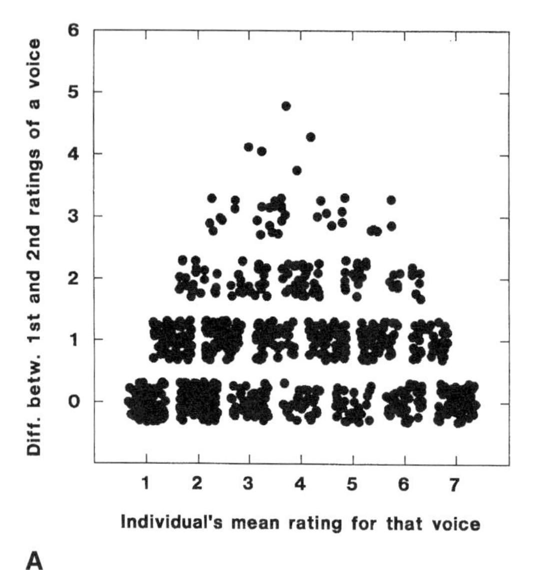

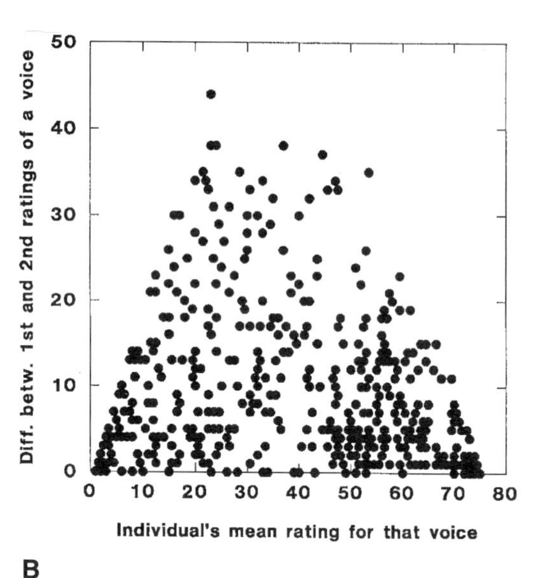

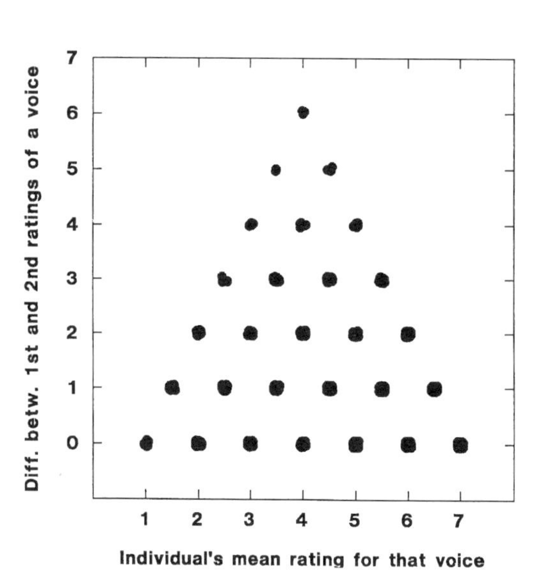

Figure 7–1. Test-retest agreement for individual stimuli. A value of 0 on the y axis indicates that a rater gave that voice the same score both times it was rated (i.e., the difference between the first and second ratings was 0); a value of 1 indicates that the first and second ratings differed by 1; and so on. Values on the x axis represent the mean of a single individual's two ratings of that stimulus. Points have been jittered slightly to show overlapping values. **A.** Test-retest agreement for EAI ratings of roughness (Kreiman et al., 1993). **B.** Test-retest agreement for visual analog ratings of roughness (Rabinov et al., 1995). **C.** Test-retest agreement for similarity ratings (Kreiman & Gerratt, 1996).

6.2. Pairwise Agreement Among Raters

6.2.1. Overall Likelihood of Interrater Agreement

Measures of interrater agreement, like measures of intrarater agreement, usually sum across voices to provide a single measure of rater concordance. In contrast, the present analyses sum across listeners to provide a measure of the likelihood that two raters will agree in their ratings of individual stimuli. Table 7–6 lists the overall likelihood of raters agreeing exactly, within 1 scale value and so on in their ratings of a single voice or pair of voices. Across studies, pairs of listeners agreed exactly for 26.7% of trials (vs. 38.6% test-retest agreement). Ratings differed by 1 scale value or less for 63.7% of trials (vs.

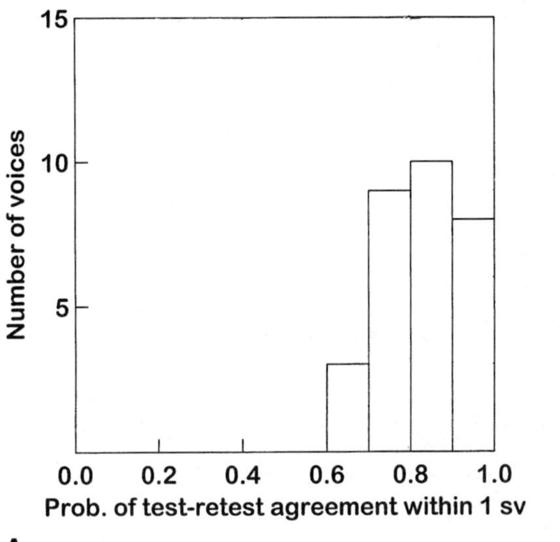

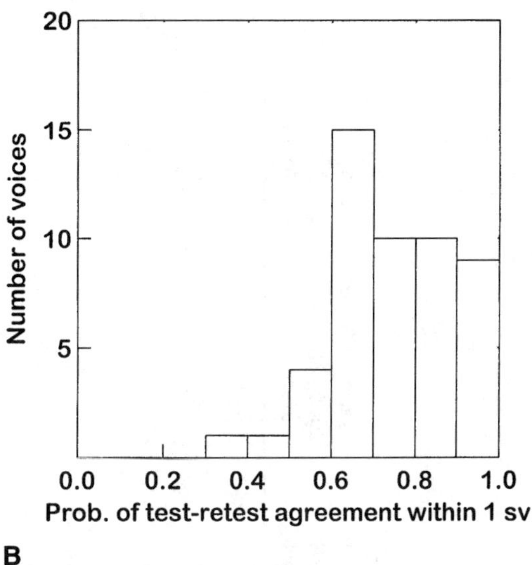

Figure 7–2. The probability of observing test-retest agreement within one scale value (or scale value equivalent) for individual voices. Each column shows the number of voices for which overall test-retest agreement occurred with the given likelihood. **A.** EAI ratings of roughness (Kreiman et al., 1993). **B.** Visual analog ratings of roughness (Rabinov et al., 1995).

76.8% test-retest agreement). Gross disagreements (ratings differing by 3 or more scale values on a 7-point scale) occurred for a total of 15.6% of trials (cf. Mackey, Finn, & Ingham, 1997, who reported similar values for ratings of speech naturalness).

6.2.2. Patterns of Interrater Agreement for Traditional Rating Scales

Patterns of interrater agreement depended on the listening task. For ratings of breathiness, roughness, and severity, interrater agreement levels were consistently poor in the midrange of the rating scales. Figure 7–3 shows the likelihood of two raters agreeing exactly (Figure 7–3A, 7–3C) or within 1 scale value (Figure 7–3B, 7–3D) for each voice in two representative data sets. Because we were interested in the extent to which mean ratings represent the underlying raw data, the probability of agreement is plotted against the group mean rating for each voice. As previously discussed, agreement near scale endpoints must be high in these plots, because average values can only approach scale endpoints when listeners agree. However, average values away from scale endpoints can result from agreement that voices are moderately pathologic or from disagreement about the extent of pathology.

In the present data, the likelihood that two raters would agree exactly for voices with mean ratings between 2.5 and 5.5 on a 7-point EAI scale averaged .21 (range = .19–.24; chance agreement for independent ratings on a 7-point scale = .14), although individual listeners were self-consistent in the same scale range. The likelihood of agreement within 1 scale value averaged .57 (range = .50–.61; chance = .39). Although these values significantly exceed chance levels of agreement (one-sample t-tests; $p < .05$), they are very low. Further, across all the data examined here, we did not find a single voice that listeners consistently agreed was moderately deviant in quality. Thus, the present data suggest that mean ratings in the midrange of the scale do not arise from a consensus among raters that the voice is moderately deviant, but indicate instead that

Table 7–6. Likelihood of pairwise agreement among raters.*

Study/Scale	*N***	*Exact Agreement*	*Ratings Differ by 1 Scale Value*	*Ratings Differ by 2 Scale Values*	*Ratings Differ by 3 or More Scale Values*
Kreiman et al. (1993) (EAI/Roughness)	26,100	31.7%	40.2%	17.7%	10.4%
Kreiman et al. (1994) (EAI/Roughness)	1,008	20.7%	35.5%	22.2%	21.5%
Kreiman et al. (1994) (EAI/Breathiness)	1,008	25.4%	41.7%	21.0%	11.9%
Kreiman et al. (1994) (Dissimilarity/Roughness)	3,060	24.4%	34.9%	21.3%	19.3%
Kreiman et al. (1994) (Dissimilarity/Breathiness)	3,060	20.9%	31.7%	20.4%	27.0%
Kreiman & Gerratt (1996) (Dissimilarity/Male voices)	88,480	24.9%	35.2%	21.4%	18.5%
Kreiman & Gerratt (1996) (Dissimilarity/Female voices)	88,480	26.2%	39.0%	21.5%	13.3%
Kreiman et al. (1993) (VA/Roughness)	26,100	30.6%	33.3%	18.7%	17.4%
Rabinov et al. (1995) (VA/Roughness)	4,500	27.0%	37.9%	17.6%	17.4%
Chhetri (1997) (EAI/Severity)	1,152	32.2%	35.3%	22.3%	10.2%
Pooled data	242,948	26.7%	37.0%	20.7%	15.6%

*EAI = equal-appearing interval scale; VA = visual analog scale.

***N* = (# possible pairs of listeners) * (number of stimuli). Differences between VA ratings were converted to scale value equivalents, as described in the text.

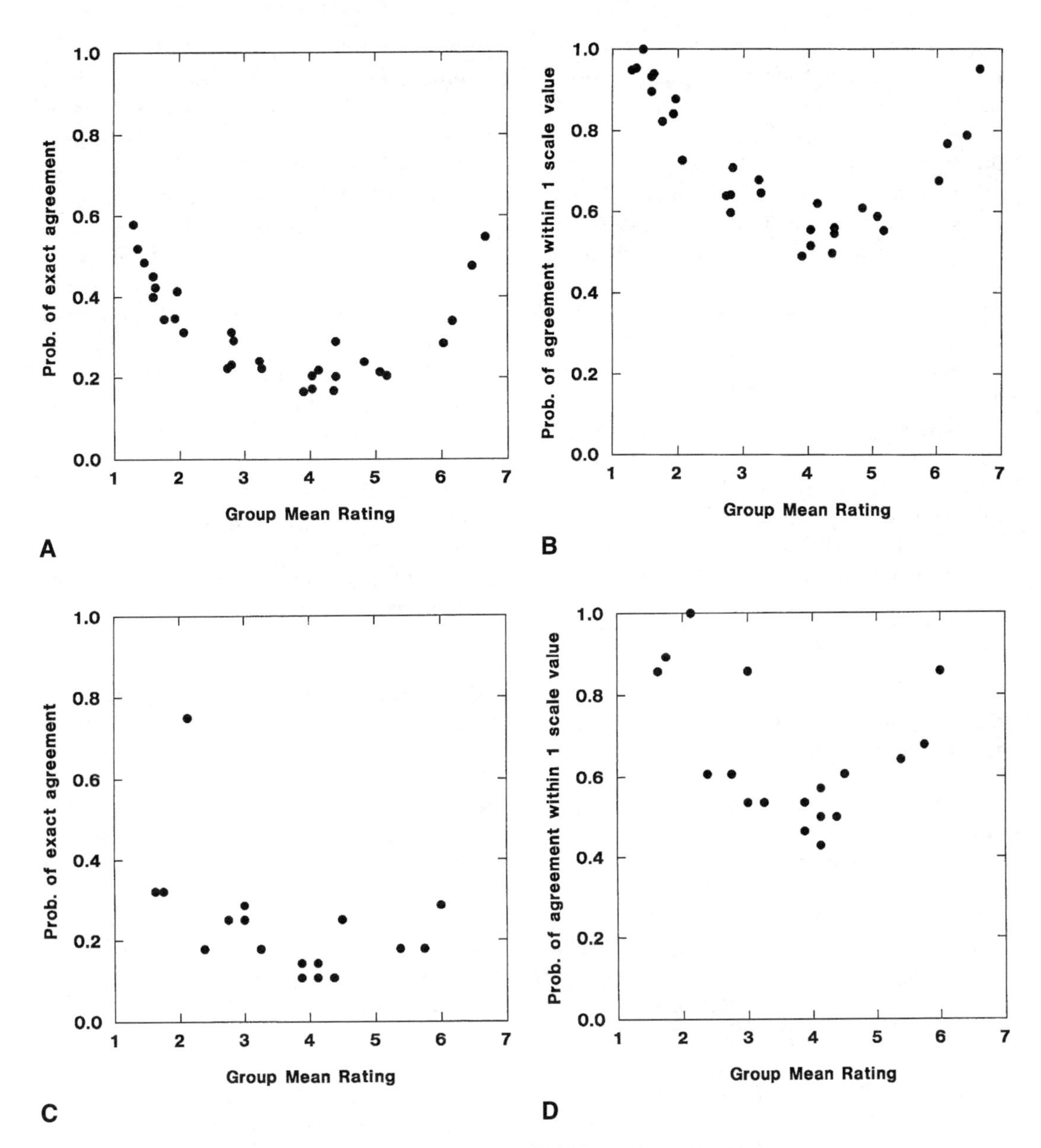

Figure 7–3. For each voice in a data set, the probability that two raters agreed in their ratings of that voice versus the overall mean rating for that voice. Results reflect only the first rating given each voice by each rater; the second rating was discarded. **A.** The likelihood of exact agreement for EAI ratings of roughness; data from Kreiman et al. (1993). **B.** The likelihood of agreement within 1 scale value for the same data. **C.** The likelihood of exact agreement for EAI ratings of breathiness; data from Kreiman et al. (1994). **D.** The likelihood of agreement within 1 scale value for the same data.

raters disagreed about the extent of deviation on that scale.

Because a significant statistical result does not necessarily indicate the size of the effect (especially when *n* is large, as it is here), we also calculated the amount of variance in quality ratings that is attributable to differences among voices. Variance accounted for was estimated by one-way analyses of variance for the different sets of ratings (e.g., Young, 1993). The independent variable in these analyses was the voice being rated, and the dependent variable was the rating received; the error term reflects all other sources of variability in quality ratings, including (but not limited to) interrater variability and random error. Because agreement near scale endpoints is in part artifactual, analyses included only voices with mean ratings between 2.5 and 5.5 (inclusive).

Results are given in Table 7–7. Differences among voices with average ratings in the "moderately pathologic" range accounted for an average of 32% of the variance in ratings (range = 22%–42%). In other words, for the midrange of the scales examined here, on average more than 60% (and as much as 78%) of the variance in ratings of voices was related to factors other than differences among voices in the quality being rated.

6.2.3. Patterns of Interrater Agreement for Similarity Ratings

The pattern of pairwise agreement among listeners for ratings of the similarity of pairs of voices was different from that for ratings of roughness, breathiness, and severity. Although agreement levels varied substantially across voice pairs, perfect or near-perfect agreement among raters was more common for ratings of overall similarity (Figure 7–4A, 7–4B; Kreiman & Gerratt, 1996) than for ratings of traditional qualities (where the likelihood of two raters agreeing perfectly never exceeded .8). Good agreement occurred across the entire scale. In particular, listeners did agree that some pairs of voices were moderately similar.

Patterns of agreement for ratings of the similarity of voices with respect to specific vocal qualities (Figure 7–4C, 7–4D; Kreiman et al., 1994) shared characteristics of both similarity ratings and ratings of specific qualities. Although levels of agreement were lower than for ratings of overall similarity, listeners did consistently agree in their ratings of at least some voices in the midrange of the scale.

6.3. Conventional Measures of Rater Reliability

Conventional measures of rating reliability, such as Cronbach's alpha (Cronbach, 1951) and the intraclass correlation for the reliability of mean ratings (Berk, 1979; Ebel, 1951; Shrout &

Table 7–7. Variance in voice ratings accounted for by differences among voices with mean ratings in the midrange of a scale.*

Study/Scale	R^2
Kreiman et al. (1993) (EAI/Roughness)	.30
Kreiman et al. (1993) (VA/Roughness)	.37
Kreiman et al. (1994) (EAI/Breathiness)	.29
Kreiman et al. (1994) (EAI/Roughness)	.22
Rabinov et al. (1995) (VA/Roughness)	.42
Chhetri (1997) (EAI/Severity)	.34

*EAI = equal-appearing interval scale; VA = visual analog scale. Midrange of a 7-point EAI scale is defined as the segment between 2.5 and 5.5, inclusive. VA scales were truncated proportionally.

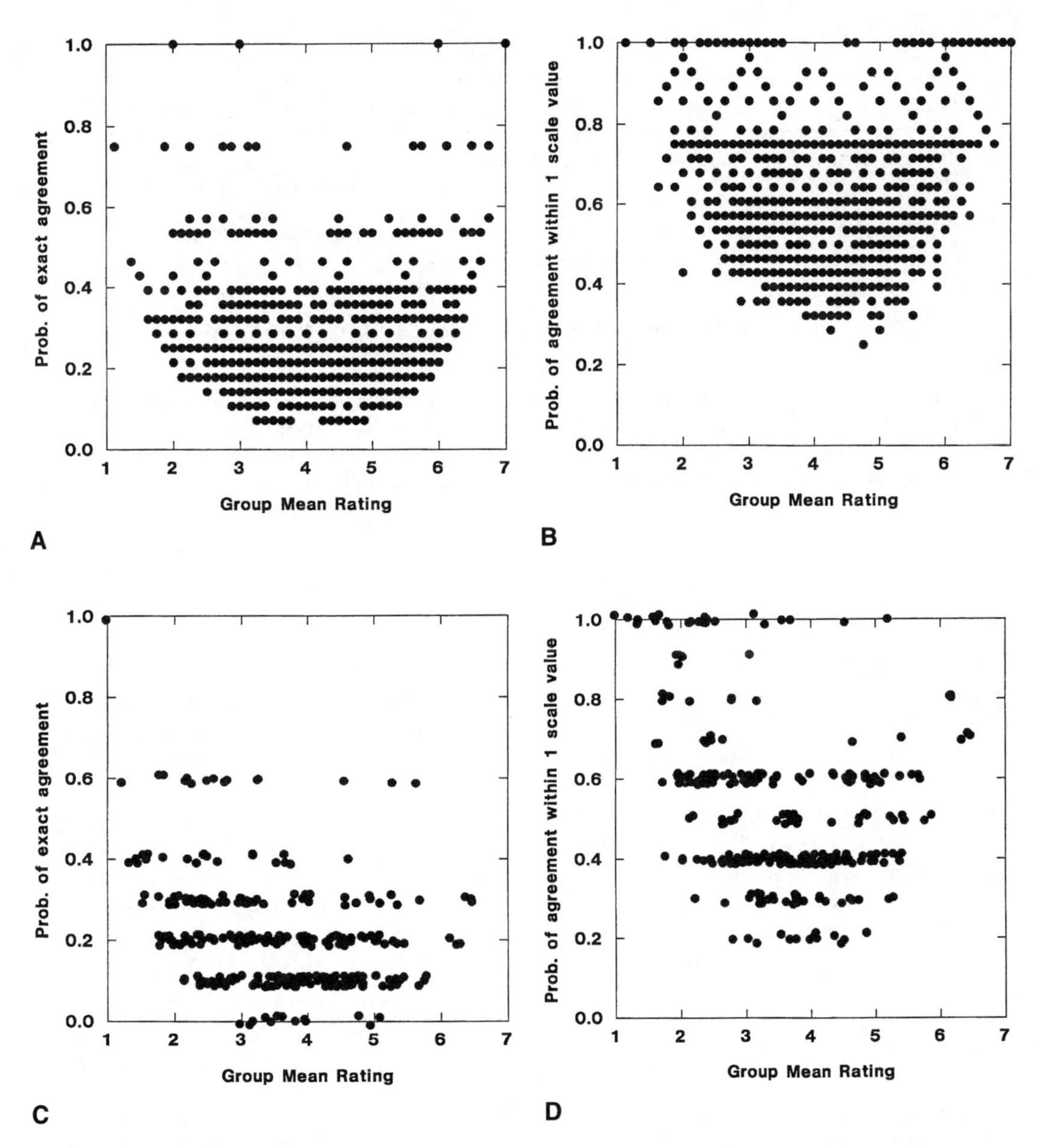

Figure 7–4. For each pair of voices in a data set, the probability that two raters agreed in their ratings of the similarity of that pair of voices versus the overall mean rating for that voice. Points have been jittered slightly to show overlapping values. **A.** The likelihood of exact agreement for ratings of the similarity of pairs of female voices; data from Kreiman and Gerratt (1996). **B.** The likelihood of agreement within 1 scale value for the same data. **C.** The likelihood of exact agreement for ratings of the similarity of pairs of voices with respect to breathiness; data from Kreiman et al. (1994). **D.** The likelihood of agreement within 1 scale value for the same data.

Fleiss, 1979), do not reflect the variability that occurs in interrater agreement, because they cannot represent patterns of agreement among raters and they cannot indicate agreement for specific voice samples (Young & Downs, 1968). Table 7–8 lists values of these statistics for the

Table 7–8 Traditional measures of rating reliability.*

Study	*Quality Judged*	*Interrater Agreement/Reliability*
Kreiman et al. (1993)	Roughness (EAI scale)	Reliability of mean rating (ICC) = .99 Cronbach's alpha = .99
Kreiman et al. (1994)	Dissimilarity of pairs of voices with respect to	Reliability of mean rating (ICC) = .68 Cronbach's alpha = .74 breathiness (EAI scale)
	Breathiness (EAI scale)	Reliability of mean rating (ICC) = .93 Cronbach's alpha = .97
Kreiman and Gerratt (1996)	Dissimilarity of pairs of female voices (EAI scale)	Reliability of mean rating (ICC) = .89 Cronbach's alpha = .90

*ICC = intraclass correlation coefficient; EAI = equal-appearing interval scale.

data in Figures 7–3 and 7–4. Summary reliability statistics were high overall, ranging from .68–.99 across studies. Thus, these data met conventional standards for reliability (see Kreiman et al., 1993, for review), despite the great variability that appeared when agreement levels for specific voices were examined. In particular, values were very high for data sets where the likelihood of listener agreement was poor (Kreiman et al., 1993) or variable (Kreiman & Gerratt, 1996), but *n* was large.

7. DISCUSSION

The experimental tasks examined here—ratings of breathiness, roughness, and severity; similarity ratings; and ratings of similarity with respect to breathiness and roughness—showed varying patterns of agreement among listeners. For ratings of traditional vocal qualities (Chhetri, 1997; Kreiman et al., 1993, 1994; Rabinov et al., 1995), individual listeners were self-consistent in their use of EAI scales. However, there were relatively few voices about which listeners as a group consistently agreed. In particular, consistent agreement *never* occurred for voices with mean ratings in the midrange of a scale. In fact, only about 30% of the variance in quality ratings was related to differences among voices when average ratings were between 2.5 and 5.5 on a 7-point scale.

For ratings of the overall similarity of pairs of voices (Kreiman & Gerratt, 1996), listeners as a group did agree that some voices were moderately similar. Patterns of agreement for ratings of similarity with respect to breathiness or roughness (Kreiman et al., 1994) shared characteristics of both traditional breathiness/ roughness ratings and ratings of the overall similarity of pairs of voices. Unlike ratings of breathiness and roughness, listeners sometimes agreed in their ratings for voices with mean ratings in the midrange of the scale, but overall reliability was lower than for ratings of overall similarity.

Several broad issues emerge from the patterns of agreement observed and from observed differences among tasks. First, are patterns of results consistent with the assumption that traditional voice rating protocols provide valid measures of vocal quality? If these protocols are not sufficiently valid, how should vocal quality be measured? Finally, what measures of rating reliability are appropriate for evaluating data in studies of vocal quality?

7.1. Validity of Rating Scale Protocols

Paradigms for assessing vocal quality on traditional unidimensional scales like breathiness and roughness require the assumption that individual differences among listeners in ratings are noise or error, so that the "true score" for a voice on a scale is solely a function of the voice itself. Average ratings provide meaningful measures of quality only if this assumption holds. The present results are inconsistent with this assumption and thus provide evidence against the validity of many protocols for assessing voice quality. Although listeners agreed at above-chance levels, most of the variance in quality ratings was attributable to factors other than differences among voices. The extent of variability in ratings received by voices away from scale endpoints indicates that mean ratings in the midrange of such scales poorly represent the extent to which a voice possesses a quality. Instead, ironically, mean ratings in the middle of a scale serve primarily to indicate that listeners disagreed. If differences among voices are not consistently reflected by differences in ratings, then traditional rating scale protocols do not measure what they are intended to measure and their validity is not supported.

Although traditional rating protocols do not appear to provide valid measures of the quality of a given voice, scalar ratings may still provide valuable information, if used to evaluate individual differences in perceptual strategy. For example, differences in patterns of disagreement that emerged from different rating tasks may provide insight into the mechanisms underlying the observed disagreements. Both traditional ratings of specific qualities and judgments of similarity with respect to specific qualities require listeners to compare observed voice stimuli to mental representations for the selected levels of that quality. This external-to-internal comparison introduces several sources of rating variability, including short- and long-term changes in mental representations, differences across listeners in how they define a quality or in standards for particular scale values, and variations in the importance of a cue in the context of variations in other cues (e.g., Kreiman et al., 1992, 1993). In contrast, similarity rating tasks require listeners to compare stimuli globally and directly, without the need to refer to mental standards or assess particular attributes. Thus, such tasks are not subject to error related to internal representations of a quality or drift in standards for particular levels of that quality. However, all tasks are subject to errors due to individual differences, perceptual biases, influences of perceptual context, mistakes, and changes over time in attention to these complex multidimensional stimuli.

Hypotheses regarding the effects of unstable internal standards for nonextreme levels of a quality are supported by data from a rating protocol using explicit anchors for each scale point (Gerratt et al., 1993). When listeners made their ratings with reference to external "anchor" stimuli (instead of presumed internal criteria), good agreement occurred when stimuli were identical to the anchors. However, agreement dropped sharply between anchors, again suggesting that listeners cannot maintain internal standards for different levels of traditional vocal qualities. These results also demonstrate the major weakness of anchored protocols. The increase in agreement gained by including an external anchor was limited to the stimuli identical to the anchor, and listener agreement quickly decreased when stimuli fell between anchors. These data indicate that unless a protocol includes a large number of anchors spaced closely together, reference stimuli will not solve the problem of listener disagreements in ratings of particular voices. Further, providing anchors for a traditional quality scale circumvents the issue of the scale's validity, which must be established by some other means.

It remains possible that listener training may provide a partial solution to these difficulties. Although short-term training has not been shown to consistently improve overall listener agreement (see Kreiman et al., 1993, for review), with extensive training listeners may learn to focus selectively on different aspects of complex auditory stimuli. Whether this is in fact the case and whether the effec ts of training persist after training ceases remain as issues for future research. In any case, the scales and stimuli with which listeners are trained must be viewed as arbitrarily chosen, unless independent evidence supports their validity.

7.2. How Should Vocal Quality Be Measured?

If traditional unidimensional rating scales are abandoned, a large gap in the conventional approach to clinical voice assessment will result. Obviously, much study is necessary to evaluate alternative strategies. Novel approaches to quality assessment should address the problems that appear to underlie listener disagreements. First, the present findings are consistent with the view that listener disagreements result in part from comparing external stimuli to idiosyncratic and/or unstable internal standards when attempting to use traditional rating scales. Second, it appears that listeners are unable to selectively attend to individual elements or dimensions of quality as required by traditional voice assessment paradigms.

Measurement of overall vocal quality offers an alternative to traditional unidimensional ratings of specific vocal qualities. In this view, quality is not a function of a fixed set of features, but instead is defined as those vocal characteristics that make it possible to determine that two signals are different.[4] Many approaches to measurement of overall quality are possible. Techniques using analysis by synthesis and/or similarity ratings have long histories in psychometric research and issues of their validity have been addressed in some detail (e.g., Gregson, 1975). Such tasks involve explicit comparisons between stimuli, rather than mappings between stimuli and internal standards, and they do not require listeners to focus attention on single dimensions of quality. Thus, in theory, they should eliminate the two causes of listener disagreement already described.

We have previously suggested that analysis by synthesis could be used to determine how listeners manipulate acoustic or other parameters to construct a synthetic token that matches the quality of a natural voice of interest (Kreiman & Gerratt, 1996). The values of these parameters would then directly represent a listener's perceptual response, rather than only having a statistical association with that response as in current correlative approaches. Although synthesizer parameters are manipulated individually, listeners still judge quality as a whole when evaluating the success of the synthesis. Thus analysis by synthesis combines unidimensional and overall approaches to quality.

Further, with the addition of multivariate or multidimensional statistical techniques, analysis by synthesis may allow development and testing of specific hypotheses about the nature and direction of changes in quality. For example, single acoustic parameters can be manipulated systematically and the resulting quality changes evaluated with similarity judgments. If the acoustic parameter in question predicts patterns of perceived similarity, a strong case for its importance to perception can be made. Note that this approach allows hypotheses about perceptual dimensions and their correlates to be investigated without the use of traditional scales for single qualities.

[4]From this it follows that when modeling overall quality, aspects of voice that signal the presence of pathology are not theoretically different from aspects that allow listeners to discriminate among speakers (for example, differences in fundamental frequency, vocal tract resonances, and so on). It further follows that perception of personal vocal quality should not be categorically separated from perception of pathological vocal quality: In this framework, both tasks involve modeling decisions that are based on global comparisons among stimuli. This contrasts to traditional approaches to these areas of study, which typically treat speaker recognition and voice discrimination as areas of study separate from perception of pathologic quality.

7.3. Reliability and the Measurement of Vocal Quality

Although the minimum "acceptable" level for listener agreement and reliability varies from study to study, a consensus exists that for most statistics, a value above .7 (or 49% variance in common) is "good" to "excellent," but that a value above .5 is adequate (e.g., de Bodt, Wuyts, Van de Heyning, & Croux, 1997; Fleiss, 1981; Hammarberg & Gauffin, 1995; Kazdin, 1977). The present results highlight several difficulties with this view. Measures of overall reliability (such as intraclass correlations and Cronbach's alpha) can mask large and predictable differences in agreement levels for different voices. For example, a data set for which Cronbach's alpha equals .9 or better may include individual voices for which agreement levels do not exceed chance. The presence or absence of normal and/or extremely severely pathologic voices in the stimulus set inflates or deflates these statistics (Kearns & Simmons, 1988). For example, ratings of roughness in the present data were more reliable overall for studies that included normal voices (Kreiman et al., 1993) than for studies that did not (Kreiman et al., 1994; Rabinov et al., 1995). The number of raters in a study also affects overall reliability. For example, a mean interrater correlation of .4 will produce Cronbach's alpha of .87, given an n of only 10 raters (Carmines & Zeller, 1979). Thus, such measures depend on differences in experimental design, as well as differences in ratings.

If averaging ratings is inappropriate, as argued previously, it follows that unaveraged data must be analyzed—in other words, individual differences in quality perception must be modeled (Kreiman & Gerratt, 1996). With individual differences models of perception there is no expectation that listeners will agree, so mean ratings are without interest. In this case, the reliability of the mean rating and the extent to which listeners agree in their ratings become moot points. Measures of variance accounted for may provide an alternative method of assessing the usefulness of a set of listener judgments. Such measures are particularly useful, because they make explicit the factors being used to predict variance in ratings. In this way, the statistical model and its fit to the data are precisely specified, rather than implied (as in the past).

For example, in the present data, overall reliability was slightly lower for similarity ratings than for ratings of traditional qualities. However, multidimensional scaling analyses accounted for much of this increased variability by quantifying the contributions of presentation order and/or individual differences in perceptual strategy to rating variability (Kreiman et al., 1994; Kreiman & Gerratt, 1996). R^2 values for individual listeners' data in Kreiman and Gerratt (1996) ranged from .56–.83; r^2 due to differences between voices in the unidimensional rating tasks reviewed here ranged from .22–.42.

Finally, patterns of listener agreement provide information not available from measures of overall reliability and thus may serve as useful supplements to measures of total variance accounted for. For example, understanding which voices listeners consistently agree about and which they cannot agree about may provide clues to the factors underlying judgments of vocal quality (see Kreiman & Gerratt, 1997, for an example of this kind of analysis). In voice studies, exact listener agreement is often held to be too strict a criterion for rating acceptability (Sheard, Adams, & Davis, 1991), and agreement within 1 scale value is a more common standard. However in the present data, the likelihood of two listeners agreeing within 1 scale value in their ratings of a single voice was significantly correlated with the likelihood of their agreeing exactly (Pearson's r averaged across studies = .76; range = .54–.93, $p < .05$). This indicates that the general pattern of listener agreement can be determined by examining either levels of exact agreement *or* patterns of agreement within 1 scale value. Broadening the definition of agreement raises the baseline of the function that describes listener performance (e.g., Figure 7–3A versus Figure 7–3B), and provides the appearance of better overall agreement among listeners, but does not change the pattern of listener performance indicated by exact agreement levels.

8. CONCLUSIONS

Accurate modeling of voice perception is essential to the success of many endeavors, including development of instrumental measures of voice, refinement of speech synthesizers, and evaluation of the effectiveness of treatments for voice disorders. The low levels of listener agreement reported here indicate that traditional continuous protocols for assessing qualities such as breathiness and roughness are not useful for measuring perceived vocal quality. More detailed analyses of listeners' performance in voice evaluation tasks and better quantification of the adequacy of models of voice perception will contribute to improved measurement of voice quality.

Acknowledgments

We thank Ted Bell, James Hillenbrand and Don Dirks for discussions of many statistical and nonstatistical aspects of this work. Dinesh Chhetri, MD, generously provided his severity rating data. This research was supported by grant DC01797 from the National Institute on Deafness and Other Communication Disorders.

REFERENCES

Allen, M. J., & Yen, W. M. (1979). *Introduction to measurement theory.* Monterey, CA: Brooks/Cole.

Anders, L., Hollien, H., Hurme, P., Sonninen, A., & Wendler, J. (1988). Perception of hoarseness by several classes of listeners. *Folia Phoniatrica, 40,* 91–100.

ANSI. (1960). *USA standard: Acoustical terminology (S1.1).* New York: American National Standards Institute, Inc.

Arends, N., Povel, D., von Os, E., & Speth, L. (1990). Predicting voice quality of deaf speakers on the basis of glottal characteristics. *Journal of Speech and Hearing Research, 33,* 116–122.

Askenfelt, A. G., & Hammarberg, B. (1986). Speech waveform perturbation analysis: A perceptual-acoustical comparison of seven measures. *Journal of Speech and Hearing Research, 29,* 50–64.

Baken, R. J. (1987). *Clinical measurement of speech and voice.* Boston: College-Hill Press.

Bassich, C., & Ludlow, C. L. (1986). The use of perceptual methods by new clinicians for assessing voice quality. *Journal of Speech and Hearing Disorders, 51,* 125–133.

Berk, R. (1979). Generalizability of behavioral observations: A clarification of interobserver agreement and interobserver reliability. *American Journal of Mental Deficiency, 83,* 460–472.

Bielamowicz, S., Kreiman, J., Gerratt, B. R., Dauer, M. S., & Berke, G. S. (1996). Comparison of voice analysis systems for perturbation measurement. *Journal of Speech and Hearing Research, 39,* 126–134.

Carmines, E. G., & Zeller, R. A. (1979). *Reliability and validity assessment.* Sage University Paper series on Quantitative Applications in the Social Sciences, 07–017. Newbury Park, CA: Sage Publications.

Chhetri, D. K. (1997). *Treatment of voice disorders related to unilateral paralysis of the vocal cord.* Unpublished senior medical student thesis, University of California, Los Angeles.

Coleman, R. F., & Wendahl, R. W. (1967). Vocal roughness and stimulus duration. *Speech Monographs, 34,* 85–92.

Cone, J. D. (1977). The relevance of reliability and validity for behavioral assessment. *Behavior Therapy, 8,* 411–426.

Crocker, L., & Algina, J. (1986). *Introduction to classical and modern test theory.* New York: Holt, Rinehart and Winston.

Cronbach, L. J. (1951). Coefficient alpha and the internal structure of tests. *Psychometrika, 16,* 297–334.

Cronbach, L. J., & Meehl, P. E. (1955). Construct validity in psychological tests. *Psychological Bulletin, 52,* 281–302.

Deal, R., & Emanuel, F. W. (1978). Some waveform and spectral features of vowel roughness. *Journal of Speech and Hearing Research, 21,* 250–264.

De Bodt, M. S., Wuyts, F. L., Van de Heyning, P. H., & Croux, C. (1997). Test-retest study of the GRBAS scale: Influence of experience and professional background on perceptual rating of voice quality. *Journal of Voice, 11,* 74–80.

Deem, J. F., Manning, W. H., Knack, J. V., & Matesich, J. S. (1989). The automatic extraction of pitch perturbation using microcomputers: Some methodological considerations. *Journal of Speech and Hearing Research, 32,* 689–697.

Dejonckere, P. H., & Lebacq, J. (1996). Acoustic, perceptual, aerodynamic and anatomical correlations in voice pathology. *Otology Rhinology Laryngology, 58,* 326–332.

Dejonckere, P. H., Obbens, C., de Moor, G. M., & Wieneke, G. H. (1993). Perceptual evaluation of dysphonia: reliability and relevance. *Folia Phoniatrica, 45,* 76–83.

de Krom, G. (1989). Voice quality: A few comments on terminology. In P. Coopmans, B. Schouten, & W. Zonneveld (Eds.), *OTS yearbook* (pp. 53–62). Utrecht: Research Institute for Language and Speech.

de Krom, G. (1994). *Acoustic correlates of breathiness and roughness: Experiments on voice quality.* Utrecht: OTS.

de Krom, G. (1995). Some spectral correlates of pathological breathy and rough voice quality for different types of vowel fragments. *Journal of Speech and Hearing Research, 38,* 794–811.

Doherty, E. T., & Shipp, T. (1988). Tape recorder effects on jitter and shimmer extraction. *Journal of Speech and Hearing Research,* 31, 485–490.

Ebel, R. (1951). Estimation of the reliability of ratings. *Psychometrica, 16,* 407–424.

Eskenazi, L., Childers, D. G., & Hicks, D. M. (1990). Acoustic correlates of vocal quality. *Journal of Speech and Hearing Research, 33,* 298–306.

Ethington, R., & Punch, B. (1994). Seawave—A system for musical timbre description. *Computer Music Journal, 18,* 30–39.

Fagel, W. P. F., van Herpt, L. W. A., & Boves, L. (1983). Analysis of the perceptual qualities of Dutch speakers' voice and pronunciation. *Speech Communication, 2,* 315–326.

Fairbanks, G. (1940). *Voice and articulation drillbook.* New York: Harper and Brothers.

Feijoo, S., & Hernandez, C. (1990). Short-term stability measures for the evaluation of vocal quality. *Journal of Speech and Hearing Research, 33,* 324–334.

Fleiss, J. L. (1981). *Statistical methods for rates and proportions.* New York: Wiley.

Fritzell, B., Hammarberg, B., Gauffin, J., Karlsson, I., & Sundberg, J. (1986). Breathiness and insufficient vocal fold closure. *Journal of Phonetics, 14,* 549–553.

Fukazawa, T., El-Assuooty, A., & Honjo, I. (1988). A new index for evaluation of the turbulent noise in pathological voice. *Journal of the Acoustical Society of America, 83,* 1189–1193.

Gelfer, M. P. (1988). Perceptual attributes of voice: Development and use of rating scales. *Journal of Voice, 2,* 320–326.

Gerratt, B. R., & Kreiman, J. (1995). The utility of acoustic voice measures. In D. Wong (Ed.), *Proceedings of the workshop on standardization in acoustic voice analysis* (pp. GER1-GER7). Denver: National Center for Voice and Speech.

Gerratt, B. R., Kreiman, J., Antonanzas-Barroso, N., & Berke, G. S. (1993). Comparing internal and external standards in voice quality judgments. *Journal of Speech and Hearing Research, 36,* 14–20.

Gerratt, B. R., Till, J., Rosenbek, J. C., Wertz, R. T., & Boysen, A. E. (1991). Use and perceived value of perceptual and instrumental measures in dysarthria management. In C. A. Moore, K. M. Yorkston, & D. R. Beukelman (Eds.), *Dysarthria and apraxia of speech* (pp. 77–93). Baltimore: Brookes.

Gregson, R. A. (1975). *Psychometrics of similarity.* New York: Academic.

Hammarberg, B., Fritzell, B., Gauffin, J., Sundberg, J., & Wedin, L. (1980). Perceptual and acoustic correlates of abnormal voice qualities. *Acta Otolaryngologica (Stockholm), 90,* 441–451.

Hammarberg, B., & Gauffin, J. (1995). Perceptual and acoustic characteristics of quality differences in pathological voices as related to physiological aspects. In O. Fujimura & M. Hirano (Eds.), *Vocal fold physiology: Voice quality control* (pp. 283–303). San Diego: Singular.

Hanson, H. M. (1995). *Glottal characteristics of female speakers.* Unpublished doctoral dissertation, Harvard University.

Hecker, M. H. L., & Kreul, E. J. (1971). Descriptions of the speech of patients with cancer of the vocal folds. Part I: Measures of fundamental frequency. *Journal of the Acoustical Society of America, 49,* 1275–1282.

Heiberger, V. L., & Horii, Y. (1982). Jitter and shimmer in sustained phonation. In N.J. Lass (Ed.), *Speech and language: Advances in basic research and practice* (Vol. 7, pp. 299–332). New York: Academic.

Helmholtz, H. (1885; reprinted 1954). *On the sensations of tone.* New York: Dover.

Hillenbrand, J. (1988). Perception of aperiodicities in synthetically generated voices. *Journal of the Acoustical Society of America, 83,* 2361–2371.

Hillenbrand, J., Cleveland, R. A., & Erickson, R. L. (1994). Acoustic correlates of breathy vocal quality. *Journal of Speech and Hearing Research, 37,* 769–778.

Hillenbrand, J., & Houde, R. A. (1996). Acoustic correlates of breathy vocal quality: Dysphonic voices and continuous speech. *Journal of Speech and Hearing Research, 39,* 311–321.

Hirano, M. (1981). *Clinical examination of voice.* New York: Springer-Verlag.

Hirano, M., Hibi, S., Yoshida, T., Hirade, Y., Kasuya, H., & Kikuchi, Y. (1988). Acoustic analysis of pathological voice. *Acta Otolaryngologica (Stockholm), 105,* 432–438.

Hiraoka, N., Kitazoe, Y., Ueta, H., Tanaka, S., & Tanabe, M. (1984). Harmonic-intensity analysis of normal and hoarse voices. *Journal of the Acoustical Society of America, 76,* 1648–1651.

Hollien, H., Michel, J., & Doherty, E. T. (1973). A method for analyzing vocal jitter in sustained phonation. *Journal of Phonetics,* 1, 85–91.

Holmgren, G. L. (1967). Physical and psychological correlates of speaker recognition. *Journal of Speech and Hearing Research, 10,* 57–66.

Horiguchi, S., Haji, T., Baer, T., & Gould, W. J. (1987). Comparison of electroglottographic and acoustic waveform perturbation measures. In T. Baer, C. Sasaki, & K. Harris (Eds.), *Laryngeal function in phonation and respiration* (pp. 509–518). Boston: College-Hill Press.

Isshiki, N., Okamura, H., Tanabe, M., & Morimoto, M. (1969). Differential diagnosis of hoarseness. *Folia Phoniatrica, 21,* 9–19.

Isshiki, N., & Takeuchi, Y. (1970). Factor analysis of hoarseness. *Studia Phonologica, 5,* 37–44.

Jensen, P. J. (1965). Adequacy of terminology for clinical judgment of voice quality deviation. *The Eye, Ear, Nose and Throat Monthly, 44,* 77–82.

Karnell, M. P. (1991). Laryngeal perturbation analysis: Minimum length of analysis window. *Journal of Speech and Hearing Research, 34,* 544–548.

Kazdin, A. (1977). Artifact, bias, and complexity of assessment: The ABCs of reliability. *Journal of Applied Behavior Analysis, 10,* 141–150.

Kearns, K., & Simmons, N. (1988). Interobserver reliability and perceptual ratings: More than meets the ear. *Journal of Speech and Hearing Research, 31,* 131–136.

Kempster, G. B., Kistler, D., & Hillenbrand, J. (1991). Multidimensional scaling analysis of dysphonia in two speaker groups. *Journal of Speech and Hearing Research, 34,* 534–543.

Kerlinger, F. N. (1973). *Foundations of behavioral research* (2nd ed.). New York: Holt, Rinehart, & Winston.

Klatt, D. H., & Klatt, L. C. (1990). Analysis, synthesis, and perception of voice quality variations among female and male talkers. *Journal of the Acoustical Society of America, 87,* 820–857.

Klich, R. (1982). Relationships of vowel characteristics to listener ratings of breathiness. *Journal of Speech and Hearing Research, 25,* 574–580.

Kreiman, J. (1997). Listening to voices: Theory and practice in voice perception research. In K. Johnson & J. W. Mullennix (Eds.), *Talker variability in speech processing* (pp. 85–108). San Diego: Academic.

Kreiman, J., & Gerratt, B. R. (1996). The perceptual structure of pathologic voice quality. *Journal of the Acoustical Society of America, 100,* 1787–1795.

Kreiman, J., & Gerratt, B. R. (1997, December). *Categorical judgments of vocal quality.* Presented at the 134th Meeting of the Acoustical Society of America, San Diego.

Kreiman, J., Gerratt, B. R., & Berke, G. S. (1994). The multidimensional nature of pathologic vocal quality. *Journal of the Acoustical Society of America, 96,* 1291–1302.

Kreiman, J., Gerratt, B. R., Kempster, G. B., Erman, A., & Berke, G. S. (1993). Perceptual evaluation of voice quality: Review, tutorial, and a framework for future research. *Journal of Speech and Hearing Research, 36,* 21–40.

Kreiman, J., Gerratt, B. R., & Precoda, K. (1990). Listener experience and perception of voice quality. *Journal of Speech and Hearing Research, 33,* 103–115.

Kreiman, J., Gerratt, B. R., Precoda, K., & Berke, G. S. (1992). Individual differences in voice quality perception. *Journal of Speech and Hearing Research, 35,* 512–520.

Krumhansl, C. L., & Iverson, P. (1992). Perceptual interactions between musical pitch and timbre. *Journal of Experimental Psychology: Human Perception and Performance, 18,* 739–751.

Lieberman, P. (1961). Perturbations in vocal pitch. *Journal of the Acoustical Society of America, 35,* 344–353.

Mackey, L. S., Finn, P., & Ingham, R. J. (1997). Effect of speech dialect on speech naturalness ratings: A systematic replication of Martin, Haroldson, and Triden (1984). *Journal of Speech, Language, and Hearing Research, 40,* 349–360.

Martin, D., Fitch, J., & Wolfe, V. (1995). Pathologic voice type and the acoustic prediction of severity. *Journal of Speech and Hearing Research, 38,* 765–771.

Matsumoto, H., Hiki, S., Sone, T., & Nimura, T. (1973). Multidimensional representation of personal quality of vowels and its acoustical correlates. *IEEE Transactions on Audio and Electroacoustics, AU-21,* 428–436.

McAllister, A., Sederholm, E., Ternstrom, S., & Sundberg, J. (1996). Perturbation and hoarseness: A pilot study of six children's voices. *Journal of Voice, 10,* 252–261.

Melara, R. D., & Marks, L. E. (1990). Interaction among auditory dimensions: Timbre, pitch, and loudness. *Perception and Psychophysics, 48,* 169–178.

Michaelis, D., Gramss, T., & Strube, H. W. (1997). Glottal-to-noise excitation ratio—A new measure for describing pathological voices. *Acustica, 83,* 700–706.

Moody, D. K., Montague, J., & Bradley, B. (1979). Preliminary validity and reliability data on the Wilson Voice Profile System. *Language, Speech, and Hearing Services in Schools, 10,* 231–240.

Mori, K., Blaugrund, S. M., & Yu, J. D. (1994). The turbulent noise ratio: An estimation of noise power of the breathy voice using PARCOR analysis. *Laryngoscope, 104,* 153–158.

Murry, T., & Singh, S. (1980). Multidimensional analysis of male and female voices. *Journal of the Acoustical Society of America, 68,* 1294–1300.

Murry, T., Singh, S., & Sargent, M. (1977). Multidimensional classification of abnormal voice qualities. *Journal of the Acoustical Society of America, 61,* 1630–1635.

Nieboer, G. L., De Graaf, T., & Schutte, H. K. (1988). Esophageal voice quality judgments by means of the semantic differential. *Journal of Phonetics, 16,* 417–436.

Osgood, C. E., Suci, G. J., & Tannenbaum, P. H. (1957). *The measurement of meaning.* Urbana: University of Illinois Press.

Pannbacker, M. (1984). Classification systems of voice disorders: A review of the literature. *Language, Speech, and Hearing Services in Schools, 15,* 169–174.

Pavlovic, C., Rossi, M., & Espesser, R. (1990). Use of the magnitude estimation technique for assessing the performance of text-to-speech synthesis systems. *Journal of the Acoustical Society of America, 87,* 373–382.

Perkins, W. (1971). Vocal function: A behavioral analysis. In L. Travis (Ed.), *Handbook of speech pathology and audiology* (pp. 481–504). New York: Appleton Century Croft.

Perry, C. K., Ingrisano, D., & Scott, S. (1996). Accuracy of jitter estimates using different filter settings on Visi-Pitch: A preliminary report. *Journal of Voice, 10,* 337–341.

Plomp, R. (1976). *Aspects of tone sensation.* London: Academic.

Prosek, R. A., Montgomery, A. A., Walden, B. E., & Hawkins, D. B. (1987). An evaluation of residue features as correlates of voice disorders. *Journal of Communication Disorders, 20,* 105–117.

Rabinov, C. R., Kreiman, J., Gerratt, B. R., & Bielamowicz, S. (1995). Comparing reliability of perceptual ratings of roughness and acoustic measures of jitter. *Journal of Speech and Hearing Research, 38,* 26–32.

Rammage, L. A., Peppard, R., & Bless, D. M. (1992). Aerodynamic, laryngoscopic, and perceptual-acoustic characteristics in dysphonic females with posterior glottal chinks: A retrospective study. *Journal of Voice, 6,* 64–78.

Sederholm, E., McAllister, A., Sundberg, J., & Dalkvist, J. (1993). Perceptual analysis of child hoarseness using continuous scales. *Scandinavian Journal of Logopedics and Phoniatrics, 18,* 73–82.

Sheard, C., Adams, R. D., & Davis, P. J. (1991). Reliability and agreement of ratings of ataxic dysarthric speech samples with varying intelligibility. *Journal of Speech and Hearing Research, 34,* 285–293.

Shoji, K., Regenbogen, E., Yu, J. D., & Blaugrund, S. M. (1992). H-Index: A new measure of glottal efficiency for the pathologic voice. *Laryngoscope, 102,* 1113–1117.

Shrout, P., & Fleiss, J. (1979). Intraclass correlations: Uses in assessing rater reliability. *Psychological Bulletin, 86,* 420–428.

Silverman, F.H. (1977). *Research design in speech pathology and audiology.* Englewood Cliffs, NJ: Prentice-Hall.

Sodersten, M., Hertegard, S., & Hammarberg, B. (1995). Glottal closure, transglottal airflow, and voice quality in healthy middle-aged women. *Journal of Voice, 9,* 182–197.

Sodersten, M., & Lindestad, P. (1990). Glottal closure and perceived breathiness during phonation in normally speaking subjects. *Journal of Speech and Hearing Research, 33,* 601–611.

Sonninen, A. (1970). Phoniatric viewpoints on hoarseness. *Acta Otolaryngologica (Stockholm), 263* (Suppl.), 68–81.

Sonninen, A., & Hurme, P. (1992). On the terminology of voice research. *Journal of Voice, 6,* 188–193.

Stewart, C. F., Allen, E. L., Tureen, P., Diamond, B. E., Blitzer, A., & Brin, M. F. (1997). Adductor spasmodic dysphonia: Standard evaluation of symptoms and severity. *Journal of Voice, 11,* 95–103.

Suen, H. K., & Ary, D. (1989). *Analyzing quantitative behavioral observation data.* Hillsdale, NJ: Lawrence Erlbaum Associates.

Takahashi, H., & Koike, Y. (1975). Some perceptual dimensions and acoustic correlates of pathological voices. *Acta Otolaryngologica (Stockholm), 338* (Suppl.), 2–24.

Titze, I. R. (1995). *Workshop on acoustic voice analysis: Summary statement.* Denver, CO: National Center for Voice and Speech.

Titze, I. R., Horii, Y., & Scherer, R. C. (1987). Some technical considerations in voice perturbation measurements. *Journal of Speech and Hearing Research, 30,* 252–260.

Titze, I. R., & Winholtz, W. S. (1993). Effect of microphone type and placement on voice perturbation measurements. *Journal of Speech and Hearing Research, 36,* 1177–1190.

Toner, M. A., & Emanuel, F. W. (1989). Direct magnitude estimation and equal appearing interval scaling of vowel roughness. *Journal of Speech and Hearing Research, 32,* 78–82.

Ventry, I. M., & Schiavetti, N. (1980). *Evaluating research in speech pathology and audiology.* Reading, MA: Addison-Wesley.

Vieira, M. N., McInnes, F. R., & Jack, M. A. (1997). Comparative assessment of electroglottographic and acoustic measures of jitter in pathological voices. *Journal of Speech, Language, and Hearing Research, 40,* 170–182.

Voiers, W. D. (1964). Perceptual bases of speaker identity. *Journal of the Acoustical Society of America, 36,* 1065–1073.

Wagner, I. (1995). A new jitter algorithm to quantify hoarseness. *Forensic Linguistics, 2,* 18–27.

Wendahl, R. W. (1963). Laryngeal analog synthesis of harsh voice quality. *Folia Phoniatrica, 15,* 241–250.

Wendahl, R. W. (1966a). Laryngeal analog synthesis of jitter and shimmer auditory parameters of harshness. *Folia Phoniatrica, 18,* 98–108.

Wendahl, R. W. (1966b). Some parameters of auditory roughness. *Folia Phoniatrica, 18,* 26–32.

Wilson, F. B. (1977). *Voice disorders.* Austin, TX: Learning Concepts.

Yanagihara, N. (1967). Significance of harmonic changes and noise components in hoarseness. *Journal of Speech and Hearing Research, 10,* 531–541.

Young, M. A. (1993). Supplementing tests of statistical significance: Variation accounted for. *Journal of Speech and Hearing Research, 36,* 644–656.

Young, M. A., & Downs, T. D. (1968). Testing the significance of the agreement among observers. *Journal of Speech and Hearing Research, 11,* 5–17.

Yumoto, E., Gould, W. J., & Baer, T. (1982). Harmonics-to-noise ratio as an index of the degree of hoarseness. *Journal of the Acoustical Society of America, 71,* 1544–1550.

Yumoto, E., Sasaki, Y., & Okamura, H. (1984). Harmonics-to-noise ratio and psychophysical measurement of the degree of hoarseness. *Journal of Speech and Hearing Research, 27,* 2–6.

Zwirner, P., Murry, T., & Woodson, G. E. (1993). Perceptual-acoustic relationships in spasmodic dysphonia. *Journal of Voice, 7,* 165–171.

APPENDIX 7–1
DEFINITIONS OF TRADITIONAL VOICE QUALITIES

breathiness:

"Audible escape of air resulting in a thin, weak phonation, related to a functional inability to firmly adduct the vocal folds" (Bassich & Ludlow, 1986, p. 133).

"Audible noise created at the glottis, probably because of insufficient glottal closure; vocal folds are vibrating, but somewhat abducted" (Askenfelt & Hammarberg, 1986, p. 53; Hammarberg & Gauffin, 1995, p. 291).

"Breathiness is believed to be generated from the turbulent noise produced at the glottis. . . This assumption seems to be reasonable if one thinks of a whisper that is made from turbulent noise at the glottis and gives a very breathy impression" (Fukazawa et al., 1988; p. 1189).

"Audible escapage of air through the glottis due to insufficient glottal closure; the degree of breathiness severity is inversely proportional to the length of the closed glottal phase" (Eskenazi, Childers, & Hicks, 1990, p. 301).

"Breathy phonation is characterized by a glottal source with (1) an increased open quotient, resulting in an increased relative amplitude of the fundamental component in the spectrum and (2) a tendency for higher harmonics to be replaced by aspiration noise" (Klatt & Klatt, 1990, p. 825).

"Audible escape of air through the glottis due to insufficient closure" (Sodersten & Lindestad, 1990, p. 605; Zwirner, Murry, & Woodson, 1993, p. 166).

"Impression of glottal air leakage and turbulence noise during phonation" (de Krom, 1995, p. 798).

"The combination of vocal tone and turbulent airflow derived from a partially open glottis" (Martin et al., 1995, p. 767).

"Containing the sound of breathing (expiration) during phonation; acoustically, breathy voice. . . has most of its energy in the fundamental, but a significant component of noise is present because of turbulence in or near the glottis" (Titze, 1995, p. 336).

harshness:

(gratings/harsh) "High-pitched noise, presumably due to irregular vocal fold vibrations" (Askenfelt & Hammarberg, 1986, p. 53).

(harsh-shrill) "A rough or unpleasant strident, metallic, or grating voice quality occurring in relatively high-pitched phonations, sometimes associated with a hard glottal attack" (Bassich & Ludlow, 1986, p. 133).

hoarseness:

(wet-hoarse) "A wet, liquid-sounding, unpleasant, and rough voice quality" (Bassich & Ludlow, 1986, p. 133).

"A voice quality which clearly contains noise components, and that can be labeled rough and breathy (i.e., source noise elements plus friction noise); its perceived pitch tends to vary substantially; common descriptors of this quality are 'noisy', harsh', 'wet'" (Anders, Hollien, Hurme, Sonninen, & Wendler, 1988, p. 91).

"Breathy plus rough; it is, therefore, a result of a combination of excessive air escapage and an aperiodicity of vocal fold vibration" (Eskenazi et al., 1990, p. 301).

"A combination of rough and breathy—that is, irregular vocal fold vibrations along with additive noise" (Martin et al., 1995, p. 767).

roughness:

"A psycho-acoustic impression of the irregularity of vocal fold vibrations. It corresponds to the irregular fluctuations in the fundamental frequency and/or the amplitude of the glottal sound source" (Hirano, 1981, p. 83).

"Low-frequency aperiodic noise, presumably related to some kind of irregular vocal fold vibrations" (Askenfelt & Hammarberg, 1986, p. 53; Eskenazi et al., 1990, p. 301; Hammarberg & Gauffin, 1995, p. 291).

(rough-fry) "A rough or unpleasant voice quality in low-pitched phonations. May or may not be associated with a rhythmic beating or crackling phenomenon of glottal fry" (Bassich & Ludlow, 1986, p. 133).

"The voice quality related to the impression of irregular pulses, of random fluctuations of the glottal pulse, with a wide F_0 range" (Dejonckere et al., 1993, p. 78).

"Presence of a low-frequency noise component" (de Krom, 1995, p. 798).

(gratings/high-frequency roughness) "High-frequency aperiodic noise, presumably related to some kind of irregular vocal fold vibrations" (Hammarberg & Gauffin, 1995, p. 291).

"Irregular vocal fold vibrations" (Martin et al., 1995, p. 767).

"An uneven, bumpy quality that appears to be unsteady in the short term, but stationary in the long term; acoustically, the waveform is chaotic, with the modes of vibration lacking synchrony" (Titze, 1995, p. 339).

CHAPTER 8

The Use of Self-Organizing Maps for the Classification of Voice Disorders

Daniel E. Callan, Ray D. Kent, Nelson Roy, and Stephen M. Tasko

The investigation of voice disorders has traditionally involved the use of multiple perceptual rating scales (e.g., degree of breathiness, strain, roughness) and more recently the use of multiple acoustic measures. One of the challenges involved in using multidimensional data is determining a way of classifying it. One way in which multidimensional data has been successfully classified is through the use of self-organizing maps (SOM). The self-organizing map was developed by Tuevo Kohonen (1982) and is a neural network algorithm that creates topologically correct feature maps. Recently, self-organizing maps have been used as a new method to characterize voice disorders.

Self-organizing maps provide three main advantages in analyzing multidimensional data compared to more traditional approaches: (1) Self-organizing maps are able to take multidimensional data and represent it along its two-dimensional surface. This provides for an easy way to visualize the relative distribution of the exemplars of the various groups across the surface of the self-organizing map. (2) The nonlinear nature of the self-organizing map allows for better classification performance than traditional multivariate statistical techniques in some cases. (3) The relative weighting of the input dimensions responsible for defining the distribution of exemplars into groups across a self-organizing map can be easily discerned. This allows for determining which input dimensions are responsible for the distribution of exemplars of the various groups across the surface of a self-organizing map.

Self-organizing maps provide for a two-dimensional representational mapping over an array of processing units (called nodes) of the multidimensional nonlinear regularities inherent in the input data space (Kohonen, 1995). Self-organizing maps can be thought of as consisting of an input layer, a representational layer, and a weight matrix connecting the two (see Figure 8–1). The input layer is a vector in which the elements correspond to the various input dimensions. The representational layer is made up of a two-dimensional array of processing units (called nodes) that have a neighborhood structure. The weight matrix connects each of the elements in the input layer to each of the nodes in the representational layer. The strengths of each of the weights is determined by an unsupervised learning algorithm that projects the probability distribution inherent in the multidimensional input space onto the two-dimensional array of nodes composing the representational layer (Kohonen, Hynninen, Kangas, & Laaksonen, 1996).

One advantage of unsupervised learning is that a gold standard target is not necessary for training. Map formation is accomplished by iteratively presenting input and allowing for the weighted connections from the representational layer to be corrected toward the input value. The values of the input nodes for each exemplar denote a vector (let's call it x [input vector]) that defines some point in an *n*-dimensional space; *n* corresponding to the number of input nodes. The weighted connections projecting from each of the nodes in the representational layer to the nodes in the input layer also denotes a vector (let's call it *m* [weight vector]) that defines some point in an *n*-dimensional space. The self-organizing map is initially set with random values for the weighted connections. Training of the self-organizing map occurs by iteratively presenting the input vectors such that each time step *t* corresponds to a separate exemplar. During each iterative step, a winning node in the representational layer is determined. This is accomplished by determining which of the nodes in the representational layer has the associated weight vector that is closest in Euclidean distance (in the *n*-dimensional space) to the input vector. This can be expressed as follows with *c* signifying the closest or winning node and *i* signifying the node identifier in the representational layer (taken from Kohonen et al., 1996):

$$\|x(t) - m_c(t)\| = \min_i\{\|x - m_i\|\}$$

which is the same as

$$c = \arg\min_i\{\|x - m_i\|\}$$

Where: $x(t)$ = input vector for time step t
$m_c(t)$ = connection weights of the winning node c for time step t
$m_i(t)$ = connection weights of node i for time step t
i = node identifier
c = winning node

After the winning node has been determined the value of the connection weights of the winning node (m_c) and its neighboring nodes are corrected toward the value of the input vector. The magnitude of the correction change is determined in part by a parameter called the learning rate (α).

$$m_i(t+1) = m_i(t) + \alpha(t)[x(t) - m_i(t)],$$

if node m_i is within the neighborhood radius of m_c; otherwise

$$m_i(t+1) = m_i(t).$$

Where: $x(t)$ = input vector for time step t
$m_i(t)$ = connection weights of node i for time step t
$\alpha(t)$ = learning rate parameter for time step

The value of the learning rate parameter monotonically decreases as training progresses ($0<\alpha(t)<1$). The learning rate is kept relatively large during initial training to ensure that a large number of weight vectors from the representational nodes will begin to approximate the input space in a rapid manner (Kohonen, 1995). Decreasing learning rate with training assures that the weight changes will not overshoot the input space (Kohonen, 1995). During initial training, the neighborhood radius is kept large to allow for the weight vectors of the representational layer to be globally ordered in relation to the input space (Kohonen, 1995). For category formation to occur across the representational map, the neighborhood radius is decreased during training. By following these procedures, a self-organizing map can be formed that approximates the nonlinear regularities inherent in the input data space.

1. SELF-ORGANIZING MAPS AND CLASSIFICATION OF VOICE DISORDERS (SPECTRAL MEASURES)

Self-organizing maps have been used to characterize various aspects of both normal and disordered voice. Several studies using self-organizing maps to detect characteristics of dysphonic voice have been conducted by Leinonen and colleagues (Leinonen, Hiltunen, Kangas, Juvas, & Rihkanen, 1993; Leinonen, Hiltunen, Laakso, Rihkanen, & Poppius, 1997; Leinonen, Kangas, Torkkola, & Juvas, 1992; Rihkanen, Leinonen, Hiltunen, & Kangas; 1994). In the first study (Leinonen et al., 1992), a self-organizing map was trained to detect characteristics of dysphonic voice by recognition of spectral composition. This was accomplished by first training a SOM using normal voices to form an acoustic map across the node array. The input used to form this map consisted of 200 Finnish words. These words were presented to the self-organizing map as 15-dimensional spectral vectors, each corresponding to a different frequency between 50 Hz and 5 kHz. The amplitudes of the values that compose the spectral vectors were calculated from short-time power spectra at 9.83-ms intervals. After training, the nodes of the map came to represent different consonants and vowels. When presented with a word, one could then trace the trajectory pattern across the map. To determine how this map would characterize disordered voice, samples were taken from individuals classified with varying degrees of dysphonia using a method derived from the GRBAS (Grade [severity], Roughness, Breathiness, Asthenia, Strain) perceptual rating scale (Hirano, 1981). The voices were classified based on the degree of dysphonia, roughness, breathiness, and strain. Samples of the Finnish vowel [a:] from both normal and disordered voices were presented to the self-organizing map. It was found that the trajectory pattern across the map differed for dysphonic and normal voices. It was also found that rough and breathy voices had different trajectory patterns. However, the self-organizing map was not able to distinguish the degree of pathology.

To better distinguish normal from disordered voices and to increase spectral resolution across the self-organizing map, a second study was conducted in which the self-organizing map was enlarged and was trained using both dysphonic and normal voice samples (Leinonen et al., 1993). The input used to form the self-organizing map consisted of 19 component spectral vectors of both normal and dysphonic voice samples.

Each of the input vectors was calculated by a 512-point FFT every 10 ms through the first syllable of the Finnish words [sa:ri], [ka:ri], [va:ri], and [la:ri]. After training, the self-organizing map was able to statistically differentiate between healthy and dysphonic voices as well as between rough and breathy voices. Analysis of the weightings of the spectral vectors across the self-organizing map revealed that the groups were differentiated based on the relative spectral energy between 1–2 kHz and 7–9 kHz. The self-organizing map in this study, as in the first study, was not able to distinguish the degree of pathology.

In a study conducted by Rihkanen et al. (1994), the self-organizing map was trained using a similar procedure as the Leinonen et al. (1993) study, with the exception of a modified input set, to determine if changes in voice quality due to laryngeal surgery as well as the relative degree of pathology could be represented. In this study, 1-s samples of the sustained Finnish vowel [a:] for both normal and dysphonic individuals were used to train the self-organizing map. The input vectors consisted of 19 component spectral vectors calculated by a 512-point FFT every 10 ms through the entire 1-s samples. After training, the self-organizing map was able to distinguish (1) normal from dysphonic voices, (2) the relative improvement in voice after treatment, and (3) the degree of pathology.

2. SELF-ORGANIZING MAPS AND CLASSIFICATION OF VOICE DISORDERS (PERCEPTUAL RATING MEASURES)

In a study conducted by Leinonen et al. (1997), instead of using acoustic data as input, the self-organizing map was trained using the dimensions of a perceptual rating scale to categorize normal from dysphonic voice. The categorization of various forms and degrees of dysphonia was accomplished by using perceptual ratings of pathology, roughness, breathiness, strain, and asthenia as input dimensions to train the SOM. Five different categories of voice quality were formed across the SOM. The categories were organized from right to left across the SOM depending on the relative degree of severity. Class A was located on the right side of the map and included individuals ranked as having good voices; class B was located adjacent to class A and included individuals ranked as healthy or slightly pathological; class C was located on the lower part of the map adjacent to class B and included individuals ranked as pathological and predominantly rough; class D was located above class C and adjacent to class B and included individuals ranked as pathological and predominantly breathy; class E was located toward the upper left corner of the map bordering with both class C and class B and it included individuals ranked as having extremely pathological voices. The SOM trained on various dimensions of a perceptual rating scale was successful in categorizing both the degree of pathology as well as the ratio of breathiness and roughness across the map.

3. SELF-ORGANIZING MAPS AND CLASSIFICATION OF VOICE DISORDERS (MULTIPLE ACOUSTIC MEASURES)

Overall, the self-organizing maps used by Leinonen and Rihkanen and colleagues are very successful in providing a two-dimensional visual representation of characteristics of normal and dysphonic voice that is easy to understand. One of the disadvantages of using multiple spectral dimensions as input is that it is difficult to evaluate which acoustic properties (other than spectral) are important in map organization that make classification of normal and dysphonic voice possible.

Another method used to train a self-organizing map to classify various aspects of voice is to use as input the value of various acoustic measures made over speech samples. This was the method used in a study conducted by Callan, Kent, Roy, and Tasko (1999). The goal of that study was to classify females with spasmodic dysphonia (SD), pretreatment functional dysphonia (PR), posttreatment functional dysphonia (PS), and individuals with normal voice (NR) across the surface of a self-organizing map using various acoustic measures as input parameters. The acoustic measures were taken using Kay Elemetrics multidimensional voice profile (MDVP) as well as cepstral analysis using the Kay Elemetrics Computerized Speech Lab (CSL). The acoustic measures were made over the central 1 s of the sustained vowel /a/. Of the 22 acoustic measures taken, 6 were selected based on a priori predictions and the results of a stepwise discriminate analysis as good independent predictors at distinguishing between the various groups. The six acoustic parameters selected were:

APQ: amplitude perturbation quotient gives a measure in percentage of the variability of the peak-to-peak amplitude within the analyzed voice sample at a smoothing factor of 11 periods (taken from the Voice Disorders Database, Kay Elemetrics Corp., 1994).

DVB: degree of voice breaks (in percentage) the ratio of the total duration where the fundamental frequency cannot be tracked to the time of the complete voice sample (taken from the Voice Disorders Database, Kay Elemetrics Corp., 1994).

RAM: rahmonic amplitude denotes the amplitude of the first dominant peak in the cepstral analysis, which corresponds to the harmonic peak of the spectrum of the signal (taken from CSL, Kay Elemetrics Corp., 1994).

SPI: soft phonation index is an average ratio of the lower-frequency to the higher frequency harmonic energy (taken from the Voice Disorders Database, Kay Elemetrics Corp., 1994).

STD: standard deviation of the fundamental frequency (in hertz) of the vocalization. This measure consisted of the standard deviation of all extracted period-to-period fundamental frequency values within the 1-s sample (taken from the Voice Disorders Database, Kay Elemetrics Corp., 1994).

VAM: coefficient of variation of the peak-to-peak amplitude (in percentage) for the voice sample (taken from the Voice Disorders Database, Kay Elemetrics Corp., 1994).

The self-organizing map was trained on 30 exemplars from each of the groups (SD, PR, PS, and NR) using the 6 acoustic parameters: APQ, DVB, RAM, SPI, STD, and VAM. After training was finished, a Sammon mapping of the weights of the SOM was conducted to represent the relative separation of the nodes in two dimensions (Sammon, 1969).

The resulting distribution of exemplars across the self-organizing map for each of the four groups (SD, PR, PS, and NR) is displayed in Figure 8–2. The position of the nodes is determined by the x and y Euclidean coordinates given by the Sammon (1969) mapping. The lines connecting the nodes in Figure 8–2 represent the underlying hexagonal neighborhood lattice. Visual inspection of the map (shown in Figure 8–2) indicates that the SOM does a fairly good job at separating the four different groups across its surface. The NR exemplars are represented mainly in the top left corner of the SOM and are densely clustered. The PS exemplars share a fair degree of overlap with the NR exemplars and are mainly clustered in the middle and bottom left side of the SOM. The PR exemplars are represented across the bottom of the SOM. The SD exemplars are represented across the top right side of the SOM. The PR and SD exemplars are more sparsely represented across the SOM than the NR and PR exemplars.

Classification performance was determined by first assigning a group representation to each node. The node representations were assigned based on the maximum number of exemplars from a group that fall on a node. When the number of exemplars falling on a single node is the same, or the case in which no exemplars fall on a node, representation is determined by majority voting of the group membership of the five nearest exemplars (in Euclidean space) to the node in question. Node representations are displayed as the big circles in Figure 8–3. Classification performance for a stepwise discriminant analysis over the same acoustic dimensions as were used to train the SOM, and the classification performance of the self-organizing map is given in Tables 8–1 and 8–2, respectively. The overall classification performance for the SOM is superior to the stepwise discriminant analysis. The SOM identified 75.8% of the exemplars correctly, whereas, the stepwise discriminant analysis correctly identified only 68.3% of the exemplars. The SOM had better predictive performance at classifying SD, PR, and PS groups (SD = 73.3%, PR = 73.3%, PS = 73.3%) compared to that of the stepwise discriminant analysis (SD = 66.7%, PR = 50%, PS = 70%). Only the NR group was classified better by the stepwise discriminant analysis (NR = 86.7%) than by the SOM (NR = 83.3%).

The weight values for each of the input parameters projecting to each of the nodes are displayed in Figure 8–3. The weight values cross the self-organizing map are displayed as small bar plots on top of each node (see Figure 8–3). The following generalizations regarding the weights of the acoustic parameters for characterizing the various groups is taken from Callan et al. (1999): SD node representations are characterized by relatively high values of VAM, APQ, and DVB, as well as low values of RAM. Most of the nodes with spasmodic dysphonia representations are characterized by relatively high values of STD and VAM, with low values of RAM. Two nodes with PR representations in the region of node (1,1) have high SPI levels. PS node representations are characterized by midrange values of RAM and SPI, as well as low values of APQ and VAM. NR node representations are characterized by high RAM values and relatively low values of all other acoustic parameters. Overall, it appears that disordered voice (SD and PR) is characterized by greater variability in amplitude (both long term [APQ, smoothing factor 11 periods] and short term [VAM, period-to-period]), as well as fundamental frequency (STD). Voice that is considered nonpathologic (NR and PS) is characterized by a low degree of variability in amplitude (APQ and VAM) and fundamental frequency (STD), as well as a high degree of harmonic energy (RAM) (see Callan et al., 1999, for further details).

The self-organizing map trained with acoustic parameters provided for three main advantages over more traditional statistical methods: (1) The SOM provided an easy way to visualize the separation of the different groups, (2) The SOM provided for at least as good statistical predictability at classifying the data as that of traditional stepwise discriminant analysis, and (3) The SOM provided for the relative contribution of the underlying acoustic parameters in distinguishing between the different groups. It is important to note that the acoustic data were obtained from a relatively brief sample of a very simple phonation task. The fact that classification appears at all in the SOM is remarkable, given the likely heterogeneity among speakers and given the short sample selected for analysis. One might achieve even better performance, if it were trained on different sets of acoustic measures from more complex tasks, such as conversation.

Although the SOM was able to distinguish between normal and pathologic voice, a further step in analysis that needs to be taken is a comparison between nodes on which exemplars of the various groups fall and their corresponding perceptual ratings of severity. With perceptual rating scores of severity, it will be possible to determine if the SOM codes for degree of pathology and/or efficacy of treatment.

To explore if degree of pathology and/or efficacy of treatment can be represented across the surface of a SOM trained on several acoustic parameters, a data set of 50 female functional dysphonic individuals pre- and posttreatment with corresponding perceptual ratings of voice quality was used for training. Data from 30 of these individuals were input for the PR and PS groups to train the previous SOM. As in the previous study, the acoustic measures were taken using Kay Elemetrics multidimensional voice protocol (MDVP) as well as cepstral analysis using CSL. The acoustic measures were made over the central 1 s of the sustained vowel /a/. The same six acoustic measures were selected to use as input to train the SOM. The six measures included APQ, DVB, RAM, SPI, STD, and VAM.

The perceptual ratings of voice quality were made pre- and posttreatment for each of the 50 individuals diagnosed with functional dysphonia. The samples used were taken from audiotape recordings of functionally dysphonic patients obtained prior to and immediately following a single treatment session. Each stimulus used in the experiment consisted of the middle 1 s of the sustained vowel /a/. Each 1-s sample was digitized (22 kHz sampling rate), and a raised cosine taper was applied to the initial and final 20 ms of the sample to eliminate any audible "clicks" associated with abrupt onset and offset of the acoustic signal. Six subjects participated in the listening experiment. However, one subject was dropped from the subsequent analysis because of technical difficulties. Each subject participated in two separate, but identical, listening sessions separated by approximately 2 weeks. Subjects were seated in an audiometric listening booth, and the stimuli were randomly presented at a comfortable loudness from a loudspeaker placed 1 meter from the subject. The subjects were instructed to rate each voice sample on the severity of the voice quality disturbance using a free-modulus method of direct magnitude estimation (Engen, 1971). Briefly, such a procedure allows the subject to select his or her own modulus and rating system. Although such a method requires an additional transformation to eliminate individual differences in modulus choice, it is believed to reduce potential bias associated with the use of a standard modulus. The subject was allowed to listen to each stimulus up to three times before assigning a rating. The rate of stimulus presentation was controlled by the subject. To allow direct comparison of ratings within and across subjects and stimuli, the raw data were transformed according to a standard method outlined by Engen (1971). In summary, the average severity ratings from five different subjects on two separate occasions across pre- and posttreatment voice samples were obtained and used to evaluate the performance of the self-organizing map.

The SOM contained a 6-node input layer, corresponding to each of the input parameters, and a 6-by-5-node representational layer. A hexagonal neighborhood lattice was used in training, as recommended by Kohonen (1995) for better visual inspection of the map. Ten self-organizing maps were trained using different initial random weights. The SOM with the lowest overall quantization error was selected for further analysis. The self-organizing maps were trained in two steps. The first step was for 2,000 iterations through the entire data set with a neighborhood radius that decreased from 6 to 0 and a learning rate that decreased from .09 to 0 over training. The second step was for 12,000 iterations through the entire data set with a neighborhood radius that decreased from 2 to 0 and a learning rate that decreased from .02 to 0 over training. This method of training in two steps, the first with a larger initial neighborhood radius and learning rate, is recommended by Kohonen (1995) for proper ordering of the weight strengths in a self-organizing map.

The resulting distribution of exemplars across the self-organizing map for the pre- and posttreatment functional dysphonia groups are displayed in Figure 8–4. The map does a good job at separating the pretreatment functional dysphonia group (red) from the posttreatment functional dysphonia group (yellow). Visualization of the SOM in Figure 8–4 shows that the pretreatment functional dysphonia group (PR) is widely distributed throughout the map, except in the extreme right top side of the map, which is the area mainly representing the posttreatment functional dysphonia group (PS). It can be easily seen that the PR group is much more spread out across the SOM than is the PS group.

Classification performance was determined by first assigning a group representation to each node. This was accomplished in the same manner as for the previous SOM. Classification performance for a stepwise discriminant analysis over the same acoustic dimensions as were used to train the SOM, and the classification performance of the self-organizing map are given in Tables 8–3 and 8–4, respectively (Table 8–5 displays the results of the stepwise discriminant analysis: RAM and APQ are the variables entered). The overall classification performance for the SOM is only marginally better than that of the stepwise discriminant analysis. The SOM correctly identified 88% of the exemplars correctly, whereas the stepwise discriminant analysis correctly identified 86% of the exemplars correctly. The SOM had marginally better predictive performance at classifying PR exemplars (PR = 92%) compared to that of the stepwise discriminant analysis over the original data (PR = 88%). The classification performance for PS exemplars was the same for both the SOM and the stepwise discriminant analysis (PS = 84%).

To determine how well the SOM codes for degree of pathology and efficacy of treatment, comparisons were made with perceptual ratings of voice quality. The mean perceptual rating scores of voice quality across the SOM are

Table 8–1. Classification results: Stepwise discriminant analysis over original data.

Total Correct	*82 68.3%*	***Predicted***							
		SD		***PR***		***PS***		***NR***	
N = 120		*No.*	*%*	*No.*	*%*	*No.*	*%*	*No.*	*%*
Actual	**SD** N = 30	**20**	**66.7**	3	10.0	7	23.3	0	0
	PR N = 30	5	16.7	**15**	**50.0**	9	30.0	1	3.3
	PS N = 30	1	3.3	2	6.7	**21**	**70.0**	6	20
	NR N = 30	0	0	0	0	4	13.3	**26**	**86.7**

Table 8-2. Classification results: Self-organizing map.

Total Correct	*82 68.3%*	***Predicted***							
		SD		***PR***		***PS***		***NR***	
N = 120		*No.*	*%*	*No.*	*%*	*NO.*	*%*	*No.*	*%*
Actual	**SD** N = 30	**22**	**73.3**	4	13.3	4	13.3	0	0
	PR N = 30	5	16.7	**22**	**73.3**	3	10	0	0
	PS N = 30	1	3.3	4	13.3	**22**	**73.3**	3	10
	NR N = 30	0	0	1	3.3	4	13.3	**25**	**83.3**

presented as a surface map in Figure 8–4. High values on the surface map (purple) denote good voice quality, whereas low values on the surface map (cyan) denote poor voice quality. Visualization of the map indicates that the highest voice quality ratings are in the region of the nodes that encode the PS exemplars, and the lowest voice quality ratings are in the region of the nodes that encode the PR exemplars with moderate voice quality ratings along bordering regions.

To determine if location on the map correlates with degree of voice quality, the distance of each exemplar on the SOM to the node with the highest voice quality rating was compared with the value of the highest voice quality rating minus the corresponding voice quality rating of the exemplar at hand. The results of a Pearson correlation indicate a significant relationship between position on the map and degree of voice quality ($r = .6$, $p < .001$). These results suggest that the SOM

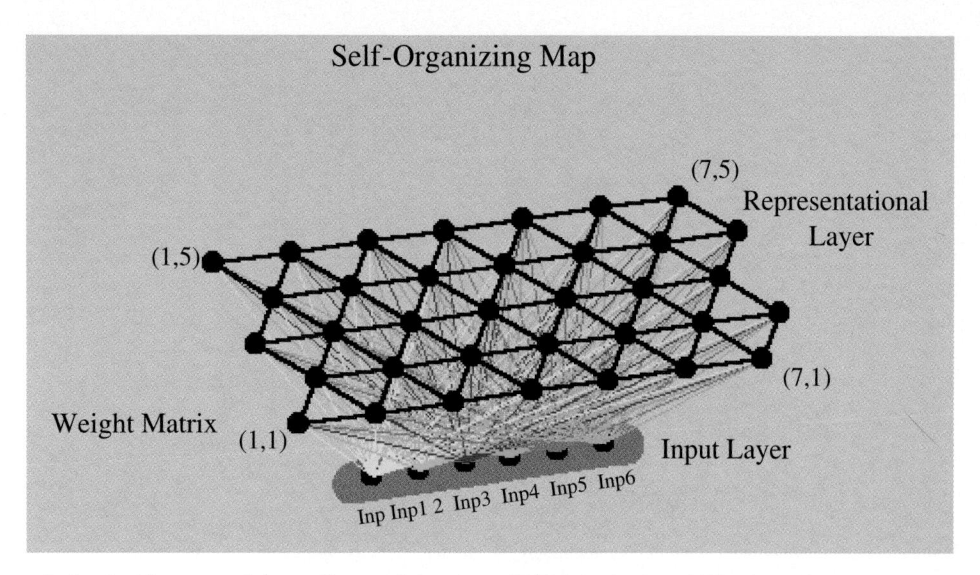

Figure 8–1. Architecture of the self-organizing map (SOM) is depicted. The input layer is composed of nodes (processing units) that encode the values of each of the input data parameters.

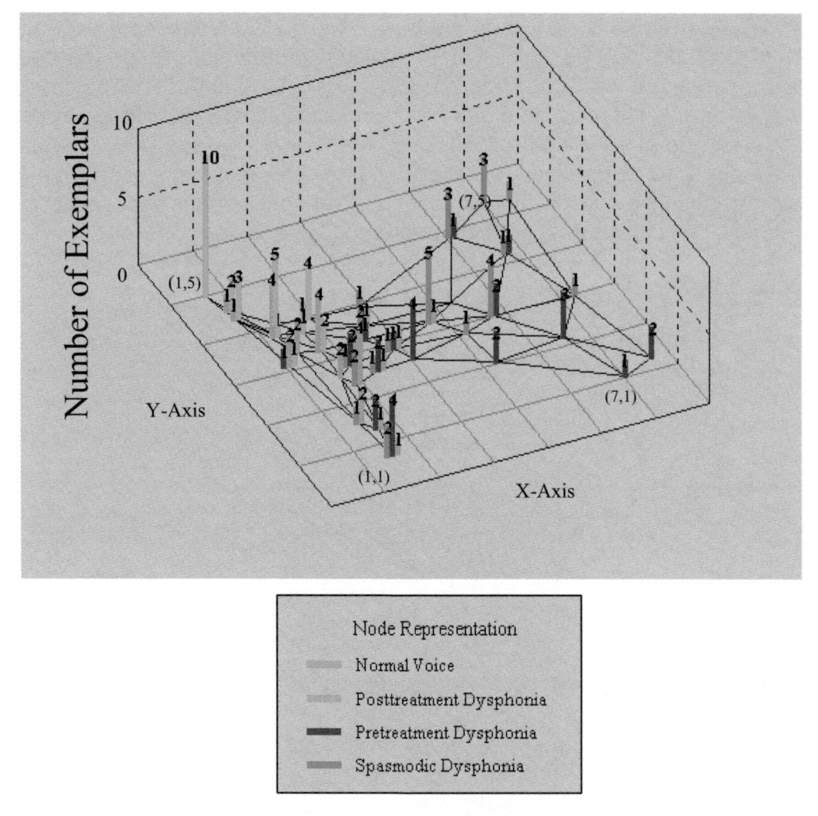

Figure 8–2. Figure two depicts the number of exemplars for each group across the nodes of the self-organizing map (blue = spasmodic dysphonia SD; red = pretreatment functional dysphonia PR; yellow = posttreatment functional dysphonia PS; green = normal voice NR) (Numeric values are given at the top of each bar). The x and y axes represent the Euclidean coordinates for each of the nodes defined by the Sammon mapping (Sammon, 1969). The node identifiers for each of the four corners of the SOM are given (1,1), (1,5), (7,5), and (7,1). See text for details. Figure 2 from Callan, Kent, Roy, and Tasko (1999).

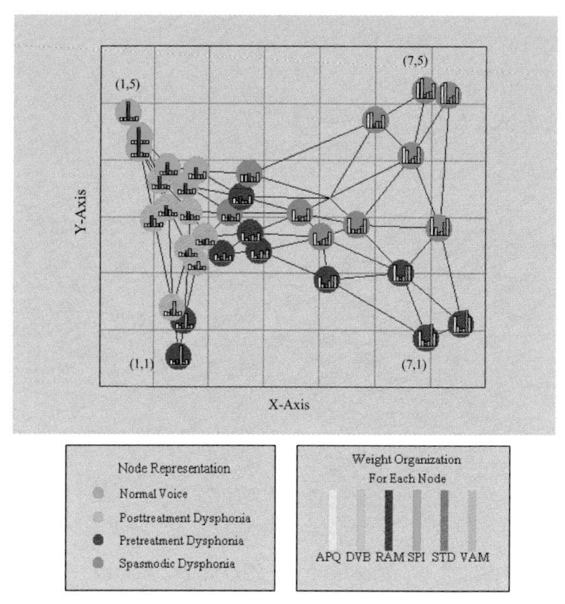

Figure 8–3. The strength of the weight values across the group node representations is shown, with (blue = spasmodic dysphonia SD; red = pre-treatment functional dysphonia PR; yellow = posttreatment functional dysphonia PS; green = normal voice NR) the SOM for each of the six underlying acoustic parameters (APQ, DVB, RAM, SPI, STD, and VAM). The x and y axes represent the Euclidean coordinates for each of the nodes defined by the Sammon mapping (Sammon, 1969). The node identifiers for each of the four corners of the SOM are given (1,1), (1,5), (7,5), and (7,1). The small bar plot on top of each node represents the strength of the corresponding weight values for each of the underlying acoustic parameters (from left to right—APQ, DVB, RAM, SPI, STD, and VAM). The relative importance of the underlying acoustic parameters in classifying the various groups across the SOM can be determined by comparing the pattern of the corresponding weight strengths to the regions of the SOM that represent the four groups. Figure 3 from Callan, Kent, Roy, and Tasko (1999).

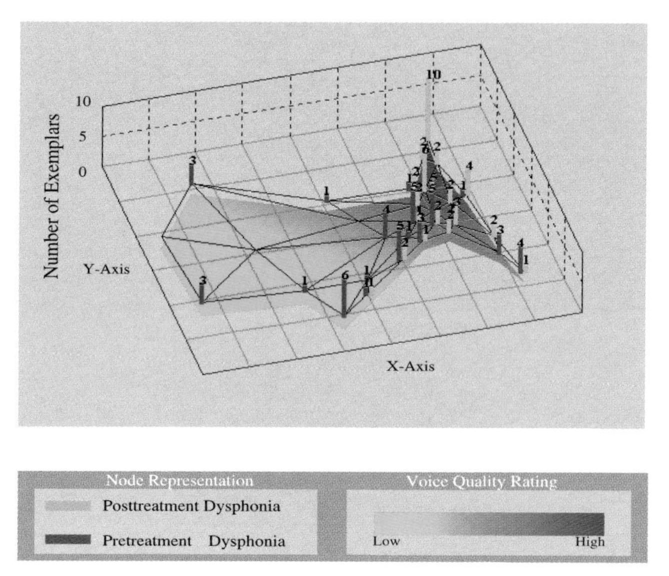

Figure 8–4. The number of exemplars are depicted for each group across the nodes of the self-organizing map (blue = spasmodic dysphonia SD; red = pretreatment functional dysphonia PR; yellow = posttreatment functional dysphonia PS; green = normal voice NR) (Numeric values are given at the top of each bar). The x and y axes represent the Euclidean coordinates for each of the nodes defined by the Sammon mapping (Sammon, 1969). The underlying surface map represents the mean voice quality rating for that node.

Table 8–3. Classification results: Stepwise discriminant analysis over original data.

Total Correct	*86 86%*	***Predicted***			
		PR		***PS***	
(N = 100)		*No.*	*%*	*No.*	*%*
Actual	**PR** N = 50	**44**	**88**	6	12
	PS N = 50	8	16	**42**	**84**

Table 8–4. Classification results self-organizing map.

Total Correct	*88 88%*	***Predicted***			
		PR		***PS***	
(N = 100)		*No.*	*%*	*No.*	*%*
Actual	**PR** N = 50	**46**	**92**	4	8
	PS N = 50	8	16	**42**	**84**

Table 8–5. Stepwise discriminant analysis of the original data for prefunctional and postfunctional groups ($N = 120$).

Step Entered	***Variable Entered***	***Wilks' Lambda***	***df***	***F***	***df1***	***Df2***	***Sig.***
1	RAM	.675	98	47.1	1	98	.001
2	APQ	.569	98	36.8	2	97	.001

At each step, the variable that minimizes the overall Wilks' Lambda is entered.

Minimum partial F to enter is 3.84.

Maximum partial F to remove is 2.71.

can code for degree of pathology across its surface.

To determine if the SOM codes for efficacy of treatment, the distance traveled across the map for each exemplar pretreatment to post-treatment was compared with the value of the post-treatment voice quality rating minus the pre-treatment voice quality rating. The results of a Pearson correlation indicate a significant relationship between distance traveled across the

SOM pre- to posttreatment and the improvement in voice quality ($r = .359$, $p < .05$). These results suggest that the SOM can code for efficacy of treatment across its surface.

The relative contribution of the six input parameters in the organization of nodes across the SOM is given by their corresponding weight strengths (see Figure 8–5). The small bar charts above each node representation in Figure 8–5 denote the strength of each of the corresponding weights (APQ, DVB, RAM, SPI, STD, and VAM). The region of the map that represents posttreatment functional dysphonic exemplars is characterized by high weight strengths for RAM and low strength values for most other weights. There are a couple nodes in the lower bordering region that have only moderate RAM values and moderate SPI values. The region of the map that represents prefunctional dysphonic exemplars is characterized by low weight strengths for RAM and high weight strengths for APQ and VAM. The closer the node is to the bordering region the lower are the relative APQ and VAM values. Nodes that classify PR that are farthest away from the bordering region are characterized by high APQ, DVB, STD, and VAM weight strengths. Nodes in the lower mid portion of the map that classify PR are characterized by high weight strengths for APQ, VAM, and moderate strengths for STD. Another region that contains nodes that classify PR is characterized by high SPI weight strengths and low strengths for all other parameters. To determine which of the weights accounted for most of the variance in predicting the mean voice quality rating for each node across the SOM, a stepwise multiple regression was carried out (see Tables 8–6 and 8–7). The results of the stepwise multiple regression indicate that APQ and RAM are the

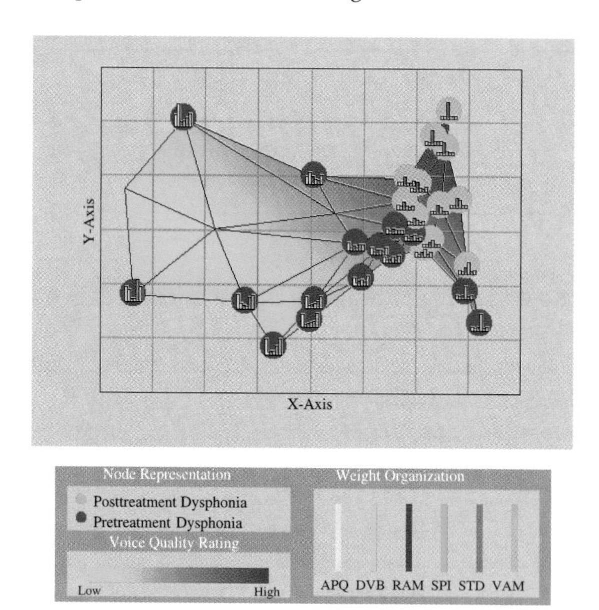

Figure 8–5. The strength is shown of the weight values across the group node, representations, (red = pretreatment functional dysphonia PR; yellow = posttreatment functional dysphonia PS) of the SOM for each of the 6 underlying acoustic parameters (APQ, DVB, RAM, SPI, STD, and VAM). The x and y axes represent the Euclidean coordinates for each of the nodes defined by the Sammon mapping (Sammon, 1969). The underlying surface map represents the mean voice quality rating for that node. The small bar plot on top of each node represents the strength of the corresponding weight values for each of the underlying acoustic parameters (from left to right—APQ, DVB, RAM, SPI, STD, and VAM). The relative importance of the underlying acoustic parameters in classifying the various groups across the SOM can be determined by comparing the pattern of the corresponding weight strengths to the regions of the SOM that represent the two groups.

Table 8–6. Stepwise linear regression of the node weights for mean voice quality ratings across the SOM.

Step Entered	*Variable Entered*	*R*	*df*	*F*	*df1*	*Df2*	*Sig.*
1	APQ	.817	28	56.1	1	28	.001
2	RAM	.843	28	4.1	2	27	.053

Minimum partial F to enter is 3.84.
Maximum partial F to remove is 2.71.

Table 8–7. Stepwise discriminant analysis of the node weights for prefunctional and postfunctional classifications across the SOM.

Step Entered	*Variable Entered*	*Wilks' Lambda*	*df*	*F*	*df1*	*Df2*	*Sig.*
1	RAM	.495	28	28.6	1	28	.001
2	APQ	.397	28	20.5	2	27	.001

At each step the variable that minimizes the overall Wilks' Lambda is entered.
Minimum partial F to enter is 3.84.
Maximum partial F to remove is 2.71.

best independent predictors of mean voice quality rating across the nodes of the SOM.

The self-organizing map trained on acoustic parameters with corresponding voice quality ratings provided for a means to evaluate how well the SOM codes for degree of pathology and efficacy of treatment. Besides the normal advantages afforded by the use of self-organizing maps (e.g., ease of visualization of the various groups, relative contribution of the acoustic parameters in distinguishing between the different groups, and at least as good statistical predictability as stepwise discriminant analysis) perceptual ratings of voice quality for each exemplar pre- and posttreatment allowed for several statistical analyses to be conducted. Correlation analyses indicated significant relationships between position on the map and degree of voice quality as well as distance traveled across the SOM pre- to posttreatment and the corresponding improvement in voice quality. The results of these analyses demonstrate the ability of a SOM trained on acoustic parameters to encode both the degree of voice pathology and efficacy of treatment across its surface.

4. CONCLUSION

It has been demonstrated that self-organizing maps are an informative tool in the analysis of voice disorders. The work summarized in this chapter complements earlier research by showing that self-organizing maps based on acoustic measures of a brief sample of vowel phonation reveal interesting features of voice disorders and have good potential for classification of these disorders. In addition, it has been demonstrated through a combined use of acoustic and perceptual data, that an acoustic interpretation can be given to perceptual judgments of voice quality. Self-organizing maps are a useful form of analysis for both acoustic measures and voice quality ratings. The classification performance of these maps is at least as good as stepwise discriminant analysis procedures, and the maps offer other advantages, especially visualization of the analysis results. Research in the use of self-organizing maps with other acoustic measures, other voice pathologies, and other vocal tasks should further define the potential of this method.

It has been demonstrated that self-organizing maps are a beneficial tool in the analysis of voice disorders. Most of the application of self-organizing maps to the classification of voice disorders has been conducted using very small databases. To achieve optimal results at classification across a SOM, it is necessary to use a much larger database for training and then to evaluate the performance of the map with a novel data set. In the case of the SOM trained on multiple acoustic measures it can be seen that, from the 24 possible measures available, only a few were used as input parameters. With a larger database it will be possible to use more input parameters for training. One of the problems of selecting the acoustic measures used in training the SOM is the great deal of correlation between the acoustic measures. With a larger database one might avoid this problem by carrying out a principle components analysis over all of the 24 acoustic measures to reduce the input dimensions to the SOM and preserve the independent relationships among all the acoustic measures. The use of larger databases that incorporate both acoustic measures and perceptual rating scales will allow for self-organizing maps to be trained on both types of data. The resultant SOM formation trained on both types of data may provide enhanced performance at classification of voice disorders than either type of data alone. It is import ant to note that these SOM were trained only using acoustic parameters of sustained phonation. The addition of acoustic parameters of continuous speech should enhance the predictive power of the SOM at classifying individuals with voice disorders.

Acknowledgment

Many portions of this article appear in Callan, Kent, Roy, and Tasko (1999). This work was supported in part by NIH research grant number 5 R01 DC 00319-11, as well as by the National Center for Voice and Speech Grant number P60 00976 from the National Institute on Deafness and Other Communication Disorders.

REFERENCES

Callan, D., Kent, R., Roy, N., & Tasko, S. (1999). Self-organizing map for the classification of normal and disordered female voices. *Journal of Speech, Language, and Hearing Research,* 42.

Engen, T. (1971). Psychophysics. II. Scaling methods. In J.W. Kling & L.A. Riggs; *Woodworth & Schlosberg's Experimental psychology,* New York: Holt, Rinehart and Winston.

Hirano, (1981). *Clinical examination of voice.* Wein: Springer-Verlag.

Kay Elemetrics Corp. (1994). *Disordered voice database. Version 1.03.* Boston, MA: Massachusetts Eye and Ear Infirmary, Voice and Speech Lab.

Kohonen, T. (1982). Self-organized formation of topologically correct feature maps. *Biological Cybernetics, 43,* 59–69.

Kohonen, T. (1995). *Self-organizing maps.* Berlin: Springer, 77–127.

Kohonen, T., Hynninen, J., Kangas, J., & Laaksonen, J. (1996). *SOM_PAK: The Self-Organizing Map Program Package: Report A31.* Helsinki: Helsinki University of Technology, Laboratory of Computer and Information Science.

Leinonen, L., Hiltunen, T., Kangas, J., Juvas, A., & Rihkanen, H. (1993). Detection of dysphonia by pattern recognition of speech spectra. *Scandinavian Journal of Logopedie Phoniatrica, 18,* 159–167.

Leinonen, L., Hiltunen, T., Laakso, M., Rihkanen, H., & Poppius, H. (1997). Categorization of voice disorders with six perceptual dimensions. *Folia Phoniatrica und Logopedie, 49,* 9–20.

Leinonen, L., Kangas, J., Torkkola, K., & Juvas, A. (1992). Dysphonia detected by pattern recognition of spectral compostion. *Journal of Speech and Hearing Research, 35,* 287–295.

Rihkanen, H., Leinonen, L., Hiltunen, T., & Kangas, J. (1994). Spectral pattern recognition of improved voice quality. *Journal of Voice, 8,* 320–326.

Sammon, J. (1969). A non-linear mapping for data structure analysis. *IEEE Transactions on Computers, 18,* 401–409.

PART II

Instrumental Assessments

In Part I of this book, contributors explored advances in the auditory-perceptual description of voice quality. However, as we pointed out in Chapter 1, it is generally accepted in current research that the impressionistic nature of perceptual description should be augmented by the more "objective" nature of instrumental analysis where possible. (It is important, however, not to assume that instrumental approaches are somehow "correct" or "infallible." Limits on accuracy exist with all techniques, and the interpretation of results is not always straightforward.)

Instrumental techniques in speech analysis break down into three main areas: those that are used to investigate speech production (for example, airstream initiation, vocal fold activity, nasal/oral airflow, and articulator movement and placement); those that are used to examine the sound waves that result from speech production activity (for example, frequency, intensity, and duration measures and how they alter during specific parts of the utterance under investigation); and those that can be employed to look at the perception of speech (for example, to ascertain the most important acoustic cues used to discriminate between sound classes).

The techniques described in this part of the book cover these three areas of investigation, as applied specifically to the study of voice quality. Eugene Buder provides a most thorough coverage of acoustic measures that have been used in voice analysis (using any of the many readily available acoustic analysis systems now on the market). Each of the measures dealt with is provided with the algorithm that is used to produce it, and with a description and set of references to studies that have used this particular measure. Acoustic approaches to voice quality measurement have been widely used in the literature, and Buder's chapter will allow readers access to definitions of most measures they will encounter.

Articulatory studies of voice need to cover a range of topics: airflow and vocal fold activity being the main ones. In Robert Hillman and James Kobler's chapter, the main aerodynamic parameters important in voice analysis, and how they can be measured by modern airflow instrumentation, are described. The chapter also discusses how aerodynamic measures can be incorporated into the routine clinical assessment of patients with speech disorders: it is clearly important that instrumental techniques are made accessible to the clinician wherever possible.

The two chapters by Bert Cranen and F. de Jong and by Shigeru Kiritani look at methods for directly imaging the vocal folds. Cranen and de

Jong discuss stroboscopy, where recent developments with flexible endoscopes have allowed clinicians to image vocal fold activity during connected speech with minimal disruption to the articulators. Stroboscopic light sources have normally been used with endoscopic investigations of vocal fold vibration, as otherwise the movement of the folds is not possible to see due to the high frequency of their vibratory cycle. Kiritani describes in his chapter a high speed camera system that allows individual frames to be recorded without the need for stroboscopy. Forty-five hundred frames per second are recorded via this system, allowing for detailed examination of vocal fold movement. Other imaging techniques are not described in this collection: x-radiography is much less commonly encountered today due to the inherent dangers of exposure to radiation, and newer techniques are either rarely available, or have yet to be applied to voice research to any extent.

Indirect imaging of vocal fold activity is possible through the use of the electroglottograph (EGG). This has become an established technique in voice research, and Evelyn Abberton and Adrian Fourcin describe the latest versions of EGG equipment in their chapter, together with a discussion of different measures EGG systems provide. The authors illustrate their chapter with a range of clinical examples, showing the type of readings one would expect for the different voice types.

The final chapter in this section looks at speech synthesis techniques and how they can be applied to voice quality measurement. Analysis by synthesis has long been used as a method of examining listeners' perceptions of speech and which aspects are most important. In this chapter, Bangayan and colleagues describe an experiment in which the voice qualities of a range of speakers with voice disorders were synthesized. Perceptual evaluation by trained judges allowed the authors to discuss how their synthesizer might be improved to include parameters important in the perception of voice quality.

Part II completes a survey of how we can describe and measure voice quality and sets the scene for the final part where specific voice disorder types are dealt with.

CHAPTER

9

Acoustic Analysis of Voice Quality: A Tabulation of Algorithms 1902–1990

Eugene H. Buder

This chapter documents algorithms for the acoustic analysis of voice quality. The algorithms are presented in tables, with the goal of organizing them into a small set of optimally comprehensive and mutually exclusive categories. Accordingly, the tables are nested under categories corresponding to acoustic representations or parameters : (1) F_0, (2) amplitude, (3) F_0/amplitude (4) waveform, (5) spectrum, (6) glottal waveform, and (7) dynamic aspect. Within most of these categories, smaller methodological divisions are defined as subtables, and the perturbation divisions of Tables 9–1.2 and 9–2.2 are further divided into short- and long-term subtables. Some studies employed voice quality algorithms to evaluate methodological, theoretical, psychoacoustic, or synthesis matters rather than empirically obtained voice qualities. Such studies falling within the covered period are tabulated in Appendix 9–A. Appendix 9–B summarizes algorithmic expressions devised by Pinto and Titze (1990) for unifying short-term perturbation measures. The 15 tables and 2 appendixes appear as:

The chapter also includes a reference list representing as broadly as possible the scientific literature including acoustic analysis of voice quality: Well over 500 such references are listed in this chapter. Many of the studies are described in notes associated with the specific algorithms employed, but those not described at that level are cited at the head of the appropriate table (including citations after 1990). Some of the most informative acoustic studies of voice quality have used a complement of measures spanning several of the tables defined here, yet virtually all algorithms developed between 1902 and 1990 could be assigned to a specific table by this scheme. Some algorithms, however, might easily have been assigned to more than one table. For example, the F_0 statistics, long-term F_0 perturbation, and dynamics categories tend to compete for certain simple algorithms. In such cases, assignments were based on the time-sampling nature of the result: F_0 statistics are reserved for quantities that summarize in a stochastic or ergodic manner entire production units at least as large as the utterance, such as mean speaking fundamental frequency. Long-term F_0 measures may apply to sample segments of utterances but can still be summarized over some short-term time span, such as tremor measures. The dynamics category is reserved for deterministic moment-to-moment trajectories described in terms of onsets/offsets, continuities/noncontinuities, or in dynamic systems terminology, such as fractal dimension.

In nearly each table, four columnar entries appear per algorithm: "measure," "unit," "algorithm," and "notes." "Measure" assigns a name to an algorithm, usually giving deference to the chronologically first published report describing that algorithm, although sometimes expanding names as necessary to resolve conflicts and clarify distinctions. "Unit" presents the dimension or dimensions of the quantity produced by the algorithm. In cases for which this was difficult to determine, descriptions from the original report are quoted. "Algorithm" specifies the steps, formula, or formulas defining a given measure. Although many readers may use these tables without exploring the internal details of the algorithm entry, the algorithm entries are the core information on which this chapter is based. To facilitate comparisons and a fluent "reading" of the algorithms, virtually all the algorithms have been more or less recast from their original publication into a codified notation system. The symbols and abbreviations of this system are keyed in the section following these introductory remarks.

The final general entry, "Notes," may be where most readers will dwell in these tables, as it includes brief synopses of sample studies employing the tabulated algorithm. The notes represent a quasiconsistent summary of the studies' subject group composition and size, task types, and general success of results. To facilitate visual scanning of the section for specific measure interpretations and previous applications groups, all words indicating a group characteristic (e.g., gender, pathology) and all words indicating a general voice quality (e.g., breathy, hoarse) are in bold print. Other comments in this section compare algorithms and their applications via links to other tables, discuss (unsystematically) aspects of the decision rule or statistical criterion by which algorithm success was determined, or review notable statements by specific authors.

The tables encompass the broadest possible construal of what may constitute voice quality. Given that real phonation is never naturally produced or heard simply as the product of vocal fold vibration in isolation from aerodynamic and acoustic coupling with the other structures of the vocal tract, it is undesirable to restrict acoustic analysis strategies exclusively to vocal fold action. Moreover, acoustic analysis per se must always operate in the domain of signal processing from which one-to-one associations with the physiology of voice production will generally not be possible. Therefore, from the point of view of acoustic analysis, any laryngeal *or* vocal tract movements or settings that may affect voiced sounds must be included (a fine distinction may be drawn, however, between those supralaryngeal settings to which a sonorant is susceptible, for example, "nasal," from those to which nonphonatory speech sounds may also be vulnerable, for example, "spirantized"—the latter do not fall within the purview of this chapter). Nor is it possible, given that natural voices are heard dynamically, to restrict naturally occurring voice quality to a static conception of tonal quality. Therefore, long-term dynamic and modulated voice movements, such as "hard onset" or "tremor," must be included along with the acoustic phenomena associated with more static percepts such as "harsh" or "breathy."

It may be important to state what this chapter does *not* do. First, as indicated by the title, the dates are circumscribed. Some justification of the onset at 1902 is provided in the next section of this introduction, but the cutoff at 1990 somewhat arbitrarily defines an "elbow," or point of rapid increase, in the growth of voice quality literature that includes acoustic analysis. This date could be seen to coincide with the first impact on the archival literature of personal computers on productivity in the application of acoustic algorithms to speech samples, stimulating productivity by both academic researchers and the speech and natural language processing industries. Although a reasonably comprehensive representation of the century's literature is provided in the bibliography of this chapter, a tabulation covering the 1990–1998 period with application notes was simply not possible in a chapter format. However, references from this period are listed and organized by table. Additionally, some notes overviewing major recent developments are offered in introductory sections to the tables, and developments of a few of the most widely used algorithm sets developed in the late 1980s are "grandfathered" and tracked into the 1990s (e.g., the new jitter algorithms found in the CSpeechSP [Milenkovic, 1997] program and the Kay Elemetrics [1993] Multi-Dimensional Voice Program [MDVP] set, but also some of the basic elements of nonlinear dynamic modeling that had been developed by 1990 but not yet applied to voice quality in the literature). Generally, where algorithms developed past 1990 are tabulated, no "notes" section is included. The availability in the early 1990s of software such as MDVP (Kay Elemetrics, 1993) has helped produce studies that assess a broad array of acoustic voice quality measures. Studies using MDVP that were therefore not easily assigned to a small subset of the tables are: Hertrich, Spieker, and Ackermann, 1998; Kent, Vorperian, and Duffy, 1999; Mendoza and Carballo, 1998; Morsomme, Orban, Remacle, and Jamart, 1997; Roy, Tasko, Callan, and Bless, 1997; Souaid, Tewfik, and Pelland-Blais, 1998; Van Lierde, Morerman, and Van Cauwenberge, 1996; Verdonck-de Leeuw, Koopsmans-van Beinum, Hilgers, and Keus, 1997; Wuyts, De Bodt, Bruckers, and Molenberghs, 1996.

As a second, and perhaps more disappointing limitation of this chapter, virtually no normative values or firm methodological prescriptions are provided other than general comments and caveats regarding broad interpretations in the table introductions and conclusion section. A decision not to offer such seemingly valuable and fundamental advice was based on the impression that the state-of-the-art is still in considerable flux, that is, the tabulated studies indicate an excessive diversity of possible methodological effects on most acoustic voice quality measures. A fuller understanding of real quantitative bedrock amidst the plethora of methods, materials, decision criteria, and algorithms that have been implemented for voice quality measurement awaits further developments and a truly comprehensive overview. This chapter may at least provide the framework under which such an overview could be conducted. The National Center for Voice and Speech (NCVS) workshop recommendations issued for application of short-term perturbation measures (Titze, 1995) is exemplary, but its implementation is still underway (pending, among other things, independent means for voice typing and less periodicity-dependence in signal processing). Moreover, similar developments for the whole complement of measures represented here are needed within the community of voice quality researchers. It therefore seems premature and lacking the authority of consensus to issue specific recommendations in this chapter.

Finally, as mentioned, notes on decision rules and interpretation of algorithm success are unsystematic in this chapter, meaning that many important observations of a statistical nature are available in the literature, but not fully summarized in the tables. When possible, algorithm successes are reported in terms of percentage correct classification for the target group, although statistics that account for variance are also occasionally reported when they represent measure validity. Other than a general attempt to include interesting correlations of a given measure with other variables, no other statistics are systematically included or discussed.

This chapter may be used in a variety of ways. Probably the most general function of the tables will be to guide the interested reader to the literature listed in the Reference list. The information in these tables is detailed and, hopefully, accurate, but any serious scholar in the area should check the original references using the table entries and references as leads to relevant sources. Such an approach would be especially useful for the investigator planning a study and wishing to identify prior research with similar measures, populations, voice quality type, and so on. The chapter should function, however, for more than resource location, perhaps leading an investigator to explore measures that have *not* been employed for a given population or to explore populations or voice qualities with measurement approaches borrowed from other topic areas.

Scientists with signal processing and programming skills who are motivated to develop or adapt their own algorithms should find the tables stimulating as a source of ideas. General readers may find the tables interesting as a sort of census, representing, by simple relative bulk in the following pages, the demographics and topography of the field. This approach might lead to a deeper understanding of how traditions and trends have caused certain measures to be widely and routinely applied over many decades, with others lying underutilized over the same period. Some older and relatively forgotten algorithms are certainly due for rediscovery and fruitful application. The classification of extant algorithms into 15 more-or-less distinct categories defined by acoustic parameter and/or analytic model, not to mention the variety of adaptations that have been explored within these categories, emphasizes the rich and multifaceted acoustic nature of voice quality. This array will hopefully encourage future studies in the area to consider the phenomenon from as many of these facets as possible, using as many of the appropriate tools as possible, and avoiding the fallacy that a single given measure or model can ever completely capture the essence of so rich an object of study.

In the remainder of this introduction, some historical notes are presented to overview the period that preceded the relatively vigorous and programmatic voice quality research that began in the 1960s and a listing of general references is provided. Other brief overviews are presented for each of the seven major table groups, including notes on the major developments of the current decade and a brief offering of some suggested directions for further developing the efficacy of acoustic analysis of voice quality.

1. THE FIRST SIX DECADES

Voice science certainly existed in the previous century (e.g., Garcia, 1855), but 1902 was an inaugural year for acoustic measures of voice quality with the publication of Scripture's *The Elements of Experimental Phonetics*. As described in his text, the preceding century had also seen important developments in sound reproduction (Thomas Alva Edison); harmonic resonance and theories of tone perception (Hermann Helmholtz); Fourier analysis of speech waveforms (Schneebeli); several French, German, Swedish, Dutch, and British acoustic phonetic investigations (most notably Rouselot and Koenig in France and Hermann in Germany); and a preliminary methodological report by Scripture in 1897 describing the "smoked drum" methods for tracing waveforms from gramophone recordings. However, Scripture's 1902 text, followed by his detailed empirical investigation in 1906 (*Researches in Experimental Phonetics: The Study of Speech Curves*), identified for programmatic application several measurement strategies for identifying vocal regularity and tone of voice in artistic speech. For example, Scripture's review of expiratory measures included a review of German work by Vietor examining variations in expiratory pressures accompanying "irritation, assertion, warning, and question" (Scripture, 1902, p. 218). Scripture was also seminal in introducing acoustic criteria for the study of speech melody and rhythm (e.g., through the extraction from waveforms of intonation contour; see also Scripture [1906] for a wealth of examples), referring to them as elements of speech quality. Some notes in his book about the study of waveforms were almost so specific as to constitute "algorithms." However, as they were developed on the basis of inadequate distinctions between source versus filter characteristics, they are not tabulated in this chapter's tables. Nonetheless, the acoustic phonetic approach to "paralinguistic" aspects of speech, such as "tone of voice" documented by Scripture supports retention of 1902 as the initial year of the traditions reviewed in this chapter. The publication of Castex's *Maladie de la voix* lent further inaugural weight to 1902 as an advent year in the development of empirical studies in voice quality. This text highlighted numerous objective techniques pertinent to voice measurement, such as early laryngography and spirometry, and discussed head versus chest registers and nasality in acoustic terms.

The ensuing decades of the century are punctuated by the world wars. Winckel (1965) summarizes early voice-dedicated (primarily European, i.e.,"phoniatric") instrumental analyses, including early spectrometer output in the 1920s and time-frequency spectrometry in the 1930s. Many sources from this period retain earlier confusions regarding formant/cavity affiliation, but the period also presages the inception of modern spectrographic analysis. Work in America, such as by Seashore and colleagues (e.g., wavelength variability work by Simon, 1927), Metfessal (1926), and Curtis, whose dissertation (1942) employed the Henrici analyzer to assess nasality, were paralleled by developments in Germany that culminated in Luchsinger and Arnold's 1949 clinical text (Luchsinger & Arnold, 1949, 1965). Arnold's 1955 review situates concepts such as median pitch, musical versus physiological range, and register in measured F_0 (Hz) terms. In the 1940s, Fairbanks framed the concepts of "harshness" and "breathiness" as separate contributors to "hoarseness" (1940).

As electronic instrumentation became more widely available to linguists as well as communication engineers, acoustic assessments of phonological rules for voice quality came into play (Pandit, 1957). Having measured natural period-to-period fluctuations, Schroeder and David (1960) used control over consecutive pitch periods to provide a more "natural" voice quality within the bandwidth constraints of the Vocoder. In related developments: the negative intraglottal pressure components of phonation were measured (van den Berg, Zantema, & Doornenbal 1957) and interpreted (van den Berg, 1958). Stroboscopy came into clinical use (Schönhärl, 1960) and high-speed films clarifying aspects of lateral vocal fold motion were summarized algorithmically by *open* and *speed* quotients (Timke, von Leden & Moore, 1959, see also Dunker & Schlosshauer, 1961). These quantities apply also to "acoustic" glottal flow waveforms recovered via inverse filtering methods—see Tables 9–6.1 and 9–6.2. Phonellegrams were still in use in the early sixties (Coleman, 1960;

Wendahl, Moore & Hollien, 1963), but Lieberman's 1961 report on perturbation measures inaugurated digital algorithmic analysis of voice quality.

2. GENERAL REFERENCES

A number of references pertinent to the acoustic analysis of voice quality have reviewed the literature, provided theoretical perspectives too broad to be listed in Appendix 9–A, or simply provide useful background information. These are recommended for further reading or historical interest: Baken, 1987; Baken and Orlikoff, 1992; Boves, 1984; Catford, 1964; Colton and Estill, 1981; Estill, Fujimura, Sawada, and Beechler, 1996; Fant, 1960; Fant, 1993; Fujimura, 1990; Fujimura and Hirano, 1995; Gerratt and Kreiman, 1994; Gould and Korovin, 1994; Hammarberg and Gauffin, 1995; Helfrich, 1979; Helfrich and Wallbott, 1986; Howard, 1998; Kent, 1993; Laver, 1980; Nolan, 1983; Pittam, 1994; Ramig and Ringel, 1983; Schoentgen and Bucella, 1997; Stevens, 1977; Strik and Boves, 1992a; Sundberg, 1987; Titze, 1992, 1994a, 1994b, 1995; Van Bezooyen, 1984; Winckel, 1974; Wirz and Mackenzie Beck, 1995; Zwicker and Fastl, 1990.

3. FORMULAS EMPLOYED IN THE CHAPTER TABLES

autocorrelation function (ACF)

$$r_\tau = \sum_{t=0}^{N-1-\tau} x_t x_{t+\tau},\ \tau = 0,1,\ldots, N-1$$

Hanning window

$hn(x) = 0.5 - \cos(2\pi x/N),\ x = 0,1,\ldots,N-1$

Hamming window

$hm(x) = 0.54 - 0.46\cos(2\pi x/N),\ x = 0,1,\ldots,N-1$

semitones for given f with respect to referent f_1:

$12\times\log(f/f_1)/0.30103$ [H. Fletcher's (1934) standard for f_1: 16.35 Hz (C^{-3}).]

4. SYMBOLS

x_t = acoustic voice signal (e.g., recordings of radiated or accelerometric speech sounds).

e_t = "error" signals (e.g., inverse filtered, LPC residual, or aperiodic noise residual).

t = discrete time sampling index, also sampling interval in ms.

f = frequency in hertz.

F_s = sampling frequency (1/t)

F0, F_0 = fundamental frequency.

f_c = critical frequency (e.g. of filter).

T0 = a fundamental period

A0 = amplitude (energy, or intensity if expressed on dB scale) integrated over a fundamental period.

A_i = amplitude (energy, or intensity if expressed on dB scale) integrated over a fixed frame.

P_i = any serial parameter (e.g., one of the above).

x_{t0} = samples comprising a fundamental period T0.

i,n = general time or frequency domain indexing variables.

$X_{n,i \text{ or } h}$ = Component(s) of discrete Fourier transform of xt.

h = frequency-domain indexing variable for harmonic components.

$X_{i \text{ or } h}(n)$ = Component(s) of discrete Fourier transform of xt from nth frame of data.

$W_{n \text{ or } i}$ = Selected component(s) of a discrete Fourier transform.

$H_{n \text{ or } i}$ = Harmonic component in frequency-domain.

B_n = Bandwidth of harmonic component in frequency-domain.

H_t = Harmonic component in time-domain.

$Noise_t$ = Noise component in time-domain.

K = Frame size, in samples.

Q = Frame shift value, in samples.

N = Sample size (sampled data points or frames of data).

T – Number of pitch periods.

N_i = Number of Frames.

k = smoothing factor.

m,r = variables representing partial counts of k.

α = filter coefficient.
M = filter order or point size of discrete Fourier transform.
τ = lag or offset.
r_τ = correlation at lag τ
j = imaginary number ( )
p_i = perturbation (differenced parameter) functions
σ = gain constant
Δ = difference

5. ABBREVIATIONS

s = seconds
ms = milliseconds
μs = microseconds
sps = samples per second
cps = cycles per second
Hz = hertz (cycles per second)
L = liters
$\log_{db}(y) = 10 \times \log_{10}(y)$, if y = signal power or intensity, and
$20 \times \log_{10}(y)$, if y = signal amplitude or energy (sound pressure or volts).
F1, 2, . . . = Formant Frequencies
A1, 2, . . . = Formant Amplitudes
BW = bandwidth
ACF = autocorrelation function (see Formulas [3.])
DC = direct current (0 Hz)
FIR = finite impulse response
FFT = Fast Fourier Transform
LPC = Linear Prediction Coefficients
HNR = Harmonics-to-Noise Ratio
SNR = Signal-to-Noise Ratio
NSR = Noise-to-Signal Ratio
RMS = Root Mean Square
MDVP = Multi-Dimensional Voice Program (Model 4305, Kay Elemetrics [1993])
P&T = Pinto and Titze's (1990) unification system

Table 9–1.1. F_0 Statistics.

It is impossible to overestimate the importance of fundamental frequency as a primary determinant of voice quality. Pitch and intonation are perhaps the most salient of all voice characteristics and changes in pitch bring concomitant changes in quality, even within register. Furthermore, the determination of fundamental frequency is usually (although not always) the basis upon which voice quality algorithms proceed; virtually all 15 tables in this chapter contain algorithms depending on the prior identification of fundamental period. Indeed, this is often a serious liability, as many voices deviate from periodicity so suddenly or drastically that algorithms tracking such deviations are doomed to fail, despite elaborate efforts to prevent such failures. See Hess (1983, 1994) and Titze and Liang (1993) for reviews. One widely used program, MDVP (Kay Elemetrics, 1993), makes use of the following steps to track F_0 (D. Deliyski, personal communication, October 1997):

1. Perform autocorrelation analysis (ACF) with user-selected analysis range parameters (default autocorrelation frame length of 30 ms).
2. Perform verification:
   a. Plot F_0 results;
   b. Check for results deviating >55% from preceding and following values;
   c. Examine whether deviating results are either a multiple of or division by an integer of either 2 or 3 of surrounding points:
      i. If integer multiple, divide back to restore continuity with surrounding results;
      ii. If integer division, multiply back to restore continuity with surrounding results, but update subharmonic frame count;
      iii. If not in integer relationship, reject result and update voiceless frame count.
3. Using expected results from steps 1 and 2, rerun autocorrelation analysis with frame length selected to fall short of two pitch periods.
4. Run peak-picking algorithm to search for glottal epochs consistent with results from step 3.
5. Perform linear interpolation for peak locations to surpass precision of sampling grid.

Even these elaborate steps yield vocal F_0 data that are sometimes plagued by tracking at subharmonics or complete drop-outs. It is therefore best to remember two basic caveats when considering results that depend on F_0 determination: (1) Acoustic-based fundamental frequency determination is virtually always designed to detect repeating cycles in a signal, and the results may therefore lack a useful correspondence to either perceptual pitch or to physiological vocal fold vibration. (2) Visual inspection of algorithm results is virtually always necessary as a precaution in any measures utilizing F_0 data, especially in disordered voices, and, even with the best algorithms, hand correction may be necessary for sensible results.

Table 9–1.1 lists measures that describe central tendency, dispersion, and distributional characteristics of F_0. These are generally obtained for entire speech unit productions, such as a sustained phonation, read passage, or a spontaneous speech sample lasting on the order of minutes. Intonation contours are also F_0 measures ($F_0 \times$ time) that have been correlated with voice qualities such as attitude and emotion since the beginning of the century (Scripture, 1906), but as their qualitative aspects are difficult to quantify algorithmically, they do not appear as a table entry. Nonetheless, the acoustic basis for the lay expression "tone of voice" certainly includes the intonation contour in conjunction with amplitude, duration, rhythm, and so on, suggesting that complex algorithms combining such parameters may yet be developed (at least within given language communities).

References reporting F_0 statistics that are not specifically noted in the following table are listed after the table.

Table 9–1.1. Continued

Measure	*Algorithm*	*Notes*
Central Tendency of F_0:		
Mean (often called SFF, or speaking fundamental frequency, when obtained from long-term connected speech samples)	$\frac{1}{N}\sum_{i=1}^{N} F0_i\,,\ (=\overline{F0}\,).$	Horii (1975) reports on sampling characteristics of means, medians, and variability measures (from speakers without pathology). He suggests that single sentence measures may be representative of larger sample means, but not of larger sample variabilities. The work also reports somewhat slow convergence of central tendency standard errors with successively larger time units; with 1-minute samples, however, standard deviations of the mean are approximately 1 Hz. Takahashi and Koike (1975) associated mean fundamental frequency with semantic differential terms "sharp, fast, small, light"— Cf. notes for FPQ and APQ. Hammarberg, Fritzell, Gauffin, Sundberg, and Wedin (1980), in a factor analytic perceptual summary of 17 read speech samples representing various **organic** and **functional** disorders, obtained moderately strong prediction for factor poles titled **coarse** (for females only) and **head register** using mean F_0. Hammarberg, Fritzell, Gauffin, and Sundberg (1986), in a similar study of 26 pathologic voices, explained 57% of variance in the **coarse** factor. Murry and Doherty (1980) found significant variance explained by lowered F_0 in a discriminant function analysis of 5 subjects with **vocal fold cancer**, although two of these subjects had F_0 means higher than the controls' average. Ludlow, Coulter, and Gentges (1983) found elevated F_0 for **Parkinson's disease**, but no effects in F_0 perturbation measures (see deviation from linear trend, Table 9–1.2a). Hufnagle and Hufnagle (1984) detected no change in speaking F_0 (SFF) after therapy for 8 females with **dysphonia** due to **nodules**. Sorensen and Horii (1984a) found no difference between F_0 central tendency and range between **male versus female pulse** registers. Linville and Fisher (1985) obtained a strong negative correlation of mean F_0 and **perceived age** and **chronological age** in sustained phonations by females aged 25 to 80, even though speakers were attempting to match a 210 Hz tone and stayed within a 200–220 Hz range (see also SD notes below and jitter ratio, Table 9–1.2a). Hirano, Hibi, Terasawa, and Fujiu (1986), in a study of 68 pathologic voice samples, obtained positive correlations of habitual F_0 with stroboscopically assessed regularity and (in polyp cases) symmetry of vibration, which they explained as gender effects. These researchers also observed an overall negative relation of habitual F_0 to perceived **hoarseness** on the GRBAS scale (see Hirano, 1981) and positive correlations with **breathy** and **strained** qualities in **carcinoma** cases. K.R. Scherer (1981, 1986a) reviews literature on vocal indicators of emotional states in which high pitch levels tend to indicate **happiness/joy, confidence, anger,** and **fear,** low pitch levels tending to indicate **indifference, contempt, boredom,** and **grief/sadness.** See Baken (1987) for additional information on normative F_0 values for adults with and without pathology, children, and infants. Garrett and Healy (1987) measured connected speech F_0 samples from 10 women and 10 men during morning, early afternoon,
Median	value that divides a histogram such that the number of observations above equals the number of observations below.	
Interquartile range	range that spans the central half of the observed values.	
Geometric (Preserves ratios among values; the geometric mean of two numbers is in the same proportion to the lower number as the higher number is to the mean.)	$\sqrt[N]{\prod_{i=1}^{N} F0_i}\,,$ or $\exp\left(\frac{1}{N}\sum_{i=1}^{N}\log_e F0_i\right)$	

Table 9–1.1. Continued

Measure	Algorithm	Notes
Central Tendency of F_0:		
RMS (root mean square).	$\sqrt{\frac{1}{N}\sum_{i=1}^{N} F0_i^2}$	and late afternoon, finding an increase across these times for men but not for women. W.S. Brown, Jr., Morris, and Michel (1990) measured SFF in readings by 19 **female aged professional singers** finding no significant differences in comparison to young women, but a significantly lower SFF for **aged women** without vocal training (but with no significant differences in sustained vowel phonation jitter between the three groups—see also SFF SD notes, below). This is an engineering definition for RMS as energy. In statistical contexts, the values entered into this formula may be deviations from mean, as in P&T system, Appendix 9–B.
Dispersion of F_0:		
Max, min, range(max–min)	Hz or semitones	Hollien and Michel (1968) defined **register** as "a series of or range of consecutive (vocal) fundamental frequencies of similar quality; in addition, there should be little or no overlap in fundamental frequency between adjacent registers" (p. 600). The authors demonstrated that fry was a register below modal by this criterion (cf. Hollien [1977] for re-labeling of this register as "pulse"). Hirano, Hibi, Terasawa, and Fujiu (1986), in a study of 68 pathologic voice samples, obtained a negative correlation of F_0 range with stroboscopically assessed regularity of vibration. They also observed a negative relation to perceived **asthenic** quality and (apparently as a mediated effect) a positive relation to **roughness** (GRBAS scale—Hirano, 1981). Ray (1986), in a study of one male voice with 214 listeners, found that increased pitch variation was predictive of 14% of variance in perceptions of **benevolence** and 4% of **competence**. K.R. Scherer (1981, 1986a) reviews literature on vocal indicators of emotional states in which wide pitch ranges tend to indicate **anger, fear,** and **contempt**, with narrow pitch ranges tending to indicate **indifference, boredom,** and **grief/sadness**. See Baken (1987) for additional information on normative F_0 variability and range values for adults with and without pathology, children, and infants. Mowrer, LaPointe, and Case (1987) found a significant difference between habitual speech F_0 and peak **laugh** F_0, although not for mean laugh initiation F_0.

Table 9–1.1. Continued

Measure	***Algorithm***	***Notes***
Dispersion of F_0:		
Standard deviation (SD)	$\sqrt{\frac{1}{N-1}\sum_{i=1}^{N}(F0_i - \overline{F0})^2}$	See Horii (1975) note for mean and median above. Murry and Doherty (1980) reported succesful discriminant function analysis of **vocal fold cancer** incorporating measurement of a higher F_0 SD (cf. mean F_0, this table, and DPF and JF notes, Table 9–1.2a). Horii (1985) reported an F_0 SD 5 times higher in **fry** than in modal register. Hammarberg et al. (1986) — see previous note for central tendency — obtained significant correlations for SD of F_0 with a perceptual **instability** factor (0.46) and with a perceptual **"overtight"** factor (0.32). Linville and Fisher (1985) obtained a positive correlation of F_0 SD and **perceived age**; this variable also had the highest loading on a discriminant function for **chronological age** in their study. K.R. Scherer (1981, 1986a) reviews literature on vocal indicators of emotional states in which large pitch variabilities tend to indicate **happiness/joy, anger,** and **fear**, with small pitch variabilities tending to indicate **indifference** and **grief/sadness**. Linville and Korabic (1987) measured F_0 SD (in semitones) in the sustained vowel phonations of 18 elderly women who were asked to keep the phonations as steady as possible, finding values on the order of 0.2–0.3, higher values for /a/ compared to /i/ and /u/, high intrasubject variability, and high overall variability (see also percent jitter, Table 9–1.2a, and Linville, 1987, for a review of phonatory measures on elderly women's voices). W.S. Brown, Jr., Morris, and Michel (1990) measured SFF SD in readings by 19 **female aged professional singers**, finding significantly higher SDs than in aged nonsinger women and young female speakers (with no significant differences between the latter two groups, and no significant differences in sustained vowel phonation jitter between the three groups).
Coefficient of variation (CV)	$\frac{\sqrt{\frac{1}{N-1}\sum_{i=1}^{N}(F0_i - \overline{F0})^2}}{\overline{F0}}$	This statistic normalizes SD to the mean. R.C. Scherer, Gould, Titze, Meyers, and Sataloff (1988) used CV of F_0 (in conjunction with CV of amplitude and jitter and shimmer, as well as EGG measures yielding adduction quotient data) as a "long-term perturbation" measure. They observed high CVs with low jitter and shimmer and vice versa, noting higher amplitudes at lower frequencies. Long- and short-term modulations could also be seen in plots of $F_0 \times$ amplitude from cases of **spasmodic dysphonia** and in events of **diplophonia**. Nikolov, Deliyski, Drumeva, and Boyanov (1989) describe a form of CV ("dFo") in a multidimensional program that evolved into MDVP, finding especially high values for **laryngeal cancer**.

Table 9–1.1. Continued

Measure	*Algorithm*	*Notes*
Other Basic F_0 Distribution Measures:		
Histogram	Distribution (number or percentage) of glottal pulse parameter (period or equivalent F_0).	Hecker and Kreul (1970) found reduced distribution in association with **vocal fold cancer**. Schultz-Coulon, Battmer, and Fedders (1979) determined using synthetic signals that the F_0 histogram width is independent (within limits) of noise in the signal. In analyses of **hyperfunctional dysphonia**, the authors suggested the F_0 histogram for detection of **vocal stability** (cf. their results with the "quotient histogram"). F_0 histograms are calculated and displayed as a component of the MDVP system.

Other Sources: Ackermann and Ziegler, 1994; Andrews and Schmidt, 1997; Apple, Streeter, and Krauss, 1979; Benson, 1995; Debruyne, Ostyn, Delaere, and Wellens, 1997; Deliyski, 1990; Deliyski, 1993; Deliyski, 1994; Estill, Baer, Honda, and Harris, 1985; S. Fex, Löfqvist, and Schalén, 1991; Graddol and Swann, 1983; Hachinski, Thomsen, and Buch, 1975; Hiller, Laver, and Mackenzie, 1983; Hiller, Laver, and Mackenzie, 1984; Holmberg, Perkell, Hillman, and Gress, 1994; Huffman, 1987; Kempster, Kistler, and Hillenbrand, 1991; Koike and Takahashi, 1972; Kuwabara and Ohgushi, 1984; LaBlance and Maves, 1992; Laufer and Horii, 1977; Laukkanen, Vilkman, Alku, and Oksanen, 1996; Linville, 1988; Linville, 1998; Maurer and Landis, 1996; Max and Mueller, 1996; Murry, Amundson, and Hollein, 1977; Murry, Brown, and Morris, 1995; Murry and Singh, 1980; Ng, Gilbert, and Lerman, 1997; Orlikoff and Baken, 1989b; Protopapas and Lieberman, 1995; Protopapas and Lieberman, 1997; Ptacek and Sander, 1966; L. O. Ramig, Scherer, Klasner, Titze, and Horii, 1990; Reich, Frederickson, Mason, and Schlauch, 1990; Rihkanen, Leinonen, Hiltunen, and Kangas, 1994; Risberg, 1962; Robbins, 1982; Roessler and Lester, 1979; Rosenfield, Viswanath, Herbrich, and Nudelman, 1991; Shipp and Huntington, 1965; Silbergleit, Johnson, and Jacobson, 1997; Stemple, Stanley, and Lee, 1995; Stoicheff, 1981; Strand, Buder, Yorkston, and Ramig, 1994; Sundberg and Askenfelt, 1983; Sussman and Sapienza, 1994; Traunmüller and Eriksson, 1995; Walton and Orlikoff, 1994; Whurr et al., 1993; Wieser, 1980; C.E. Williams and Stevens, 1972; C.E. Williams and Stevens, 1981; Wolfe, Cornell, and Palmer, 1991; Wolfe, Fitch, and Cornell, 1995; Wolfe and Ratusnik, 1988; Yonick, Reich, Minifie, and Fink, 1990.

Table 9–1.2a F_0 Perturbations (Short Term).

The quasiperiodic nature of the voice is perhaps its most "human" quality, as deviation from pure periodicity seems to be required for "naturalness." Scripture (1906) was probably the first to make note in print that glottal cycles are quasiperiodic, writing that "the glottal tone is never still, even within a very short vowel" (p. 41). Later, in 1916, Scripture observed excessive irregularity in waveforms of sustained phonations produced by speakers with disorders (e.g., multiple, or "disseminated," sclerosis) whose laryngeal control could be described as "ataxic." Although Lieberman is often credited with originating "perturbation" research in 1961, the first documented quantification seems to have been by Simon (1927), and in 1960 Schroeder and David measured pitch period fluctuations against a 3-point moving average to improve vocoder quality, therefore anticipating what would later become known as the relative average perturbation, or RAP measure.

The fate of F_0 perturbation, or jitter, measures for voice quality has been dramatic. The measure is historically the most widely applied, but has recently foundered on methodological and conceptual grounds. Put simply, algorithms attempting to measure deviation from periodicity reach their limits when that very periodicity becomes weak or its analysis becomes affected by other sources of fluctuation and/or modulation. A significant degree of slippage between signal characteristic and perceptual outcome has been another source of difficulty. The most authoritative statement reviewing these and other problems with jitter (and amplitude shimmer) measures is the National Center for Voice and Speech workshop statement issued in 1995 (Titze, 1995). Nonetheless, a review of this and other tables in this chapter may provide additional insight into the basic measure and its alternatives; note in particular the sporadically acknowledged observation that many instances of pitch period fluctuation are clearly not random. See also important psychophysical results in Appendix 9–A and the codification and classification of measurement procedures offered by Pinto and Titze (1990) summarized in Appendix 9–B.

Perhaps because of the very widespread use of F_0 perturbation measurement, the following table includes measure titles that have been inconsistently used, sometimes even by the same authors. The same title may be used for algorithms that begin sometime with frequency estimates and sometimes with period measurements (the latter is more correct for a potentially nonrepeating event such as a single perturbed cycle, but the difference is actually arbitrary once successive glottal cycles have been identified). Other times a given "ratio" may be multiplied by 100 to become a percentage, by 1,000 to become a measure indexing tenths of percentage points, or left as a simple ratio, all under the same title (e.g. jitter ratio). The most common currently adopted form of f0 perturbation is some measure describing single-cycle deviations from a smoothed average, but the same term, that is, RAP, may be used for a deviation from a 3-cycle or a 5-cycle moving average. The following table is offered, therefore, not necessarily as a definitive resolution of these inconsistencies, but simply as a survey of the array of measurement approaches; deference to historical precedent was attempted as a way to minimize the inconsistencies.

References reporting short-term F_0 perturbations that are not specifically noted in the following table are listed at the end of the table.

Table 9–1.2a Continued

Measure	*Unit*	*Algorithm*	*Notes*
Simon's (1927) measures of wavelength perturbation in photographic records of tonoscope waveforms	Minimal units of 0.1 mm from film moving at 2,000–2,500 mm/sec	Wavelength measures converted to Hz and summarized over 50 wavelength cycles	Simon (1927) measured **trained and untrained** vocalists' sustained ("sung") /a/ phonations, finding reduced fluctuations in trained vocalists by all 4 measures. Recognizing the need to eliminate longer-term fluctuations, Simon also measured deviations from sinusoidal and linear trends, still replicating his observations on trained voices. Measuring glide tones, he also observed smaller fluctuations on falling tones compared to rising tones for all vocalists.
	1. Number/50	1. Number of measurable wavelength changes 2. Greatest wavelength change	
	2. % of dominant tone	3. Sum of changes/50	
	3. Average of wavelength changes in total sample 4. Average of wavelength change	4. Sum of changes/number of measured changes	
Percentual variability and coefficient of consistency (Scripture, 1933)	%	From film records of phonation waveforms, translate mm into time, measure glottal pulse epochs by noting "sharp upward jerks," translate into Hz to obtain $F0_i$. percentual variability $= \frac{\frac{1}{N}\sum_{i=1}^{N}\lvert F0_i - \overline{F0}\rvert}{\overline{F0}}$ coefficient of consistency $= \frac{\overline{F0}}{\frac{1}{N}\sum_{i=1}^{N}\lvert F0_i - \overline{F0}\rvert}$	In a reanalysis of Janvrin's (1933) data, Scripture proposed percentual variability as a measure of **laryngeal ataxia** and its inverse coefficient of consistency as a measure of laryngeal eutaxia, finding variability measure of 4% for her control subject and measures of 17% and 33% for her two subjects with **disseminated (i.e., multiple) sclerosis**.

Table 9–1.2a Continued

Measure	*Unit*	*Algorithm*	*Notes*
Pitch perturbation ($\Delta T0$)	ms	$\lvert T0_i - T0_{i-1} \rvert$ Series of $\Delta T0$ over i represented in P&T system by first order perturbation function p_i^k	Lieberman (1961) instituted programmatic research into "perturbations" in a hand analysis of oscillographic display of sentence material (of 7,000 cycles). He noted correlation with period up to 6 ms and reduction during emotional modes "that seemed to require greater conscious vocal control in their production." He also noted a "hysteresis" effect of alternating long and short cycles, investigated by lag 1 and lag 2 serial correlation coefficients.
Mean absolute period jitter	ms or µs	$\frac{1}{N-1}\sum_{i=1}^{N-1} \lvert T0_i - T0_{i+1} \rvert$	Implemented in Horii's SEARP program (Horii, 1975) F_0 which uses a peak-picking method of F_0 detection. Horii (1979), analyzed synthetic and actual male nonpathological phonations with F_0 values ranging from 98–298 Hz digitized at 40 kHz sampling rates to obtain a µs order of precision, and found a linear increase in absolute jitter with increasing F_0 to 210 Hz and level values above, but level jitter ratios to 210 Hz and increasing values above. This work also found variable errors with differences in sampling rate (although not always overestimation of jitter with lower F_s). Ludlow, Bassich, Connor, Coulter, and Lee (1987), measuring jitter in long sustained phonation samples, obtained significant discrimination between 34 patients with **laryngeal pathology** and 99 control subjects only in males and not in females, with an overall correct classification of about 79%, and 100% classification of **carcinoma** and **partial laryngectomy**, but relatively poor classification of **polyps** or **nodules, edema,** or **unilateral**

Table 9–1.2a Continued

Measure	***Unit***	***Algorithm***	***Notes***
			paralysis (see also absolute shimmer, Table 9–2.2a). Orlikoff (1989) reviews cardiovascular and neuromuscular jitter-inducing mechanisms that may help explain nonlinear relations between absolute jitter and F_0. He postulates cardiovascular influence as a deterministic influence and motor unit noise as a random influence, both likely to have varying degrees of influence at different F_0 levels.
Normalized mean absolute period jitter, (Feijoo & Hernández, 1990)	μs	$\frac{1}{MXP}\frac{1}{N}\sum_{i=1}^{N}\lvert T0_{i+1} - T0_i\rvert$, where $MXP = \max(T0_i)$	Feijoo and Hernández (1990) measured this form of jitter in sustained /e/ phonations by 56 individuals with **glottic cancer** (stages T1–T4) and 64 control speakers, obtaining 77% classification success and correlations of 0.75 with both **hoarseness** and **breathiness** ratings. All other measures applied to this dataset were superior in classification (normalized mean absolute shimmer [Table 9–2.2a], VF [Table 9–4.0], D and NNE [Table 9–5.2], and CE [Table 9–5.4]).
Mean absolute frequency jitter		$\frac{1}{N-1}\sum_{i=1}^{N-1}\lvert F0_i - F0_{i+1}\rvert$	Horiguchi, Haji, Baer, and Gould (1987) compared acoustic to electroglottographic sustained phonation sources for absolute jitter in semitones, finding superior detection for EGG-jitter for discrimination of normal and **dysphonic** speakers (58% correct detection for EGG v. 16% for acoustic). See also notes on EGG-shimmer, Table 9–2.2a, absolute shimmer entry.
Percent Jitter	100 × ratio of deviation in *T0* to mean T0		Horii (1985) demonstrated greater percent jitter in **fry** (mean value of 2.47) than in modal register (mean 0.87) in healthy speakers—absolute

Table 9–1.2a Continued

Measure	Unit	Algorithm	Notes
		$100 \times \frac{\frac{1}{N-1}\sum_{i=1}^{N-1}\lvert T0_i - T0_{i+1}\rvert}{\frac{1}{N}\sum_{i=1}^{N} T0_i}$, or $100 \times \frac{\frac{1}{N-1}\sum_{i=1}^{N-1}\lvert F0_i - F0_{i+1}\rvert}{\frac{1}{N}\sum_{i=1}^{N} F0_i}$	jitter and F_0 SD were also greater for fry (see also absolute shimmer, Table 9-2.2a). Linville and Korabic (1987) measured percent jitter in 18 **elderly** women's sustained phonations, finding average values in excess of 1%, high variabilities, significantly higher values in /a/ (versus /i/ and /u/), high intra-subject variability, and high overall variability (SDs on the order of 1%–2%). (See also F_0 SD, Table 9–1.1, and Linville, 1987, for a review of phonatory measures on elderly women's voices). Also implemented in GLIMPES (R.C. Scherer et al., 1988; Titze and Liang, 1993). Ringel and Chodzko-Zajko (1987) review studies on biological age and report data comparing good and **poor physiological status in older** (c. aged 60) **speakers.** Using percent jitter, shimmer, HNR, and F_0, they obtained a significant discriminant analysis (75% classification success) and moderate but significant correlations of under-estimations of age with reduced levels of these measures. R.C. Scherer et al. (1987) measured declining trends in (by order of effect size): percent jitter, shimmer, and HNR_{Yumoto} with progression of **vocal fatigue** in a **trained singer,** but not in an untrained speaker. See R.C. Scherer et al. (1988) in Table 9–1.1, CV of F_0, for notes on long- versus short-term perturbations. Linville et al. (1990) measured percent jitter in 14 **elderly men**'s and 14 **elderly women**'s repeated sustained phonations of /i/, /a/, and /u/, comparing a fixed protocol of measuring 100 cycles after the 1st s of phonation to a protocol of measuring the steadiest 100 cycles. Although a significant reduction in jitter was obtained in the latter protocol, the authors observed that intertrial variability

Table 9–1.2a Continued

Measure	*Unit*	*Algorithm*	*Notes*
Normalized jitter, or 100 × PM ("perturbation magnitude" in Kasuya, Ogawa, Kikuchi, & Ebihara, 1986)	%, or proportion for PM.	$100 \times \frac{1}{N-1}\sum_{i=1}^{N-1}\left\|\frac{T0_i - T0_{i+1}}{T0_i}\right\|$ or $100 \times \frac{1}{N-1}\sum_{i=1}^{N-1}\frac{\|F0_i - F0_{i+1}\|}{F0_i}$	was still so large as to require multiple tokens for reliable estimation, especially for women. Zyski, Bull, McDonald, and Johns (1984) compared this "locally" normed measure (cf. the "globally" normed jitter factor, this table) with absolute jitter, RAP, PPF, and also four amplitude perturbation measures (shimmer, normalized amplitude perturbation, absolute amplitude perturbation, and 3-point smoothed amplitude perturbation; see Table–2.2a,) for discrimination of 52 **organic** and **functional dysphonias** from 20 controls (0.2 s samples of sustained "ahs" recorded with pretracheal accelerometers and digitized at 100 kHz), finding good performance on all measures except PPF, which suffered from a floor effect. Optimum discrimination was obtained with the remaining 3 pitch-based measures and absolute amplitude perturbation. Hammarberg et al. (1986), in a factor analytic perceptual summary of 17 read speech samples representing various **organic** and **functional** disorders, obtained significant correlations for normalized jitter with an **instability** factor (0.39).
Pitch perturbation factor (PPF)Lieberman (1961)	relative frequency	$\frac{\text{frequency of } \Delta T0 \geq 0.5 \text{ ms}}{\text{total number of } \Delta T0 \text{ in sample}}$	Lieberman (1963) applied this metric (following upon Lieberman, 1961) to laryngeal pathologies (changes in vocal fold morphology, e.g., tumors and polyps). Coupled with high-speed motion pictures, suggested cause: "transients in the air-pressure drop across the glottis"(Lieberman, 1963, p. 351). He devised the perturbation factor and observed correlations with larger growths but not smaller. He was also unable to measure periodicity in some extreme cases (advanced cancer, mul-

Table 9–1.2a Continued

Measure	*Unit*	*Algorithm*	*Notes*
Jitter ratio (JR) Jacob (1968)	1,000 × ratio of deviation in period to mean period	$1000 \times \frac{\frac{1}{N-1}\sum_{i=1}^{N-1}\lvert T0_i - T0_{i+1}\rvert}{\frac{1}{N}\sum_{i=1}^{N} T0_i}$	tiple polyps on both folds, large cysts). See PPQ_{EVX} entry following for Schoentgen's (1989) use of PPF. Calculated by SEARP program (see previous Horii [1979] note for absolute jitter). Jitter ratio was the less effective than mean or SD of F_0 in discriminating perceived or chronological age in a study of female voices by Linville and Fisher (1985)—compare with Table 9–1.1 notes.
Jitter factor (JF), also called percent jitter	100 × ratio of deviation in F_0 to mean F_0	$100 \times \frac{\frac{1}{N-1}\sum_{i=1}^{N-1}\lvert F0_i - F0_{i+1}\rvert}{\frac{1}{N}\sum_{i=1}^{N} F0_i}$	Implemented in Hollien et al. (1975). Murry and Doherty (1980) obtained JF with hand measurements to 0.1ms precision of wavforms; compare to following note for DPF. Horii (1982), using SEARP with accelerometer signals, obtained no significant difference across vowels in nonpathological phonations (cf. absolute shimmer notes, Table 9–2.2a). Using synthetic signals in which jitter and shimmer were controlled to common % levels, Klingholz and Martin (1985) demonstrated that the spectral effect (relative portion of harmonic energy, SNR) of jitter was much stronger than with comparable shimmer. They also obtained better discrimination of **hypo**-versus **hyper-functional voice** (in 14 women) with JF than with shimmer factor (with much higher JF in hypofunctional than in hyperfunctional voices).
Directional perturbation factor (DPF)	% of pitch perturbations $\Delta T0$ that change sign	as defined in unit, left. In P&T system, DPF/100 = ZCR[1], or first order zero crossing rate.	Hecker and Kreul (1970) applied DPF to **vocal fold cancer**, finding correlation with pathology not found with Lieberman's (1963) PPF. Murry and Doherty (1980) also found useful discrimination of vocal fold cancer using DPF, but found nonredundant information for JR, mean and SD of F_0 as well. Sorensen and Horii (1984a) obtained

Table 9–1.2a Continued

Measure	*Unit*	*Algorithm*	*Notes*
Relative average perturbation(RAP) in Koike (1973)	%	$\frac{\frac{1}{N-2}\sum_{i=2}^{N-1}\left\|\frac{T0_{i-1}+T0_i-T0_{i+1}}{3}-T0_i\right\|}{\frac{1}{N}\sum_{i=1}^{N}T0_i}$ $\left(=\frac{MR^2}{3\times\overline{F0}}\text{ in P\&T system}\right)$	values for normal voices ranging from 35% to 63%. Koike (1973) originated the widespread practice of 3-point smoothing and normalization to average period. Hirano (1981) advocated use of RAP over other pitch perturbation indices. Applications of this measure can be found passim throughout the tables of this chapter.
Frequency perturbation quotient (FPQ) in Takahashi & Koike (1975), and Koike, Takahashi, & Calcaterra (1977)	%	$\frac{\frac{1}{N-2}\sum_{i=2}^{N-1}\left\|\frac{F0_{i-1}+F0_i-F0_{i+1}}{3}-F0_i\right\|}{\frac{1}{N}\sum_{i=1}^{N}F0_i}$ $\left(=\frac{MR^2}{3\times\overline{F0}}\text{ in P\&T system}\right)$	See Takahashi and Koike (1975) notes for APQ; FPQ related to both **breathy** and **rough** scores, and with terms "awful, sour, and dirty." Koike et al. (1977) observed that FPQ was not linearly related to F_0, but rather that it was found to be minimum near "comfortable" pitch and increased with higher and lower F_0. For statistical analyses peformed with 10 $\log_e$(FPQ × 1000), see note in Table 9–2.2a for APQ. Nikolov et al. (1989) describe an implementation of FPQ in a multidimensional program precursor to MDVP, finding especially high values for **laryngeal cancer**.
Deviation from linear trend (DLT)	μs	$\frac{1}{N-5}\sum_{i=3}^{N-2}\left\|\frac{T0_{i-2}+T0_{i+2}}{2}-T0_i\right\|$, Ludlow et al. (1983) Ludlow et al. (1986) $\left(=\frac{MR^2}{2\times\overline{T0}}\text{ in P\&T system}\right)$	Ludlow et al. (1983) compared mean absolute perturbation, mean DLT, jitter ratio, DR, and mean F_0 in **laryngeal neoplasms, Parkinson's disease, Shy-Drager syndrome,** and normal controls. Increased frequency perturbation was distinctive only of the neoplasms. Neoplasm group effects were ordered in significance: JR>Abs. Perturb.>DLT.

Table 9–1.2a Continued

Measure	*Unit*	*Algorithm*	*Notes*
Perturbation factor without linear trend (Ramig & Shipp, 1987)	%	$100 \times \frac{\frac{1}{N-2}\sum_{i=2}^{N-1}\left\|\frac{T0_{i-1}+T0_{i+1}}{2} - T0_i\right\|}{\frac{1}{N}\sum_{i=1}^{N}T0_i}$	Ramig and Shipp (1987), in an investigation with the primary goal of comparing vibrato and tremor, investigated perturbations in F_0 and amplitude (cf. companion entry in Table 9–2.2a) with and without linear trend to assess if perturbations distinctive of **nerogenically pathological** voices with **tremor** remained after removal of tremor. Results indicated that perturbation, while reduced, remained higher in the patients than in the singers. L.O. Ramig, Scherer, Titze, and Ringel (1988) used this algorithm implemented in GLIMPES (R.C. Scherer et al., 1988; Titze & Liang, 1984) for jitter and shimmer measures along with HNR_{Yumoto} in an attempt to identify sub-clinical signs distinguishing short- and long-term **neurogenic** vocal instabilities in patients with **myotonic dystrophy (MD), Huntington's disease (HD), Parkinson's disease (PD), and amyotrophic lateral sclerosis (ALS)**. Although the perturbation measures were useful for distinguishing **MD** and **PD** and for tracking disease progression (e.g., in **ALS**), long–term instabilities such as amplitude tremor in **PD** and dynamic phenomena such as low-frequency segments in **HD** (see Table 9–7.0) were also important.

Table 9–1.2a Continued

Measure	***Unit***	***Algorithm***	***Notes***
Diplophonia ratio (Mean DR in Ludlow et al., 1983)	Ratio of μs	$\dfrac{\frac{1}{N-3}\sum_{i=2}^{N-1}\left\lvert\frac{T0_{i-1}+T0_{i+1}}{2}-T0_i\right\rvert}{\frac{1}{N-5}\sum_{i=3}^{N-2}\left\lvert\frac{T0_{i-2}+T0_{i+2}}{2}-T0_i\right\rvert}$	Ludlow et al. (1983) found heightened DR in 2 of 10 patients with **Shy-Drager syndrome**, but not in other groups (see DLT note, this table). Ludlow and Bassich (1983) employed absolute perturbation, jitter ratio, DR, and a variety of other acoustic and perceptual measures of **Parkinson's disease** and **Shy-Drager syndrome**, finding only moderate utility for jitter ratio and DR even though many perceptual measures of voice quality were distinctive of these dysarthrias.
Pitch variability index (PVI in Deal & Emanuel [1978])	% × 1,000	$1000 \times \dfrac{\frac{1}{N}\sum_{i=1}^{N}(T0_i-\overline{T0})^2}{\overline{T0}^2}$, in which *T0* is extracted from signal derived from a 10 Hz bandpass filter centered on the first harmonic frequency of a sustained phonation. (= $rms^0/1000\sqrt{\overline{T0}^2}$ in P&T system)	Deal and Emanuel (1978) compared PVI, AVI (q.v., Table 9–2.2a) and SNL (q.v., Table 9–5.2) in analysis of 1 s normal, **simulated rough**, and **clinically hoarse** sustained vowel samples, finding comparatively poor correlation of PVI with roughness ratings.
Pitch period perturbation quotient (PPQ)		$\dfrac{\frac{1}{N-4}\sum_{i=1}^{N-4}\left\lvert\frac{1}{5}\sum_{r=0}^{4}T0_{i+r}-T0_{i+2}\right\rvert}{\frac{1}{N}\sum_{i=1}^{N}T0_i}$	This algorithm is widely applied and is included in MDVP. See Schoentgen (1989) notes for PPQ_{EVS} (this table, following) for comparison of several preprocessing procedures for PPQ measurement.

Table 9–1.2a Continued

Measure	*Unit*	*Algorithm*	*Notes*
Smoothed pitch period perturbation quotient (sPPQ in MDVP [Kay Elemetrics, 1993])		$\dfrac{\dfrac{1}{N-k+1}\sum_{i=1}^{N-k+1}\left\|\dfrac{1}{k}\sum_{r=0}^{k-1}T0_{i+r} - T0_{i+m}\right\|}{\dfrac{1}{N}\sum_{i=1}^{N}T0_i}$, k (= smoothing factor) must be odd integer greater than one, and $m = (k-1)/2$.	A general formula for pitch perturbation incorporating normalization and variable smoothing, sPPQ is reported in most studies using MDVP (see a listing of MDVP references in the introduction to this chapter).
Pulse jitter (Cavallo, Baken, & Shaiman, 1984)	both absolute and %; performed over doubled waveform units when present	as for absolute jitter and jitter ratio above.	Cavallo et al. (1984) found extremely high (about 20%–50%) perturbations, even over doubled (**dicrotic**) waveforms, and no normalizing effect from jitter ratio, in nonpathological **pulse**.
Fundamental period perturbation (PP in Hartmann & von Cramon, 1984)	%	$\left(\dfrac{100}{n-2}\right)\sum_{i=2}^{n-1}\dfrac{\left\|T0_i - [(T0_{i-1} + 2T0_i + T0_{i+1})/4]\right\|}{[(T0_{i-1} + 2T0_i + T0_{i+1})/4]}$	Hartmann and von Cramon (1984) found significant discrimination in this parameter of **rough** voice quality (from breathy, tense, or normal) in central dysphonias due to **traumatic brain injury** and **cerebrovascular accident** (see also Tables 9–5.3 and 9–7.0).

Table 9–1.2a Continued

Measure	***Unit***	***Algorithm***	***Notes***
PPQ_{Kasuya} (Kasuya, Masubuchi, Ebihara, & Yoshida, 1986) = 100 × PQR (Kasuya, Ogawa, et al., 1986)	% or proportion, for PQR	$\frac{100}{N-k+1}\sum_{i=1}^{N-k+1}\left\lvert\frac{1-T0_{i+m}}{\frac{1}{k}\sum_{n=1}^{k}T0_{i+n-1}}\right\rvert,$ $k=3,\ m=1$	Kasuya, Masubuchi, et al. (1986) describe a screening protocol that begins with thresholds for MPPQ and a nonzero RUV criterion (see Table 9–7.0, followed by PPQ_{Kasuya}, APQ_{Kasuya} (see Table 9–2.2a), and NNE (see Table 9–5.2), resulting in a "**hoarseness** grade" statistic. Applied in a multiphasic protocol (including perceptual and stroboscopic assessments) to 991 voice samples, the system proved to be of clinical value but showed larger numbers of false positives on "weak" (low intensity) phonation samples.
MPPQ (Kasuya, Masubuchi, et al., 1986)	%	PPQKasuya (see previous), measured over mean pitch periods (*T0*) obtained from 40 ms frames updated at 20 ms intervals	
NHE_{Pitch} (Normalized high frequency energy—Kasuya, Ogawa, et al. 1986)	ratio of energies	$\frac{\sum_{t=3}^{N}(T0_t-2T0_{t-1}-T0_{t-2})^2}{\sum_{t=1}^{N}T0_t^2}$	See Kasuya, Ogawa, et al. (1986) for a mathematical derivation demonstrating similarity between this measure and RAP. These authors measured this value on 250 voices (same set described for NNE, Table 9–5.2), finding virtually identical discrimination performance as with RAP, PPQ_{Kasuya}, and normalized jitter, but clearly better than with DPF (cf. these measures, this table), and overall somewhat better than the cognate measures for amplitude perturbation (see Table 9-2.2a). See also notes on NNE, Table 9-5.2 for a spectral measure that had the best overall success with this dataset.
J-DEVEX	SD	"standard deviation of (signed) excursions from [F_0] trendline" (Laver, Hiller, Mackenzie, & Rooney, 1986, p. 518)	See notes for DPF, Table 9–2.2a, for a description of Laver et al. (1986) pre- and postprocessing steps for pitch determination. J-DEVEX was their second best parameter for discriminant function based classification for females (after shimmer DPF), fourth for males.

Table 9–1.2a Continued

Measure	***Unit***	***Algorithm***	***Notes***
Differences distribution (quotient histogram in Schultz-Coulon et al., [1979])	graph	Absolute or % frequency (histograms) or cumulative frequency (ogive curves) sorted into $\Delta T0$ ms bins	Lieberman (1961, 1963) used histograms of pitch periods extracted from acoustic signals to develop PPF (q.v., this table). Iwata and von Leden (1970a) also examined cumulative frequency ogive curves for pitch periods from throat microphones (advocating this source over radiated acoustic signals) and found significant variations among pathologic groups (e.g., **chronic laryngitis** vs. **vocal nodules**, **laryngeal carcinoma** vs. **paralysis**, and pre- vs. post-**Teflon injection in unilateral vocal fold paralysis**) by comparing cumulative frequencies within specific $\Delta T0$ bins. Schultz-Coulon et al., (1979) found, using synthetic signals, sensitivity to stochastic noise as well as the width and velocity of pitch modulation (in comparison to a simple F_0 histogram, q.v.). Both types of distributions distinguished **hyperfunctional dysphonia** from normal phonations, but this work suggested that the quotient histogram was superior for detecting **hoarseness**.

Table 9–1.2a Continued

Measure	*Unit*	*Algorithm*	*Notes*
PPQ_{EVS} (PPQ of signal preprocessed with envelope variation criterion, Schoentgen ([1989])	%	The EVS preprocessing steps are designed to model the glottal waveform plus single-formant resonance as a signal with cycles marked by single positive and negative extrema (see original report for further details): 1. Bandpass filtering of signal with FIR filter of 400 Hz bandwidth and variable center frequency (optimal results obtained with center frequency = F1, window length and first differencing interval varying according to center frequency) 2. Envelope extraction by Hilbert transform 3. Smoothing by window with length varying as function of center frequency set in step 1 4. Finite differencing at interval varying as a function of center frequency (step 1) and window length (step 3)	Schoentgen (1989) studied PPQ jitter with EVS preprocessing and two other standard conditioning processes (whitening by LPC inverse-filtering and low-pass filtering) designed to enhance pitch-period detection. The basic assessment criterion was the discrimination (by "merit factor;" see Schoentgen, 1982) of 30 **dysphonic male** speakers and 33 male control subjects. Discrimination was difficult for low-pass filtering but good for the other preprocessing measures (though dysphonic values for PPQ_{EVS} were often quite high, apparently due to the differencing over longer intervals). Schoentgen (1989) attributed significant vowel differences (i.e., between sustained French /i/, /a/, and /e/) in his results to variations in intrinsic F_0, and postulated that other differences in the literature were caused similarly, especially due to the use of absolute jitter. In a second experiment described in this report, incorporating female speakers and connected speech samples, enhanced performance was obtained for EVS preprocessing. Lieberman's PPF (preceding) was also employed, requiring an increase of the standard 0.5 ms threshold to accommodate female speakers. For his subjects and measures, connected speech samples discriminated dysphonia no better than sustained phonations, though absolute perturbations were larger and hence more easily measured.

Table 9–1.2a Continued

Measure	***Unit***	***Algorithm***	***Notes***
DSH — degree of subharmonic components (Deliyski, 1994; Kay Elemetrics, 1993)	% of sample	$\frac{100 \times \text{time of intervals with subharmonics}}{\text{total phonation time}}$ (see MDVP pitch determination procedures in introduction to Table 9-1.1 for subharmonic detection protocols)	First implementation described in Nikolov et al. (1989).

Other Sources: Ackermann and Ziegler, 1994; Baer, 1980; Beckett, 1969; Blomgren, Chen, Ng, and Gilbert, 1998; Dejonckere and Wieneke, 1994; Deliyski, 1990, 1993, 1994; Ferrand, 1995, 1998; B. Fex, Fex, Shiromoto, and Hirano, 1994; Fröhlich, Michaelis, Strube, and Kruse, 1997; Fujimura, 1968; Gamboa et al., 1997; Gubrynowicz, Kacprowski, Mikiel, and Zarnecki, 1981; Gubrynowicz, Mikiel, and Zarnecki, 1980; Hartelius, Nord, and Buder, 1995; Heiberger and Horii, 1982; Hertrich and Ackermann, 1995; Hiller et al., 1983; Hirose, Imaizumi, and Yamori, 1995; Hollien, Michel, and Doherty, 1975; Kasuya and Ando, 1991; Kasuya and Endô, 1995; Kasuya, Endô, and Saliu, 1993; Kempster, 1984; Kempster et al., 1991; Kitajima, Tanabe, and Isshiki, 1975; Koike and Takahashi, 1972; LaBlance and Maves, 1992; Laver, Hiller, and Beck, 1992; Linville, 1988; Linville, Korabic, and Rosera, 1990; Mackenzie, Laver, and Hiller, 1984; McAllister, Sederholm, Ternström, and Sundberg, 1996; Moore and Thompson, 1965; Murry and Large, 1979; Ng et al., 1997; Novák, Dlouha, Capkova, and Vohradnik, 1991; Omori, Kojima, Kakani, Slavit, and Blaugrund, 1997; Orlikoff, 1989, 1995; Orlikoff and Baken, 1989a; 1990; Orlikoff and Kahane, 1991; Protopapas and Lieberman, 1995, 1997; Rabinov, Kreiman, and Gerratt, 1994; Rabinov, Kreiman, Gerratt, and Bielamowicz, 1995; Ramig et al., 1990; Rasch, 1983; Robbins, 1982; Schoentgen and De Guchteneere, 1991, 1995, 1996, 1997; Smith, Weinberg, Feth, and Horii, 1978; Stemple et al., 1995; Sussman and Sapienza, 1994; Thompson, 1962; Wilcox and Horii, 1980; C.E. Williams and Stevens, 1972, 1981; Wolfe et al., 1991; Wolfe, Fitch, and Cornell, 1995; Wolfe and Ratusnik, 1988; Wong, Ito, Cox, and Titze, 1991; Yonick et al., 1990; Zemlin, 1962.

Table 9–1.2b F_0 Pertubations (Long-Term).

From a purely methodological point of view, the distinction between long-term and short term perturbation is somewhat arbitrary, based merely on frequency domain. Psychophysically, however, modulations from pure periodicity that are themselves perceptible as fluctuations in pitch (or loudness) are quite distinct from those that are perceived as a change in tonal quality. Study of the vocal arts has long been concerned with modulations and fluctuations from the long-term frequency domain, so vibrato, for example, was and continues to be an important object of voice quality analysis (Dejonckere, 1995). Historically, the distinction between short-term and long-term perturbations has actually been far clearer than that between F_0 perturbations versus amplitude perturbations. These notes serve therefore as an introduction to both this table and its companion Table 9–2.2b; in fact, the precise analysis of long-term modulations of F_0 as a separate parameter seems to be remarkably recent (although singers have undoubtedly been at least partially aware of the distinction for some time). The measures included in these tables assume prior extraction of frequency and/or amplitude records from speech waveforms; as fundamental frequency fluctuations may also be evident spectrographically, some additional long-term F_0 measures are grouped with other spectrographic measures in Table 9–5.1, for example, Imaizumi's (1980) spectrographic analysis measures 3 and 4.

References reporting long-term F_0 perturbations that are not specifically noted in the following table are listed at the end of the table.

Measure	***Unit***	***Algorithm***	***Notes***
Time-domain F_0 oscillation rate	Hz (subsonic), or cycles per second	Determined by inspection of F_0 contour (or by inspection of waveform only for vibrato [Bartholomew, 1934] or gross tremor [Ramig & Shipp, 1987])	Bartholomew (1934) listed **vibrato** at a 6–7 cycle per second rate (including intensity and timbre oscillation in addition to F_0) as one physical criterion of "**good**" voice quality in the male **singing** voice. L.A. Ramig and Shipp (1987) compared vibrato produced by 9 professional (opera) singers with **neurogenic** tremor produced by 6 patients, observing statistically insignificant higher rates for tremor (cf. L.A. Ramig and Shipp [1987] entries in Table 9–2.2b: these investigators described occurrences of oscillations in F_0 only or in both F_0 and amplitude, but did not in the latter case identify distinct rates for the parameters.) They also observed statistically insignificant greater F_0 oscillation extent in tremor. (See, however, significant results for jitter and shimmer, Tables 9–1.2a and 9–2.2a). L.A. Ramig et al. (1988) observed 4–7 Hz tremor in waveforms of sustained phonations by patients with **Parkinson's Disease**. Hakes, Doherty and Shipp (1990) measured nine
Time domain F_0 oscillation extent	range (semitones or Hz)	Determined by inspection of F_0 contour	

Table 9–1.2b Continued

Measure	*Unit*	*Algorithm*	*Notes*
			singers' trillo (a kind of pulsed vowel repetition) at rates of 2.0–6.9 Hz for slow trillo and 7.5–12.4 Hz for fast trillo.
Slew rate algorithm (Ludlow, Bassich, Connor, and Coulter, 1986)	μs for range of F_0 tremor Hz for frequency % cycles for "regularity"	From hardware-generated F_0 series, apply sliding linear regression analysis over 9 cycles for men (11–13 for women) to identify maximum slopes in alternative negative and positive directions. Compute range of tremor as mean maximum slope, and average tremor frequency as the average inverse period between maxima. For regularity, find mode of histogram of all cycles and calculate the percentage of all cycles represented by that mode	Ludlow et al. (1986) used this algorithm on sustained /a/ phonations by 4 patients with **benign essential tremor** (BET), 5 patients with **vocal tremor** (associated with dystonias, myoclonus, or spasmodic dysphonia) and 20 control subjects. The results were among the first to assess F_0 variation separately from amplitude, finding yet more widespread involvement of F_0 than amplitude in the tremor cases. All speakers with tremor exhibited higher F_0 ranges. Although the frequencies of these tremors did not distinguish any of the groups, the BET group had the highest F_0 range and the most regular tremor.
Flutter spectrum (Ternström and Friberg, 1989) Hz_f A_f	dB × Hz plot Hz (F_0 × time cycles) Log scale, for example, cents relative to mean F_0	1. Obtain F_0 contour of sustained phonation signal by epoch analysis, for example, zero-crossing with interpolation 2. Convert signal to standard deviations around zero mean and pass analog form at 50 times true speed to narrowband spectrum analyzer (e.g., Hewlett-Packard 3580A set to 0.6 Hz resolution)	Ternström and Friberg (1989) obtained flutter spectra from 8 **singers'** sustained phonations of /a/, /i/, and /u/, finding distinctive peak Hz_f values for each subject that were stable within subjects' vowel samples and ranged from 4 to 7 cps. The authors suggest a rough categorization of fluctuations < 5 cps as **wow**, > 5 cps but < 20 cps as **flutter**, and > 20 cps as jitter. They also measured A_f values ranging around 10 cents, with /a/ > /u/, and bass singers > sopranos.

Table 9–1.2b Continued

Measure	*Unit*	*Algorithm*	*Notes*
frequency-domain F_0 variation:		General approach is to obtain F_0 data in the form of a time-series (e.g., by hand measurement of zero-crossings or by digitizing the output of a Kay Elemetrics Visi-Pitch), apply a Fourier transform, and inspect spectrum for peaks	Rothman and Arroyo (1987) inspected 1024-point Hamming-windowed spectra for dominant peaks representing **professional opera singers' vibrato, tremolo,** and **wobble,** and suggested that magnitude and the copresence of amplitude variations were more important than rate when distinguishing among these qualities. Philippbar, Robin, and Luschei (1989) used Fourier analysis to measure tremor in the sustained phonations of 8 men with **Parkinson's disease** and 8 control subjects. These investigators found it difficult to identify prominent spectral peaks (between 3 Hz and 10 Hz) in most of these analyses and did not observe distinguishing characteristics between their pathologic and control groups. Peaks were observed more readily in F_0 records than in amplitude.
frequency or rate	Hz (subsonic) or cycles per second		
magnitude	Hz, semitones, or percentage deviation from mean F_0		
F_0 modulation	% (Peak deviation from mean)	$\frac{Max(T0) - Min(T0)}{Max(T0) + Min(T0)}$	Titze (1994b).

Table 9–1.2b Continued

Measure	*Unit*	*Algorithm*	*Notes*
MDVP FFTR (F_0 tremor frequency) and MDVP FTRI (frequency tremor intensity index) Kay Elemetrics, 1993	% (peak-to-peak deviation from mean)	For each 2 s frame of fundamental frequency data (see MDVP pitch detection protocol in formula section preceding Table 9–1.1): 1. Low-pass filter at 30 Hz and downsample to 400 sps 2. Calculate energy 3. Subtract DC component 4. Calculate ACF (see section 3. of introduction for ACF formula) 5. Convert ACF to % energy 6. Extract period from ACF peak 7. Report frequency and amplitude corresponding to extracted period. Average ACFs and tremor amplitudes from all frames.	

Other Sources: Abdoerrachman, Imaizumi, Hirose, and Niimi, 1993; Ackermann and Ziegler, 1991; Aronson, Ramig, Winholz, and Silber, 1992; Buder, Hartelius, and Strand, 1995) Buder and Strand, 1994; Deliyski, 1990, 1993, 1994; Ekholm, Papagiannis, and Chagnon, 1998; Gath and Yair, 1987; Hartelius, Buder, and Strand, 1997; Hartelius et al., 1995; Hirose et al., 1995; Izdebski and Dedo, 1980; Kent, Duffy, Vorperian, and Thomas, 1998; Lindsey and Vieira, 1997; Morsomme et al., 1997; Rothman, Rullman, and Arroyo, 1990; Seidner, Nawka, and Cebulla, 1995; Shipp, Doherty, and Haglund, 1990; Shipp and Izdebski, 1981; Shipp, Leanderson, and Sundberg, 1980; Sundberg, 1995; Traunmüller and Eriksson, 1995; Winholz and Ramig, 1992; Yair and Gath, 1988; Zwirner and Barnes, 1992.

Table 9–2.1. Amplitude Statistics.

Along with fundamental frequency, the control of intensity (or more generally from a descriptive point of view, amplitude) is a basic element of voice quality. Indeed, the most basic "quality"—whether there is phonation at all—is a matter of amplitude. However, although the basic descriptive quantities are essentially the same in form as for F_0, amplitude is measured quite differently and the perceptual quality correlates seem to be quite distinct. Because absolute sound pressure measures require careful procedures with relatively expensive equipment and controlled environments, it is perhaps not surprising that "loud" speech and its concomitant qualities are only now being described and understood (e.g., by Alku, Vilkman, & Laukkanen, 1998). As with F_0, investigators of voice quality have tended to overlook the basic parameter of amplitude and the associated changes in vocal fold vibration as a chief determinant of the quality of a voice. The following table also incorporates the measures describing nasal qualities; although seemingly unrelated to basic "loudness" related measures, the chief clinical measures of "nasalance" are based on intensity ratios and so are included here to accord with the parameter-based organization of these tables.

References reporting amplitude statistics that are not specifically noted in the following table are listed at the end of the table.

Measure	***Algorithm***	***Notes***
Central Tendency of Intensity:		
Mean	Analog: Most commonly and directly measured using sound pressure level meter, in dB SPL units. Digital: Values (A_I) measured using integration, such as RMS, of instantaneous amplitudes x_t (see RMS following) over successive frames of N data points. A common frame size for speech signals is 20 ms and a typical unit would be volts. The resulting values can be converted to dB scales using an arbitrary reference level. A0 = value integrated over fundamental period T0.	Bartholomew (1934) listed "total intensity" as one of four criteria for "**good**" voice quality in adult male **singers** (see Table 9–5.2 for a listing of the other three). Hirano et al. (1986) in a study of 68 pathologic voice samples observed a negative correlation between mean SPL and **mean flow rate** (as measured using aerodynamic transducer) a negative correlation between habitual SPL and F_0 range, and among **carcinoma** samples a positive correlation between habitual SPL and habitual F_0. In comparisons with stroboscopic observations, this group obtained a negative correlation of habitual SPL and extent of normal mucosal wave. These researchers obtained a positive relation of habitual SPL with **hoarseness** (GRBAS scale—Hirano, 1981). See also intensity dispersion entries following and Table 9–5.1 entries for other Hirano et al. (1986) results incorporating SPL
Median	Value that divides a histogram such that the number of observations above equals the number of observations below.	
Interquartile range	Range that spans the central half of the observed values.	
Geometric	Digital:	

Table 9–2.1. Amplitude Statistics (Continued)

Measure	Algorithm	Notes
Central Tendency of Intensity (Continued):		
	$\sqrt[N]{\prod_{t=1}^{N} x_t}$, or $\exp\left(\frac{1}{N}\sum_{t=1}^{N}\log_e x_t\right)$; either may be applied to A_i.	measures. Ray (1986), in a study of one male voice with 214 listeners, found that loudness increases were predictive of higher **competence** ratings, but of lower **benevolence**. K.R. Scherer (1981, 1986a) reviews literature on vocal indicators of emotional states in which loud voice levels tend to indicate **happiness/joy**, **confidence**, **anger**, and **contempt**, soft voice levels tending to indicate **boredom** and **grief/sadness**.
RMS	Digital: $\sqrt{\frac{1}{N}\sum_{t=1}^{N} x_t^2}$ Also available as output of analog devices.	

Table 9–2.1. Amplitude Statistics (Continued)

Measure	*Algorithm*	*Notes*
Dispersion of Intensity:		
Max, min, range (max–min)	volts or dB	Hirano et al. (1986), in a study of 68 pathologic voice samples, obtained a negative correlation of SPL range with habitual F_0 and a positive correlation with stroboscopically assessed glottic closure. They also obtained a negative correlation with perceived **asthenic** and **rough** qualities (GRBAS scale—Hirano, 1981). See also Table 9–5.1 and comments for F_0 statistics above for other SPL related observations from this work. Ludlow and Connor (1987) found a reduced range of SPL levels in nine speakers with **spasmodic dysphonia** in "soft, regular, loud, and shout" sustained /a/ phonations in comparison to speakers without this disorder.
Standard deviation	$\sqrt{\frac{1}{N-1}\sum_{i=1}^{N}(A_i-\overline{A})^2}$	
Coefficient of variation	$\frac{\sqrt{\frac{1}{N-1}\sum_{i=1}^{N}(A_i-\overline{A})^2}}{\overline{A}}$	Normalizes variation to the mean. R.C. Scherer et al. (1988) used CV of amplitude as a "long-term perturbation" measure, using plots of $F_0 \times$ amplitude to examine cases of **spasmodic dysphonia** and in events of **diplophonia** (see Table 9–1.1, CV of F_0 for additional notes).

Table 9–2.1. Amplitude Statistics (Continued)

Measure	Algorithm	Notes
Other Basic Amplitude Distribution Measures:		
Amplitude density distribution (Klingholz & Martin, 1989).	Preprocessing: Low-pass filter at F_c just over F_0 to obtain amplitude envelope, digitize, and calculate distribution for linear amplitudes normalized to RMS amplitude. Measures: Form factor ($20\times\log_{10}$[RMS amplitude/average absolute amplitude]),skewness,coefficient of excess(see formula, Table 9–6.1).	Klingholz and Martin (1989) measured amplitude density and level distribution typologies and statistics from 60-second connected speech samples obtained from 55 speakers with **laryngeal diseases** and 20 control speakers, both gender balanced. They presented density distributions typed by **hyperfunctional dysphonia**, **normal voice**, **hypofunctional dysphonia**, **large glottal chink**, **papilloma**, and **bilateral recurrent nerve paralysis**. Statistics from these distributions significantly distinguished **gender** in normal and mildly dysphonic voices. Although some disease categories could be characterized by unique measures, others produced no deviation from the normal speakers. Regarding level distributions, the authors noted 6 types, among which all normals were type 2, **hyperfunctional dysphonias** were almost exclusively type 1, and other disorders (**nerve paralysis**, **mass lesions**, **large chink**) fell into types 3–6. DA parameters represented insufficient variance, but RH measures significantly discriminated **gender** and normal versus pathologic subjects. RH was unaffected by age but could be manipulated by a normal subject in negative association with **tension**. The authors favored the use of level distributions, and interpreted the RH parameter primarily as a ratio of voiceless to voiced segments, but suggested that a similar measure be developed to focus exclusively on voiced segments.
Amplitude level distribution (Klingholz & Martin, 1989).	Preprocessing: as just stated, except distribution calculated for logarithmic amplitudes (plus moving average smoothing of frequency histogram) Measures: Graphic inspection of histogram for typology based on number and relative levels of modes (see Klingholz & Martin [1989], Figure 3, p. 25) Calculate DA (difference between loci of mode peaks) and RH (ratio of magnitudes of mode peaks).	

Table 9–2.1. Amplitude Statistics (Continued)

Measure	*Unit*	*Algorithm*	*Notes*
Other Basic Amplitude-Based Measures:			
TONAR (the oral nasal acoustic ratio, S. Fletcher, 1970; S. Fletcher & Bishop, 1970)	Ratio	1. Record sound radiation from oral and nasal acoustic cavities via two separate microphones separated physically by material providing at least 40 dB attenuation between signals 2. Pass amplified oral and nasal through wave spectrum analyzers to select specific frequency bands for comparison (e.g., 1 kHz wideband analysis in a frequency sweep [Fletcher, 1970], or in 200 Hz narrowband analyses covering a 150–3350 Hz range [Fletcher & Bishop, 1970]) 3. Analyze spectrum analyzer outputs via custom analog ratio computer to obtain nasal/oral energy ratios, displaying original signals, ratio, and analysis center frequency on a paper oscillograph	S. Fletcher (1970) describes the development of TONAR and reviews previous literature assessing the psychophysical properties of similar measures. S. Fletcher and Bishop (1970) performed psychophysical studies with TONAR on a set of speech samples by **children with repaired clefts**, obtaining significant Spearman rho correlation coefficients between wideband (1 kHz) with perceived **nasality** ranging from 0.6 to 0.84 depending on listening condition (e.g., better results were obtained with ratings of speech played backwards). Narrowband analyses suggested that the dominant effects occured in the 250–850 Hz range.
Nasalance (parameter produced by Nasometer™ equipment, Kay Elemetrics, 1988)	%	Based on TONAR (see previous entry, this table), microcomputer-based Nasometer™ equipment provides 25 dB attenuation between oral and nasal channels, filters the signals with a 300 Hz bandpass filter centered at 500 Hz, and calculates nasalance as the nasal energy divided by nasal-plus-oral energy multiplied by 100. Associated software displays the resulting values in several formats, and hardware outputs a voltage signal representing nasalance.	Kay Elemetrics (1991) has compiled a set of references applying nasalance as a metric for **nasal** voice quality, primarily for applications to cases of **cleft lip** and **palate**, but also for **tonsillectomy**, **adenoidectomy**, and **velopharyngeal insufficiency**.

Table 9–2.1. Amplitude Statistics (Continued)

Measure	Unit	Algorithm	Notes
Other Basic Amplitude-Based Measures:			
HONC (Horii oral-nasal coupling index, Horii, 1980a)	Ratio or, alternatively, % or dB.	RMS amplitude(nasal) is measured from a nasal accelerometer applied to the external surface of one of the nostrils and RMS amplitude (vocal) is obtained from a neck accelerometer applied between the thyroid and the sternal notch. HONC = RMS (nasal) / k × RMS (vocal),in which k is a correction factor unique to each application. HONC in % is HONC × 100, and HONC in dB is $20 \times \log_{10}$(HONC)	Horii (1980a) describes an analog implementation of HONC that displays nasal and vocal levels and their ratio whenever the vocal signal is above a threshold level. This introductory paper also presented connected speech examples illustrating **hyponasality** and **hypernasality**.

Other Sources: Cleveland and Sundberg, 1983; Dromey and Ramig, 1998; Dromey, Ramig, and Johnson, 1995; S. Fex et al., 1991; Gelfer and Young, 1997; Holmberg et al., 1994; Horii and Lang, 1981; Howell and Williams, 1988; Kempster et al., 1991; Klich, 1982; Laukkanen et al., 1996; Morris and Brown, 1987; Niederjohn and Haworth, 1983; Ptacek and Sander, 1966; Ramig et al., 1990; Redenbaugh and Reich, 1985; Robbins, 1982; Seaver, Dalston, Leeper, and Adams, 1991; Stevens, Nickerson, Boothroyd, and Rollins, 1976; R.G. Williams, Eccles, and Hutchings, 1990; Winholtz and Titze, 1997; Yonick et al., 1990.

Table 9–2.2a. Amplitude Perturbations (Short-Term).

The forms of most cycle-to-cycle amplitude perturbation (or "shimmer") measures are quite similar to parallel jitter measures, and many of the measurement issues and interpretations are similar. Indeed, in the modern literature, the two perturbation types are usually measured in tandem. Many of the studies listed in the following table have found, however, that shimmer is often statistically more powerful than jitter for distinguishing pathological voice qualities. Methodological studies reviewed in Appendix 9-A have delineated other important theoretical differences between jitter and shimmer, including, for example, that pure shimmer will distort or broaden frequency-domain distributions (e.g., harmonic width) less severely than pure jitter, and other studies have revealed why the two types of perturbation are difficult to distinguish in practice. For purely empirical reasons that have an unclear physiological basis (if any), the preferred moving average against which amplitude perturbations are measured are often longer than for frequency perturbations, for example "APQ" (11-point baseline) versus "RAP" (3-point baseline). See the introduction to Table 9-1.2a for other general comments regarding historical trends in the development and use of short-term perturbation measures, and also for comments regarding inconsistencies in the published nomenclature.

References reporting short amplitude perturbations that are not specifically noted in the following table are listed at the end of the table.

Measure	***Unit***	***Algorithm***	***Notes***
Absolute shimmer	dB	$\frac{1}{N-1}\sum_{i=1}^{N-1}\lvert 20\log_{10}(A0_{i+1}/A0_i)\rvert$	Horii (1982) obtained no significant differences in absolute shimmer (or jitter, see Table 9–1.2a) **across vowels** produced at comfortable levels and durations by subjects without pathology. The average value of 0.17 dB, obtained from throat contact accelerometer, was approximately half that obtained from airborne radiated speech signals. Horii (1985) found greater shimmer in **fry** (mean value 1.15) than in modal register (mean 0.48) in healthy speakers (cf. percent jitter, Table 9–1.1a). Horiguchi et al. (1987) compared acoustic to electroglottographic sustained phonation sources for absolute shimmer, finding somewhat superior detection for EGG shimmer for discrimination of normal and **dysphonic** speakers (68% correct detection for EGG vs. 51% for acoustic). See also notes on EGG-jitter, Table 9–1.2a, Absolute frequency jitter entry. Ludlow et al.

Table 9–2.2a. Continued

Measure	*Unit*	*Algorithm*	*Notes*
			(1987), measuring shimmer in long sustained phonation samples, obtained significant discrimination between 34 patients with **laryngeal pathology** and 99 control subjects in both males and females, with an overall correct classification of 78%–80%, and 100% classification of **carcinoma** and **partial laryngectomy**, but relatively poor classification of **polyps** or **nodules**, **edema**, or **unilateral paralysis** (see also absolute period jitter, Table 9–1.2a). Implemented in GLIMPES (R.C. Scherer et al. 1988; Titze and Liang, 1993). See Ringel and Chodzko-Zajco (1987) notes in percent jitter, Table 9–1.2a, for associations of shimmer with **poor physiological status in older speakers**. Among the variables correlating with a **trained singer's fatigue** (see Table 9–1.2a, percent jitter), R.C. Scherer et al. (1987) obtained the best correlations to self-assessments with shimmer. See Scherer et al. (1988) in Table 1.1, CV of F_0 for notes on long- versus short-term perturbations. Newman, Harris, and Hilton (1989) found significantly greater shimmer for a group of 14 **stutterers** (12 male, 2 female) on sustained vowel phonation shimmer (but no differences for jitter).
Absolute amplitude perturbation	sound pressure (or comparable waveform unit, e.g., volts)	$\frac{1}{N-1}\sum_{i=1}^{N-1}\lvert A0_i - A0_{i+1}\rvert$	See notes on Zyski et al. (1984) application in Table 9–1.2a, normalized jitter.

Table 9–2.2a. Continued

Measure	*Unit*	*Algorithm*	*Notes*
Normalized mean absolute period shimmer (Feijoo & Hernández, 1990)	sound pressure (or comparable waveform unit, e.g., volts)	$\frac{1}{MXA}\frac{1}{N}\sum_{i=1}^{N}\lvert A0_{i+1} - A0_i\rvert$, where $MXA = \max(A0_i)$	Feijoo and Hernández (1990) measured this form of shimmer in sustained /e/ phonations by 56 individuals with **glottic cancer** (stages T1–T4) and 64 control speakers, obtaining 86% classification success and correlations of approximately 0.92 with both **hoarseness** and **breathiness** ratings. Other measures applied to this dataset were superior in classification (D and NNE [Table 9–5.2], and CE [Table 9–5.4]), one was comparable (VF [Table 9–4.0]), and normalized mean absolute jitter (Table 9–1.2a) was inferior.
Normalized amplitude perturbation = 100 × PM_{Kasuya} (Kasuya et al., 1986)	%(of average amplitude)	$100 \times \frac{1}{N-1}\sum_{i=1}^{N-1}\frac{A0_i - A0_{i+1}}{A0_i}$	See notes on Zyski et al. (1984) application in Table 9–1.2a, normalized jitter.
Percent shimmer (also called shimmer factor by Klingholz & Martin [1985].)	%(of average amplitude)	$100 \times \frac{\frac{1}{N-1}\sum_{i=1}^{N-1}\lvert A0_i - A0_{i+1}\rvert}{\frac{1}{N}\sum_{i=1}^{N} A0_i}$	Using synthetic signals in which jitter and shimmer were controlled to common % levels, Klingholz and Martin demonstrated that the spectral effect (relative portion of harmonic energy, SNR) of shimmer was slight in comparison to jitter (see jitter factor, Table 9–1.2a.)
Amplitude perturbation quotient (APQ in Koike et al. [1977])	%(of average amplitude)	$\frac{\frac{1}{N-10}\sum_{i=1}^{N-10}\left\lvert\frac{1}{11}\sum_{r=0}^{10} A0_{i+r} - A0_{i+5}\right\rvert}{\frac{1}{N}\sum_{i=1}^{N} A0_i}$	Takahashi and Koike (1975) investigated (contact microphone) APQ, FPQ (see table 9–1.2a..) and mean F_0 in normal and pathologic samples rated for breathy and rough, plus 12 semantic differential items, finding association of APQ with **breathy** score and terms "awful, sour, and dirty." In general, their results indicated the strongest effects with APQ, although they noted that over-

Table 9–2.2a. Continued

Measure	*Unit*	*Algorithm*	*Notes*
			all intensity variation in otherwise identical synthetic signals also affected the semantic differential based factors. Koike et al. (1977) used 10 $\log_e$(APQ × 1000) to establish 2-dimensional (with 10 $\log_e$(FPQ × 1000)) "critical ellipse" norms to establish multidimensional statistical confidence limits for groups of pathologic and control subjects. For both APQ and FPQ, nonsignificant trends were observed to differentiate /i/ and /a/. Nikolov et al. (1989) describe an implementation of APQ in a multidimensional program precursor to MDVP, finding especially high values for **laryngeal cancer**.
Amplitude variability index (AVI in Deal & Emanuel [1978])	$\log_{10}$(1,000 × % [of average amplitude])	$\log_{10}\left(1{,}000 \times \frac{\frac{1}{N}\sum_{i=0}^{N-1}(A0_i - \overline{A0})^2}{\overline{A0}^2}\right)$, in which $A0$ is extracted from signal derived from a 10 Hz bandpass filter centered on the first harmonic frequency of a sustained phonation. ($= 10^{rms^0/1000}\sqrt{\overline{A0}^2}$ in P&T System).	Deal and Emanuel (1978) compared AVI, PVI (table 9–1.2a) and SNL (table 9–5.2) in analysis of 1 s normal, **simulated rough**, and **clinically hoarse** sustained vowel samples, finding poor correlation of AVI with roughness ratings in comparison with SNL, although better performance in comparison with PVI. The study also found variability across vowels, suggesting that high vowels evidenced greater susceptibility to amplitude perturbation. Nichols (1979) replicated the superiority of "shimmer" over "jitter" with respect to roughness ratings.

Table 9–2.2a. Continued

Measure	***Unit***	***Algorithm***	***Notes***
Directional perturbation factor (DPF, or DSF [Sorensen & Horii, 1984a] for directional shimmer factor)	% of amplitude perturbations $\Delta T0$ that change sign	As specified in definition (left). In P&T system, DPF/100 = ZCR[1], or first order zero crossing rate Laver, Hiller, Mackenzie, and Rooney (1986) preprocessed connected speech data for this and other parameters by phase compensation, low-pass filtering, and postprocessed pitch data with nonlinear smoothing and parabolic interpolation.	Sorensen and Horii (1984a) obtained values for **normal** voices ranging from 44% to 73%, higher than their results for pitch DPF (or DJF, for directional jitter factor.). Laver et al. (1986) reported that shimmer DPF was the single best basis for principle components classification of **structural** disorders of the larynx: in combination with average F_0 (their second best parameter for male subjects, seventh for females) achieving a 92% classification success. A comparable rate of success combining altogether 10 parameters was achieved using linear discriminant analysis—see J-DEVEX notes, Table 9–1.2a.
Smoothed amplitude perturbation quotient (sAPQ in MDVP, Kay Elemetrics, 1993) = PQ for amplitude (Kasuya, Ogawa, Kikuchi, et al., 1986)	% (of average amplitude)	$$\frac{\frac{1}{N-k+1}\sum_{i=1}^{N-k+1}\left\|\frac{1}{k}\sum_{r=0}^{k-1}A0_{i+r}-A0_{i+m}\right\|}{\frac{1}{N}\sum_{i=1}^{N}A0_i},$$ k (= smoothing factor) must be odd integer greater than one, and $m = (k\text{-}1)/2$.	A general formula for amplitude perturbation incorporating normalization and variable smoothing, sAPQ is reported in most studies using MDVP (see a listing of MDVP references in the introduction to this chapter).
APQ_{Kasuya} (Kasuya, Masubuchi, et al. 1986) = 100 × PQR (Kasuya, Ogawa, Kikuchi, et al., 1986)	% or proportion, for PQR	$$\frac{100}{N-k+1}\sum_{i=1}^{N-k+1}\left\|\frac{1-A0_{i+m}}{\frac{1}{k}\sum_{n-1}^{k}A0_{i+n-1}}\right\|,$$ $k = 3,\ m = 1$	See Table 9–1.2a, PPQ_{Kasuya} notes for use of APQ_{Kasuya} in Kasuya, Ogawa, Kikuchi, et al. (1986) screening protocol.

Table 9–2.2a. Continued

Measure	*Unit*	*Algorithm*	*Notes*
$NHE_{Amplitude}$ (normalized high frequency energy—Kasuya, Ogawa, Kikuchi, et al., 1986)	ratio of energies	$\frac{\sum_{t=3}^{N}(A0_i - 2A0_{t-1} - A0_{t-2})^2}{\sum_{t=1}^{N} A0_t^2}$	See Kasuya, Ogawa, Kikuchi, et al., (1986) for a mathematical derivation demonstrating similarity between this measure and APQ_{Kasuya}.
Perturbation factor without linear trend (L.A. Ramig & Shipp, 1987)	%	$100 \times \frac{\frac{1}{N-2}\sum_{i=2}^{N-1}\left\lvert\frac{A0_{i-1} + A0_{i+1}}{2} - A0_i\right\rvert}{\frac{1}{N}\sum_{i=1}^{N} A0_i}$	L.A. Ramig and Shipp (1987), in an investigation with the primary goal of comparing vibrato and tremor, investigated perturbations in amplitude and F_0 (cf. companion entry in Table 9–1.2a) with and without linear trend to assess whether perturbations distinctive of **nerogenically pathological** voices **with tremor** remained after removal of tremor. Results indicated that perturbation, although reduced, remained higher in the patients than in the singers.

Other Sources: Blomgren, Chen, et al., 1998; Deliyski, 1990, 1993, 1994; Ferrand, 1995; Ferrand, 1998; B. Fex et al., 1994; Fröhlich, Michaelis, Strube, and Kruse, 1997; Gamboa et al., 1997; Hartelius et al., 1995; Heiberger and Horii, 1982; Hertrich and Ackermann, 1995; Hirose et al., 1995; Horii, 1980b; Kasuya and Ando, 1991; Kasuya and Endô, 1995; Kasuya et al., 1993; Kempster, 1984; Kempster et al., 1991; Kitajima and Gould, 1976; LaBlance and Maves, 1992; Laver et al., 1992; Omori et al., 1997; Orlikoff, 1995; Orlikoff and Kahane, 1991; Ramig et al., 1990; Robbins, 1982; Wolfe, Fitch, and Cornell, 1995; Wong et al., 1991; Yonick et al., 1990.

Table 9–2.2b. Amplitude Perturbations (Long-Term).

See the introduction to Table 9–1.2b for general comments regarding short- versus long-term perturbations. One important distinction here is that long-term amplitude perturbations have a longer historical precedent in the literature, given the relative facility with which long-term amplitude modulations can be measured in waveform records. It seems, nonetheless, that measures of long-term F_0 modulations are more important for both measuring desirable vibrato effects as well as for many types of undesirable pathological tremors.

References reporting long-term amplitude perturbations that are not specifically noted in the following table are listed at the end of the table.

Measure	***Unit***	***Algorithm***	***Notes***
Intensity oscillation rate	Hz (subsonic), or cycles per second	Determined by inspection of waveform	Bartholomew (1934) listed **vibrato** at a 6–7 cycle per second rate (including F_0 and timbre oscillation in addition to intensity) as one physical criterion of "**good**" voice quality in the male **singing** voice. He cites Metfessel's use of the term "**sonance**" for this quality.
Peak-to-peak amplitude modulation (and frequency) (J.R. Brown & Simonson, 1963), measures called "oscillation rate" and "oscillation extent," by L.A. Ramig & Shipp, 1987)	%, (frequency in Hz)	$\frac{Max\,(Amp.) - Min\,(Amp.)}{Max\,(Amp.)}$	J.R. Brown and Simonson (1963) measured amplitudes from oscillograms and used this measure in one of the first clinical studies of **organic voice tremor**, reporting from 40%–100% change in amplitude at frequencies of 4 Hz–9 Hz. L.A. Ramig and Shipp (1987) compared vibrato produced by 9 professional (opera) singers with **neurogenic** tremor produced by 6 patients as determined by hand inspection of 1-s sample waveform extracted from sustained /a/ phonation observing statistically insignificant higher rates for tremor (cf. L.A. Ramig and Shipp [1987] "F_0 oscillation" entries in Table 9–1.2b: these investigators found no instances of "amplitude only" oscillations). They also observed statistically insignificant greater amplitude oscillation extent in tremor. (See, however, significant results for jitter and shimmer, Tables 9–1.2a and 9–2.2a.)

Table 9–2.2b. Continued

Measure	***Unit***	***Algorithm***	***Notes***
Slew rate algorithm (Ludlow et al., 1986)	amplitude units for range of amplitude tremor, Hz for tremor rate	From hardware-generated *A0* series, apply sliding linear regression analysis over 9 cycles for men (11–13 for women) to identify maximum slopes in alternative negative and positive directions. Compute range of tremor as mean maximum slope and average tremor frequency as the average inverse period between maxima.	
Frequency-domain amplitude tremor frequency magnitude	Hz (subsonic)Hz (deviation from mean F_0)	General approach is to obtain amplitude data in the form a time-series (e.g., by digitizing the output of a Kay Elemetrics VisiPitch) and apply a Fourier transform	See note for Philippbar et al. (1989), Table 9–1.2b, for analysis of **vocal tremor** in **Parkinson's disease**: Peaks were observed more readily in F_0 records than in amplitude, but failed to distinguish the pathologic group from control subjects.
Peak amplitude modulation	%	$\frac{Max\,(A0) - Min\,(A0)}{Max\,(A0) + Min\,(A0)}$	Titze (1994b). See also spectrographic analysis measures 1 and 2, Imaizumi, Hiki, Hirano, and Matsushita (1980), Table 9–5.1.
MDVP FATR (amplitude tremor frequency) and MDVP ATRI (amplitude tremor intensity index).	% (within-period peak-to-peak deviation from mean)	A. For each 2 s frame of amplitude data: 1. a. Using 30 ms frame and 2.5 ms shifts to do averaging, retaining thereby 400 sps.b. Low-pass filter at 30 Hz. 2. Calculate energy 3. Subtract DC component 4. Calculate ACF 5. Convert ACF to % energy 6. Extract period from ACF peak	Kay Elemetrics (1993). See MDVP pitch-extraction protocol in formula section preceding Table 9-1.1.

Table 9–2.2b. Continued

Measure	*Unit*	*Algorithm*	*Notes*
		7. Report frequency and ATRI (% deviation from mean) corresponding to extracted period. 8. Allow user-selection of alternative frequency B. Average ACFs and tremor amplitudes from all frames	

Other Sources: Abdoerrachman et al., 1993; Ackermann and Ziegler, 1991; Aronson and Hartman, 1981; Aronson et al., 1992; Buder et al., 1995; Buder and Strand, 1994; Dejonckere, 1995; Deliyski, 1990, 1993, 1994; Hachinski et al., 1975; Hartelius et al., 1997; Hartelius et al., 1995; Hartman, Abbs, and Vishwanat, 1988; Hartman, Overholt, and Vishwanat, 1982; Hirose et al., 1995; Izdebski and Dedo, 1980; Kent et al., 1998; Lindsey and Vieira, 1997; Morsomme et al., 1997; Sundberg, 1995; Winholz and Ramig, 1992.

Table 9–3.0. F_0/Amplitude Covariations.

Plots mapping a speaker's dynamic range over fundamental frequencies have been more widely used in Europe than in the USA or Japan, and may be relatively uncommon primarily because of the time and effort required for both administrator and subject. Some important methodological issues have been reviewed more recently by Coleman (1993) and Titze (1994a). Given the basic importance of the two dimensions of the voice range profile and, furthermore, the dependence of many voice qualities on these dimensions, the technique seems inevitably of great value in developing a secure understanding of voice qualities.

References reporting F_0/amplitude covariations that are not specifically noted in the following table are listed at the end of the table.

Measure	***Description and Notes***
Voice range profile, phonetogram, or F_0-SPL profile	Display of vocal intensity ranges (ordinate) against fundamental frequencies (abscissa). The current tradition was initiated by Damsté (1970)—see Ohlsson and Löfqvist (1986) for an application to pathological voices.
Voice field (Hurme & Sonninen, 1986)	"an amplitude/F_0 description of connected speech . . . formed in real time on the basis of cycle-to-cycle analysis of the speech signal [used] to evaluate the results of speech therapy" (Hurme and Sonninen, 1986, p. 491).
Voice quality registration (Pabon & Plomp, 1988)	$F_0 \times$ SPL displays with density indicators for jitter (**roughness**), 0–1.5 kHz/1.5–5 kHz band ratios (**sharpness**), or > 5 kHz noise level (**breathiness**). Pabon and Plomp (1988) used a hardware-based system to achieve essentially real-time registration, using PPQ for jitter and describing sharpness as an "α-type" slope parameter (see Table 9–5.3, LTAS measures), and breathiness as Yanigahara-based (see Table 9–5.1, spectrographic measures). Much quality $\times F_0 \times$ SPL variation is seen in every phonetogram. See original report for hardware details and numerous quality phonetograms from case studies suggesting special utility for jitter and slope measures in reference to pathological voice.
Voice print ($F_0 \times$ SPL $\times$ $SNR_{Klingholz}$ distribution, Klingholz [1990])	$F_0 \times$ SPL displays with density indicators for $SNR_{Klingholz}$ (see Table 9–5.2). Klingholz (1990) discusses this display in the context of alternative distributional displays and includes samples from a normal male and speakers with **hypofunctional dysphonia**, **mutational dysyphonia**, **recurrent nerve paralysis**, and pre- versus postoperative laryngeal cancer and notes that each shows a distinguishing voice print characteristic (Klingholz acknowledges the prior use of the term voice print for contour spectrograms [cf. Table 9–5.2], but argues for readoption of the term for this voice quality display.)

Other Sources: Awan, 1991; Awan, 1993; Heylen, Wuyts, Mertens, De bodt, Pattyn, and Van de Heyning, 1996; Heylen, Wuyts, Mertens, and Pattyn, 1996; Hiki, 1967; Pabon, 1991.

Table 9–4.0. Waveform Perturbations.

Simple waveform irregularities that deviated noticeably from normal quasiperiodicity were probably the first acoustic measures of disordered voice quality—see Scripture's 1916 work. (However, see also Haggard [1969], who disputed Scripture's claims of "infallible" differential diagnosis and suggested a focus on dynamic aspects of phonation onset.) Although the early measurements, in which amplitude and period/frequency were not decomposed, were relatively crude, the concept that waveform shape is a definitive acoustic correlate of voice quality remains powerful, yet subtle and even elusive. For example, Milenkovic's sample-by-sample statistics introduced in 1987 (Leddy, Milenkovic, & Bless, 1993; Milenkovic, 1987, 1997) seem to derive descriptive power from a fundamental frequency extraction method that is waveform based (see also Titze & Liang, 1993 for indications of the superiority of this approach for F_0 determination in quality measures). Included in this table as well are many measures that relate closely to spectral noise measures but that are implemented in the time-domain, for example the widely used HNR measure introduced by Yumoto (Yumoto, Gould, & Baer, 1982). One important advantage of waveform measures in contrast to measures based on prior extraction of single-cycle F_0 and amplitude measures is the potential resolution down to the sampling interval and the concomitant reduced impact of periodicity and stationarity assumptions (cf. the "wavelet" approach of Qi & Shipp, 1992, and the newer glottal-to-noise excitation ratio measures developed by Michaelis [Michaelis, Fröhlich, & Strube, 1998; Michaelis, Gramss, & Strube, 1997; Michaelis & Strube, 1995].)

References reporting waveform perturbations that are not specifically noted in the following table are listed at the end of the table:

Measure	***Unit***	***Algorithm***	***Notes***
Glottal pulse irregularity	none	observation of smoked drum or filmed tonoscopic waveform	Janvrin (1933) and Janvrin and Worster-Drought (1932) reported that pulse irregularities, especially at the onset of sustained /a/ phonation, were diagnostic signs of **laryngeal ataxia**. They highlighted cases of **disseminated** (i.e., multiple) **sclerosis**, but reported that similar phenomema had been observed in **Friedrich's ataxia**, **cerebellar tumor**, **polyneuritis**, and "**general paralysis of the insane**." Scripture (1933) followed up these reports with a quantitative analysis of the F_0 perturbations evident in Janvrin's data (see Table 9–1.2a).

Table 9–4.0. Continued

Hardware-based threshold-detection measures (Askenfelt & Hammarberg, 1986), general notes:

Waveform perturbation measures were produced by an adaptive threshold detecting hardware device that triggered a new data point with each completed glottal cycle. Cycle-to-cycle variation in amplitude therefore yielded similar variation in cycle times in addition to the variation caused by actual cycle length changes. The data for the following groups of measures were extracted from contact microphone signals recorded during a passage reading and processed by the hardware device. To select data for perturbation analysis, pauses, unvoiced speech segments, and the first and last five periods from each voiced segment were removed. Some of the measures below were based on prior identification of perturbed sections of speech, that is, in which the rate of cycle-to-cycle change exceeded 2% for a minimum of five consecutive cycles: $N_{Perturb}$ = total number of perturbed periods in a sample. Other measures were based on the distribution of relative cycle-to-cycle differences $\Delta F0 = \frac{F0_{i+1} - F0_i}{F0_i}$.

Measure	Unit	Algorithm	Notes
Perturbation factor (PF)	proportion	$\frac{N_{Perturb}}{\text{total number of periods meeting selection criterion}}$	Askenfelt and Hammarberg (1986) assessed the 7 measures listed in this table section against perceptual profiles of 41 dysphonic voices (33 **organic**, 8 **functional**) **pre-** and **posttherapy**. The measures were assessed using a discrimination factor (DF) defined (using regression analysis) as the percentage change in the measure per perceptual scale degree, and correlation coefficients (r) between the measure and the perceptual scale; an overall usefulness index was formed from the product DF × r. By this index, DF_0SD and DF_0P were superior, followed closely by PF and PMM (though the latter measures appeared to be excessively sensitive to analysis settings such as the rate-of-change criterion—see General Notes at the top of this section). PM suffered from high dispersion in these results, and DPF and DF_0C showed high correlations but a low discrimination factors.
Perturbation magnitude (PM)	%	$\frac{1}{N_{Perturb}} \sum_{i=1}^{N_{Perturb}} \frac{\lvert F0_{i+1} - F0_i \rvert}{F0_i}$	
Perturbation magnitude mean (PMM)	proportion × %	PF × PM	
Directional perturbation factor (DPF)	% of total pitch periods $\Delta T0$ that change sign	As specified in unit (left)	
Delta-F_0 standard deviation (Df_0SD)	proportion	Standard deviation of $\Delta F0$ distribution	

Table 9–4.0. Continued

Measure	*Unit*	*Algorithm*	*Notes*
Delta-F_0 compression (DF_0C)	%	Mean height of $\Delta F0$ distribution in band of ± 1% surrounding 0	
Delta-F_0 peakedness (DF_0P)	ratio	$\frac{DF_0C}{DF_0SD}$	

Least mean square measures (Milenkovic, 1987, 1994):
Statistical steps for estimating perturbation parameters from data digitized at low sampling rates:

1. Designate a seed value for pitch period $T_{initial}$.
2. Minimize cycle-to-cycle mean square error (approximated as E_0) with respect to cycle-to-cycle amplitude change factor G and $T_{initial}$ by taking the derivative of E_0 with respect to G, setting it to 0, and solving for G
3. Search (within bounds of ±10% from the previous period) for the pitch period T (in samples) that minimizes E_0 for the value of G obtained in step 2
4. Enhance the resolution of T using an interpolated time *t(int)* by minimizing a parabolic fit to sample values of E_0 [and retain the reference sample *i(ref)* from which that time was interpolated]
5. Using *t(int)*, refine the sample value estimates of G and E_0 by parabolic interpolation of period-to-period covariance functions, retaining minimum interpolated E_0 as E_{opt}
6. Update sampled data frame length N using nearest integer fit to T.

Note: G here is K in Milenkovic 1987 and 1994.

Measure	*Unit*	*Algorithm*	*Notes*
Least mean square jitter	μs	$\lvert T0_{i(ref)} - T0_{i(ref)-N} \rvert$	Implemented in current CSpeech and CSpeechSP programs (Milenkovic, 1992; 1997). Milenkovic (1987) obtained accurate measurements of synthesized jitter at low sampling rates (8.3 kHz) but observed jitter in many samples with synthetic shimmer and no jitter. He also measured very low levels of jitter (9–37 μs) in subjects with no pathology.

Table 9–4.0. Continued

Measure	*Unit*	*Algorithm*	*Notes*
Least mean square shimmer	%	$\lvert 100(1 - G) \rvert$	Implemented in current CSpeech and CSpeechSP programs (Milenkovic, 1992; 1997). Milenkovic (1987) obtained accurate measurements of synthesized shimmer at low sampling rates (8.3 kHz) but observed shimmer in samples with synthetic jitter and no shimmer.
$SNR_{Milenkovic}$ (Milenkovic, 1987), SNR_{nujit} (Milenkovic, 1992, 1997).	dB	$10 \times \log_{10}\left(\frac{\sum_{t=0}^{t=T} x_t^2}{E_{opt}}\right)$	Using the least mean squares steps described above, Milenkovic (1987) observed some sensitivity of SNR to synthetic jitter and shimmer. In "nujit" method, the noise estimate E_{opt} is obtained by application of a low-pass"pitch prediction" filter to an interpolated signal, replacing the interpolation of covariance described in steps 4–6 of the listed steps preceding. Implemented in CSpeech program version 3.0 and older. "Nujit" method in CSpeech 4.0 and CspeechSP (Milenkovic, 1992, 1997) programs is optimal for sampling rates > 20 kHz and is reported (Leddy et al., 1994) to exhibit reduced deflation of SNR at higher jitter levels.
Cross correlation function (CCF—plot called correlogram.)	function is coefficient r × lag τ, applied to any serial parameter P_i such as fundamental periods or their amplitudes	$r_\tau = \frac{\frac{1}{N-\tau}\sum_{i=1}^{N-\tau} P_i \times P_{i+\tau} - \overline{P_1}\,\overline{P_2}}{s_1 s_2}$, where $\overline{P}_1 = \frac{\sum_{i=1}^{N-\tau} P_i}{N-\tau}$, $s_1 = \sqrt{\sum_{i=1}^{N-\tau} \frac{(P_i - \overline{P}_1)^2}{N-\tau}}$,	Koike (1968) applied CCF to epoch amplitude peaks of phonations by subjects with **laryngeal neoplasms**, **unilateral laryngeal paralysis**, and controls, finding significant correlations in approximately 50% of records from all groups, periodic (lag 3–12) modulations distinctive of neoplasm pathology, and no periodic modulation in paralysis. Used **hoarseness** as descriptor. Iwata (1972) applied to pitch perturbations of phonations by subjects with **chronic laryngitis**, **neoplasms**, and **unilateral laryngeal paralysis**,

Table 9–4.0. Continued

Measure	*Unit*	*Algorithm*	*Notes*
		$\overline{P}_2 = \frac{\sum_{i=\tau+1}^{N}}{N-\tau}, \; s_2 = \sqrt{\sum_{i=\tau+1}^{N} \frac{(P_i - \overline{P}_1)^2}{N-\tau}}$	finding significant periodic correlations at around 7 lags for those with normal voice, multiple high correlations in neoplasm, and little correlation pattern for other inflammatory conditions. The CCF plot is recommended by Hirano (1981) as a measure for fundamental frequency series. See Talkin (1994) for a grayscale display which he also calls a correlogram; in analogy to a spectrogram it displays time-varying CCFs with correlations close to 1 in black and correlations close to 0 in white.
HNR_{Yumoto}	log_{dB} (energy of harmonic signal/ energy of noise signal)	1. Extract N pitch periods T0 comprised of samples x_{t0} (t0 = 1, . ., T), and retain largest T as T_{max} 2. For all T0s with $T < T_{max}$, pad with additional 0s to yield $x_{t0(pad)}$ T to T_{max} (to eliminate variations due to jitter) 3. Derive harmonic signal estimate as average of sampled periods: $H_t = \sum_{i=1}^{N} x_{t0(pad),i} / N$ 4. Derive noise signal estimates for each of N sampled periods: $Noise_{t,i} = x_{t0(pad),i} - H_t$ 5. Compute ratio of harmonic signal energy to noise signal energy: $\frac{N \times \sum_{t=1}^{t=T_{max}} H_t^2}{\sum_{i=1}^{N} \sum_{i=1}^{t=T_{max}} Noise_{t,i}^2}$	Yumoto, et al., (1982) applied to **pre- and post-operative** phonations by speakers with a **variety of organic voice disorders** presenting with **hoarseness**, and a group of control subjects. Using semiautomatic zero-crossing pitch period detection aided by lowpass filtered signal inspection for the hoarse voices, Yumoto used 50 periods for calculation of HNR (signals digitized at 20 kHz). Normative values were 11.9 dB, preoperative mean was 1.6, postoperative 11.3. Synthetic pure tone signals yielded measures in mid to upper 30 dB range, decreasing with higher frequencies. This HNR showed high correlation with Yanigahara classification (q.v., Table 9–5.1), especially in a comparison of postoperative minus preoperative difference scores (Spearman's rank correlation coefficient = 0.944). An important distinction to frequency domain methods (e.g., HNR_{Kojima}) is the detection of noise components overlapping harmonic frequencies. Yumoto, Sasaki, and Okamura (1984) obtained

Table 9–4.0. Continued

Measure	*Unit*	*Algorithm*	*Notes*
		6. Convert expression to dB by taking $\log_{10}$ and multiply by 10	HNR_{Yumoto}, JF, Yanigahara classification, and a psychophysical 4-point scale measurement of **hoarseness** (8 trained judges), obtaining essentially identical corrrelations of 0.81 for HNR_{Yumoto} and Yanigahara classification and 0.71 for JF, also demonstrating statistically significance of the differences between these correlations. R.C. Scherer et al. (1987) measured declining trend in HNR_{Yumoto} with progression of **vocal fatigue** in a trained speaker, but not in an untrained speaker, and no significant association with these speakers' self-ratings of voice condition (see however this study's results with percent jitter, Table 9–1.2a). See also comparison of HNR_{Yumoto} to NSR_{Muta} in the entry for the latter, Table 9–5.2.
Modulation index parameters (Imaizumi, 1986)	WMI (waveform modulation index) is an averaged difference between correlation coefficients, and WMF (waveform modulation index) is a frequency. PMI and AMI are pitch and amplitude modulation indices and PMF and AMF are the frequencies of these modulations.	Using sustained phonation samples of 0.5 s duration, digitized at 20 kHz, pitch periods (*T0*) are identified and frames of data (x_{T0}) extracted. Correlations ($R(i,j)$) between i^{th} and j^{th} frames are measured from each sample up to a maximum of $i - j = 10$.WMI = the differences between the maximum and minimum R(i,j)s averaged over the samples.WMF = the inverse of the period separating the ith and j^{th} frames at which the maximum $R(i,j)$s were observed. Correlograms of lag 40 were calculated on the periods (*T0*) and amplitudes (*A0*), and the modulation indices PMI, AMI, PMF, and AMF were calculated similarly to WMI and WMF. (See Imaizumi (1986) for additional details.)	Imaizumi (1986), using 90 pathologic and 8 normal voices from an earlier perceptual study, demonstrates periodic components in the modulation of glottal waveforms and their pitches and amplitudes graphically by plots of R(i,j) and pitch and amplitude correlograms, arguing that at least one important component of perceived roughness is a periodic, multiplicative component occurring over several pitch periods. Although PPQ and APQ (see Tables 9-1.2a and 9-2.2a) were also calculated showing high values for rough voices, some rough voices received low perturbation measures.

Table 9–4.0. Continued

Measure	***Unit***	***Algorithm***	***Notes***
Br parameter (breathiness, Fukuzawa, Blaugrund, et al., 1988)	Energy ratio (energy of second derivative of preemphasized signal divided by energy of pre-emphasized waveform)	$100 \times \frac{\sum (x'_t - 2x'_{t-1} + x'_{t-2})^2}{\sum (x'_t)^2}$ where x'_t = signal with 6 dB preemphasis.	Fukuzawa, Blaugrund, El-Assuooty, and Gould. (1988) measured Br, St, and percent jitter (see Table 9–1.2a) in the sustained vowel phonations of 39 patients with **laryngeal cancer**, **recurrent nerve palsy (RNP)**, and **polyps**, and 24 control samples, demonstrating tendencies for distinctive patterns among these measures. Although more than half the patients fell within normal ranges for jitter (**RNP** never producing values more than 5 SDs off norm), Br was more sensitive to the pathologies (**polyp** cases produced significantly lower Br than the other pathologies). Many St values from the pathological voices did not fall outside of normative ranges, but some **cancer** cases were unique in doing so. Two-dimensional plots combining Br with the other parameters were especially effective in isolating **cancer**. Fukuzawa, El-Assuooty, and Honjo (1988) additionally obtained a significant rank difference correlation of Br with perceptual ratings of **breathiness** (0.73) but not with **roughness** (0.21).
St parameter ("strain," Fukuzawa, Blaugrund, et al., 1988)	Energy ratio (signal energy divided by low-pass filtered signal energy)	$\frac{\sum (x_i)^2}{\sum (lpx_t)^2}$, where lpx_t = signal lowpass filtered at f_c of 339 Hz.	See preceding notes entry.

Table 9–4.0. Continued

Measure	***Unit***	***Algorithm***	***Notes***
Correlation Factor (Cox et al., 1989b)	dB	$\mathrm{CF}(K) = 10 \times \log_{10}\left(\frac{1}{N}\sum_{i=1}^{N}\frac{1 + r_{i,i+K}}{1 - r_{i,i+K}}\right)$, where $r_{i,i+K}$ is the cross-correlation function (see previous entry in this table), and K is an integer period separation constant.	See Appendix 9–A entry, Cox, Ito, and Morrison (1989b) study, for methodological notes reviewing the performance of this algorithm. These authors suggest the use of K > 1 for measurement of periodic perturbations, that is, the use of CF(2)–CF(1) for detecting a one-half subharmonic.
VF (cycle-to-cycle variation of waveform, Feijoo & Hernández, 1990)	Normalized average per-sample cross-cycle amplitude difference.	Let MIN = the number of samples in the shortest glottal cycle considered, and $x_{t0}(n)$ = the samples comprising the nth glottal cycle. VF = , $\frac{1}{MIN}\frac{1}{\overline{\overline{A0}}}\frac{1}{N}\sum_{n=1}^{N}\sum_{t0=1}^{MIN}\frac{\lvert x_{t0}(n+1) - x_{t0}(n)\rvert}{AVG(x_{t0})}$, where $AVG(x_{t0})$ = $\frac{1}{N}\frac{1}{\max(A0)}\sum_{n=1}^{N} x_{t0}(n),\ t0 = 1, \ldots, MIN$	Feijoo and Hernández (1990) measured VF in sustained /e/ phonations by 56 individuals with **glottic cancer** (stages T1–T4) and 64 control speakers, obtaining 86% classification success and correlations of approximately 0.82 with both **hoarseness** and **breathiness** ratings. Other measures applied to this dataset were superior in classification (D and NNE [Table 9–5.2], and CE [Table 9–5.4]), one was comparable (normalized mean absolute shimmer [Table 9–2.2a]), and normalized mean absolute jitter (Table 9–1.2a) was inferior.
NOIS (Aspiration noise in the F3 region of the spectrum, Klatt & Klatt [1990])	4-point subjective scale	1. Obtain visual estimate of F3 frequency from broadband spectrogram 2. Bandpass filter vowel segment with center frequency set to F3 estimate (e.g., Klatt & Klatt [1990] used 4-pole Butterworth filter with 600 Hz BW).	Klatt and Klatt (1990) measured NOIS in 10 female and 6 males reiterant imitations of two different sentences, one set with /hɑ/ syllables, one with /ʔɑ/. They found a 0.4–1 scale point greater average for **women** consistent with **breathiness** (the difference depending on the sentence imitated), and obtained a 0.84 correlation with

Table 9–4.0. Continued

Measure	*Unit*	*Algorithm*	*Notes*
		3. Plot approximately 100 ms–150 ms of filtered waveform in synchrony with original waveform and assign judgment to filtered waveform (1) "periodic, no visible noise," (2) "periodic but occasional noise intrusion," (3) "weakly periodic, clear evidence of noise excitation," (4) "little or no periodicity, noise is prominent." (Klatt et al., 1990, p. 831)	perceived breathiness of the /hɑ/ reiterant sentence. They observed considerable intersubject variability, an increase in **unstressed** syllables, and most notably an increase in many s**entence-final F_0 drops**. Remarking on the paradox between this last observation of breathiness and the concurrent decrease of $H1_{re2}$ (see Table 9–5.1), they postulate a **breathy-laryngealized** mode of vibration for normal sentence-final phonation in many speakers (cf. results for the H1 amplitude measure $H1_{re2}$, Table 9–5.2, and notes on the synthesis portion of their work in Appendix 9–A).

Other Sources: Cairns, Hansen, and Kaiser, 1996; Dolanský and Tjernlund, 1968; Fröhlich, Michaelis, Strube, and Kruse, 1997; Hiki, 1983; Granqvist and Hammarberg, 1998; Kempster et al., 1991; Leeper, Millard, Bandur, and Hudson, 1996; Milenkovic, Bless, and Rammage, 1991; Mori, Blaugrund, and Yu, 1994; Pabon and de Krom, 1995; Qi, 1992; Qi and Shipp, 1992; Qi, Weinberg, Bi, and Hess, 1995; Ramig et al., 1990; Schoentgen, 1985; Silbergleit et al., 1997; Strand et al., 1994; Talkin, 1994; Wendahl, Moore, and Hollien, 1963; Wolfe, Fitch, and Cornell, 1995; Yumoto, 1983; Zwirner, Murry, Swenson, and Woodson, 1991; Zwirner, Murry, and Woodson, 1991.

Table 9–5.1. Spectral Measures: Spectographic Measures.

It is well known that frequency domain representations, such as the power spectrum resulting from the smoothed Fourier transformed speech waveform, have been crucial for the understanding of basic speech qualities. This truism also applies to voice quality. Indeed, the basic elements of vowel quality, that is, the frequency, amplitude, and bandwidth parameters of formant structure, are also important elements of radiated voice quality, as has been particularly evident to researchers at Massachusetts Institute of Technology (Bickley, 1982; Klatt & Klatt, 1990; Stevens & Hanson, 1995) and the Royal Institute of Technology in Stockholm (Ananthapadmanabha, 1995).

Four tables listing spectral measures follow, distinguishing between those based on inspection of the spectrogram, those based on inspection or automatic calculation using elements of traditional two-dimensional spectra (both Fourier and linear prediction coefficients [LPC]), those based on long-term averaged spectra (either continuously obtained via hardware or integrated across discrete spectra), and those based on the inverse Fourier transform of the log magnitude spectrum, or cepstrum. The spectrogram-based measures are listed first in Table 9–5.1, even though the spectrum is more elemental and historically earlier: this is because the preponderance of spectrographic measures were in use before the more elaborated automatic spectral algorithms, such as the various harmonics-to-noise ratios. The spectrogram remains nonetheless a valuable tool for exploring voice qualities, all the more so for the researcher who wisely chooses to inspect a given signal for all its potential features of interest before entrusting the signal to an automated metric that may in fact obscure or miss the most important features altogether. Table 9–5.2 lists discrete spectral based measures, of which the preponderance are Fourier based. Some LPC-based spectral measures are listed here, although others are grouped in Table 9–6.1, as they are derived in the course of analyses primarily oriented to extraction of underlying glottal excitation information from the radiated signal. Still other spectrographic representations are possible, for example, the "cone-kernel" technique (Kheirallah & Jamieson, 1994), some of which promise enhanced time resolution for nonstationary signals, but none had been implemented as the basis for voice quality measures in the time period encompassed by these tables (nor, unfortunately, have they been adopted in the meantime in substantive applications, to this author's best knowledge). The long-term averaged measures listed in Table 9–5.3 showed conceptual promise for voice quality research as a simple means of attenuating the impact of changing transfer functions associated with connected speech production. Although it is apparent that this approach is vulnerable to exogenous variables and is not very well correlated with perceptual effects, the technique is very appropriate within subjects and for guiding associated analysis. Finally, the measures listed in Table 9–5.4 indicate promising outcomes from the cepstral technique, as has been demonstrated meanwhile in work by de Krom (1993), Dejonckere and Wieneke (1992, 1994), and others.

References reporting spectrographic measures that are not specifically noted in the following table are listed at the end of the table.

Table 9–5.1. Continued

Measure	***Description***	***Application Notes***
Yanigahara classification of (standard narrowband) spectrograms (Yanigahara, 1967)	Type I: "The regular harmonic components are mixed with the noise component chiefly in the formant region of the vowels." Type II: "The noise components in the second formants of /ɛ/ and /i/ predominate over the harmonic components, and slight additional noise components appear in the high frequency region above 3000 Hz in the vowels /ɛ/ and /i/." Type III: "The second formants of /ɛ/ and /i/ are totally replaced by noise components, and the additional noise components above 3000 Hz further intensify their energy and expand their range." Type IV: "The second formants of /ɑ/, /ɛ/ and /i/ are replaced by noise components, and even the first formants of all vowels often lose their periodic components which are supplemented by noise components. In addition, more intensified high frequency additional noise components are seen." (Yanigahara, 1967, pp. 533–534.)	This system has been rather widely adopted but not often investigated as a quantitative measure. Moran and Gilbert (1984) compared the system with the Wilson Voice Profile system and found strong associations of Yanigahara-based NHR with **laryngeal tension**, and Wilson's +**2-2** (tension + air loss) **dysfunction**.
Voice prints (Iwata & von Leden, 1970b)	Display of phonation samples in contour mode displays on older analog equipment (e.g., Kay Sona-graph model 6061). The nature of this display is reproduced in some degree by the discrete gray level fields seen on digital microcomputer-based displays (e.g., MS-DOS-based versions of Kay Elemetrics' CSL). A return to virtually continuous gray-scale displays can be achieved on more recent systems (e.g., Kay Elemetrics Multispeech or CSL for Windows)	Iwata and von Leden (1970b) argued for the superiority of voice prints (especially with expanded display of DC-2 kHz range) over sonagrams for detection of energy fluctuations and subclassification of **severe hoarseness**.
Imaizumi's multi-dimensional analysis of sustained vowels (Imaizumi et al., 1980, as summarized in	1. Size of F_0 variation (ΔF_0-$\bar{F}_0$) measured on narrowband spectrogram. 2. Speed of F_0 fluctuation (number of peaks in one second). 3. Size of overall amplitude fluctuation (peak-to-peak value on an amplitude display). 4. Speed of overall amplitude fluctuation (number of peaks in one second.	1: Hirano et al. (1986), in an application to 68 pathologic samples, observed a negative relation of this parameter to stroboscopically assessed amplitude of vibration.

Table 9–5.1. Continued

Measure	***Description***	***Application Notes***
Hirano, 1981)	5. Richness of high frequency harmonics (ratio of mean level in 3.5 to 4.5 kHz to that below 1 kHz, obtained from section display). 6. Relative noise level (difference between spectral envelope of harmonic peaks to harmonic troughs, measured in regions of first and second harmonics, sometimes called S/N ratio, such as by Hirano et al. 1986). 7. Rising time (on amplitude display, time required to increase from 10% to 90% of steady level). 8. Falling time (on amplitude display, time required to decrease from 90% to 10% of steady level)	3: Hirano et al. (1986) observed a negative correlation of this parameter with SPL range and in **polyp** cases with stroboscopically assessed regularity of vibration. The parameter was positively related to perceived **breathy** quality (GRBAS scale—Hirano, 1981). 5: A negative relation between this parameter and habitual F_0 obtained by Hirano et al. (1986) was presumed to be a gender effect. They also observed a negative relation with stroboscopically assessed regularity of vibration in cases of polyp. The parameter was positively related to perceived breathy quality in cases of parlysis (GRBAS scale—Hirano, 1981). 6: Hirano et al. (1986) observed a negative correlation of this parameter to size of amplitude fluctuation, richness of higher harmonics, habitual SPL, and to aerodynamically assessed mean flow rate. A positive relation to habitual F_0 was presumed to be an artifact of the technique (due to closer harmonic spacing in lower F_0). These researchers also noted a positive correlation of this S/N parameter with normalcy of mucosal wave in cases of **paralysis**. In correlation analyses with perceptual GRBAS scales (see Hirano, 1981), this parameter was negatively related to overall **hoarseness**, to **asthenic** quality, and to **breathy** quality in paralysis cases.

Table 9–5.1. Continued

Measure	***Description***	***Application Notes***
		Yoon, Kakita, and Hirano (1984) applied these eight measures plus F1 frequency to evaluate sustained phonations by 11 subjects with **glottic carcinoma** (**stages T1a** and **T3**), finding an association of measures 1, 2, 3, 5, and 6 with stage of lesion advancement.
Relative noise level (Fujiu, Hibi, & Hirano, 1988)	As in the Imaizumi et al. (1980) measure by the same name (see previous cell, this table), the dB ratio of the summed peaks to the summed troughs is measured. Digital spectrography techniques are used, with variable filter bandwidths (22.5 or 45 Hz for males, 45 or 90 Hz for females) and analysis attenuators, to include all peaks and troughs in 1.5–2 kHz range.	Fujiu, Hibi, and Hirano (1988) assessed this measure on phonations produced by normal adults, demonstrating the value of bandwidth adjustments for different vocal F_0 ranges. Analysis attenuation was seen to be effective for the narrower bandwidth settings.
Formant analysis (with averaged power spectrum of selected interval)	Narrowband spectrogram with simultaneous averaged power spectrum display of selected interval, for example, on Kay Elemetrics DSP-5500.	Yanagisawa, Estill, Kmucha, and Leder (1989) measured singer's formant at approximately 3 kHz in loud sections of messa di voce productions by male and female singers. They observed notable strength of this formant in association with endoscopically observed aryepiglottic narrowing in twang¸belting, and opera styles (as opposed to the quieter modal, falsetto, and sob styles).

Other Sources: Fischer-Jørgensen, 1967; Henton and Bladon, 1988; Hertrich and Ackermann, 1995; Isshiki, Yanagihara, and Morimoto, 1966; Kirk, Ladefoged, and Ladefoged, 1984; Murry and Singh, 1980; Murry, Singh, and Sargent, 1977; Pandit, 1957; Rontal, Rontal, and Rolnick, 1975; Sasaki, Okamura, and Yumoto, 1991; Walton and Orlikoff, 1994; Wendler, Wagner, Seidner, and Stürzebecher, 1976; Wirz, Subtelny, and Whitehead, 1981; Wolfe and Ratusnik, 1988.

Table 9–5.2. Spectral Measures: Fourier and LPC Spectra.

References reporting spectral measures that are not specifically noted in the following table are listed at the end of the table.

Measure	***Unit***	***Algorithm***	***Notes***
Timbre	Harmonic distribution	Henrici analyzer results (a mechanical form of Fourier harmonic analysis–see Kent & Read, 1991).	Bartholomew (1934) used Henrici analysis to measure "**good**" voice quality in adult male **singers**. He listed three criteria based on qualitative summaries of the resulting line spectra: (1) timbre vibrato (cf. entries in Tables 9–1.2b and 9–2.2b); (2) low formant, an emphasis of lower harmonics he attributed to a preference for open vowel qualities; and (3) high formant, a consistent resonance at about 2800 Hz now known as the singer's formant.
Spectral noise level (SNL)	dB SPL	1. 3 Hz bandwidth spectral analysis of 2-s sample of sustained vowel phonation. 2. Lowest dB SPL level in each 100 Hz section from 100–8000 Hz range. 3. Levels averaged over different frequency ranges (100–2600 Hz, 2600–5100 Hz, 5100–8000 Hz, 100-5100 Hz, and 100–8000 Hz)	Applied to normal and **simulated roughness** in females by Lively and Emanuel (1970), to males by Sansone and Emanuel (1970), and to males and females together by Emanuel, Lively, and McCoy (1973). In all, means in 100-2600 Hz range correlated best with perception. Evaluated together, males were perceived to be rougher than females Deal and Emanuel (1978) argued for superior performance of SNL in comparison to PVI and AVI (see Tables 9–1.2a and 9–2.2a.), arguing that SNL better represents the frequency range of roughness. Nichols (1979), however, indicated that SNL may be less easily obtained as a clinical measure. Compare these with the Imaizumi et al. spectrographic analysis measure 6,"Relative noise level,"Table 9–5.1.

Table 9–5.2. Continued

Measure	***Unit***	***Algorithm***	***Notes***
Number of partials	Integer count	1. Perform narrowband spectral analysis. 2. Use comb template to identify partials at least 2 dB above nosie floor.	Colton (1972) used this procedure on DC-10 kHz spectra (50 Hz analysis bandwidth) to identify quality difference between males' modal and falsetto **registers**, finding roughly 10–15 partials in falsetto, 15–20 in modal.
Formant frequencies	Hz	Generally estimated by visual inspection of DFT spectra, LPC spectra, or spectrograms.	Linville and Fisher (1985) obtained lower F1 values for **older females' whispered** phonations, correlating both with perceived and actual age. They found no such effects for F2 frequency. Mount and Salmon (1988) observed effects of postoperative speech therapy in a 63-year-old male-to-female transsexual in elevated F_0 but also, and apparently most critically, in elevated F2 frequencies.
Amplitude of first harmonic (H1–H2 difference in Henton & Bladon [1985], A_0 in Bickley & Stevens [1986, 1987], $H1_{re2}$ in Klatt & Klatt [1990]).	$dB_{re:\ RMS(vow)}$, $dB_{re:\ amp(H2)}$, or $dB_{re:\ amp(F1)}$	Measured from narrowband spectra (e.g., measured from Hamming windowed 256-point segment of 10 kHz sampled adult); against reference value (e.g., RMS amplitude of vowel, amplitude of second harmonic, or amplitude of first formant). Klatt and Klatt (1990) added 10 dB to the difference between H1 and H2 to keep all values positive.	Henton and Bladon (1985) used narrow band spectral analysis from 80 ms steady-state portion of British vowels produced by 32 women and 29 men, finding greater H1–H2 differences in **women's voices**, (ranging from 3.3 to 8.4 dB, on average about 5.5 dB more than in men's), suggesting this reflected **"desirable" breathiness**. Bickley and Stevens (1986, 1987) measured a decrease in A_0 as a result of **supraglottal constriction** (using a mechanic device at the lips), over and above that due to the attendant shift in first formant frequency, inferred to be a decrease in area of glottal pulse (DC component of flow). Klatt and Klatt (1990) measured $H1_{re2}$ in 10 female and 6 males, reiterant imitations of two different sentences, one set with phonetic /hɑ/

Table 9–5.2. Continued

Measure	*Unit*	*Algorithm*	*Notes*
			syllables, one with /ʔɑ/. They found a 5.7 dB greater intensity for **women** consistent with **breathiness**, considerable intersubject variability, and a reduction in $H1_{re2}$ amplitude in many **sentence-final F_0 drops**, consistent with **laryngealization**. They also obtained a 0.83 correlation of $H1_{re2}$ with **breathiness** perceived in excised vowel samples. See results for the NOIS measure, Table 9–4.0, the entry for this study in Appendix 9–B indicating that $H1_{re2}$ may also correlate with perceived **nasality**, and the original report for additional measures that did not reach statistically significant correlations with perceptions of breathiness.
Amplitude of first formant (A1)	dB	Measured from narrowband spectra (e.g. from Hamming windowed 256-point segment of 10 kHz sampled adult)	Bickley and Stevens (1986, 1987) measured a decrease in A1 as a result of **supraglottal constriction**, over and above that caused by the attendant shift in first and second formant frequencies, inferred as a decrease in area of glottal pulse and in slope of pulse at closure. Additional decrement in this value beyond the comparable decrements in A_0 and A2 (q.v., this table) indicated an increase in F1 bandwidth.
Amplitude of second formant (A2)	dB	Measured from narrowband spectra (e.g., from Hamming windowed 256-point segment of 10 kHz sampled adult)	Bickley and Stevens (1986, 1987) measured a decrease in A1 as a result of **supraglottal constriction**, over and above that caused by the attendant shift in first and second formant frequencies, inferred as a decrease in high frequency harmonic energy due to reduced magnitude in the slope of pulse at closure.

Table 9–5.2. Continued

Measure	***Unit***	***Algorithm***	***Notes***
Spectral tilt of high frequencies	dB change as a function of frequency (often dB/octave)	Average magnitude of upper harmonics/ average magnitude of lower harmonics.	See Stevens (1977) and Stevens and Hanson (1995) for theoretical basis. Correlates with flow declination rate; decrease of energy at higher harmonics may indicate less abrupt closure or lack of simultaneity in glottal closure along anterior-posterier length, that is, a **breathy** voice. Increase of energy at higher harmonics may indicate a "constricted" glottis with greater adducation, that is, a **creaky** voice (cf. Fant-Liljencrants's fifth parameter, Fant, 1986), and Frequency at which spectral tilt begins, this table). Also compare with Imaizumi et al.'s (1980) spectral measure 5 Richness of high frequency harmonics, Table. 9–5.1.
Frequency at which spectral tilt begins	Hz	No clear or consistent basis for measurement across speakers	See Stevens (1977) and Stevens and Hanson (1995) for theoretical basis in adjustment of adduction/abduction; a lower than normal breakpoint would be expected from "spread" arytenoids, and a higher breakpoint from a "constricted" glottis.
F1 bandwidth	Hz	Spectral envelope width (Hz) of first formant measured 3 dB below peak value	Value exceeding 60-80 Hz may indicate incomplete glottal closure.
H1–A3	dB	Difference between amplitude of first harmonic and third formant	Examined by Stevens (1977) and Stevens and Hanson (1995).
$HNR_{Kitajima}$ (noise ratio)	ratio of signal RMS values.	1. Original signal is 205 ms of sustained /a/ digitized at 5 kHz with 2.5 kHz antialias filtering	Kitajima (1981) applied the Noise ratio to 20 voice samples from patients with **various** (primarily organic) **voice disorders** and assessed its

Table 9–5.2. Continued

Measure	***Unit***	***Algorithm***	***Notes***
		2. Periodogram (magnitude plot of FFT) is smoothed with a moving average to obtain mean and SD of the magnitudes as a model of the spectral noise threshold. 3. The mean+1 SD is subtracted from periodogram magnitudes greater than this threshold, and magnitudes below the threshold are set to zero. 4. The frequency domain ratio of the resulting magnitudes to the original signal periodogram magnitudes is used to create a noise-reducing filter, which (via inverse FFT) is then applied in the time domain to the central 51.5 ms of the original signal to produce a filtered signal. 5. The filtered signal is subtracted from the 51.5 sample of the original signal to produce a residue (noise) signal. 6. The noise ratio is defined as the ratio of the RMS energy of the filtered signal to the RMS energy of the residue signal.	reliability in repeat applications and against hand-obtained average harmonic peak-noise trough dB distances (within each of five 500 Hz bands from DC–2.5 kHz), finding significant correlations in all comparisons. Kitajima argued that the performance was especially strong considering the limited signal duration and frequency bandwidth examined.
HNR_{Kojima}	$\log_{db}$(dB ratio)	$10 \times \log_{10}\left(\frac{\sum_{n=1}^{N}\sum_{h=1}^{Max(h)}\left\|X_{3\times h}(n)\right\|^2}{\sum_{n=1}^{N}\sum_{h=1}^{Max(h)}\left\|X_{3\times h-1}(n)\right\|^2 + \left\|X_{3\times h-2}(n)\right\|^2}\right)$	Kojima, Gould, Lambiase, and Isshiki (1980) obtained a correlation of –0.868 between HNR_{Kojima} and a 4-point scale of perceived **hoarseness** for 58 sustained /a/ phonations, 30 of which were from subjects with various **organic** and **neurogenic** pathologies.

Table 9–5.2. Continued

Measure	***Unit***	***Algorithm***	***Notes***
H_r (Hiraoka et al., 1984)	% (harmonic energy)	$100 \times \left(\frac{\sum_{i \geq 2} H_i}{\sum_{i \geq 1} W_i} \right);$ Hiraoka uses 4096 points (sampled at 20 kHz) for Hamming windowed FFT and uses F_0 determination by frequency-domain harmonic-picking algorithm for calculation of harmonic series H_i sum to 10 kHz.	Hiraoka, Kitazoe, Ueta, Tanaka, and Tanabe, 1984, classified **hoarse** voices (**organic**, **neurogenic**, and **spastic**) with 92.5% success using a critical Hr of 67.2%. Hiraoka's three-part model suggests separation of F_0 from harmonic and noise components.
F_0F_1Q (Banci, Monini, Falaschi, & De Sario, 1986)	ratio (of spectral magnitudes)	"quotient between spectral amplitudes corresponding to the fundamental frequency and those corresponding to the first formant" (Banci et al., 1986, p. 497)	Banci et al. (1986) applied this measure in isolation to 53 pathological (various **organic** and **functional disorders**) and 30 nonpathological sustained phonation samples and obtained an overall 71.1% classification success (using decision rules based on classification training with a Mahalanobis distance criterion). This was inferior to other LPC residue-based measures (see Table 9–6.1).
Normalized noise energy (NNE, Kasuya, Ogawa, Mashima & Ebihara, 1986; also described as frequency domain noise estimation by adaptive comb filtering.)	logdb(dB ratio)	$10 \times \log_{10} \left(\frac{\frac{1}{N} \sum_{n=M_L}^{M_N} \sum_{i=l}^{N} \lvert \hat{W}_i(n) \rvert^2}{\frac{1}{N} \sum_{n=M_L}^{M_N} \sum_{i=l}^{N} \lvert X_i(n) \rvert^2} \right)$ where $\hat{W}_i(n)$ = an estimate of the Fourier transform of $noise_t$ obtained by evaluating $X_i(n)$ at frequencies i corresponding to intervals between harmonics—these intervals are determined	(See Kasuya, Ogawa, Mashima, et al. [1986] for discussions of computational details and the selection of 1 to 5 kHz fL fH range to exclude F1 frequencies). Kasuya, Ogawa, Mashima, et al., (1986) applied the NNE measure to 250 sustained phonations, 64 normal, and 186 pathological (dominated by mass lesions, especially T1 glottic cancer cases [n = 32], but also including recurrent nerve paralysis [n = 23], and laryngitis [n =21]). A threshold value of –11.0 dB was optimal

Table 9–5.2. Continued

Measure	*Unit*	*Algorithm*	*Notes*
		by an adaptive procedure employing an autocorrelation-based estimate of f_0, a Hamming window of length $7 \times T0$ (to ensure separation of harmonics), and a comb filtering in the frequency domain using the f_0 estimate to locate harmonics. M_L = the greatest integer function of $K \times f_L \times t$, (f_L = lowest frequency at which the noise estimate $\hat{W}_i(n)$ is taken, and M_L = the greatest integer function of $K \times f_H \times t$, (f_H = highest frequency at which the noise $\hat{W}_i(n)$ estimate is taken). (See Kasuya, Ogawa, Mashima, et al. [1986] for discussions of computational details and the selection of 1 to 5 kHz $f_L f_H$ range to exclude F1 frequencies).	in this dataset, achieving a classification success rate of 84.8%, with perfect detection of T1 cancer and 91% success for paralysis, but poor detection of laryngitis (45%). Kasuya, Masubuchi, et al. (1986). See also Table 9–1.2a, PPQ_{Kasusa} notes for use of NNE in Kasuya, Masubuchi, et al. (1986) screening protocol, and NHEPitch, Table 9–1.2a, for notes on perturbation measures applied to this dataset with somewhat lower discrimination success rates. Hirano et al. (1988) assessed NNE, PPQ_{Kasuya}, and APQ_{Kasuya} in cases of cancer, polyp, and recurrent nerve paralysis (RNP) pre- and post-treatment, observing that all measures demonstrated treatment efficacy and were positively correlated with perceptual, aerodynamic, and stroboscopic measures. Although they found APQ_{Kasuya} and PPQ_{Kasuya} to be particularly distinctive of RNP, the parameters were not generally useful in differentiating the pathologies. Feijoo and Hernández (1990) measured NNE in sustained /e/ phonations by 56 individuals with **glottic cancer** (stages T1-T4) and 64 control speakers, obtaining 89% classification success and correlations of approximately 0.86 with both **hoarseness** and **breathiness** ratings. Other measures applied to this dataset were comparable in classification (D [Table 9–5.1], and CE [Table 9–5.4]), and others (VF [Table 9–4.0]), Normalized mean absolute jitter [Table 9–1.2a] and Normalized mean absolute shimmer [Table 9–2.2a]) were inferior. In addition their NNE measures were moderately correlated (0.74) with both VF and D.

Table 9–5.2. Continued

Measure	***Unit***	***Algorithm***	***Notes***
$SNR_{Klingholz}$ (an analysis-by-synthesis technique) Klingholz (1987)	$\log_{db}$(dB ratio), displayed as a contour.	1. Extract successive Gaussian windowed data frames of 80 ms length for connected speech (160 ms for sustained vowels) overlapping by 20 ms. (Klingholz [1987] used 12.5 kHz sampling rate yielding 1,000-point frames for connected speech) 2. Zero-pad to 160 ms (320 ms), FFT, and interpolate then low-pass filter spectral components X_n to enhance spectral density 3. Use product moment technique (Schroeder, 1968) to estimate F_0, and use estimate to identify frequencies and magnitudes of harmonics H_n 4. Compute bandwidths B_n of H_n by parabolic interpolation to half-width values meeting two criteria: (a) 12 < Bn < 24, (b) ratio of Hn magnitude to mean of adjacent values > 12 dB 5. Smoothed B_n distribution is rank ordered by decreasing magnitude 6. First bandwidth is used in determination of synthetic Gaussian-shaped harmonics (H_{syn} at frequencies and magnitudes of original H_n) 7. Compute harmonic energy H_{syn} (EH) and total energy ΣX_n (ET) 8. If EH>ET, select next ranked B_n, and iterate until ET>EH	Klingholz (1987) tested $SNR_{Klinholz}$ on synthetic vowels, and on connected speech and sustained /a/ vowel samples produced by 81 speakers with **laryngeal disorders** and 20 speakers with no voice disorders. Synthetic signals revealed no dependence of $SNR_{Klingholz}$ on F_0. Only a rough screening of pathologic voices was obtained, although the algorithm was seen to be effective for short speech segments and the highly variable nature of continuous speech. SNR was relatively high (>17 dB) for **hyperfunctional dysphonia** and other pathological cases with high SNR are discussed in Klingholz (1987).

Table 9–5.2. Continued

Measure	Unit	Algorithm	Notes
		9. Compute SNR = 10 $\log_{10}$ (ET/ET-EH) 10. Set SNR to 36 dB for SNR > 36 dB 11. Produce SNR contour by three-point median smoothing then linear smoothing	
NSR_{Muta} (Muta, Baer, Wagatsuma, Muraoka, & Fukuda, 1988)	$\log_{db}$(dB ratio)	1. Perform time-domain F_0 estimation: (a) obtain initial estimate of fundamental period *T0* by any method, (b) specify frame size $K = 4 \times T0$ and apply Hanning window, (c) calculate ACF over *K* and use to revise initial estimate, repeating (b) and (c) as necessary to obtain $F_0 = 1/T0$ and redefine $K = 4 \times T0$. 2. Fourier transform *K* to produce X_n with line spectrum with harmonics at every fourth *n*, and further refine F_0 estimation in the frequency domain by minimizing an error term derived from a function that describes, up to the 16th harmonic, the expected spectrum spread due to the effects of Hanning window effects on discrepancies between discrete frequency sampling of discrete F_0 and actual continuous F_0 (f_r — see original citation for further details on the error minimization procedures). 3. Redefine Hanning windowed *K* on the basis of f_r and calculate pitch synchronous power spectrum by squaring	Muta et al. (1988) developed and applied this algorithm to synthetic /u/ vowel samples with varying amounts of jitter, shimmer, additive noise, amplitude and frequency modulation, as well as to three-syllable connected speech samples of three male and three female **hoarse** voices with **benign laryngeal disease**, **pre-** and **postoperatively**. Synthetic samples demonstrated sensitivity of NSR_{Muta} to additive noise, jitter, and shimmer (although with higher variability in the latter perturbation measures). Analysis of signals with constant levels of additive noise demonstrated that both NSR_{Muta} and HNR_{Yumoto} declined with increasing F_0, though NSR_{Muta} less steeply. Analysis of modulated signals demonstrated relative insensitivity of NSR_{Muta} to amplitude modulations up to 16% and frequency modulations up to 2% at $F_0 = 110$, with higher thresholds (32% and 4%) at $F_0 = 220$. The measure also reflected improvements in all patients' voice samples.

Table 9–5.2. Continued

Measure	*Unit*	*Algorithm*	*Notes*
		absolute magnitudes of the Fourier transform ($P(i) \equiv \lvert W_i \rvert^2$). 4. Identify noise components $Pn(i)$ by locating the minimum values $\lvert W_i \rvert^2$ in regions from $4i - 1$ to $4i + 2$, and calculate $\mathrm{NSR}_{\mathrm{Muta}} = 10 \times \log_{10}\left(\frac{\sum_{i=3}^{66} Pn(i)}{\sum_{i=3}^{66} P(i)}\right)$, these ranges of i being variable but set in this case to cover up to the 16th harmonic.	
MDVP pitch-synchronous frequency-domain measures, preprocessing: For each 81.92 ms frame: 1. Low-pass filter at fc = 6 kHz with 22nd order Hamming window FIR routine, downsample to 12.5 kHz, Hilbert transform. 2. Compute 1,024 FFT power spectrum. 3. Calculate average F_0 for frame from results of pitch-adaptive autocorrelation function with postprocessing for error correction (see MDVP pitch detection protocol in Table 9–1.1). Use pitch-synchronous routine to separate harmonic from in-harmonic spectral components.			
Noise-to-harmonic ratio (NHR in MDVP)	Ratio of inharmonic to harmonic spectral magnitudes	From preprocessed frames, compute ratio of in-harmonic energy in 1500–4500 Hz range to harmonic energy in 70–4500 Hz range	
Soft phonation index (SPI in MDVP)	Ratio of low to high frequency spectral magnitudes	From preprocessed frames, compute ratio of harmonic energy in 70–1600 Hz range to harmonic energy in 1600–4500 Hz range	

Table 9–5.2. Continued

Voice turbulence index (VTI in MDVP)	Ratio of high frequency spectral magnitudes to total spectral energy	1. Select 2 to 4 of frames from preprocessed frames where frequency and amplitude perturbations are minimal and there are no voice breaks or subharmonics. 2. Compute average ratio of inharmonic energy in 2800–5800 Hz range to harmonic energy in 70–4500 Hz range for selected frames.

Measure	Unit	Algorithm	Notes
HNR_{Cox} (Cox, Ito, & Morrison, 1989c)	$\log_{dB}$(power ratio)	$\frac{10}{N} \times \sum_{n}^{N} \log_{10}\left(\frac{\sum_{h=1}^{Max(h)} \lvert X_{T\times h^{(n)}}\rvert^2}{\sum_{i=NSKIP+1}^{T-NSKIP-1} \sum_{h=1}^{Max(h)} \lvert X_{T\times h-1^{(n)}}\rvert^2}\right),$ where T = number of pitch periods in each frame n, and $NSKIP$ = number of excluded components each side of the harmonic peaks	This is a generalized formulation of HNR_{Kojima} (q.v., this table) with additional parameters designed to allow for a variable number of pitch periods per frame and Fourier components exclusion for purposes of avoiding spectral leakage effects. See Appendix 9–A, Cox et al. (1989c) entry for methodological notes.
$HNR_{Cox(sor)}$ (Cox et al., 1989c)	$\log_{dB}$(power ratio)	$\frac{10}{N} \times \sum_{n}^{N} \log_{10}\left(\sum_{h=1}^{Max(h)} \frac{\lvert X_{T\times h^{(n)}}\rvert^2}{\sum_{i=NSKIP+1}^{T-NSKIP-1} \lvert X_{T\times h-i^{(n)}}\rvert^2}\right) - 10 \times \log_{10}\left(Max\,(h)\right),$ where T = number of pitch periods in each frame n, and $NSKIP$ = number of excluded components each side of the harmonic peaks	This is a variation of HNR_{Cox} (preceding entry), which is computed as a sum of ratios (hence "sor") instead of as a ratio of sums. Summing of ratios reduces emphasis of formant regions by applying equal weighting to all spectral components. See Appendix 9–A, Cox et al. (1989c) entry for methodological notes.

Table 9–5.2. Continued

Measure	Unit	Algorithm	Notes
DH (degree of hoarseness in Nikolov, Deliyski, et al., 1989)	ratio of noise to harmonic energy sums	1. Stable phonation zones ("without variations" of F_0 or A0) are located 2. 2,048 rectangular windowed FFTs are calculated and F_0 estimates used to measure harmonic bands at multiples of $F_0 \pm 2$ frequency components 3. Ratios of summed noise (total minus harmonic bands) to summed harmonic bands are calculated for all stable zones 4. DH = average of ratios from step 3	Nikolov et al. (1989) described the implementation of this parameter in a multidimensional program leading to the development of MDVP, observing especially high values for **recurrent nerve paralysis** and **laryngeal cancer**.
D (spectral distortion, Feijoo & Hernández, 1990)	average log likelihood of spectral ratio	Let SEG_n be the nth 3 cycle segment of a sample. Let A_n be the matrix of linear prediction filter coefficients of such a segment, A_n^t be the transpose of A_n, and R_n the matrix of linear prediction autocorrelation coefficients from SEG_n. $D = \frac{1}{N}\sum_{n=1}^{N} \log\left(\frac{A_{n+1}^t R_{n+1} A_{n+1}}{A_n^t R_n A_n}\right)$	Feijoo and Hernández (1990) measured this form of jitter in sustained /e/ phonations by 56 individuals with **glottic cancer** (stages T1–T4) and 64 control speakers, obtaining 89% classification success and correlations of approximately 0.92 with both **hoarseness** and **breathiness** ratings. Other measures applied to this dataset were comparable in classification (NNE [Table 9–5.2], and CE [Table 9–5.4]) and others (VF [Table 9–4.0]), normalized mean absolute jitter [Table 9–1.2a] and normalized mean absolute shimmer [Table 9–2.2a]) were inferior.

Table 9–5.2. Continued

Other Sources: Alku, Strik, and Vilkman, 1997; Alku et al., 1998; Castellengo, 1985; Chuang and Hanson, 1996; Cleveland and Sundberg, 1983, 1985; Colton, 1973; Debruyne et al., 1997; Dejonckere and Wieneke, 1994; Deliyski, 1990, 1993, 1994; Doval, d'Alessandro, and Diard, 1997; Ekholm et al., 1998; Emanuel and Sansone, 1969; Emanuel and Smith, 1974; B. Fex et al., 1994; Fröhlich, Michaelis, Strube, and Kruse, 1997; Gamboa et al., 1997; Gerull, Giesen, Hippel, Mrowinski, and Schweers, 1977; Hanson, 1997; Henton and Bladon, 1988; Hertrich and Ackermann, 1995; Hillenbrand, Cleveland, and Erickson, 1994; Hillenbrand and Houde, 1996; Hirose et al., 1995; Holmberg, Hillman, and Perkell, 1995; Holmberg, Hillman, Perkell, Guiod, and Goldman, 1995; Holmberg et al., 1994; Howell and Williams, 1988; Huffman, 1987; Kasuya and Ando, 1991; Kempster, 1984; Klatt, 1986, 1987; Klich, 1982; Ladefoged, 1983; Lee, 1988; Lee and Childers, 1991; Lotto, Holt, and Kluender, 1997; Ní Chasaide and Gobl, 1995; Omori et al., 1997; Raphael and Scherer, 1987; Ruiz et al., 1995; Ruiz, Absil, Harmegnies, Legros, and Poch, 1996; Sasaki et al., 1991; Schutte and Miller, 1991; Scobbie, Gibbon, Hardcastle, and Fletcher, 1998; Shoji, Regenbogen, Yu, and Blaugrund, 1992; Singh and Murry, 1978; Sluijter and van Heuven, 1996; Sluijter, van Heuven, and Pacilly, 1997; Södersten and Hammarberg, 1993; Södersten, Hertegård, and Hammarberg, 1995; Södersten and Lindestad, 1990; Södersten, Lindestad, and Hammarberg, 1991; Toner, Emanuel, and Parker, 1990; Wang, 1983; C.E. Williams and Stevens, 1972; C.E. Williams and Stevens, 1981; Wolfe et al., 1991; Zwirner and Barnes, 1992.

Table 9–5.3. Spectral Measures: Long-Term Average Spectra.

References reporting long-term average spectral measures that are not specifically noted in the following table are listed at the end of the table.

Measure	Unit and Definition	Notes
Hardware Bandpass filtered speech (BW = 250 Hz, Jansson & Sundberg, 1975):		Sundberg and Nordström (1976) studied LTAS of singing with **raised** and **lowered larynx** postures, finding higher average formants for raised larynx. Hammarberg et al. (1980) accounted for 85% of the variance in a set of 28 term ratings of **various functional and organic voice disorders** by five factors they identified as: I. Unstable-Steady, II. Breathy-Overtight, III. Hyper-Hypofunctional, IV. Coarse-Light, V. Head-Chest register. They found strong prediction (i.e., R^2s of 35% or greater in multiple regression models) of these factors using the following LTAS predictors: **Breathy:** Δ1 – Δ3 (i.e.,"slope") **Overtight:** Δ3 **Hyperfunctional:** Δ2 **Hypofunctional:** Δ1 – Δ3
Formant frequencies:	Hz	
Frequency band specific maximum levels and their differences:	L_0: peak level of LTAS analysis after 36 dB/octave low-pass filtering with cutoff one octave above previously determined average sample F_0. (Hammarberg et al., 1986). L_1: level of LTAS in first formant region. L_{0-2}: Max dB(0–2 kHz) L_{2-5}: Max dB(2–5 kHz) L_{5-8}: Max dB(5–8 kHz) Δ1: Max dB(0–2 kHz) — Max dB(2–5 kHz) Δ2: Max dB(0–2 kHz) — Max dB(5–8 kHz) Δ3: Max dB(2–5 kHz) — Max dB(5–8 kHz)	Other significant predictors were found with mean F_0 (see Table 9–1.1.). The authors speculated that earlier attempts to classify voice disorders using LTAS (e.g., Prytz, 1977) may have failed due to incorporation of consonant energy and an assumption that samples from given voice disorders should be clustered for LTAS assessment. Izdebski (1984) measured an elevated Δ1 – Δ3 (and low F_0 amplitude) in the **overpressured** voice of **spasmodic dysphonia** before RLN section, with a decrease in the same parameter (and higher F_0 amplitude) in association with postsurgical **breathiness**. Hammarberg, Fritzell, Gauffin, Sundberg (1986) extended their earlier (1980) work to a new set of 26 voices, and obtained correlations with perceptual factors as follows: **unstable** with Δ1 (0.44) and with L_0 (0.32), **overtight** with L_{0-2}. (–.048) and L_{5-8} (–0.47), **sonorous** with Δ3 (0.55), and **hypofunctional** with $L_0 - L_1$ (0.43) (see also Table 9–1.1, F_0 central tendency and Table 9–1.2a, normalized jitter, for other correlations with the Hammarberg et al. [1980, 1986] factors).

Table 9–5.3. Continued

Measure	***Unit and Definition***	***Notes***
Hardware 400 channel narrowband analysis (0–5 kHz unless otherwise noted)		Histograms of α-parameter sampled every 0.04 ms from continuous speech revealed an increase in the central tendency after therapy for a speaker with unilateral vocal fold paralysis. (Summarized in Hirano, 1981.)
α-parameter (Frøkjaer-Jensen & Prytz, 1976)	$\frac{dB(>1{,}000\ Hz)}{dB(<1{,}000\ Hz)}$	
Kitzing (1986) parameters:		
$1/\alpha$	dB ratio	Kitzing (1986) applied these parameters (plus others summarized earlier in this table) to 10 speech pathologists' **simulated leaky**, **strained**, and **soft** voices.
F_{min}	Hz of lowest level between F_0 and F1	
F_{max}	Hz of maximum level	The most powerful parameters for consistently distinguishing all these qualities from the normal sonorous voices were (1) $1/\alpha$ applied to a 0–2kHz range, (2) the $F_0 \pm 50/F_{min} + 400$ ratio, (3) the L_0/L_1 ratio. In addition, L_1 was effective for distinguishing the **strained** quality. Strong correlations were noted between many of these parameters and overall SPL in all qualities, suggesting the need for intensity controls to render LTAS useful in voice comparisons.
L_{max}	dB of maximum level	
F_0/F1	Hz quotient	
300–800 Hz/1.5–3 kHz	dB quotient (1.5–2 kHz denominator for 0–2 kHz LTAS)	
$F_0 \pm 50/F_{min} + 400$	dB quotient (only for 0–2 kHz LTAS)	
Median from 0	%Hz dividing LTAS into equal areas	
Median from F_{min}	%Hz dividing LTAS>Fmin into equal areas	
Median from F_{min} normalized	%Hz(>F_{min}) dividing LTAS>F_{min} into equal areas	

Table 9–5.3. Continued

Measure	*Unit and Definition*	*Notes*
1/3 octave band analysis	DC–16 kHz, (Wendler et al., 1980): 29 (normalized) dB values. 63Hz–12.5 kHz (Wendler et al, 1986): 25 dB values	Using discriminant analysis, Wendler, Doherty, and Hollien (1980) reported strong classification success for 30 read speech samples (approx. 200 s each, with no removal of unvoiced sounds) representing **various functional and organic voice disorders** based on (single rater) scores of **hoarseness** (4 scale points), **roughness** (6 points), and **breathiness** (3 points). No details regarding particular spectral distributions were reported. Wendler, Rauhut, and Krüger (1986) assessed LTAS statistical groupings of 473 voices into perceptual (**hoarse**, **breathy**, **rough**) classes, obtaining only 25%–50% success (25% = chance), although the LTAS did show strong clustering into groups overlapping these classes.
Low frequency spectral energy (A1 in Hartmann & von Cramon, 1984)	% dB—The relative amount of energy in a lower portion of the FFT spectrum of a sustained phonation (e.g., Hartmann & von Cramon's A1 parameter measured the 1 to 5 kHz portion of the mean of 512-point Hamming-windowed frames of data sampled at 20 kHz).	Elevated levels of Hartmann and von Cramon's (1984) A1 tended to discriminate their **central dysphonic** voices perceived as **rough** from those perceived as breathy and tense (but not from the normal) and also discriminated the **tense** from the normal.
High frequency spectral energy (A5 in Hartmann & von Cramon, 1984)	% dB—The relative amount of energy in a higher portion of the FFT spectrum of a sustained phonation (e.g., Hartmann & von Cramon's A5 parameter measured the 1 to 5 kHz portion of the mean of 512-point Hamming-windowed frames of data sampled at 20 kHz)	Elevated levels of Hartmann and von Cramon's (1984) A5 tended to discriminate their **central dysphonic** voices perceived as **breathy** from those perceived as rough and normal, but also from those perceived as **tense** (when one subject whose voice was measured with high A5 is excluded whose voice was measured with high A5). They noted discrepancy with others' results with breathy phonation, suggesting that the voices of central dysphonia tended to be "whispery" but not "lax" (p. 437).
High frequency spectral variance (V5 in Hartmann & von Cramon, 1984)	dB2—The variability of energy across the frequencies in a higher portion of the FFT spectrum of a sustained phonation (e.g., Hartmann & von Cramon's A2 parameter measured the 1 to 5 kHz portion of the mean of pitch-synchronous frames of data sampled at 20 kHz)	Hartmann and von Cramon (1984) reported that their V5 parameter distinguished **male central dysphonic** voices perceived to be **tense**, but not in their female samples.

Table 9–5.3. Continued

Measure	*Unit and Definition*	*Notes*
Two-dimensional analysis: 0–1/1-5 kHz ratio × relative energy in 5–8 kHz band (Löfqvist and Mandersson, 1987).	ratio × normalized energy plot—Digitized connected speech samples are analyzed in 12 ms frames using a dB threshold to reject background noise and a user-variable criterion based on the ratio of energy >1 kHz/energy <1 kHz to discriminate unvoiced frames, and normalization of the frames to a constant 0–1 kHz energy value of 1,000. Parameters are then measured as defined at left.	Löfqvist and Mandersson (1987) applied these measures to normal speakers simulating **hyperfunctional**, **hypofunctional**, and **hyperfunctional** + **breathy** samples, finding generally good discrimination on these dimensions. They also assessed effects of voiceless sample rejection, finding a minor increase in the 0–1/1-5 kHz ratio (0.34 vs. 0.32) and a more sizable decrease in the 5–8 kHz relative energy (478 vs. 737). They also assessed the effects of reducing analyzed time from an original sample duration of approximately 20 s by successive large fractions, finding increased variability for fractions of 1/3 or less but reasonable stability in a $^1/_2$ fraction. See also following entry for discussion of intraindividual variability.

General observations on long-term averaged spectra:
Hurme & Sonninen (1986) review a program of Finnish research using long-term average spectra, noting intraindividual variations and an inverse relation between F_0 strength and SPL. Löfqvist (1986) demonstrated large intraindividual variation in females with **normal** voices measured in the morning and again in the afternoon on a work day in a two-dimensional analysis (see previous entry, this table). He also demonstrated a failure to distinguish pathologic from normal voices in a plot of these parameters, but indicated that the parameters showed value when applied to track an individual's progress in therapy.

Other Sources: Ananthapadmanabha, 1995; Frøkjær-Jensen and Prytz, 1974; Izdebski, 1984; Kitzing and Åkerlund, 1993; Linville, 1998; Mendoza, Muñoz, and Naranjo, 1996; Mendoza, Naranjo Muñoz, and Trujillo, 1996; Novák et al., 1991; Roessler and Lester, 1979; Wendler, Fischer, Seidner, Rauhut, and Wendler, 1985.

Table 9–5.4. Spectral Measures: Cepstra.

References reporting cepstral measures that are not specifically noted in the following table are listed at the end of the table.

Measure	***Unit***	***Algorithm***	***Notes***
Cepstrum	Plot of gamnitude (representing amplitude of fluctuation in spectral magnitudes) over quefrency (in ms, representing time-domain Fourier analogs of spectral frequencies).	1. Obtain log-magnitude FFT spectrum, 2. Compute Inverse FFT and retain real coefficients for cepstrum.	Koike (1986) compared cepstra of original signal and inverse-filtered residue signals from normal and pathologic voices, observing the relative lack of a gamnitude spike at the quefrency corresponding to the pitch period in **cancer** and **paralysis** cases. He advocated the residue cepstrum for removing low quefrency "noise" theoretically corresponding to the vocal tract transmission characteristics.
CE (cepstrum of excitation signal, Feijoo & Hernández, 1990)	average gamnitude	1. See previous steps 1 and 2 for Cepstrum 2. Measure gamnitudes of cepstral peaks associated with pitch periods for each of the N segments under consideration ("PC_n") 3. $CE = \frac{1}{N}\sum_{n=1}^{N} PC_n$	Feijoo and Hernández (1990) measured CE in sustained /e/ phonations by 56 individuals with **glottic cancer** (stages T1–T4) and 64 control speakers, obtaining 89% classification success and correlations of approximately –0.9 with both **hoarseness** and **breathiness** ratings. This classification success was superior to their other measures (normalized mean absolute period jitter [Table 9–1.2a], normalized mean absolute shimmer [Table 9–2.2a], VF [Table 9–4.0], D and NNE [Table 9–5.2].)

Other Sources: de Krom, 1993, 1994a, 1994b, 1995; Dejonckere and Wieneke, 1994; Fröhlich, Michaelis, Strube, and Kruse, 1997; Hillenbrand and Houde, 1996; Koike and Kohda, 1991; Max and Mueller, 1996; Roy et al., 1997.

Table 9–6.1. Inverse Filter Measures (Radiated Signal).

Despite the acknowledged importance of techniques that describe voice quality as a product of the entire speech production apparatus, any analytic decomposition that enables the researcher to focus specifically on the laryngeal source provides valuable information. Such techniques strengthen the researcher's ability to bridge the acoustics/physiology gap. An early aeromechanical technique for recovering the glottal flow waveform was via coupling of a reflectionless tube to the lips, which when applied during phonation through an essentially unconstricted vocal tract, would theoretically allow recovery of the glottal waveform (Sondhi, 1975). However, although the technique revealed some interesting features (Monson, 1981; Monson & Engebretson, 1977), difficulties with calibration and other constraints have prevented its useful application for the study of voice quality. Signal processing techniques have employed analog hardware filtering to recover the glottal flow waveform and, with the advent of LPC algorithms, such techniques have become more widespread. The latter approach, in particular, has encouraged researchers to derive a mathematically more pure (but physiologically fictitious) "residue" signal, the train of impulses theoretically marking the instant of vocal tract acoustic excitation provided by glottal closure. Those purely acoustic techniques that operate on the radiated acoustic signal are listed in Table 9–6.1. A second set of glottal flow measures is provided in Table 9–6.2, which lists those measures derived via inverse filtering of a flow signal at the lips obtained by use of the Rothenberg mask (Rothenberg, 1973). These aerodynamic techniques, described in Chapter 10 of this handbook, are not strictly speaking acoustic but are nonetheless descriptive of the volume velocity source by which the glottis acoustically excites the vocal tract. One key distinction in contrast to the measures listed in Table 9–6.1 is the ability to measure the non-acoustic DC flow that might occur during the "closed" portion of the glottal cycle (although see Alku et al. [1998] for calibration steps that may be taken to estimate absolute flow from radiated signals). The flow mask techniques and derivative measures have provided important perspectives on acoustic voice qualities, especially regarding functional voice disorders, and are included here for completeness.

References reporting radiated signal inverse filtered measures that are not specifically noted in the following table are listed at the end of the table.

Davis (1976) method processing steps (see also Davis 1975, 1978, 1979, 1981)

1. Select steady-state sample of sustained /a/, between 77 and 308 ms (i.e., $500 < N < 2{,}000$ at $F_s = 6{,}500$) in duration, beginning at least 400 ms past voice onset (optimal results obtained for most measures with approximately 120–140 ms windows (800–900 samples at $F_s = 6{,}500$).
2. Digitize at 6500 Hz sampling rate with analog anti-alias filtering at 3200 Hz.
3. Multiply signal by Hamming window (see formula in "key")
4. Preemphasize by first-differencing signal (although optimal pathology detection was subsequently found with 0–0.2 preemphasis, therefore this step may be omitted). (*Note:* in subsequent steps, x_t is the windowed preemphasized signal.)
5. Compute inverse filter coefficients a_i using linear prediction model (optimal results obtained with 8th order [M = 8] filter), by iterative (Levinson's method

   [Davis, 1976, p. 71]) solution of $\sum_{i=1}^{M} a\, r_{\tau=i-k} = -\, r_{\tau=k}$, where $r_\tau \sum_{t=0}^{N-1-\tau} x_t x_{t+\tau}$, and $k = 1, 2, \ldots, M$

Table 9–6.1. Continued

6. Calculate spectral flatness of filter (see SFF, following) and spectral flatness of residue signal (see SFR, following).
7. Obtain residue signal $e_t = \frac{1}{\sigma}\sum_{i=0}^{M} a_i x_{t-1}$ for window samples.
8. Calculate Coefficient of Excess on residue signal.
9. Obtain autocorrelation of Hamming-windowed residue signal $r_\tau = \sum_{t=0}^{N-1-\tau} e_t h_t e_{t+\tau}$, $\tau = 0, 1, \ldots, N-1$, and h_t is Hamming window (see formula in section 3 of introduction, "Formulas Employed in the Chapter Tables").
10. Apply peak detector to autocorrelation series to obtain first peak in series, reporting its lag as the pitch period T0 and its correlation value as pitch amplitude (PA).
11. Locate pitch periods and amplitudes in residual signal with following rules:
    a. Locate maximum positive peak.
    b. Search for positive peak in interval preceding current location by T0 ±0.3T0.
    c. Iterate search to beginning of frame
    d. Invert series following initial positive peak and repeat steps a–c.
    e. Apply parabolic interpolation to refine pitch period durations ($T0_t$) and amplitudes ($A0_t$).
12. Calculate PPQ and APQ with variable smoothing factors, using sPPQ and sAPQ formulas in Tables 9–1.2a and 9–2.2a (optimal results obtained with $sf = 5$ for both).
13. Recalculate step 11 for negative residual peaks and retain these perturbation quotients if APQ is smaller than in step 12.

Measure	***Unit***	***Algorithm***
SFF (spectral flatness of inverse filter)	$\log_{dB}$ of ratio of spectral dB magnitudes (ratio of geometric to arithmetic mean); maximum value is 0 for a constant spectrum.	$10 \times \log_{10} \frac{\exp\left(\frac{1}{N}\sum_{k=0}^{N-1}\log_e\left(\frac{1}{\sum_{i=0}^{M} a_i e^{-j2\pi k/N}}\right)\right)}{\frac{1}{N}\sum_{k=0}^{N-1}\left(\frac{1}{\sum_{i=0}^{M} a_i e^{-j2\pi k/N}}\right)}$, for window length N.

Table 9–6.1. Continued

Measure	*Unit*	*Algorithm*
SFR (spectral flatness of residue signal)	dB difference (Spectral flatness of data minus SFF); maximum value is 0 for a constant spectrum.	$10 \times \log_{10}\left(\frac{\exp\left[\frac{1}{N}\sum_{k=0}^{N-1}\log_e x_k\right]}{\frac{1}{N}\sum_{k=0}^{N-1} x_k}\right) - SFF,$ window length N.
EX (coefficient of excess)	dimensionless distribution parameter (ratio of 4th moment to 2nd moment) calibrated to 0 for univariate normal distribution.	$\frac{\frac{1}{N}\sum_{i=0}^{N-1}\left(x_i - \bar{x}\right)^4}{\frac{1}{N}\sum_{i=0}^{N-1}\left(x_i - \bar{x}\right)^2} - 3,$ where $\bar{x} = \frac{1}{N}\sum_{i=0}^{N-1} x_i$.
PA (pitch amplitude)	autocorrelation coefficient between successive pitch periods.	See steps 9 and 10 in processing steps at top of this table.
$PPQ_{residuals}$	% (of average residual pitch period)	See processing steps 11–13.
$APQ_{residuals}$	% (of average residual amplitude)	See processing steps 11–13.

General comments on Davis method:
Davis (1976, 1979) provides physiological interpretations for these measures: SFF—masking of formants by noise; SFR—masking of harmonics by noise; EX—the degree of noise (and lack of closure) at the glottis; PA—strength of perioidic voicing; PPQ and APQ—degree of aperiodicity in glottal

Table 9–6.1. Continued

period and amplitude, respectively. Davis (1976) implemented and tested these measures on 123 recorded sustained phonations by control subjects and speakers with pathologies of a **wide variety of functional, organic, neurogenic, and unknown etiologies**. Using maximum likelihood pathology detection classification on feature vectors with training on a reference group of 38 speakers and closed (same test group) and open (different test group, 69 speakers) tests, Davis (1976) examined algorithm control parameters of filter order, preemphasis, window length, and perturbation smoothing factors (results adopted as parameter settings described in the processing steps at the top of this table), with overall detection probability of 94.7%. Student's *t*-tests indicated significant group differences on all measures, and one-dimensional classification assessment indicated the ranking (best to worst): PPQ, APQ, SFR, PA, EX, SFF. However, the EX measure was distinctive in its sensitivity to the pathologic samples, with the other measures being relatively better at classifying normal samples than pathologic. Multivariate normal distribution assumptions seemed to be borne out for all measures except PPQ and APQ, which appeared to be log normal in distribution. Schoentgen (1982) explored the possibility that multimodal distributions of the measures might prevent their accurate assessment under a standard statistical decision model. He applied a cluster analysis to sustained phonation samples from 37 control subjects and from 24 speakers with a **wide variety of functional, organic, neurogenic, and unknown etiologies**. This approach yielded clear superiority for PPQ, APQ, and PA, followed by far less discrimination for EX, SFR, and SFF. Schoentgen argued that the poor performance of the latter measures was because of their dependence on the assumptions of the LPC model, suggesting that residue analysis was inappropriate for disordered voice types chiefly because of artificial enhancement of speaker variability. He also observed that (1) SFF was reduced in many disordered voice samples, not elevated, (2) PA was highly F_0 dependent and potentially enhanced by normalization, and (3) that EX and SFF were highly vulnerable to changes in recording conditions.

Prosek, Montgomery, Walden, and Hawkins (1987) measured SFF, SFR, $PPQ_{residuals}$, $APQ_{residuals}$, PA and EX on sustained /a/ phonations by 90 patients with **a wide variety of functional, organic, neurogenic, and unknown etiologies** and assessed their predictiveness of a 7-point perceptual **severity** rating, obtaining a multiple R^2 of 0.65 with the largest simple correlation (–0.75) from PA but the largest unique contributions (squared semipartial correlations) from SFF and SFR. They also assessed the measures against 10 voice quality scales, finding high interdependence among the scales, high multiple R^2 with **breathiness** (0.74), **adequacy** (0.66), **strained-strangled** (0.58), **hoarseness** (0.56), and **harshness** (0.52), with the strongest correlations in each being with PA (–0.68 to –0.76) and the lowest with SFF (0.08 – 0.24).

Eskenazi, Childers, and Hicks (1990), proceeding on the basis of pilot results in a doctoral dissertation by Eskenazi (1988), measured SFR, PA, PPQ, APQ, and percent jitter in LPC residue signals, and HNR_{Yumoto} in direct waveforms in 2-s samples of sustained /i/ phonations by 25 male and 25 female speakers with no history of laryngeal disease and 16 speakers with **various organic and functional vocal disorders**. The speech samples were rated for **overall severity**, **hoarseness**, **breathiness**, **roughness**, and **vocal fry**, and the measures assessed against these ratings using a prediction sum of squares (PRESS) criterion. No clear trends among ratings or measure-rating regressions emerged for the normal speakers. Results were summarized as follows: **overall quality** predicted by low PA and HNR (R^2 = 0.57); **hoarseness** by low PA and high percent jitter (R^2 = 0.56); **breathiness** by high percent jitter (R^2 = 0.30); **roughness** by low SFR and HNR (R^2 = 0.59); and **vocal fry** by low PA and HNR (R^2 = 0.54).

Table 9–6.1. Continued

Measure	***Unit***	***Algorithm***	***Notes***
IPI (inversion of pitch period index, Banci et al., 1986)	%	"the normalized number of algebraic sign inversion of the differences (greater than a pre-established threshold) between each pitch period and the previous one in the residue." (Banci et al., 1986, p. 497)	Banci et al. (1986) applied these measures (plus residue-based PPQ and APQ, Cf. Tables 9–6.1, 9–1.2a and 9–2.2a and a spectral measure F_0F_1Q, see Table 9–5.2) to 53 pathological (various **organic** and **functional disorders**) and 30 nonpathological sustaned phonation samples. Using decision rules based on classification training with a Mahalanobis distance criterion, individual measures ranked in overall success APQ (86.7% success) >PPQ > RAE > IPI > SIG > APD > AWM > F_0F_1Q, (71.1% success), and obtained a multivariate classification success of 91.6%.
SIG	Hz^2	"pitch variance normalized to the average pitch in the analyzed residue frame." (Banci et al., 1986, p. 497)	
RAE (Residue Anomalous Energy, Banci et al., 1986).	?	"a measure of the noise-like energy present between pitch peaks of the residue." (Banci et al., 1986, p. 497)	
APD	difference between autocorrelation coefficiants.	1. Calculate autocorrelation function of window used to weight residue signal (R'). 2. Calculate autocorrelation function of residue signal (R); identify first peak (R_1) and corresponding R (R'_1). APD = $(R'_1 - R_1)$.	
AWM	difference between autocorrelation coefficiants.	See steps 1 and 2 for APD preceding; obtain weighted mean of first three peaks of R (R_1) and corresponding R (R'_1). (weights unspecified) AWM = $(R'_1 - R_1)$.	
Residue NS (Noise-to-Signal) Ratio (Muta et al. 1987)	$\log_{db}$ (power ratio)	1. Obtain residues of 12 coefficient LPC analysis of 8 kHz sampled vowel phonations. 2. Calculate 1,024-point overlapping FFTs (X_n). 3. For each X_n series, use autocorrelation based estimate of F_0 from residuals to determine harmonic, a) by searching for peaks at $F_0 \pm \Delta(8kHz/1{,}024)$, i.e. ±FFT frequency resolution, then b) employ FFT of	Muta et al. (1987) analyzed sustained vowel samples from nine patients with **hoarse** voices due primarily due to **polyps** and **nodules** **pre-** and **postoperatively**,

Table 9–6.1. Continued

Measure	*Unit*	*Algorithm*	*Notes*
	%	Hanning window as an interpolation tool to improve resolution of harmonic amplitude estimates H_n (up to 3 kHz or $X_{1..384}$). 4. Calculate total residue power by summing the squared absolute magnitudes of X_{1-384} (P_T). 5. Calculate total harmonic power by summing the squared harmonic amplitude estimates H_n (P_H) and obtain Noise power (P_N) = $P_T - P_H$. 6. Obtain NS ratio $10 \times \log10(P_N/P_T)$.	finding significant improvements in NS ratio for all but one patient in the sustained /e/ vowel (i.e. dB values ranging –2.9 . . . –6.5 prior to, and ranging –3.7 . . . –12.5 following), but more variability in other vowels..
Inverse filter spectrum envelope (Muta et al., 1987)	Waterfall display of running LPC spectra	Use standard procedures for Fourier transforming LPC predictive coefficients into frequency-domain representation (see, e.g., Rabiner & Schafer, 1978).	Muta et al. (1987) observed more prominent and less variable formant peaks **post-operatively** in patients with **hoarse** voice (see details in previous cell).

Other Sources: Alku and Vilkman, 1995, 1995b, 1996; Alku et al., 1998; Alku, Vilkman, and Laukkanen, 1997, Childers and Lee, 1991; Cleveland and Sundberg, 1983; Cumming and Clements, 1995; Eskenazi, 1988; Gobl and Ní Chasaide, 1992; Imaizumi, 1986; Koike and Markel, 1975; Laukkanen et al., 1996; Lee, 1988; Lee and Childers, 1991; Mori et al., 1994; Ní Chasaide and Gobl, 1995; Plant, Hillel, and Waugh, 1997; Plante, Salian, Scholder, Cheetham, and Earis, 1997; Strik and Boves, 1992a, 1992b; Waters, Nunn, Gillcrist, and VonColln, 1995; Yonick et al., 1990.

Table 9–6.2. Inverse Filter Measures (Flow-Mask Signals).

References reporting flow-mask inverse filtered measures that are not specifically noted in the following table are listed at the end of the table.

Measure	Notes
1. Po amplitude of second crest of ACF 2. WI width of second crest of ACF 3. MP amplitude of first trough of ACF 4. PDEV standard deviation of fundamental period 5. ADEV standard deviation of peak amplitude 6. PPER period of fluctuation of the correlogram of peak amplitude (see Table 9–4.0 for correlogram formula) 7. APER period of fluctuation of the correlogram of peak amplitude 8. P1 correlation coefficient between adjacent periods 9. P10 correlation coefficient between fundamental periods separated by ten intervals 10. PINC rate of declination of the correlogram of fundamental period 11. A1 correlation coefficient between adjacent peak amplitudes 12. A10 correlation coefficient between peak amplitudes separated by ten intervals 13. AINC rate of declination of the correlogram of peak amplitude 14. SPINC rate of declination of spectral envelope Hirano (1981, p. 75)	Parameters investigated by Hiki, Hirano and co-workers (Hiki, Imaizumi, Hirano, Matsushita, and Kakita, 1976; Hirano, 1975; Hirano, Kakita, Matsushita, Hiki, and Imaizumi, 1977a, 1977b; Kakita, Hirano, Matsushita, Hiki, and Imaizumi, 1977a,1977b), summarized in Hirano (1981). Canonical correlation analysis using these 14 parameters successfully classified 70%–80% phonations by normal subjects and by persons with **carcinoma**, **recurrent laryngeal nerve paralysis**, **polyp**, and **sulcus vocalis**.

Measure	Unit	Algorithm	Notes
Glottal insufficiency (Fritzell, Hammarberg, Gauffin, Karlsson, & Sundberg, 1986)	mm^2	Perform Rothenberg acoustic inverse filtering (Rothenberg, 1973) to obtain "glottogram" (estimated glottal flow waveform), obtain simultaneous readings of subglottal pressure, and calculate minimum glottal area from minimum flow in glottogram.	Fritzell et al. (1986) measured these parameters in 8 patients with **breathy** voice due to **organic** disorders (4 **pre-** and **postsurgical**), finding a better correlation with perceptual ratings and greater consistency of improvement with surgery for the minimum/maximum flow quotient measure. (See

Table 9–6.2. Continued

Measure	*Unit*	*Algorithm*	*Notes*
Minimum/maximum air flow quotient (Fritzell, et al. 1986)	ratio	Obtain Rothenberg glottogram (as in previous measure) and measure ratio of minimum flow to maximum flow	also high bandwidth measures, following.)
Y, peak-to-peak amplitude of the flow glottogram and its derivation EPA (Estimated Glottal Peak Area, Fritzell et al., 1986; Gauffin & Sundberg, 1989).	cm^3/s for Y cm^3/s for U3 for EPA	From glottogram and subglottal pressure (P), measure peak volume velocity in cm^3/s (Y) and approximate EPA by formula: $\sqrt{0.5 \times k \times \rho}\left(\frac{\hat{U}}{\sqrt{P}}\right)$, where ρ = air density and k = correction factor that can be set to 1.	Gauffin and Sundberg (1989) noted in sustained vowel phonations a strong correlation of *Y* and peak amplitude of the source spectrum fundamental and observed a singer's reduction of this amplitude for **pressed** phonation, maximizing of this amplitude for **breathy** and **whisper** phonations, and defined **flow** mode of phonation as the highest flow amplitude that could be achieved while maintaining complete closure in the same cycle. (See also high bandwidth measures, following.)
Negative peak amplitude of the differentiated flow glottogram (dU_G/dt in Gauffin & Sundberg, 1989; E_e in Gobl,	dB	Differentiate flow glottogram, measure amplitude of negative peak (in $liters/s^2$), and convert to dB against arbitrary reference.	Gauffin and Sundberg (1989) noted a strong correlation of dU_G/dt with sound pressure level and (via theory) the total energy of overtones of the fundamental. They noted that

Table 9–6.2. Continued

Measure	*Unit*	*Algorithm*	*Notes*
1989 as based on theoretical point defined by Fant, Liljencrants, & Lin, 1985).			nonsingers tended to decrease Y (see previous), that is, alter sustained vowel phonation towards a **pressed** mode when increasing **loudness**, with trained singers able to increase loudness without altering Y. The authors discussed the concordance of their measures with theoretical features of Fant's LF glottal source model (Fant, 1986; Fant et al., 1985). (See also high bandwidth measures, following.)
Time-domain measured LF model parameters (Gobl, 1989, based on Fant et al. 1985 model):		Measured from glottograms:	Gobl (1989) measured these parameters in the first vowel of the nonsense word /bæbə/ in a carrier phrase spoken by a single male British phonetician in **modal**, **breathy**, **whispery**, and **creaky** voice qualities (as defined by Laver, 1980). He also measured from original signals the dB levels of harmonic H1, formant amplitudes A1, A2, A3, A4 and formant bandwidths B1, B2, B3, and B4. The following patterns were observed:
R_a and its frequency-domain equivalent F_a	Ratio of times and equivalent low-pass filter f_c (Hz).	$R_a = t_a/T0$, where t_a is the time constant defined by projection on the time axis of the slope of the flow derivative immediately after the negative peak discontinuity at time t_e, and $F_a = 1/2\pi t_a$.	
R_g	Ratio of frequencies.	$R_g = F_g/f_0$, where $F_g = 1/2t_p$ and t_p is time from glottal opening to peak flow.	
R_k (pulse assymetry)	Ratio of times.	$R_k = (t_e - t_p)/t_p$.	

Table 9–6.2. Continued

Measure	Unit	Algorithm	Notes
O_q (open quotient)	Ratio of times.	$O_q = te/T0$.	**breathy**: high R_a and low F_a, low R_g, high O_q, high U_p, somewhat higher E_i, and moderately higher R_k; high attenuation of frequencies above F_0, weak A1 and A2, large B1-3. **whispery**: weak E_e, very high R_z and very low F_a, low R_g, high O_q, low E_e/E_i and slightly lower E_i; high attenuation above F_0 and very high attenuation above 1 kHz, slightly lower H1, weak formants, and large B1 and B2. **creaky**: moderately stronger E_e, low R_a and high F_a, low R_k, low E_i, low U_p and high E_e/E_i; small boost of frequencies 0–2 kHz, some attenuation above 3 kHz, slightly lower H1, strong formants with slightly reduced B1-4. See original report for discussion of some unexpected results and the need for further study of voice quality in dynamic, connected speech contexts.
E_i	dB	positive peak of flow derivative, that is, maximum slope of opening phase.	
U_p (=Y).	dB	flow maximum.	
E_e/E_i	ratio of amplitudes.	absolute value of negative flow derivative peak divided by positive flow peak	
Frequency domain measures:		Measured from narrow-band spectra of glottograms normalized for F_0 by first-order differentiation at F_0	
0–1, 1–2, 2–3, 3–4 kHz band deviations	dB differences	deviations from –12 dB/octave slope	

Table 9–6.2. Continued

Measure	***Unit***	***Algorithm***	***Notes***
High-bandwidth measures (Hillman, Holmberg, Perkell, Walsh, & Vaughan, 1989; Holmberg, Hillman & Perkell, 1988)		Preprocessing steps: flow-signal from Rothenberg mask is low-pass filtered at f_c = 900 Hz twice to ensure removal of resonances >F1, digitized at 8192 Hz and inverse filtered at F1 frequency measured by LPC and DFT spectra. Time periods t_1 = opening phase, t_2 = closing phase, and t_3 = closed phase are measured, and a first-differenced signal U_G' is also obtained.	Hillman et al. (1989) assessed these, other (low bandwidth) aerodynamic measures, F_0, and SPL in the vowel portions of five /pæ/ syllables spoken at normal, soft, and loud levels from patients with **hyperfunctional** disorders. The subjects were chosen to represent different types and stages of the disorder within a theoretical framework distinguishing **adducted hyperfunction** (with organic pathologies due to impact trauma such as **nodules**, **polyps**, and **contact ulcers**) from **non-adducted hyperfunction** (cases presenting with **hoarseness** or **breathiness** but normal laryngeal exams). Including 45 normal voices, the investigators demonstrated distinctively high AC flow and maximum flow declination rates in the **adducted** group and distinctively high levels of DC flow in the **nonadducted** group. Further distinctions based on these measures were drawn in the report, and suggestions regarding the relative merits of the measurement set were provided.
Open quotient	ratio of times	$(t_1 + t_2)/T0$	
Speed quotient	ratio of times	t_1/t_2	
Closing quotient	ratio of times	$t_2/T0$	
AC flow	L/s	Peak flow above closed phase DC offset	
Minimum flow	L/s	closed phase DC offset	
Peak flow	L/s	Sum of AC flow and minimum flow	
AC–DC ratio	ratio of L/s flows	Mean of flow above closed phase DC offset, RMS of flow is taken around this mean and divided by the mean.	
Maximum flow declination rate	L/s^2	Measured at negative peak of U_G'.	

Table 9–6.2. Continued

Measure	***Unit***	***Algorithm***	***Notes***
Z score profiles		multiple normalized dimensions (F_0, SPL, estimated transglottal pressure and flow, AC flow, minimum flow and maximum flow declination rate [MFDR]—see cell above for descriptions) expressed as $\frac{\text{observed value} - \text{normal group mean}}{\text{normal group standard deviation}}$, displayed in Hillman et al. (1990) as histograms in conjunction with flow glottograms	See Hillman et al. (1989) for notes on use of Z_R versus Z; Z_R appeared to be more sensitive to pathologies but was applied with certain limitations. Hillman, Holmberg, Perkell, Walsh, and Vaughan (1990) obtained further support for the claims of Hillman et al. (1989), providing multiple Z score histograms from 10 subjects. The scores were assessed with a ±2 SD criterion to support the following general conclusions regarding acoustical differentiation of **hyperfunctional** voice disorders (< meaning more than 2 SDs below normal, > more than 2 SDs above normal, and = meaning normal): **nodules**: = F_0 and > MFDR; **polypoid**: < F_0 and = MFDR; **contact ulcer**: < F_0, and > MFDR.
Z_R		pressure and flow measures regressed on f0 and SPL, then expressed as $\frac{\text{observed value} - \text{predicted value}}{\text{standard error of estimate from regression}}$	

Other Sources: Holmberg, Hillman, and Perkell, 1995; Holmberg, Perkell, Guiod, et al., 1995; Holmberg et al., 1994; Huffman, 1987; Ng et al., 1997; Perkell, Hillman, and Holmberg, 1994; Raes and Clement, 1996; Sapienza and Stathopoulos, 1994; Södersten et al., 1995; Sulter and Wit, 1996.

Table 9–7.0. Dynamics.

The first six table categories in this chapter all have an acoustic parameter or set of parameters as their measurement basis; this seventh table is instead defined by the temporal basis against which such parameters are measured. Because traditional frameworks for speech and voice analysis assume that the statistical nature of an acoustic characteristic is stationary, and because the notion of quality implies a static characteristic whose duration or evolving nature may be secondary, it is possible for a student of the literature to overlook basic dynamic aspects of voice quality. For example, studies of sustained phonation will frequently excise phonatory onsets and offsets in an effort to obtain "representative" samples. Indeed, these onsets and offsets are often highly idiosyncratic and rich with phenomena that may be challenging to summarize quantitatively. Note that even simple terms such as pitch break and voice break are defined quite differently by different authors; as an example, Coleman's pitch break = Bowler's frequency break = Fairbank's voice break. Nonetheless, rapid changes and transient phenomena are especially salient perceptually and potentially highly revealing of the underlying physiology, particularly its motility, flexibility, robustness, and other distinctively biological characteristics. As with many other measurement categories summarized in this chapter, this table includes very early and apparently simple measures, yet also reveals that the measurement approach still seems to have fallen short of its ultimate potential. Although voice quality research has been performed in both segment specific and suprasegmental contexts, general investigations of how voice quality is revealed in the course of spontaneous connected speech production seem to have begun only recently (Fant, 1997; Strik & Boves, 1992b). More fundamentally, the descriptive apparatus of non-linear dynamic theory, some of which is evident by 1990 and therefore listed in the following table, seems yet to be adopted by the general voice analyst. See, however, additional work by Herzel, Berry, and others (Berry, Herzel, Titze, & Krischer, 1994; Berry, Herzel, Titze, & Story, 1996; Boek, Wieneke, & Dejonckere, 1997; Herzel, 1996; Herzel, Berry, Titze, & Saleh, 1994; Herzel, Berry, Titze, & Steinecke, 1995; Herzel, Steinecke, Mende, & Wermke, 1991; Kakita & Okamoto, 1995; Mergell & Herzel, 1997; Titze, Baken, & Herzel, 1993). For a highly accessible graphic introduction to the descriptive concepts of nonlinear dynamic systems analysis, see also the four volume set developed by Abraham and Shaw (1983, 1984, 1985, 1988; also compiled and republished as Abraham & Shaw, 1992).

References reporting dynamic measures that are not specifically noted in the following table are listed at the end of the table.

Measure	***Unit***	***Algorithm***	***Notes***
Breaks (Coleman, 1960):	critical ΔP/time		Coleman (1960) measured these in sustained /i/, /ɑ/, /æ/, and /u/ phonations by 15 speakers with varying degrees of **hoarseness** (ranging from **laryngitis** to **recurrent laryngeal nerve paralysis**). Coleman defines
Pitch break		ΔF_0 >1 octave/>7 cycles	
Frequency break		ΔF_0 >1 octave/<7 cycles	
Voice break		ΔF_0 <1 octave/"aperiodically on a cycle-to-cycle basis" (p. 16).	
Amplitude break		"relatively large change in amplitude, occurring aperiodically on a cycle-to-cycle basis" (p. 16)	

Table 9–7.0. Continued

Measure	*Unit*	*Algorithm*	*Notes*
			the breaks perceptually as: pitch break—"a variation in pitch," frequency break—"a pitch change, "voice break—"a voice quality deviation," amplitude break—"a voice quality deviation. " In contrast to earlier findings with adolescent male speech, no pitch or frequency breaks, but a predominance of voice and amplitude breaks was found in perceptibly hoarser voices.
Maximum rate of F_0 change	Pitch change/unit time	As specified in unit definition (left), but also requires specification of (a) frequency scale (e.g., Hz or tone), (b) unit of time, (c) direction, (d) task type, and (e) eligible segment (see illustrative choices to right).	Hecker and Kruel (1970) found reduced rate in association with **vocal fold cancer**, most notably in Hz rises over 50 ms time unit and Hz falls over 100 ms time unit from sentence material, excluding phonatory initiations and terminations.
Vocal rise time	ms	Time from vocal onset to time when mean steady-state vowel energy is achieved.	Koike, Hirano, and von Leden (1967) measured average **hard attack** at 29 ms, **breathy attack** at 121 ms, and **soft attack** at 247 ms. See also the Imaizumi et al. (1980) amplitude display measure 7, rising time and falling time, Table 9–5.1.

Table 9–7.0. Continued

Measure	***Unit***	***Algorithm***	***Notes***
Consonant perturbation	Pitch change/unit time	Select obstruent consonant such as stop or fricative, measure F_0 change over frame aligned with consonant.	Hecker and Kruel (1970) found trend for greater perturbation (in tones) with voiced stops (50 ms frame) and voiced fricatives (100 ms frame) in association with **vocal fold cancer**.
Turbulent preexhalation noise (Hartmann & von Cramon, 1984)	ms	Duration of turbulent noise preceding first fundamental period in a sustained phonation.	Hartmann & von Cramon (1984) found significant discrimination in this parameter of **breathy** voice quality (from rough, tense, or normal) in central dysphonias due to **traumatic brain injury** and **cerebrovascular accident** (see also Tables 9–1.2a and 9–5.3).
Voice initiation perturbation (PP1 in Hartmann & von Cramon, 1984)	%	PP (see Table 9–1.2a) applied to first 10 pitch periods.	Hartmann and von Cramon (1984) found significant discrimination with this parameter of **rough** voice quality in males with central dysphonia (cf. note above).
Low frequency segments	number, duration, F_0 preceding, during, and following	"abrupt drops in fundamental frequency of at least five cycles in duration followed by a return to modal frequency [occurring] after at least 250 ms of modal phonation and 250 ms preceding termination of phonation" (L.A. Ramig, 1986, p. 289).	L.A. Ramig (1986) observed low frequency segments in sustained phonations by 7 of 8 patients with **Huntington's disease**. See also L.A. Ramig, Scherer, Titze, and Ringel, 1988, Table 9–1.2a, Perturbation factor without linear trend.

Table 9–7.0. Continued

Measure	***Unit***	***Algorithm***	***Notes***
Maximum duration of sustained phonation	seconds	as defined	L.A. Ramig (1986) observed reduced durations in more severe cases of **Huntington's disease**.
Abnormal phonatory terminations	qualitative observations of waveforms and/or spectrograms	"strain-strangled": low frequency pulsatile glottal waveforms persisting at the ends of phonations. "breathy": low intensity high turbulent waveforms persisting at the ends of phonations.	L.A. Ramig (1986) observed both **strain-strangled** and **breathy** terminations in **Huntington's disease**, suggesting a subclassification of the disorder in terms of adductory versus abductory arrest episodes, respectively.
Laryngeal dynamics in diadochokinesis tasks (Ludlow & Connor, 1987)	syllable rates, absolute times in ms for on times and off times, percent of total DDK time for percent off time, and- percent of syllable time for percent on time.	Waveforms of repeated productions of mono- or di-syllables like /a/, /pa/, or /pata/ are measured for syllable repetition rates, times of voiced intervals (phonatory on times) and intervening stop gaps (phonatory off times).	Ludlow and Connor (1987) measured significantly reduced rates and shortened percentage on times in /a/ DDK, and significantly prolonged absolute and percentage off times in /a/ DDK in nine speakers with **spasmodic dysphonia** compared to normal control speakers.
DI (Degree of pitch amplitude interruptions, Nikolov, et al., 1989)	% of total sample time containing voiced A0 £ 0.18 of the preceding average A0.		Nikolov et al. (1989) described the implementation of this parameter in a multidimensional program leading to the development of MDVP, observing especially high values for **laryngeal cancer** and **recurrent nerve paralysis**.

Table 9–7.0. Continued

Measure	***Unit***	***Algorithm***	***Notes***
Unvoiced Intervals (e.g., RUV—rate of unvoiced interval [Kasuya, Masubuchi, et al., 1986], DVB — Degree of Voice Breaks [Deliyski, 1994; Kay Elemetrics, 1993])	% of sample	$100 \times \frac{\text{time of unvoiced intervals}}{\text{total phonation time}}$	In MDVP, includes only unvoiced portions internal to phonation sample (not intervals outside of phonated portion of total digitized sample). See Table 9–1.2a, PPQ_{Kasusa} notes for use of RUV in Kasuya, Masubuchi, et al. (1986) screening protocol. L.A. Ramig (1986) observed vocal arrests in **Huntington's disease**. (See also abnormal phonatory terminations, this table).
DUV—degree of unvoiced (Deliyski, 1994; Kay Elemetrics, 1993)	% of sample time	$100 \times \frac{\text{time of unvoiced intervals}}{\text{total sample time}}$	Nikolov et al. (1989) describe an implementation of DUV in a multidimensional program precursor to MDVP, finding especially high values for **laryngeal cancer** and **laryngitis**. In MDVP Includes all unvoiced portions of record.
DV (Degree of pitch frequency interruptions, Nikolov, et al., 1989)	% of total sample time containing T0 deviating from the preceding mean by more		Nikolov et al. (1989) described the implementation of this parameter in a multidimensional program leading to the development of MDVP, observing especially

Table 9–7.0. Continued

Measure	*Unit*	*Algorithm*	*Notes*
	than 25% of that mean.		high values for **laryngeal cancer** and **functional dysphonia**.
Fractal dimension (e.g., D_F in Baken, 1990).	Noninteger dimension, for example, 1.46 (the dimension of a line is 1.0 and the dimension of a plane is 2.0)	Box-counting method (one of many estimation methods): 1. Map a time-series P_t as a line plot onto a grid surface. 2. Begin with a rough grid divisor, for example, 5 × 5, and count the number of grid boxes occupied by the line. 3. Increase the grid density at least twice, for example, to divisors 10 and 15, again counting the number of occupied grid boxes. 4. Calculate the slope with which the logarithm of the number of occupied boxes increases as the logarithm of the grid divisor increase. The resulting slope is D_f.	Baken (1990) introduced the box-counting method as a procedure for measuring irregularity in vocal period and amplitude time-series data. This report demonstrated that divisors ranging from 15 to 55 were adequate for male and female modal and male pulse registers, and that the D_f measure did not appear sensitive to simple changes in F_0 variability. An application to four men and four women's sustained /a/ phonations at three pitch levels yielded a mean D_f of 1.46 for period and 1.54 for amplitude, with no significant differences in D_f between gender or pitch level. No significant correlations were obtained between D_f and absolute or RAP jitter (Table 9–1.2a) or absolute shimmer (Table 9–2.2a), but reduced variability in comparison to the perturbation measures was noted.

Table 9–7.0. Continued

Measure	***Unit***	***Algorithm***	***Notes***
Phase portrait	graphic display of attractor (in variant point, period limit-cycle, or chaotic strange).		Graph time series against one or more delay coordinates P_{t-1}, P_{t-2}.
Bifurcations	change in system behavior, for example, from one attractor to another, as some control parameter is changed		Observe virtually instantaneous changes in voice waveform or spectrographic display, for example, from stationary F_0 to subharmonic or noisy structure in sustained phonation or cry.
Poincaré section	graphic display of discrete states of a behavior upon cyclic returns, also tending to show attractor structure		One example is a next amplitude map, with coordinates At and At-1.

Other Sources: Aronson and Hartman, 1981; Behrman and Baken, 1997; Bowler, 1957; Bowler, 1964; Dejonckere and Lebacq, 1983; Deliyski, 1990; Deliyski, 1993; Deliyski, 1994; Fletcher, 1996; Gubrynowicz et al., 1981; Haggard, 1969; Hirose et al., 1995; Mergell, Herzel, Wittenberg, Tigges, and Eysholdt, 1998; Reuter and Herzel, 1998; Sapienza, Murry, and Brown, 1998.

Appendix 9–A. Methodological, Theoretical, Psychacoustic, and Synthesis-Based Studies.

Other methodological references not specifically noted in the following appendix are listed at the end of the appendix.

Signal Type	***Investigation***	***Notes***
Flutter index testing	Comerci (1955)	Comerci reviews the empirically based "flutter index" promulgated by the Society of Motion Picture and Television Engineers (SMPTE). The index is intended to quantify thresholds for perception of periodic frequency perturbations between .5 and 100 cps. Comerci reviews literature suggesting that flutter in carrier tones below 500 Hz is perceptible at fixed frequency excursions, but that this threshold increases as a percentage of the carrier tone frequency above 500 Hz. He also suggests that modulation rates below 5 cps yield the perception of a modulating tone, at 5–15 cps this effect is heard as modulating intensity and at higher cps the flutter is heard as a low-frequency tone. Thresholds seem lowest for 1 to 3 cycles. Comerci used standardized mechanical devices to introduce flutter into pure tone, music, and speech materials. Perceived flutter scores ranked closely with the intermodulation distortion and flutter index measures (the latter index is calculated by dividing a measured flutter amplitude by a reference threshold amplitude). He also replicated the U-shaped threshold curve (with a minimum on approximately 2 cps) obtained in earlier studies and presents evidence that (1) music and speech flutter effects are basically similar to those obtained with pure tones and (2) an RMS integration of flutter modulation energy may be superior to a peak or peak-to-peak measure.
Analog perturbation synthesis	Wendahl (1963)	Investigating **harsh** voice quality, Wendahl synthesized (via a system dubbed LADIC) quasi-sawtooth waveforms at 100 and 200 Hz median rates, with variable pulse timing deviating up to 10 Hz, evaluated perceptually. Results suggested sensitivity to **roughness** even at 1 Hz deviation with greater sensitivity to low frequency voices (suggesting appropriateness of % deviation metric). In a footnote, he suggested that term "fundamental frequency" is erroneous, and preferably would be replaced with a concept of successive cycle periods.
Analog open-quotient synthesis	Coleman (1971)	Investigating **rough** voice quality, Coleman used Wendahl's LADIC apparatus to vary the duty cycle of 100 Hz sawtooth waves (i.e., simulating open quotient range from maximum [100% duty cycle] to minimum [pulse]) to prepare five waveform types: (1) pulse, (2) variability between 25%–100% duty cycle, (3) variability between 50%–100% duty cycle, (4) variability between 75%–100% duty cycle, and (5) 100% duty cycle. A second set also used a fixed jitter pattern with 10% variation. Results indicated strong effects of waveform duty cycle variation on roughness, with virtually no additional increase on addition of jitter. Frequency domain effects of the duty cycle effect can be summarized as an increase in lower partial amplitudes, suggesting a commonality with perturbation.

Appendix 9–A. Continued

Signal Type	***Investigation***	***Notes***
Audiometric evaluation of periodic modulation	Terhardt (1974)	Investigating perception of **roughness** in periodically modulated tones, Terhardt's investigations, although not oriented to voice specifically, suggest that "envelope fluctuations which are present in spectral regions corresponding to the critical bands of the ear" as evaluated by the appropriately windowed short-time amplitude spectra constitutes "the physical parameter which has to be considered when the perception of roughness is discussed" (1974, p. 211). This work furthermore suggests that auditory sensitivity to such roughness should be regarded as a low-pass filtering with a cutoff frequency around 250–300 Hz.
Relations between measures of pitch perturbation, amplitude perturbation, and additive noise	Hillenbrand (1987)	Hillenbrand (1987) constructed test signals using Klatt formant synthesis (Klatt, 1980) to create 5-formant vowels. HNR test signals ranged from –22dB to 32 dB and were tested with the Yumuto method (see Table 9–4.0). Jitter test signals varied from 0 to 8 Hz standard deviations centering on 130 Hz (absolute jitter; 0 to 500 μs, percent jitter; 0% to 6.4%) and were measured for absolute jitter (see Table 9–1.2a), and shimmer signals ranged from 0 to 2.6 dB, tested for absolute shimmer (see Table 9–2.2a). Results demonstrated that changes in any one parameter affected measures of the other two. Effects of jitter on shimmer were partly explained by the variations in decay times between successive pulses, and the effects of additive noise were explained by the concomitant pulse period and amplitude determinations. Hillenbrand suggested some remediative steps for the Yumoto algorithm, but suggested caution in interpreting perturbation measures, especially at low levels.
Relations between perceived dysphonia and variation in pitch perturbation, amplitude perturbation, and additive noise	Hillenbrand (1988)	Hillenbrand (1988) constructed test signals using pitch-synchronous synthesis to create 5-formant [a] vowels: Jitter test signals with F_0 centering on 130 Hz ranged from 0 to 461 μs (0 to 6.0% relative jitter). Two continua were developed: one with uncorrelated perturbations (period sequences generated by a white noise generator) and one with correlated perturbations (period sequences generated by a 1/f noise generator). Direct magnitude perceptual estimations of **roughness** by 10 listeners revealed a "compression" beyond approximately 2.0% beyond which increasing jitter yielded smaller increases in perceived roughness. Correlated sequences were perceived as more rough, although this difference was attenuated when the sequences were measured using relative average perturbation measures such as RAP or PPQ (see Table 9–1.2a). Two continua of shimmer continua were developed (correlated and uncorrelated), with absolute shimmer ranging from 0 to 2.6 dB. Perceived **roughness** in correlated sequences was also greater than with the uncorrelated sequences, and this difference was not attenuated by use of relative average perturbation measures such as RAP or APQ (see Table 9–2.2a). At moderate and

Appendix 9–A. Continued

Signal Type	***Investigation***	***Notes***
		high levels of perturbations, listeners were able to discriminate between pitch and amplitude perturbation sequences. To construct additive noise continua with spectral slope variations, Hillenbrand added Klatt synthesis aspiration noise and varied spectral slope in two ways: (1) by altering the bandwidths of glottal resonance between 75 and 300 Hz or (2) by adjusting formant amplitudes. A strong relationship was found between perceived **breathiness** and additive noise, but virtually no effects were found in association with slope differences.
Effects of frequency and amplitude resolution, interpolation, filtering, and sample size on jitter and shimmer	Titze, Horii, and Scherer (1987)	The investigators derived theoretical functions defining maximum normalized percentage shimmer ($50\ R/2^N$, where R is the amplitude reduction factor of a given signal relative to the full scale of the analog–digital converting hardware and N is the number of bits used for amplitude quantization) and percentage jitter ($50\ F_0/F_s$), revealing that 9 bits of resolution may generally give good accuracy for shimmer but that 500 samples per glottal cycle may be needed for good jitter measurement. Using synthetic triangular and sinusoidal waveforms along with natural male and female sustained /a/ phonations, the investigators compared different sampling rates, and two cycle-identifying procedures: (a) negative and positive peak-picking with no interpolation and (b) zerocrossing with interpolation. Results indicated that interpolation methods were required to produce good jitter estimates at sampling rates lower than 500 samples per cycle. Low-pass and bandpass were also deleterious to jitter but only when performed in ranges close to F_0. A second study investigated peak interpolation techniques and filter effects for cycle detection, finding again that interpolation was critical for accurate jitter detection at less than 500 samples per cycle and again revealing that low-pass filtering began to deteriorate accuracy when cutoff frequencies fell below 1 kHz. Additional results suggested that approximately 20–30 cycles are needed in a sample for stable results and that multiple productions may be necessary.
Effects of voice quality on pitch judgment	Wolfe and Ratusnik (1988)	The investigators used a pure-tone pitch matching paradigm on one-second /i/ and /a/ sustained vowel samples produced by patients with **dysphonia**, grouped as either clear/mild or moderate/severe. They measured Yanigahara classification (Table 9–5.1) and absolute jitter and jitter ratio (Table 9–1.2a). They found pitch underestimation associated with level of dysphonia and in significant negative correlation with all variables.

Appendix 9–A. Continued

Signal Type	***Investigation***	***Notes***
Effects of sampling rate, quantization, and pitch determination errors on RAP and DPQ jitter and shimmer	Cox, Ito, and Morrison (1989a)	The investigators derive RAP (see Table 9–1.2a) from a more generalized formulation that includes potential features not exemplified by either algorithm. Using mathematical analysis of this formulation with probability theory, they derive expected values, expected effects of period measurement errors and demonstrate that quantization and other error sources cause RAP to overestimate true jitter and shimmer. They demonstrate that a center-limit on perturbations, bringing a value to zero when its absolute value is below this limit, can compensate for bias in such errors but not for excess variance. They proceed to demonstrate the sampling rates at which rounding errors will have negligible effects, finding, for example, that to detect absolute RAP down to 0.001 ms and maintain a maximum error of 10% at an F_0 of 200 Hz, 41 kHz sampling is required. At higher F_0, sampling rates in excess of 50 kHz are needed even to maintain a maximum error of 15% down to a RAP of 0.003. Although rates for minimizing shimmer were lower for /u/, they were again quite high (>40 kHz) for /i/. Similar analyses were applied to a generalized formulation of DPQ (see Table 9–1.2a)—demonstrating an underestimation of DPQ resulting from errors, with some amelioration but a concomitant increase in the range of underestimation when a center limit strategy is employed. By these analyses, DPQ is even more demanding of high sampling rates than RAP, but a 12-bit quantization or better was seen to be adequate. Without error control measures in place DPQ scores are influenced in part by simple perturbation magnitude. Overall, although interpolations may help, pitch period demarcation errors, even at relatively high sampling rates, are a significant problem in perturbation measures.
Effects of sampling rate and pitch period measurement errors on time-domain HNR measures	Cox et al. (1989b)	The investigators present formulations based on HNR_{Yumoto} (see Table 9–4.0) designed to include terms for variable integration ranges, data offset (DC bias), and multipliers for modeling shimmer. They show how the formulation can be implemented for a single pass through the data, and also how the formulation can be used to represent $HNR_{Milenkovic}$ (see Table 9–4.0) and why the latter tends to overestimate HNR in comparison to procedures that inspect more than two pitch periods. They also present a correlation factor noise measure (q.v., Table 9–4.0). A mathematical demonstration of HNR underestimation due to pitch period measurement errors is presented showing that the effects are relatively minor for vowels dominated by low-frequencies (/u/) but serious for other vowels such as /i/ and /a/, even at higher sampling rates (e.g., 30 kHz). An optimization procedure for pitch period measurement utilizing interpolation of crosscorrelation functions between adjacent pitch periods is presented and compared to the similar procedure employed by Milenkovic (1987) for perturbation measures (see Table 9–4.0). Evaluations on synthetic and actual vowel samples demonstrate that nonoptimized pitch period demarcation (e.g., use of pitch period peaks or

Appendix 9–A. Continued

Signal Type	*Investigation*	*Notes*
		negative zero-crossings) can cause HNR underestimation. Overall recommendations include the use of high sampling rates, period measurement optimization, and interpolation procedures.
Effects of pitch period measurement, Fourier processing, algorithm parameter settings, and sample characteristics on frequency–domain HNR measures.	Cox et al. (1989c)	The investigators present HNR_{Cox} and $HNR_{Cox(sor)}$ based on HNR_{Kojima} (see algorithm details Table 9–4.0). They present and discuss the merits of digital resampling with Lagrange interpolation as an alternative to zero-padding for FFT processing of variable sample lengths and proceed to implement a high-frequency adaptation of vowel synthesis appropriate for their algorithm calibration studies. Overall results included: observations that oversampling could be important for accurate measurement in samples without perturbation, observations that FFT algorithms with interpolated resampling were as effective as DFTs with continuously variable sample lengths for generating frequency-domain HNRs, observations that pitch period quantization and other demarcation offsets had relatively low effects on HNRs even with rectangular windowing with demarcation errors having high impact somewhat reduced by Hanning windows, that $HNR_{Cox(sor)}$ was highly effective for reducing vowel artifactual formant structure impact on other HNRs and somewhat effective for reducing F_0 impact, that jitter affected HNR for all types, and that shimmer and noise were not deleterious to HNR accuracy. Recommendations included the use of windowing and NSKIP parameters (see algorithm, Table 9–4.0) for reducing problems associated with pitch-asynchronous framing and period measurement errors and the incorporation of larger numbers of pitch periods when possible.
Effects of waveform event criteria in jitter analysis of sinusoidal signals.	Deem, Manning, Knack, and Matesich (1989)	The investigators implemented 12 different fundamental period measurement strategies by incorporating negative and positive peak-picking, zero-crossing, and variable baseline crossing approaches with and without the interpolation techniques also investigated by Titze et al. (1987) (q.v., this appendix). Best results on sinusoidal samples (i.e., lowest absolute and percent jitter values) sampled at 100 kHz directly and off reel-to-reel tape recordings were obtained with interpolated zero crossing measures, with measurable accuracy decreases due to tape recording. No clear benefits of these period measurement strategies appeared for actual nondisordered male and female sustained vowel phonation samples, although vowel differences did appear (higher jitter values consistently measured for /a/ vs. /i/ or /u/, especially in males).

Appendix 9–A. Continued

Signal Type	***Investigation***	***Notes***
Perceptual and analysis-by-synthesis studies of breathiness and laryngealization in connected speech using KLSYN88 synthesis.	Klatt & Klatt (1990)	Klatt and Klatt (1990) varied a set of parameters newly implemented in the KLSYN88 program to model a woman's reiterant imitations of a sentence using /hɑ/ and /ʔɑ/ syllables, successfully capturing voice quality dominated by aspects of **breathiness** and **laryngealization**. Parameters used for glottal source quality modeling in this program include OQ (open quotient), TL (spectral tilt), AH (aspiration noise), FL (flutter, or slowly varying statistical fluctuations to the glottal period), and DI (for diplophonia, or double pulsing, in which temporal offset and reduced amplitude is introduced in alternate periods). In a study manipulating these and other parameters to assess 11 variations of sustained (female) vowel quality, the investigators found, among other things: (1) that manipulations of OQ and TL parameters to boost first harmonic amplitude often produced nasality perceptions instead of merely breathiness, (2) that aspiration noise appeared to be the single strongest parameter to produce breathiness percepts by itself, and (3) that complex interactions among parameters obtained, with strongest breathiness percepts resulting from the combination of increased AH, TL, OQ, and bandwidths of F1 and F2.

Other Sources: Alwan, Bangayan, Kreiman, and Long, 1995; Ananthapadmanabha, 1984; Askenfelt, Gauffin, Sundberg, and Kitzing, 1980; Behrman, Agresti, Blumstein, and Lee, 1998; Bielamowicz, Kreiman, Gerratt, Dauer, and Berke, 1996; Boyanov, Hadjitodorov, Teston, and Doskov, 1997; Carlson, Granström, and Karlsson, 1991; Cranen and Schroeter, 1995, 1996; Doherty and Shipp, 1988; Dwire and McCauley, 1995; Fant et al., 1985; Flanagan, Rabiner, Christopher, Bock, and Shipp, 1976; Gauffin, Granqvist, Hammarberg, and Hertegard, 1996; Gauffin, Granqvist, Hammarberg, Hertegard, and Hakansson, 1995; Gelfer and Fendel, 1995; Green, Buder, Rodda, and Moore, 1998; Hermes, 1991; Isshiki et al., 1966; Jiang, Lin, and Hanson, 1998; Kacprowski, 1979; Karlsson, 1992; Karnell et al., 1995; Laver, Hiller, and Hanson, 1982; Liljencrants, 1996; Lippman, 1981; Pabon and de Krom, 1995; Pawlowski, Pawluczyk, and Kraska, 1985; Perry, Ingrisano, and Scott, 1996; Pollack, 1971; Quackenbush, Barnwell, and Clements, 1988; Rosenberg, 1971; Rossiter and Howard, 1996; Rozsypal and Millar, 1979; Schoentgen, 1988; Titze and Winholtz, 1993; Van Bezooyen, 1986; Wendahl, 1966a; Wendahl, 1966b; Winholtz and Titze, 1997; Wong et al., 1991.

Appendix 9–B. Pinto and Titze's Unified Perturbation System.

Measure	*Unit*	*Algorithm*
0-order perturbation function (p_i^0)	differenced parameter (e.g., difference in ms if parameter is pitch period)	$P_i - \overline{P}$
higher-order perturbation functions (p_i^k)	multiply differenced parameter (i.e., differences taken k times)	$p_i^{k-1} - p_{i-1}^{k-1}$, *k odd*, $p_{i+1}^{k-1} - p_1^{k-1}$, *k even.* $k_1 + 1 \le i \le N - k_2$, k odd: $k_1 = (k + 1)/2$, $k_2 = (k + 1)/2$, k even: $k_1 = k/2$, $k_2 = k/2$,
Measures of extent (order k):		
Mean Rectified (MR^k)	original parameter (mean)	$\frac{1}{N-k}\sum \lvert p_i^k \rvert$
Root mean squared (RMS^k [statistical])	original parameter (deviation)	$\left[\frac{1}{N-k}\sum (p_i^k)^2\right]^{1/2}$
		RMS^0 = incorporates standard deviations, but note that RMS as an engineering operation incorporates absolute values.
Median Rectified (MER^k)	original parameter	p_i^k such that the number of values greater equals the number of values lesser.

6. CONCLUSION: FUTURE DIRECTIONS

As is evident from a scan of the reference list dates appearing at the end of this chapter, many algorithm developments and applications have appeared since 1990. However, as should also be obvious from the preceding tables, the number of algorithms and selected applications up to 1990 were already voluminous. Practical limitations prevent an expansion of these tables here to include all the citations listed, but the listing of these references preceding individual tables may provide some rough guidance. There are several directions that are open for further review and development in acoustic analysis:

1. Despite intensive efforts dedicated to enhanced and reliable automatic F_0 extraction, it still appears that users need to be continually vigilant when utilizing voice quality measures that depend on prior extraction of periodicity. More interactive interfaces, perhaps implementing artificial intelligence and expert systems approaches, guided by user selection of perceptual or physiologic orientations, may become available; but, in the meantime, the community must continue to distrust and double-check such measures. The situation is ironically exacerbated in "deviant" qualities (although many such qualities are as likely to be encountered in nondisordered spontaneous and conversational speech samples), especially those voice qualities marked by voice and pitch breaks and subharmonic modulations. Any developments leading to truly useful normative values must account for these phenomena.
2. Voice quality measures need to be normed against vocal F_0 and amplitude, ideally incorporating both dimensions in voice range profile format (see Table 9–3.0).
3. More comprehensive application of Pinto and Titze's (1990) system would help to reduce the terminological proliferation and the attendant confusion of measurement values. Such an effort might follow from the tabulation presented here, but this standardization would need to be adopted by the community of researchers and practitioners using the measures. Furthermore, comparable efforts are needed in other areas of voice quality measurement in addition to the perturbation measures. Note, for example, the preponderance of measures utilizing spectral (Table 9–5.2) and inverse filtering of acoustic signals (Table 9–6.1).
4. The essential epistemological gaps between acoustics, physiology, and perception need to be respected. Perhaps the ultimate direction to which acoustic measures of voice quality should be oriented—perceptual or physiological—may not need to be resolved so long as it is clear in a given application or research program. It seems to have been assumed historically that the basic orientation should be perceptual; this may be based on desires to press acoustic measures into service as aids to the clinical ear. However, given the conclusions of Kreiman and Gerratt (1996), further efforts in this regard may be futile. It might be more useful in the long run to attempt a better grounding of acoustic measures in physiological mechanisms. Research oriented in this direction is still surprisingly sparse, perhaps because of the difficult and interdisciplinary nature of such an enterprise. It is probable that multivariate (and multitask) descriptions will be needed; here again the paucity of such efforts is striking. One hope is that the array of tables presented in this chapter will stimulate more comprehensive efforts. The payoff may be clinical, as well as in basic scientific understanding, as one potential benefit of acoustic analysis may be to guide the detection of physiological effects that are difficult or impossible to pick up with the clinical ear alone.
5. Many exciting avenues for basic application are still open for pursuit, for example, the study of voice dynamics in spontaneous connected speech (Fant, 1997) and the study of emotion and attitude in nondisordered

speech, singing, and other "real-world" domains. The variety of voice types both within and across individual speakers presents sufficient grounds for the realization that the enterprise of understanding voice qualities has only begun.

Acknowledgments

I wish to thank Joe Clark for his dedication in assisting with reference location and management and Brenda Bender for her close proofreading skills, but I accept full responsibility for any remaining errors or omissions.

Commercial software systems featuring multiple acoustic voice quality measures:

AVAAZ Innovations (1995b). Interactive Voice Analysis System (IVANS).
Kay Elemetrics (1993). Multi-Dimensional Voice Program.
Tiger DRS (1995). Dr. Speech.

Other microcomputer-based commercial systems including acoustic voice quality measures:

AVAAZ Innovations (1995a). Computerized Speech Research Environment (CSRE).
GW Instruments (1997). SoundScope.
Kay Elemetrics (1991) Computerized Speech Laboratory (CSL).
InfoSignal (1994). Signalyze.
Entropic Research Laboratory (1997). ESPS+/Waves.
Milenkovic, P. (1997). CSpeechSP.
Sensimetrics Corp. (1998). SpeechStation2.
Scicon (1998). Pcquirer, Macquirer.
Soundswell Music Acoustics (1999). Swell.

REFERENCES

Abdoerrachman, H., Imaizumi, S., Hirose, H., & Niimi, S. (1993). Slow and fast perturbations in voice—A preliminary report. *Research Institute of Logopedics and Phoniatrics (RILP) Annual Bulletin, 27,* 125–134.

Abraham, R. H., & Shaw, C. D. (1983). *Dynamics, the geometry of behavior. Part one: Periodic behavior.* Santa Cruz, CA: Aerial Press.

Abraham, R. H., & Shaw, C. D. (1984). *Dynamics, the geometry of behavior. Part two: Chaotic behavior.* Santa Cruz, CA: Aerial Press.

Abraham, R. H., & Shaw, C. D. (1985). *Dynamics, the geometry of behavior. Part three: Global behavior.* Santa Cruz, CA: Aerial Press.

Abraham, R. H., & Shaw, C. D. (1988). *Dynamics, the geometry of behavior. Part four: Bifurcation behavior.* Santa Cruz, CA: Aerial Press.

Abraham, R. H., & Shaw, C. D. (1992). *Dynamics, the geometry of behavior.* Redwood City, CA: Addison-Wesley.

Ackermann, H., & Ziegler, W. (1991). Cerebellar voice tremor: an acoustic analysis. *Journal of Neurology, Neurosurgery, and Psychiatry, 54,* 74–76.

Ackermann, H., & Ziegler, W. (1994). Acoustic analysis of vocal instability in cerebellar dysfunctions. *Annals of Otology, Rhinology & Laryngology, 103,* 98–104.

Alku, P., Strik, H., & Vilkman, E. (1997). Parabolic spectral parameter-A new method for quantification of the glottal flow. *Speech Communication, 22,* 67–79.

Alku, P., & Vilkman, E. (1995a). Comparing methods for quantifying the voice source of different phonation types inverse filtered from acoustic speech signals. In K. Elenius & P. Branderud (Eds.), *Proceedings of the XIIIth International Congress of Phonetic Sciences* (Vol. 2, pp. 422–425). Stockholm, Sweden: KTH and Stockholm University.

Alku, P., & Vilkman, E. (1995b). Effects of bandwidth on glottal airflow waveforms estimated by inverse filtering. *Journal of the Acoustical Society of America, 98,* 763–767.

Alku, P., & Vilkman, E. (1996). A comparison of glottal voice source quantification parameters in breathy, normal and pressed phonation of female and male speakers. *Folia Phoniatrica et Logopaedica, 48,* 240–254.

Alku, P., Vilkman, E., & Laukkanen, A. (1998). Parameterization of the voice source by combining spectral decay and amplitude features of the glottal flow. *Journal of Speech Language and Hearing Research, 41,* 990–1002.

Alku, P., Vilkman, E., & Laukkanen, A.-M. (1997). Estimation of the amplitude features of the glottal flow by inverse filtering speech pressure signals. *Speech Communication, 24,* 123–132.

Alwan, A., Bangayan, P., Kreiman, J., & Long, C. (1995). Time and frequency synthesis parameters of severely pathological voice qualities. In K. Elenius & P. Branderud (Eds.), *Proceedings of the XIIIth International Congress of Phonetic Sciences* (Vol. 2, pp. 250–253). Stockholm, Sweden: KTH and Stockholm University.

Ananthapadmanabha, T. V. (1984). Acoustic analysis of voice source dynamics. *Speech Transmission Laboratory Quarterly Progress and Status Report, 2–3,* 1–24.

Ananthapadmanabha, T. V. (1995). Acoustic factors determining perceived voice quality. In O. Fujimura & M. Hirano (Eds.), *Vocal fold physiology: Voice quality control* (pp. 113–126). San Diego, CA: Singular Publishing Group.

Andrews, M. L., & Schmidt, C. P. (1997). Gender presentation: Perceptual and acoustical analyses of voice. *Journal of Voice, 11,* 307–313.

Apple, W., Streeter, L. A., & Krauss, R. M. (1979). Effects of pitch and speech rate on personal attributions. *Journal of Personality and Social Psychology, 37,* 715–727.

Arnold, G. E. (1955). Vocal rehabilitation of paralytic dysphonia. *A. M. A. Archives of Otolaryngology, 62,* 593–601.

Aronson, A. E., & Hartman, D. E. (1981). Adductor spastic dysphonia as a sign of essential (voice) tremor. *Journal of Speech and Hearing Disorders, 46,* 52–58.

Aronson, A. E., Ramig, L. O., Winholz, W. S., & Silber, S. R. (1992). Rapid voice tremor, or "flutter," in amyotrophic lateral sclerosis. *Annals of Otology, Rhinology & Laryngology, 101,* 511–518.

Askenfelt, A., Gauffin, J., Sundberg, J., & Kitzing, P. (1980). A comparison of contact microphone and electroglottograph for the measurement of vocal fundamental frequency. *Journal of Speech Research, 23,* 258–273.

Askenfelt, A., & Hammarberg, B. (1986). Speech waveform perturbation analysis: A perceptual-acoustic comparison of seven measures. *Journal of Speech and Hearing Research, 29,* 50–64.

Awan, S. N. (1991). Phonetographic profiles of F_0–SPL characteristics of untrained versus trained vocal groups. *Journal of Voice, 5,* 41–50.

Awan, S. N. (1993). Superimposition of speaking voice characteristics and phonetograms in untrained and trained vocal groups. *Journal of Voice, 7,* 30–37.

Awan, S. N., & Frenkel, M. L. (1994). Improvements in estimating the harmonics-to-noise ratio of the voice. *Journal of Voice, 8,* 255–262.

Baer, T. (1980). Vocal jitter: A neuromuscular explanation. In V. Lawrence & B. Weinberg (Eds.), *Transcripts of the Eighth Symposium: Care of the Professional Voice. Part I: Physical factors in voice, vibrato, registers* (pp. 19–24). New York: The Voice Foundation.

Baken, R. J. (1987). *Clinical measurement of speech and voice.* Boston, MA: Allyn and Bacon.

Baken, R. J. (1990). Irregularity of vocal period and amplitude: A first approach to the fractal analysis of voice. *Journal of Voice, 4,* 185–197.

Baken, R. J., & Orlikoff, R. F. (1992). Acoustic assessment of vocal function. In A. Blitzer, M. F. Brin, C. T. Sasaki, S. Fahn, & K. S. Harris (Eds.), *Neurologic disorders of the larynx* (pp. 124–134). New York: Thieme Medical Publishers, Inc.

Banci, G., Monini, S., Falaschi, A., & De Sario, N. (1986). Vocal fold disorder evaluation by digital speech analysis. *Journal of Phonetics, 14,* 495–499.

Bartholomew, W. T. (1934). A physical definition of "good voice-quality" in the male voice. *Journal of the Acoustical Society of America, 6,* 25–33.

Beckett, R. L. (1969). Pitch perturbation as a function of subjective vocal constriction. *Folia Phoniatrica, 21,* 416–425.

Behrman, A., Agresti, C. J., Blumstein, E., & Lee, N. (1998). Microphone and electroglottographic data from dysphonic patients: Type 1, 2 and 3 signals. *Journal of Voice, 12,* 249–260.

Behrman, A., & Baken, R. J. (1997). Correlation dimension of electroglottographic data from healthy and pathologic subjects. *Journal of the Acoustical Society of America, 102,* 2371–2739.

Benson, P. (1995). Analysis of the acoustic correlates of stress from an operational aviation emergency. In I. Trancoso & R. Moore (Eds.), *ESCA – NATO tutorial and research workshop on speech under stress* (pp. 61–64). Lisbon, Portugal: ESCA.

Berry, D., Herzel, H., Titze, I., & Krischer, K. (1994). Interpretation of biomechanical simulations of normal and chaotic vocal fold oscillations with empirical eigenfunctions. *Journal of the Accoustical Society of America, 95,* 3595–3604.

Berry, D., Herzel, H., Titze, I., & Story, B. (1996). Bifurcations in excised larynx experiments. *Journal of Voice, 10,* 129–138.

Bickley, C. (1982). Acoustic analysis and perception of breathy vowels, *Speech Communication Group Working Papers* (Vol. 1, pp. 71–81). Cambridge, MA: Research Laboratory of Electronics, MIT.

Bickley, C. A., & Stevens, K. N. (1986). Effects of a vocal-tract constriction on the glottal source: Experimental and modeling studies. *Journal of Phonetics, 14,* 373–382.

Bickley, C. A., & Stevens, K. N. (1987). Effects of a vocal tract constriction on the glottal source: Data from voiced consonants. In T. Baer, C. Sasaki, & K. Harris (Eds.), *Laryngeal function in phonation and respiration* (pp. 239–253). Boston: College-Hill.

Bielamowicz, S., Kreiman, J., Gerratt, B. R., Dauer, M. S., & Berke, G. S. (1996). Comparison of voice analysis systems for perturbation measurement. *Journal of Speech and Hearing Research, 39,* 126–134.

Blomgren, M., Chen, Y., Ng, M. L., & Gilbert, H. R. (1998). Acoustic, aerodynamic, physiologic, and perceptual properties of modal and vocal fry registers. *Journal of the Acoustical Society of America, 103,* 2649–2658.

Boek, W., Wieneke, G. H., & Dejonckere, P. H. (1997). Clinical relevance of the fractal dimension of F_0 perturbations computed by the box-counting method. *Journal of Voice, 11,* 437–442.

Boves, L. (1984). *The phonetic basis of perceptual ratings of running speech.* Dordrecht, Holland: Foris.

Bowler, N. W. (1957). *A fundamental frequency analysis of harsh vocal quality.* Unpublished doctoral dissertation, Stanford University.

Bowler, N. W. (1964). A fundamental frequency analysis of harsh vocal quality. *Speech Monographs, 31,* 128–134.

Boyanov, B., Hadjitodorov, S., Teston, B., & Doskov, D. (1997). Software system for pathological voice analysis. *Larynx 97* (pp. 139–142). Aix en Provence, France: Universite de Provence.

Brown, J. R., & Simonson, J. (1963). Organic voice tremor. *Neurology, 13,* 520–525.

Brown, W. S., Jr., Morris, R. J., & Michel, J. F. (1990). Vocal jitter and fundamental frequency characteristics in aged, female professional singers. *Journal of Voice, 4,* 135–141.

Buder, E. H., Hartelius, L., & Strand, E. A. (1995). Phonatory instabilities in ALS and MS dysarthrias: Graphic and quantitative analyses. In K. Elenius & P. Branderud (Eds.), *Proceedings of the XIIIth International Congress of Phonetic Sciences* (Vol. 4, pp. 472–479). Stockholm, Sweden: KTH and Stockholm University.

Buder, E. H., & Strand, E. A. (1994). Phonatory instability in ALS dysarthria: A case study. *The Journal of the Acoustical Society of America, 94,* 1782.

Cairns, D., Hansen, J., & Kaiser, J. (1996, October). *Recent advances in hypernasal speech detection using the nonlinear teager energy operator.* Paper presented at The Fourth International Conference on Spoken Language Processing, Philadephia.

Campbell, W. (1995). Loudness, spectral tilt, and perceived prominence in dialogues. In K. Elenius & P. Branderud (Eds.), *Proceedings of the XIIIth International Congress of Phonetic Sciences* (Vol. 3, pp. 676–679). Stockholm, Sweden: KTH and Stockholm University.

Carlson, R., Granström, B., & Karlsson, I. (1991). Experiments with voice modelling in speech synthesis. *Speech Communication, 10,* 481–489.

Castellengo, M., Roubeau, B., & Valette, C. (1985). Study of the acoustical phenomena characteristic of the transition between chest, voice and falsetto. In A. Askenfelt, S. Felicetti, E. Jansson, & J. Sundberg (Eds.), *SMAC 83 — Proceedings of the Stockholm Music Acoustics Conference* (pp. 113–124). Stockholm.

Castex, A. (1902). *Maladies de la voix.* Paris: Masson et Cie.

Catford, J. C. (1964). Phonation types: The classification of some laryngeal components of speech production. In D. Abercrombie, D. B. Fry, P. A. D. MacCarthy, N. C. Scott, & J. L. M. Trim (Eds.), *In honour of Daniel Jones. Papers contributed on the occasion of his eightieth birthday 12 September 1961* (pp. 26–37). London: Longmans.

Cavallo, S. A., Baken, R. J., & Shaiman, S. (1984). Frequency perturbation characteristics of pulse register phonation. *Journal of Communication Disorders, 17,* 231–243.

Childers, D. G., & Lee, C. K. (1991). Voice quality factors: Analysis, synthesis, and perception. *Journal of the Acoustical Society of America, 90,* 2394–2410.

Chuang, E. S., & Hanson, H. M. (1996). Glottal characteristics of male speakers: Acoustic correlates and comparison with female data. *Journal of the Acoustical Society of America, 100,* 2657.

Cleveland, T., & Sundberg, J. (1983). Acoustic analysis of three male voices of different quality. *Speech Transmission Laboratory Quarterly Progress and Status Report, 4,* 27–38.

Cleveland, T., & Sundberg, J. (1985). Acoustic analysis of three male voices of different quality. In A. Askenfelt, S. Felicetti, E. Jansson, & J. Sundberg (Eds.), *SMAC 83 — Proceedings of the Stockholm Music Acoustics Conference* (pp. 143–156). Stockholm.

Coleman, R. (1969). Effect of median frequency levels upon the roughness of jittered simuli. *Journal of Speech and Hearing Research, 12,* 330–336.

Coleman, R. F. (1960). *Some acoustic correlates of hoarseness.* Unpublished master's thesis, Vanderbilt University, Nashville.

Coleman, R. F. (1971). Effect of waveform changes upon roughness perception. *Folia Phoniatrica, 23,* 314–322.

Coleman, R. F. (1993). Sources of variation in phonetograms. *Journal of Voice, 7,* 1–14.

Colton, R. H. (1972). Spectral characteristics of the modal and falsetto registers. *Folia Phoniatrica, 24,* 337–344.

Colton, R. H. (1973). Some acoustic parameters related to the perception of modal-falsetto voice quality. *Folia Phoniatrica, 25,* 302–311.

Colton, R. H., & Estill, J. A. (1981). Elements of voice quality: Perceptual, acoustic, and physiologic aspects. In N. J. Lass (Ed.), *Speech and language: Advances in basic research and practice* (Vol. 5, pp. 311–403). New York: Academic Press.

Comerci, F. A. (1955). Perceptibility of flutter in speech and music. *Journal of the Society of Motion Picture and Television Engineers, 64,* 117–122.

Cox, N. B., Ito, M. R., & Morrison, M. D. (1989a). Quantization and measurement errors in the analysis of short-time perturbations in sampled data. *Journal of the Acoustical Society of America, 85,* 42–54.

Cox, N. B., Ito, M. R., & Morrison, M. D. (1989b). Data labeling and sampling effects in harmonic-to-noise ratios. *Journal of the Acoustical Society of America, 85,* 2165–2178.

Cox, N. B., Ito, M. R., & Morrison, M. D. (1989c). Technical considerations in computation of spectral harmonics-to-noise ratios for sustained vowels. *Journal of Speech and Hearing Research, 32,* 203–218.

Cranen, B., & Schroeter, J. (1995). Modeling a leaky glottis. *Journal of Phonetics, 23,* 165–177.

Cranen, B., & Schroeter, J. (1996). Physiologically motivated modelling of the voice source in articulatory analysis/synthesis. *Speech Communication, 19,* 1–19.

Cummings, K., & Clements, M. (1995). Analysis of the glottal excitation of emotionally styled and stressed speech. *Journal of the Acoustical Society of America, 98,* 88–98.

Curtis, J. F. (1942). *An experimental study of the wave-composition of nasal voice quality.* Unpublished doctoral dissertation, The University of Iowa, Iowa City.

Damsté, H. (1970). The phonetogram. *Practica Oto-Rhino-Laryngologica, 32,* 185–187.

Davis, S. B. (1975). Preliminary results using inverse filtering of speech for automatic evaluation of laryngeal pathology. *The Journal of the Acoustical Society of America, 58,* SIII.

Davis, S. B. (1976). *Computer evaluation of laryngeal pathology based on inverse filtering of speech.* Unpublished doctoral dissertation, University of California, Santa Barbara. (Also SCRL Monograph No. 13. Santa Barbara, CA: Speech Communications Research Laboratory, 1976.)

Davis, S. B. (1978). Acoustic characteristics of normal and pathological voices. *Status Report on Speech Research, 54,* 133–163.

Davis, S. B. (1979). Acoustic characteristics of normal and pathological voices. In N. J. Lass (Ed.), *Speech and language: Advances in basic research and practice* (Vol. 1, pp. 271–335). New York: Academic Press.

Davis, S. B. (1981). Acoustical characteristics of normal and pathological voices. *ASHA Reports, 11,* 97–115.

Deal, R. E., & Emanuel, F. W. (1978). Some waveform and spectral features of vowel roughness. *Journal of Speech and Hearing Research, 21,* 250–264.

Debruyne, F., Ostyn, F., Delaere, P., & Wellens, W. (1997). Acoustic analysis of the speaking voice after thyroidectomy. *Journal of Voice, 11,* 479–482.

Deem, J. F., Manning, W. H., Knack, J. V., & Matesich, J. S. (1989). The automatic extraction of pitch perturbation using microcomputers: Some methodological considerations. *Journal of Speech and Hearing Research,* 32, 689–697.

de Krom, G. (1993). A cepstrum-based technique for determining a harmonics-to-noise ratio in speech signals. *Journal of Speech and Hearing Research, 36,* 254–266.

de Krom, G. (1994a). *Acoustic correlates of breathiness and roughness (Doctoral Dissertation, Utrecht University, 1994).* Utrecht, Netherlands: Onderzoeksinstituut voor Taal en Spraak.

de Krom, G. (1994b). Consistency and reliability of voice quality ratings for different types of speech fragments. *Journal of Speech and Hearing Research, 37,* 985–1000.

de Krom, G. (1995). Some spectral correlates of pathological breathy and rough voice quality for different types of vowel fragments. *Journal of Speech and Hearing Research, 38,* 794–811.

Dejonckere, P. H. (1995). Caruso's vibrato: An acoustic study. In P. H. Dejonckere, M. Hirano, & J. Sundberg (Eds.), *Vibrato* (pp. 111–120). San Diego: Singular Publishing Group.

Dejonckere, P. H., & Lebacq, J. (1984). Damping coefficient of oscillating vocal folds in relation with pitch perturbations. *Speech Communication, 3,* 89–92.

Dejonckere, P. H., & Lebacq, J. (1983). An analysis of the diplophonia phenomenon. *Speech Communication, 2,* 47–56.

Dejonckere, P., & Wieneke, G. (1994). Spectral, cepstral and aperiodicity characteristics of pathological voices before and after phonosurgical treatment. *Clinical Linguistics and Phonetics, 8,* 161–169.

Deliyski, D. (1990). *Digital processing of voice signals in the diagnosis of laryngeal diseases.* Unpublished doctoral dissertation, Bulgarian Academy of Sciences, Institute of Industrial Cybernetics and Robotics, Sofia, Bulgaria. (Text written in Bulgarian.)

Deliyski, D. (1993). *Acoustic model and evaluation of pathological voice production.* Paper presented at The Third Conference on Speech Communication and Technology, Berlin, Germany.

Deliyski, D. D. (1994). Suggestion for a pitch extraction method and file format for pathological voice data. In D. Wong (Ed.), *Proceedings of the Workshop on Acoustic Voice Analysis.* Iowa City, IA: National Center for Voice and Speech.

Doherty, E. T., & Shipp, T. (1988). Tape recorder effects on jitter and shimmer extraction. *Journal of Speech and Hearing Research, 31,* 485–490.

Dolansk´y, L., & Tjernlund, P. (1968). On certain irregularities of voiced-speech waveforms. *IEEE Transactions on Audio and Electroacoustics, AU-16,* 51–56.

Doval, B., d'Alessandro, C., & Diard, B. (1997). Spectral methods for voice source parameters estimation. In G. Kokkinakis, N. Fakotakis, & E. Dermatas (Eds.), *Eurospeech '97 proceedings* (Vol. 1, pp. 533–536). Grenoble, France: European Speech Communication Association.

Dromey, C., & Ramig, L. (1998). Intentional changes in sound pressure level and rate: Their impact on measures of respiration, phonation, and articulation. *Journal of Speech, Language and Hearing Research, 41,* 1003–1018.

Dromey, C., Ramig, L. O., & Johnson, A. B. (1995). Phonatory and articulatory changes associated with increased vocal intensity in Parkinson Disease: A case study. *Journal of Speech and Hearing Research, 38,* 751–764.

Dunker, E., & Schlosshauer, B. (1961). Unregelmässige stimmlippenschwingungen bei funktionellen stimmstörungen. *Zeitschrift für Laryngologie, Rhinologie, Otologie und ihre Grenzgebiete, 40,* 919–934.

Dwire, A., & McCauley, R. (1995). Repeated measures of vocal fundamental frequency perturbation obtained using the Visi-Pitch. *Journal of Voice, 9,* 156–162.

Ekholm, E., Papagiannis, G. C., & Chagnon, F. P. (1998). Relating objective measurements to expert evaluation of voice quality in western classical singing: Critical perceptual parameters. *Journal of Voice, 12,* 182–196.

Emanuel, F. W., Lively, M. A., & McCoy, J. F. (1973). Spectral noise levels and roughness ratings for vowels produced by males and females. *Folia Phoniatrica, 25,* 110–120.

Emanuel, F. W., & Sansone Jr., F. E. (1969). Some spectral features of "normal" and simulated "rough" vowels. *Folia Phoniatrica, 21,* 401–415.

Emanuel, F. W., & Smith, W. F. (1974). Pitch effects on vowel roughness and spectral noise. *Journal of Phonetics, 2,* 247–253.

Eskenazi, L. (1988). *Acoustic correlates of voice quality and distortion measure for speech processing.* Unpublished doctoral dissertation, University of Florida, Gainesville.

Eskenazi, L., Childers, D. B., & Hicks, D. M. (1990). Acoustic correlates of vocal quality. *Journal of Speech and Hearing Research, 33,* 298–306.

Estill, J., Baer, T., Honda, K., & Harris, K. S. (1985). Supralaryngeal activity in a study of six voice qualities. In A. Askenfelt, S. Felicetti, E. Jansson, & J. Sundberg (Eds.), *SMAC 83—Proceedings of the Stockholm Music Acoustics Conference* (pp. 157–174).

Estill, J., Fujimura, O., Sawada, M., & Beechler, K. (1996). Temporal perturbation and voice qualities. In P. Davis & N. Fletcher (Eds.), *Vocal fold physiology: Controlling complexity and chaos* (pp. 237–252). San Diego, CA: Singular Publishing Group.

Fairbanks, G. (1940). *Voice and articulation drillbook.* New York: Harper and Brothers.

Fant, G. (1960). *Acoustic theory of speech production.* s'Gravenhage: Mouton.

Fant, G. (1986). Glottal Flow: Models and interaction. *Journal of Phonetics, 14,* 393–399. (Reprinted in Kent, R. D., Atal, B. S., & Miller, J. L. [Eds.], [1991]. *Papers in speech communication: Speech production* [pp. 139–146]. Woodbury, NY: Acoustical Society of America.)

Fant, G. (1993). Some problems in voice source analysis. *Speech Communication, 13,* 7–22.

Fant, G. (1997). The voice source in connected speech. *Speech Communication, 22,* 125–139.

Fant, G., Liljencrants, J., & Lin, Q. (1985). A four-parameter model of glottal flow. *Speech Transmission Laboratory Quarterly Progress and Status Report, 4,* 1–13.

Feijoo, S., & Hernández, C. (1990). Short-term stability measures for the evaluation of vocal quality. *Journal of Speech and Hearing Research, 33,* 324–334.

Ferrand, C. T. (1995). Effects of practice with and without knowledge of results on jitter and shimmer levels in normally speaking women. *Journal of Voice, 9,* 419–423.

Ferrand, C. T. (1998). The effects of time constraints on phonatory stability in normally speaking adult women. *Journal of Voice, 12*, 175–181.

Fex, B., Fex, S., Shiromoto, O., & Hirano, M. (1994). Acoustic analysis of functional dysphonia: Before and after voice therapy (accent method). *Journal of Voice, 8*, 163–167.

Fex, S., Löfqvist, A., & Schalén, L. (1991). Videostroboscopic evaluation of glottal open quotient, related to some acoustic parameters. In J. Gauffin & B. Hammarberg (Eds.), *Vocal fold physiology: Acoustic, perceptual and physiological aspects of voice mechanisms* (pp. 273–278). San Diego: Singular Publishing Group, Inc.

Fischer-Jørgensen, E. (1967). Phonetic analysis of breathy (murmured) vowels in Gujarati. *Indian Linguistics, 28*, 71–139.

Flanagan, J. L., Rabiner, L. R., Christopher, D., Bock, D. E., & Shipp, T. (1976). Digital analysis of laryngeal control in speech production. *Journal of the Acoustical Society of America, 60*, 446–455.

Fletcher, H. (1934). Loudness, pitch, and the timbre of musical tones and their relation to the intensity, the frequency, and the overtone structure. *Journal of the Acoustical Society of America, 6*, 59–69.

Fletcher, N. H. (1996). Nonlinearity, complexity, and control in vocal systems. In P. Davis & N. Fletcher (Eds.), *Vocal fold physiology: Controlling complexity and chaos* (pp. 3–16). San Diego: Singular Publishing Group.

Fletcher, S. (1970). Theory and instrumentation for quantitative measurement of nasality. *Cleft Palate Journal, 7*, 601–609.

Fletcher, S., & Bishop, M. (1970). Measurement of nasality by TONAR. *Cleft Palate Journal, 7*, 610–621.

Fritzell, B., Hammarberg, B., Gauffin, J., Karlsson, I., & Sundberg, J. (1986). Breathiness and insufficient vocal fold closure. *Journal of Phonetics, 14*, 549–553.

Fröhlich, M., Michaelis, D., Strube, H. W., & Kruse, E. (1997). Acoustic voice quality description: Case studies for different regions of the hoarseness diagram. In T. Wittneberg, P. Mergell, M. Tigges, & U. Eysholdt (Eds.), *Advances in Quantitative Laryngoscopy, 2nd 'Round Table'* (pp. 143–150). Erlanger.

Frøkjær-Jensen, B., & Prytz, S. (1974). Evaluation of speech disorders by means of long-time-average spectra, *Annual report of the Institute of Phonetics of the University of Copenhagen (ARIPUC)* (Vol. 8, pp. 227–237). Copenhagen.

Frøkjær-Jensen, B., & Prytz, S. (1976). Registration of voice quality. *Bruel and Kjar Technical Review, 3*, 3–17.

Fujimura, O. (1968). An approximation to voice aperiodicity. *IEEE Transactions on Audio and Electroacoustics, AU-16*, 68–72.

Fujimura, O. (1990). Methods and goals of speech production research. *Language and Speech, 33*, 195–258.

Fujimura, O., & Hirano, M. (1995). *Vocal fold physiology: voice quality control*. San Diego: Singular.

Fujiu, M., Hibi, S. R., & Hirano, M. (1988). An improved technique for measurement of the relative noise level using a sound spectrograph. *Folia Phoniatrica, 40*, 53–57.

Fukazawa, T., Blaugrund, S. M., El-Assuooty, A., & Gould, W. J. (1988). Acoustic analysis of hoarse voice: A preliminary report. *Journal of Voice, 2*, 127–131.

Fukazawa, T., El-Assuooty, A., & Honjo, I. (1988). A new index for evaluation of the turbulent noise in pathological voice. *Journal of the Acoustical Society of America, 83*, 1189–1193.

Gamboa, J., Jimenez-Jimenez, F. J., Nieto, A., Montojo, J., Orti-Pareja, M., Molina, J. A., Garcia-Albea, E., & Cobeta, I. (1997). Acoustic voice analysis in patients with Parkinson's disease treated with dopaminergic drugs. *Journal of Voice, 11*, 314–320.

Garcia, M. (1855). Observations of the human voice. *Proceedings of the Royal Society of London, 7*, 399–410.

Garret, K. L., & Healey, E. C. (1987). An acoustic analysis of fluctuations in the voices of normal adult speakers across three times of day. *Journal of the Acoustical Society of America, 82*, 58–62.

Gath, I., & Yair, E. (1987). Comparative evaluation of several pitch process models in the detection of vocal tremor. *IEEE Transactions Biomedical Engineering BME, 34*, 532–538.

Gauffin, J., Granqvist, S., Hammarberg, B., & Hertegård, S. (1996). Irregularities in the voice: A perceptual experiment using synthetic voices with subharmonics. In P. Davis & N. Fletcher (Eds.), *Vocal fold physiology: Controlling complexity and chaos* (pp. 253–261). San Diego: Singular Publishing Group.

Gauffin, J., Granqvist, S., Hammarberg, B., Hertegård, S., & Hakansson, A. (1995). Irregularities in the voice: Some perceptual experiments using synthetic voices. In K. Elenius & P. Branderud (Eds.), *Proceedings of the XIIIth International Congress of Phonetic Sciences* (Vol. 2, pp. 242–245). Stockholm, Sweden: KTH and Stockholm Universtiy.

Gauffin, J., & Sundberg, J. (1989). Spectral correlates of glottal voice source waveform characteristics. *Journal of Speech and Hearing Research, 32*,

556–565. (Reprinted in Kent, R. D., Atal, B. S., & Miller, J. L. [Eds.], [1991]. *Papers in speech communication: Speech production* [pp. 147–156]. Woodbury, NY: Acoustical Society of America.)

Gelfer, M. P., & Fendel, D. M. (1995). Comparisons of jitter, shimmer, and signal-to-noise ratio from directly digitized versus taped voice samples. *Journal of Voice, 9*, 378–382.

Gelfer, M. P., & Young, S. R. (1997). Comparisons of intensity measures and their stability in male and female speakers. *Journal of Voice, 11*, 178–186.

Gerratt, B. R., & Kreiman, J. (1994). The utility of acoustic measures of voice quality. In D. Wong (Ed.), *Proceedings of the Workshop on Acoustic Voice Analysis* . Iowa City, IA.

Gerull, G., Giesen, M., Hippel, K., Mrowinski, D., & Schweers, H. (1977). Untersuchung verschiedener gruppen von stimmstörungen durch statistische spektralanalyse. *HNO, 25*, 14–22. (In German)

Gobl, C. (1989). A preliminary study of acoustic voice quality correlates. *Speech Transmission Laboratory Quarterly Progress and Status Report, 4*, 9–22.

Gobl, C., & Ní Chasaide, A. (1992). Acoustic characteristics of voice quality. *Speech Communication, 11*, 481–490.

Gould, W. J., & Korovin, G. S. (1994). Laboratory advances for voice measurements. *Journal of Voice, 8*, 8–17.

Graddol, D., & Swann, J. (1983). Speaking fundamental frequency: some physical and social correlates. *Language and Speech, 26*, 351–366.

Granqvist, S., & Hammarberg, B. (1998). The Correlogram: a visual disply of periodicity. *Speech, Music and Hearing Quarterly Progress and Status Report, 4*, 13–22.

Green, J. R., Buder, E. H., Rodda, P. R., & Moore, C. A. (1998). Reliability of measurements across several acoustic voice analysis systems. In M. P. Cannito, K. M. Yorkston, & D. R. Beukelman (Ed.), *Neuromotor speech disorders: Nature, assessment, and management* (pp. 275–292). Baltimore, MD: Paul H. Brookes.

Gubrynowicz, R., Kacprowski, B., Mikiel, W., & Zarnecki, P. (1981). Detection and evaluation of laryngeal pathology based on pitch period measurements in continuous speech, *Proceedings of the Fourth Symposium of the Federation of the Acoustical Societies of Europe* (pp. 131–134). Venice.

Gubrynowicz, R., Mikiel, W., & Zarnecki, P. (1980). An acoustic method for the evaluation of the state of larynx source in cases involving pathological changes in the vocal folds. *Archives of Acoustics, 5*, 3–30.

Hachinski, V. C., Thomsen, I. V., & Buch, N. H. (1975). The nature of primary vocal tremor. *Canadian Journal of Neurological Sciences, 2*, 195–197.

Haggard, M. P. (1969). Speech waveform measurements in multiple sclerosis. *Folia Phoniatrica, 21*, 307–312.

Hakes, J., Doherty, E. T., & Shipp, T. (1990). Trillo rates exhibited by professional early music singers. *Journal of Voice, 4*, 305–308.

Hammarberg, B., Fritzell, B., Gauffin, J., & Sundberg, J. (1986). Acoustic and perceptual analysis of vocal dysfunction. *Journal of Phonetics, 14*, 533–547.

Hammarberg, B., Fritzell, B., Gauffin, J., Sundberg, J., & Wedin, L. (1980). Perceptual and acoustic correlates of abnormal voice qualities. *Acta Otolaryngologica, 90*, 441–451.

Hammarberg, B., & Gauffin, J. (1995). Perceptual and acoustic characteristics of quality differences in pathological voices as related to physiological aspects. In O. Fujimura & M. Hirano (Eds.), *Vocal fold physiology: Voice quality control* (pp. 283–304). San Diego, Singular Publishing Group, Inc.

Hanson, H. M. (1997). Glottal characteristics of female speakers: Acoustic correlates. *Journal of the Acoustical Society of America, 101*, 466–481.

Hartelius, L., Buder, E. H., & Strand, E. A. (1997). Long-term phonatory instability in individuals with Multiple Sclerosis. *Journal of Speech, Language, and Hearing Research, 40*, 1056–1072.

Hartelius, L., Nord, L., & Buder, E. H. (1995). Acoustic analysis of dysarthria associated with multiple sclerosis. *Clinical Linguistics and Phonetics, 9*, 95–120.

Hartman, D. E., Abbs, J. H., & Vishwanat, B. (1988). Clinical investigations of adductor spastic dysphonia. *Annals of Otology, Rhinology and Laryngology, 97*, 247–252.

Hartman, D. E., Overholt, S. L., & Vishwanat, B. (1982). A case of vocal cord nodules masking essential (voice) tremor. *Archives of Otolaryngology, 108*, 52–53.

Hartmann, E., & von Cramon, D. (1984). Acoustic measurement of voice quality in central dysphonia. *Journal of Communication Disorders, 17*, 425–440.

Hecker, M. H. L., & Kreul, E. J. (1970). Descriptions of the speech of patients with cancer of the vocal folds. Part I: Measures of fundamental frequency. *The Journal of the Acoustical Society of America, 49*, 1275–1282.

Heiberger, V. L., & Horii, Y. (1982). Jitter and shimmer in sustained phonation. In N. J. Lass (Ed.), *Speech and language: Advances in basic research and practice* (Vol. 7, pp. 299–332). New York: Academic Press.

Helfrich, H. (1979). Age markers in speech. In K. R. Scherer & H. Giles (Eds.), *Social markers in speech.* Cambridge, UK: Cambridge University Press.

Helfrich, H., & Wallbott, H. G. (1986). Contributions of the German"Expression Psychology"to nonverbal behavior research, Part IV: The voice. *Journal of Nonverbal Behavior, 10,* 187–204.

Henton, C., & Bladon, A. (1988). Creak as a sociophonetic marker. In L. Hyman & C. N. Li (Eds.), *Language, speech, and mind: Studies in honour of Victoria A. Fromkin* (pp. 3–29). London: Routledge.

Henton, C. G., & Bladon, R. A. W. (1985). Breathiness in normal female speech: inefficiency versus desirability. *Language & Communication, 5,* 221–227.

Hermes, D. J. (1991). Synthesis of breathy vowels: Some research methods. *Speech Communication, 10,* 497–502.

Hertrich, I., & Ackermann, H. (1995). Gender-specific vocal dysfunctions in Parkinson's Disease: Electroglottographic and acoustic analyses. *Annals of Otology, Rhinology & Laryngology, 104,* 197–202.

Hertrich, I., Spieker, S., & Ackermann, H. (1998). Gender-specific phonatory dysfunctions in disorders of the basal ganglia and the cerebellum: Acoustic and perceptual characteristics. In W. Ziegler & K. Deger (Eds.), *Clinical phonetics and linguistics* (pp. 448–457). London: Whurr Publishers, Ltd.

Herzel, H. (1996). Possible mechanisms of vocal instabilities. In P. Davis & N. Fletcher (Eds.), *Vocal fold physiology: Controlling complexity and chaos* (pp. 63–75). San Diego: Singular Publishing Group.

Herzel, H., Berry, D., Titze, I. R., & Saleh, M. (1994). Analysis of vocal disorders with methods from nonlinear dynamics. *Journal of Speech and Hearing Research, 37,* 1008–1019.

Herzel, H., Berry, D., Titze, I., & Steinecke, I. (1995). Nonlinear dynamics of the voice: Signal analysis and biomechanical modeling. *Chaos, 5,* 30–34.

Herzel, H., Steinecke, I., Mende, W., & Wermke, K. (1991). Chaos and bifurcations during voiced speech. In E. Mosekilde & L. Mosekilde (Eds.), *Complexity, chaos, and biological evolution* (pp. 41–50). New York: Plenum Press.

Hess, W. (1983). *Pitch determination of speech signals: Algorithms and devices.* Berlin: Springer-Verlag.

Hess, W. J. (1994). Pitch determination of speech signals, with special emphasis on time-domain method. In D. Wong (Ed.), *Proceedings of the Workshop on Acoustic Voice Analysis.* Iowa City, IA: National Center for Voice and Speech.

Heylen, L., Wuyts, F. L., Mertens, F., De Bodt, M., Pattyn, J., & Van de Heyning, P. H. (1996a). Comparison of the results of the frequency and the intensity data of the BSGVD with phonetogram characteristics. *Acta Oto-Rhino-Laryngologica Belgica, 50,* 353–360.

Heylen, L. G., Wuyts, F. L., Mertens, F. W., & Pattyn, J. E. (1996b). Phonetography in voice diagnoses. *Acta Oto-Rhino-Laryngologica Belgica, 50,* 299–308.

Hiki, S. (1967). Correlation between increments of voice pitch and glottal sound intensity. *Journal of Acoustical Society of Japan, 23,* 20–22. Text in Japanese.

Hiki, S. (1983). Relationship between efficiency of phonation and the tonal quality of speech. In D. M. Bless & J. H. Abbs (Eds.), *Vocal fold physiology: Contemporary research and clinical issues* (pp. 333–343). San Diego, CA: College-Hill Press.

Hiki, S., Imaizumi, S., Hirano, M., Matsushita, H., & Kakita,Y. (1976). Acoustical analysis for voice disorders, Conference record, 1976 *IEEE International Conference on Acoustics, Speech, and Signal Processing* (pp. 613–616). Rome, NY: Canterbury Press.

Hillenbrand, J. (1987). A methodological study of perturbation and additive noise in synthetically generated voice signals. *Journal of Speech and Hearing Research, 30,* 448–461.

Hillenbrand, J. (1988). Perception of aperiodicities in synthetically generated voices. *Journal of the Acoustical Society of America, 83,* 2361–2371.

Hillenbrand, J., Cleveland, R. A., & Erickson, R. L. (1994). Acoustic correlates of breathy vocal quality. *Journal of Speech and Hearing Research, 37,* 769–778.

Hillenbrand, J., & Houde, R. A. (1996). Acoustic correlates of breathy vocal quality: Dysphonic voices and continuous speech. *Journal of Speech and Hearing Research, 39,* 311–321.

Hiller, S., Laver, J., & Mackenzie, J. (1983). *Automatic analysis of waveform perturbations in connected speech* (Work in Progress 16). University of Edinburgh.

Hiller, S., Laver, J., & Mackenzie, J. (1984). *Durational aspects of long-term measurements of fundamental frequency perturbations in connected speech* (Work in Progress 13). Edinburgh: University of Edinburgh.

Hillman, R., Oesterle, E., & Feth, L. (1983). Characteristics of the glottal turbulent noise source. *Journal of Accoustical Society of America,* 691–694.

Hillman, R. E., Holmberg, E. B., Perkell, J. S., Walsh, M., & Vaughan, C. (1989). Objective assessment of vocal hyperfunction: An experimental framework and initial results. *Journal of Speech and Hearing Research, 32,* 373–392.

Hillman, R. E., Holmberg, E. B., Perkell, J. S., Walsh, M., & Vaughan, C. (1990). Phonatory function associated with hyperfunctionally related vocal fold lesions. *Journal of Voice, 4,* 52–63.

Hirano, M. (1975). Phonosurgery: Basic and clinical investigations. *Otologia (Fukuoka), 21,* 239–440. (Text in Japanese)

Hirano, M. (1981). *Clinical examination of voice.* Vienna: Springer-Verlag.

Hirano, M., Hibi, S., Terasawa, R., & Fujiu, M. (1986). Relationship between aerodynamic, vibratory, acoustic and psychoacoustic correlates in dysphonia. *Journal of Phonetics, 14,* 445–456.

Hirano, M., Hibi, S., Yoshida, T., Hirade, Y., Kasuya, H., & Kikuchi, Y. (1988). Acoustic analysis of pathological voice. *Acta Otolaryngologica, 105,* 432–438.

Hirano, M., Kakita, Y., Matsushita, H., Hiki, S., & Imaizumi, S. (1977a). Correlation between parameters related to vocal vibration and acoustical parameters in voice disorders. *Practica Otologia (Kyoto), 70,* 393–403. (Text in Japanese)

Hirano, M., Kakita, Y., Matsushita, H., Hiki, S., & Imaizumi, S. (1977b). Psychoacoustic parameters in voice disorders. *Practica Otologia (Kyoto), 70,* 525–531. (Text in Japanese)

Hiraoka, N., Kitazoe, Y., Ueta, H., Tanaka, S., & Tanabe, M. (1984). Harmonic-intensity analysis of normal and hoarse voices. *Journal of the Acoustical Society of America, 76,* 1648–1651.

Hirose, H., Imaizumi, S., & Yamori, M. (1995). Voice quality in patients with neurological disorders. In O. Fujimura & M. Hirano (Eds.), *Vocal fold physiology: Voice quality control* (pp. 235–248). San Diego, CA: Singular Publishing Group, Inc.

Hollien, H. (1977). The registers and ranges of the voice. In M. Cooper & J. H. Cooper (Eds.), *Approaches to vocal rehabilitation* (pp. 76-121). Springfield, IL: C. C. Thomas.

Hollien, H., Michel, J., & Doherty, E. T. (1975). A method for analyzing vocal jitter in sustained phonation. *Journal of Phonetics, 1,* 85–91.

Hollien, H., & Michel, J. F. (1968). Vocal fry as a phonational register. *Journal of Speech and Hearing Research, 11,* 600–604.

Holmberg, E. B., Hillman, R. E., & Perkell, J. S. (1988). Glottal airflow and transglottal air pressure measurements for male and female speakers in soft, normal and loud voice. *Journal of the Acoustical Society of America, 84,* 511–529.

Holmberg, E., Hillman, R., & Perkell, J. (1995). Measures of the glottal airflow waveform, egg, and acoustic spectral slope for female voice. In K. Elenius & P. Branderud (Eds.), *Proceedings of the XIIIth International Congress of Phonetic Sciences* (Vol. 3, pp. 178–181). Stockholm, Sweden: KTH and Stockholm University.

Holmberg, E., Hillman, R., Perkell, J., Guiod, P., & Goldman, S. (1995). Comparisons among aerodynamic, electroglottographic, and acoustic spectral measures of female voice. *Journal of Speech and Hearing Research, 38,* 1212–1223.

Holmberg, E. B., Perkell, J. S., Hillman, R. E., & Gress, C. (1994). Individual variation in measures of voice. *Phonetica, 51,* 30-37.

Horiguchi, S., Haji, T., Baer, T., & Gould, W. J. (1987). Comparison of electroglottographic and acoustic waveform perturbation measures. In T. Baer, C. Sasaki, & K. Harris (Eds.), *Laryngeal function in phonation and respiration* (pp. 509–518). Boston: College-Hill Press.

Horii, Y. (1975). Some statistical characteristics of voice fundamental frequency. *Journal of Speech and Hearing Research, 18,* 192–201.

Horii, Y. (1979). Fundamental frequency perturbation observed in sustained phonation. *Journal of Speech and Hearing Research, 22,* 5–19.

Horii, Y. (1980a). An accelerometric approach to nasality measurement: A preliminary report. *Cleft Palate Journal, 17,* 254–261.

Horii, Y. (1980b). Vocal shimmer in sustained phonation. *Journal of Speech and Hearing Research, 23,* 202–209.

Horii, Y. (1982). Jitter and shimmer differences among sustained vowel phonations. *Journal of Speech and Hearing Research, 25,* 12–14.

Horii, Y. (1985). Jitter and shimmer in sustained vocal fry phonation. *Folia Phoniatrica, 37,* 81–86.

Horii, Y., & Lang, J. (1981). Distributional analyses of an index of nasal coupling in simulated hypernasal speech. *Cleft Palate Journal, 18,* 279–285.

Howard, D. M. (1998). Practical voice measurement. In T. Harris, S. Harris, J. S. Rubin, & D. M. Howard (Eds.), *The voice clinic handbook* (pp. 323–382). London: Whurr Publishers.

Howell, P., & Williams, M. (1988). The contribution of the excitatory source to the perception of neutral vowels in stuttered speech. *Journal of the Accoustical Society of America, 84,* 80–89.

Huffman, M. K. (1987). Measures of phonation type in Hmong. *Journal of the Acoustical Society of America, 81,* 495–504.

Hufnagle, J., & Hufnagle, K. (1984). An investigation of the relationship between speaking fundamental frequency and vocal quality improvement. *Journal of Communication Disorders, 17,* 95–100.

Hurme, P., & Sonninen, A. (1986). Acoustic, perceptual and clinical studies of normal and dysphonic voice. *Journal of Phonetics, 14,* 489–492.

Imaizumi, S. (1986). Acoustic measures of roughness in pathological voice. *Journal of Phonetics, 14,* 457–462.

Imaizumi, S., Hiki, S., Hirano, M., & Matsushita, H. (1980). Analysis of pathological voices with a sound spectrograph. *Journal of Acoustical Society of Japan, 36,* 9–16. (Text in Japanese)

Isshiki, N., Kitajima, K., Kojima, H., & Harita, Y. (1978). Turbulent noise in dysphonia. *Folia Phoniatrica, 30,* 214–224.

Isshiki, N., Yanagihara, N., & Morimoto, M. (1966). Approach to the objective diagnosis of hoarseness. *Folia Phoniatrica, 18,* 393-400.

Iwata, S. (1972). Periodicities of pitch perturbations in normal and pathologic larynges. *The Laryngoscope, 82,* 87–96.

Iwata, S., & von Leden, H. (1970a). Pitch perturbations in normal and pathologic voices. *Folia Phoniatrica, 22,* 413–424.

Iwata, S., & von Leden, H. (1970b). Voice prints in laryngeal disease. *Archives of Otolaryngology, 91,* 346–351.

Izdebski, K. (1984). Overpressure and breathiness in spastic dysphonia. *Acta Otolaryngologica, 97,* 373–378.

Izdebski, K., & Dedo, H. (1980). Characteristics of vocal tremor in spastic dysphonia: A preliminary study. In V. Lawrence (Ed.), *Transcripts of the Eighth Symposium, Care of the Professional Voice. Part III: Medical/surgical therapy* (pp. 17–23). New York: The Voice Foundation.

Jacob, L. J. (1968). *A normative study of laryngeal jitter.* Unpublished master's thesis, University of Kansas, Lawrence, KS.

Jansson, E., & Sundberg, J. (1975). Long-time-average-spectra applied to analysis of music. Part I: Method and general applications. *Acustica, 34,* 15–19.

Janvrin, F. (1933). Diagnosis of a nervous disease by sound tracks. *Nature, 132,* 642.

Janvrin, F., & Worster-Drought, C. (1932). Diagnosis of disseminated sclerosis by graphic registration and film tracks. *Lancet, Dec 24,* 1384.

Jiang, J., Lin, E., & Hanson, D. (1998). Effect of tape recording on perturbation measures. *Journal of Speech, Language and Hearing Research, 41,* 1031–1041.

Kakita, Y., Hirano, M., Matsushita, H., Hiki, S., & Imaizumi, S. (1977a). Acoustical parameters relevant to diagnosis in voice disorders. *Practica Otologia (Kyoto), 70,* 269–276.

Kakita, Y., Hirano, M., Matsushita, H., Hiki, S., & Imaizumi, S. (1977b). Differentiation of laryngeal diseases using acoustical analysis. *Practica Otologia (Kyoto), 70,* 729–739.

Kakita, Y., & Okamoto, H. (1995). Visualizing the characteristics of vocal fluctuation from the viewpoint of chaos: An attempt toward "qualitative quantification." In O. Fujimura & M. Hirano (Eds.), *Vocal fold physiology: Voice quality control* (pp. 79–96). San Diego: Singular Publishing Group, Inc.

Karlsson, I. (1992). Modelling voice variations in female speech synthesis. *Speech Communication, 11,* 491–495.

Karnell, M. P., Hall, K. D., & Landahl, K. L. (1995). Comparison of fundamental frequency and perturbation measurements among three analysis systems. *Journal of Voice, 9,* 383–393.

Kasuya, H., & Ando, Y. (1991). Acoustic analysis, synthesis, and perception of breathy voice. In J. Gauffin & B. Hammarberg (Eds.), *Vocal fold physiology* (pp. 251–258). San Diego: Singular Publishing Group, Inc.

Kasuya, H., & Endô, Y. (1995). Acoustic analysis, conversion, and synthesis of the pathological voice. In O. Fujimura & M. Hirano (Eds.), *Vocal fold physiology: Voice quality control* (pp. 305–320). San Diego, CA: Singular Publishing Group, Inc.

Kasuya, H., Endô, Y., & Saliu, S. (1993). *Novel acoustic measurements of jitter and shimmer characteristics from pathological voice.* Paper presented at The Eurospeech '93, Berlin.

Kasuya, H., Masubuchi, K., Ebihara, S., & Yoshida, H. (1986). Preliminary experiments on voice screening. *Journal of Phonetics, 14,* 463–468.

Kasuya, H., Ogawa, S., Kikuchi, Y., & Ebihara, S. (1986). An acoustic analysis of pathological voice and its application to the evaluation of laryngeal pathology. *Speech Communication, 5,* 171–181.

Kasuya, H., Ogawa, S., Mashima, K., & Ebihara, S. (1986). Normalized noise energy as an acoustic measure to evaluate pathologic voice. *Journal of the Acoustical Society of America, 80,* 1329–1334.

Kay Elemetrics. (1988). Nasometer Model 6200 IBM. Pine Brook, NJ: Kay Elemetrics Corp.

Kay Elemetrics. (1991). *Nasometer application notes model 6200.* Pine Brook, NJ: Kay Elemetrics Corp.

Kay Elemetrics. (1993). Multi-Dimensional Voice Program (MDVP), Model 4305 [Computer software]. Lincoln Park, NJ: Kay Elemetrics Corporation.

Kempster, G. B. (1984). *A multidimensional analysis of vocal quality in two dysphonic groups.* Unpublished doctoral dissertation, Northwestern University, Evanston, IL.

Kempster, G. B., Kistler, D. J., & Hillenbrand, J. (1991). Multidimensional scaling analysis of dysphonia in two speaker groups. *Journal of Speech and Hearing Research, 34*, 534–543.

Kent, R. D. (1993). Vocal tract acoustics. *Journal of Voice, 7*, 97–117.

Kent, R. D., Duffy, J. R., Vorperian, H. K., & Thomas, J. E. (1998). Severe essential vocal and oromandibular tremor: a case report. *Phonosurgery, 1*, 237–253.

Kent, R. D., & Read, W. C. (1992). *The acoustic analysis of speech*. San Diego: Singular Publishing Group.

Kent, R. D., Vorperian, H. K., & Duffy, J. R. (1999). Reliability of the multi-dimensional voice program. *American Journal of Speech-Language Pathology, 8*, 129–136.

Kheirallah, I., & Jamieson, D. G. (1994). High resolution spectral estimation. In D. Wong (Ed.), *Proceedings of the Workshop on Acoustic Voice Analysis*. Iowa City, IA: National Center for Voice and Speech.

Kirk, P., Ladefoged, P., & Ladefoged, J. (1984). The linguistic use of different phonation types. *UCLA Working Papers in Phonetics, 59*, 102–113. University of California at Los Angeles.

Kitajima, K. (1981). Quantitative evaluation of the noise level in pathologic voice. *Folia Phoniatrica, 33*, 115–124.

Kitajima, K., & Gould, W. J. (1976). Vocal shimmer in sustained phonation of normal and pathologic voice. *Annals of Otology, Rhinology and Laryngology, 85*, 337–381.

Kitajima, K., Tanabe, M., & Isshiki, N. (1975). Pitch perturbations in normal and pathologic voice. *Studia Phonologica, 9*, 25–32.

Kitzing, P. (1986). LTAS criteria pertinent to the measurement of voice quality. *Journal of Phonetics, 14*, 477–482.

Kitzing, P., & Åkerlund, L. (1993). Long-time average spectrograms of dysphonic voices before and after therapy. *Folia Phoniatrica, 45*, 53–61.

Klatt, D. H. (1980). Software for a cascase/parallel formant synthesizer. *Journal of the Acoustical Society of America, 67*, 971–995. (Reprinted in Kent, R. D., Atal, B. S., & Miller, J. L. [Eds.], [1991]. *Papers in speech communication: Speech production* [pp. 765–790]. Woodbury, NY: Acoustical Society of America.)

Klatt, D. H. (1986). Detailed spectral analysis of a female voice. *Journal of the Acoustical Society of America, 81* (Suppl.1), S80.

Klatt, D. H. (1987, November). *Acoustic correlates of breathiness: First harmonic amplitude, turbulence noise, and tracheal coupling*. Paper presented at The 114th Meeting of the Acoustical Society of America, Miami.

Klatt, D. H., & Klatt, L. C. (1990). Analysis, synthesis, and perception of voice quality variations among female and male talkers. *Journal of the Acoustical Society of America, 87*, 820–857. (Reprinted in Kent, R. D., Atal, B. S., & Miller, J. L. [Eds.], [1991]. *Papers in speech communication: Speech production* [pp. 791–828]. Woodbury, NY: Acoustical Society of America.)

Klich, R. J. (1982). Relationships of vowel characteristics to listener ratings of breathiness. *Journal of Speech and Hearing Research, 25*, 574–580.

Klingholz, F. (1987). The measurement of the signal-to-noise ratio (SNR) in continuous speech. *Speech Communication, 6*, 15–26.

Klingholz, F. (1990). Acoustic representation of speaking-voice quality. *Journal of Voice, 4*, 213–219.

Klingholz, F., & Martin, F. (1985). Quantitative spectral evaluation of shimmer and jitter. *Journal of Speech and Hearing Research, 28*, 169–174.

Klingholz, F., & Martin, F. (1989). Distribution of the amplitude in the pathologic voice signal. *Folia Phoniatrica, 41*, 23–29.

Koike, Y. (1968). Vowel amplitude modulations in patients with laryngeal diseases. *Journal of the Acoustical Society of America, 45*, 839–844.

Koike, Y. (1973). Application of some acoustic measures for the evaluation of laryngeal dysfunction. *Studia Phonologica, 7*, 17–23.

Koike, Y. (1986). Cepstrum analysis of pathologic voices. *Journal of Phonetics, 14*, 501–507.

Koike, Y., Hirano, M., & von Leden, H. (1967). Vocal Initiation: Acoustic and aerodynamic investigations of normal subjects. *Folia Phoniatrica, 19*, 173–182.

Koike, Y., & Kohda, J. (1991). The effect of vocal fold surgery on the speech cepstrum. In J. Gauffin & B. Hammarberg (Eds.), *Vocal fold physiology: Acoustic, perceptual and physiological aspects of voice mechanisms* (pp. 259–264). San Diego: Singular Publishing Group, Inc.

Koike, Y., & Markel, J. (1975). Application of inverse filtering for detecting laryngeal pathology. *Annals of Otology, Rhinology & Laryngology, 84*, 117–124.

Koike, Y., & Takahashi, H. (1972). Glottal parameters and some acoustic measures in patients with laryngeal pathology. *Studia Phonologica, 6*, 45–50.

Koike, Y., Takahashi, H., & Calcaterra, T. C. (1977). Acoustic measures for detecting laryngeal pathology. *Acta Otolaryngologica, 84*, 105–117.

Kojima, H., Gould, W. J., Lambiase, A., & Isshiki, N. (1980). Computer analysis of hoarseness. *Acta Otolaryngologica, 89*, 547–554.

Kreiman, J., & Gerratt, B. R. (1996). The perceptual structure of pathologic voice quality. *Journal of the Acoustical Society of America, 100,* 1787–1795.

Kuwabara, H., & Ohgushi, K. (1984). Experiments on voice qualities of vowels in males and females and correlation with acoustic features. *Language and Speech, 27,* 135–145.

LaBlance, G. R., & Maves, M. D. (1992). Acoustic characteristics of post-thyroplasty patients. *Otolaryngology-Head and Neck Surgery, 107,* 558–563.

Ladefoged, P. (1983). The linguistic use of different phonation types. In D. M. Bless & J. H. Abbs (Eds.), *Vocal fold physiology: Contemporary research and clinical issues* (pp. 351–360). San Diego: College-Hill Press.

Laufer, M. Z., & Horii, Y. (1977). Fundamental frequency characteristics of infant non-distress vocalizations during the first twenty-four weeks. *Journal of Child Language, 4,* 171–184.

Laver, J. (1980). *The phonetic description of voice quality.* Cambridge, England: Cambridge University Press.

Laver, J., Hiller, S., & Beck, J. M. (1992). Acoustic waveform perturbations and voice disorders. *Journal of Voice, 6,* 115–126.

Laver, J., Hiller, S., & Hanson, R. (1982). Comparative performance of pitch detection algorithms on dysphonic voices, *Proceedings of the IEEE International Conference on Acoustics, Speech, and Signal Processing* (pp. 192–195).

Laver, J., Hiller, S., Mackenzie, J., & Rooney, E. (1986). An acoustic screening system for the detection of laryngeal pathology. *Journal of Phonetics, 14,* 517–524.

Leddy, M., Milenkovic, P., & Bless, D. M. (1993). A two-tap pitch predictor for measuring voice aperiodicity noise at high SNR. *Journal of the Acoustical Society of America, 94,* 1783.

Lee, C. K. (1988). *Voice quality: Analysis and synthesis.* Unpublished doctoral dissertation, University of Florida, Gainesville.

Leeper, H. A., Millard, K. M., Bandur, D. L., & Hudson, A. J. (1996). An investigation of deterioration of vocal function in subgroups of individuals with ALS. *Journal of Medical Speech-Language Pathology, 4,* 163–181.

Lieberman, P. (1961). Perturbations in vocal pitch. *The Journal of the Acoustical Society of America, 33,* 597–603.

Lieberman, P. (1963). Some acoustic measures of the fundamental periodicity of normal and pathologic larynges. *The Journal of the Acoustical Society of America, 35,* 344–353.

Liljencrants, J. (1996, October). *Experiments with analysis by synthesis of glottal airflow.* Paper presented at The Fourth International Conference on Spoken Language Processing, Philadelphia.

Lindsey, L. A., & Vieira, M. N. (1997). Modulation analysis-A new method for modelling and measurement of both the production and perception of vocal fold cycle perturbation, *Larynx 97* (pp. 65–68). Aix en Provence, France: Universite de Provence.

Linville, S. E. (1987). Acoustic-perceptual studies of aging voice in women. *Journal of Voice, 1,* 44–48.

Linville, S. E. (1988). Intraspeaker variability in fundamental frequency stability: An age-related phenomenon? *Journal of the Acoustical Society of America, 83,* 741–745.

Linville, S. E. (1998). Acoustic correlates of perceived versus actual sexual orientation in men's speech. *Folia Phoniatrica et Logopaedica, 50,* 35–48.

Linville, S. E., & Fisher, H. B. (1985). Acoustic characteristics of perceived versus actual vocal age in controlled phonation by adult females. *Journal of the Acoustical Society of America, 78,* 40–48.

Linville, S. E., & Korabic, E. W. (1987). Fundamental frequency stability characteristics of elderly women's voices. *Journal of the Acoustical Society of America, 81,* 1196–1199.

Linville, S. E., Korabic, E. W., & Rosera, M. (1990). Intraproduction variability in jitter measures from elderly speakers. *Journal of Voice, 4,* 45–51.

Lippman, R. P. (1981). Detecting nasalization using a low-cost miniature accelerometer. *Journal of Speech and Hearing Research, 24,* 314–317.

Lively, M. A., & Emanuel, F. W. (1970). Spectral noise levels and roughness severity ratings for normal and simulated rough vowels produced by adult females. *Journal of Speech and Hearing Research, 13,* 503–517.

Löfqvist, A. (1986). The long-term-average spectrum as a tool in voice research. *Journal of Phonetics, 14,* 471–475.

Löfqvist, A., & Mandersson, B. (1987). Long-time average spectrum of speech and voice analysis. *Folia Phoniatrica et Logopaedica, 39,* 221–229.

Lotto, A. J., Holt, L. L., & Kluender, K. R. (1997). Effect of voice quality on perceived height of English vowels. *Phonetica, 54,* 76–93.

Luchsinger, R., & Arnold, G. E. (1949). *Lehrbuch der stimm- und sprachheilkunde.* Wien: Springer-Verlag.

Luchsinger, R., & Arnold, G. E. (1965). *Voice-speech-language — Clinical communicology: Its physiology and pathology* (G. E. Arnold & E. R. Finkbeiner, Trans.). Belmont, CA: Wadsworth Publishing Company.

(Originally published in German under the title *Lehrbuch der Stimm- und Sprachheilkunde*, 1949.)

Ludlow, C. L., & Bassich, C. J. (1983). The results of acoustic and perceptual assessment of two types of dysarthria. In W. R. Berry (Ed.), *Clinical dysarthria* (pp. 121–153). San Diego: College Hill Press.

Ludlow, C. L., Bassich, C. J., Connor, N. P., & Coulter, D. C. (1986). Phonatory characteristics of vocal fold tremor. *Journal of Phonetics, 14*, 509–515.

Ludlow, C. L., Bassich, C. J., Connor, N. P., Coulter, D. C., & Lee, Y. J. (1987). The validity of using phonatory jitter and shimmer to detect laryngeal pathology. In T. Baer, C. Sasaki, & K. Harris (Eds.), *Laryngeal Function in Phonation and Respiration* (pp. 492–508). Boston: College-Hill.

Ludlow, C., & Connor, N. P. (1987). Dynamic aspects of phonatory control in spasmodic dysphonia. *Journal of Speech and Hearing Research, 30*, 197–206.

Ludlow, C. L., Coulter, D. C., & Gentges, F. (1983). The differential sensitivity of frequency perturbation to laryngeal neoplasms and neuropathologies. In D. Bless & L. Abbs (Eds.), *Vocal fold physiology conference: Contemporary research and clinical issues* (pp. 381–392). San Diego, CA: College-Hill Press.

Mackenzie, J., Laver, J., & Hiller, S. (1984). *Acoustic screening for vocal pathology: Preliminary results* (Work in Progress 17). University of Edinburgh.

Martin, D., Fitch, J., & Wolfe, V. (1995). Pathological voice type and the acoustic prediction of severity. *Jouranl of Speech and Hearing Research, 38*, 765–771.

Maurer, D., & Landis, T. (1996). Intelligibility and spectral differences in high-pitched vowels. *Folia Phoniatrica et Logopaedica, 48*, 1–10.

Max, L., & Mueller, P. B. (1996). Speaking F_0 and cepstral periodicity analysis of conversational speech in a 105-year-old woman: Variability of aging effects. *Journal of Voice, 10*, 245–251.

McAllister, A., Sederholm, E., Ternström, S., & Sundberg, J. (1996). Perturbation and hoarseness: A pilot study of six children's voices. *Journal of Voice, 10*, 252–261.

Mendoza, E., & Carballo, G. (1998). Acoustic analysis of induced vocal stress by means of cognitive workload tasks. *Journal of Voice, 12*, 263–273.

Mendoza, E., Muñoz, J., & Naranjo, N.V. (1996). The long-term average spectrum as a measure of voice stability. *Folia Phoniatrica et Logopaedica, 48*, 57–64.

Mendoza, E., Naranjo, N.V., Muñoz, J., & Trujillo, H. (1996). Differences in voice quality between men and women: Use of the long-term average spectrum (LTAS). *Journal of Voice, 10*, 59–66.

Mergell, P., & Herzel, H. (1997). Modelling biphonation: The role of the vocal tract. *Speech Communication, 22*, 141–154.

Mergell, P., Herzel, H., Wittenberg, T., Tigges, M., & Eysholdt, U. (1998). Phonation onset: Modelling and high speed glottography. *Journal of the Accoustical Society of America, 103*.

Metfessal, M. (1926). Technique for objective studies of the vocal art. *Psychological Monographs, 36*, 1–40.

Michaelis, D., Fröhlich, M., & Strube, H. W. (1998). Selection and combination of acoustic features for the description of pathalogic voices. *Journal of the Acoustical Society of America, 103*, 1628–1638.

Michaelis, D., Gramss, T., & Strube, H. W. (1997). Glottal to noise excitation ratio—A new measure for describing patholocial voices. *Acustica, 83*, 700–706.

Michaelis, D., & Strube, H. W. (1995). Empirical study to test the independence of different acoustic voice parameters on a large voice database. *Eurospeech '95 Proceedings, 3*, 1891–1894.

Milenkovic, P. (1987). Least mean square measures of voice perturbation. *Journal of Speech and Hearing Research, 30*, 529–538.

Milenkovic, P. (1992). CSpeech (Version 4.0) [Computer software]. Madison, WI: University of Wisconsin-Madison.

Milenkovic, P. (1997). CSpeechSP [Computer software]. Madison, WI: University of Wisconsin-Madison.

Milenkovic, P. H. (1994). Rotation-based measure of voice aperiodicity. In D. Wong (Ed.), *Proceedings of the Workshop on Acoustic Voice Analysis*. Iowa City, IA: National Center for Voice and Speech.

Milenkovic, P. H., Bless, D. M., & Rammage, L. A. (1991). Acoustic and perceptual characterization of vocal nodules. In J. Gauffin & B. Hammarberg (Eds.), *Vocal fold physiology: Acoustic, perceptual and physiological aspects of voice mechanisms* (pp. 265–272). San Diego: Singular Publishing Group, Inc.

Monsen, R. B. (1981). The use of a reflectionless tube to assess vocal function. In C. L. Ludlow & M.G. Hart (Eds.), *Proceedings of the Conference on the Asssessment of Vocal Pathology* (Vol. 11, pp. 141–150). Rockville, MD: American Speech-Language-Hearing Association.

Monsen, R. B., & Engebretson, A. M. (1977). Study of variations in the male and female glottal wave. *Journal of the Acoustical Society of America, 62*, 981–993.

Moore, P., & Thompson, C. L. (1965). Comments on physiology of hoarseness. *Archives of Otolaryngology, 81*, 97–102.

Moran, M. J., & Gilbert, H. R. (1984). Relation between voice profile ratings and aerodynamic and acoustic parameters. *Journal of Communication Disorders, 17,* 245–260.

Mori, K., Blaugrund, S. M., & Yu, J. D. (1994). The turbulent noise ratio: An estimation of noise power of the breathy voice using PARCOR analysis. *Laryngoscope, 104,* 153–158.

Morris, R. J., & Brown, W. S., Jr. (1987). Age-related voice measures among adult women. *Journal of Voice, 1,* 38–43.

Morsomme, D., Orban, A., Remacle, M., & Jamart, J. (1997). Comparison of a vibrato study by a panel of judges and spectral voice analyser, *Larynx 97* (pp. 25–28). Aix en Provence, France: Universite de Provence.

Mount, K. H., & Salmon, S. J. (1988). Changing the vocal characteristics of a postoperative transsexual patient: A longitudinal study. *Journal of Communication Disorders, 21,* 229–238.

Mowrer, D. E., LaPointe, L. L., & Case, J. (1987). Analysis of five acoustic correlates of laughter. *Journal of Nonverbal Behavior, 11,* 191–199.

Murphy, P. (1999). Perturbation-free measurment of the harmonics-to-noise ratio in voice signals using pitch synchronous harmonic analysis. *Journal of the Accoustical Society of America, 105,* 2866–2881.

Murry, T., Amundson, P., & Hollien, H. (1977). Acoustical characteristics of infant cries: Fundamental frequency. *Journal of Child Language, 4,* 321–328.

Murry, T., Brown, W. S., Jr., & Morris, R. J. (1995). Patterns of fundamental frequency for three types of voice samples. *Journal of Voice, 9,* 282–289.

Murry, T., & Doherty, E. T. (1980). Selected acoustic characteristics of pathologic and normal speakers. *Journal of Speech and Hearing Research, 23,* 361–369.

Murry, T., & Large, J. (1979). Frequency perturbations in singers. In V. Lawrence (Ed.), *Transcripts of the Seventh Symposium: Care of the Professional Voice* (pp. 36–39). New York: The Voice Foundation.

Murry, T., & Singh, S. (1980). Multidimensional analysis of male and female voices. *Journal of the Acoustical Society of America, 68,* 1294–1300.

Murry, T., Singh, S., & Sargent, M. (1977). Multidimensional classification of abnormal voice qualities. *Journal of the Acoustical Society of America, 61,* 1630–1635.

Muta, H., Baer, T., Wagatsuma, K., Muraoka, T., & Fukuda, H. (1988). A pitch-synchronous analysis of hoarseness in running speech. *Journal of the Acoustical Society of America, 84,* 1292–1301.

Muta, H., Muraoka, T., Wagatsuma, K., Horiuchi, M., Fukuda, H., Takayama, E., Fujioka, T., & Kanou, S. (1987). Analysis of hoarse voices using the LPC method. In T. Baer, C. Sasaki, & K. Harris (Eds.), *Laryngeal function in phonation and respiration* (pp. 463–474). Boston: College-Hill Press.

Newman, P. W., Harris, R. W., & Hilton, L. M. (1989). Vocal jitter and shimmer in stuttering. *Journal of Fluency Disorders, 14,* 87–95.

Ng, M. L., Gilbert, H. R., & Lerman, J. W. (1997). Some aerodynamic and acoustic characteristics of acute laryngitis. *Journal of Voice, 11,* 356–363.

Ní Chasaide, A., & Gobl, C. (1995). Towards acoustic profiles of phonatory qualities. In K. Elenius & P. Branderud (Eds.), *Proceedings of the XIIIth International Congress of Phonetic Sciences* (Vol. 4, pp. 6–13). Stockholm, Sweden: KTH and Stockholm University.

Nichols, A. C. (1979). Jitter and shimmer related to vocal roughness: A comment on the Deal and Emanuel study [letter]. *Journal of Speech and Hearing Research, 22,* 670–671.

Niederjohn, R. J., & Haworth, D. G. (1983). The relationship between rms level and the average absolute magnitude of long-time continuous speech. *Journal of the Acoustical Society of America, 74,* 444–446.

Nikolov, Z., Deliyski, D., Drumeva, L., & Boyanov, B. (1989). Computer system for analysis of pathological voices, *Proceedings of the 21st Congress of the International Association of Logopedics and Phoniatrics* (Vol. 2, pp. 341–343). Prague, Czechoslovakia.

Nittrouer, S., McGowan, R., Milenkovic, P., & Beehler, D. (1990). Acoustic measurements of men's and women's voices: A study of context effects and covariation. *Journal of Speech and Hearing Research, 33,* 761–775.

Nolan, F. (1983). *The phonetic bases of speaker recognition.* Cambridge, UK: Cambridge University Press.

Novák, A., Dlouha, O., Capkova, B., & Vohradnik, M. (1991). Voice fatigue after theater performance in actors. *Folia Phoniatrica, 43,* 74–78.

Novák, A., & Vokrál, J. (1993). Emotions in the sight of long-time averaged spectrum and three-dimensional analysis of periodicity. *Folia Phoniatrica, 45,* 198–203.

Ohlsson, A., & Löfqvist, A. (1986). Phonetograms of normal and pathological voices. *Working Papers in Logopedics and Phoniatrics, 3,* 94–106.

Omori, K., Kojima, H., Kakani, R., Slavit, D., & Blaugrund, S. (1997). Acoustic characteristics of rough voice: Subharmonics. *Journal of Voice, 11,* 40–47.

Orlikoff, R. F. (1989). Vocal jitter at different fundamental frequencies: A cardiovascular–neuromuscular explanation. *Journal of Voice, 3,* 104–112.

Orlikoff, R. F. (1995). Vocal stability and vocal tract configuration: An acoustic and electroglottographic investigation. *Journal of Voice, 9,* 173–181.

Orlikoff, R. F., & Baken, R. J. (1989a). The effect of the heartbeat on vocal fundamental frequency perturbation. *Journal of Speech and Hearing Research, 32,* 576–582.

Orlikoff, R. F., & Baken, R. J. (1989b). Fundamental frequency (F_0) modulation of the human voice by the heartbeat: Preliminary results and possible mechanisms. *Journal of the Acoustical Society of America, 85,* 888–893.

Orlikoff, R. F., & Baken, R. J. (1990). Consideration of the relationship between the fundamental frequency of phonation and vocal jitter. *Folia Phoniatrica, 42,* 31–40.

Orlikoff, R. F., & Kahane, J. C. (1991). Influence of mean sound pressure level on jitter and shimmer measures. *Journal of Voice, 5,* 113–119.

Pabon, J. P. H. (1991). Objective acoustic voice-quality parameters in the computer phonetogram. *Journal of Voice, 5,* 203–216.

Pabon, J. P. H., & de Krom, G. (1995). Validation of temporal and spectral noise parameters using (re)synthesis. In K. Elenius & P. Branderud (Eds.), *Proceedings of the XIIIth International Congress of Phonetic Sciences* (Vol. 2, pp. 246–249). Stockholm, Sweden: KTH and Stockholm University.

Pabon, J. P. H., & Plomp, R. (1988). Automatic phonetogram recording supplemented with acoustical voice-quality parameters. *Journal of Speech and Hearing Research, 31,* 710–722.

Pandit, P. B. (1957). Nasalization, aspiration and murmur in Gujarati. *Indian Linguistics, 17,* 165–172.

Pawlowski, Z., Pawluczyk, R., & Kraska, Z. (1985). Epiphysis vibrations of singers studied by holographic interferometry. In A. Askenfelt, S. Felicetti, E. Jansson, & J. Sundberg (Eds.), *SMAC 83—Proceedings of the Stockholm Music Acoustics Conference* (pp. 37–60).

Perkell, J., Hillman, R., & Holmberg, E. (1994). Group differences in measures of voice production and revised values of maximum airflow declination rate. *Journal of the Accoustical Society of America, 96,* 695–698.

Perry, C. K., Ingrisano, D. R., & Scott, S.R. (1996). Accuracy of jitter estimates using different filter settings on Visi-Pitch: A preliminary report. *Journal of Voice, 10,* 337–341.

Philippbar, S. A., Robin, D. A., & Luschei, E. S. (1989). Limb, jaw, and vocal tremor in Parkinson's individuals. In K. M. Yorkston & D. R. Beukelman (Eds.), *Recent advances in clinical dysarthria* (pp. 165–197). Boston: College-Hill Press.

Pinto, N. B., & Titze, I. R. (1990). Unification of perturbation measures in speech signals. *Journal of the Acoustical Society of America, 87,* 1278–1289.

Pittam, J. (1987). Discrimination of five voice qualities and prediction to perceptual ratings. *Phonetica, 44,* 38–49.

Pittam, J. (1994). *Voice in social interaction: An interdisciplinary approach.* Thousand Oaks, CA: Sage Publications.

Plant, R. L., Hillel, A. D., & Waugh, P. F. (1997). Analysis of voice changes after thyroplasty using linear predictive coding. *The Laryngoscope, 107,* 703–709.

Plante, F., Salian, S., Scholder, J., Cheetham, B. M. G., & Earis, J. (1997). Inverse filtering of voiced sounds for the study of laryngeal disease, *Larynx 97* (pp. 51–54). Aix en Provence, France: Universite de Provence.

Pollack, I. (1971). Amplitude and time jitter thresholds for rectangular wave trains. *Journal of the Acoustical Society of America, 50,* 1133–1142.

Prosek, R. A., Montgomery, A. A., Walden, B. E., & Hawkins, D. B. (1987). An evaluation of residue features as correlates of voice disorders. *Journal of Communication Disorders, 20,* 105–117.

Protopapas, A., & Lieberman, P. (1995). Effects of vocal F0 manipulations on perceived emotional stress. In I. Trancoso & R. Moore (Eds.), *ESCA - NATO tutorial and research workshop on speech under stress* (pp. 1–4). Lisbon, Portugal: ESCA.

Protopapas, A., & Lieberman, P. (1997). Fundamental frequency of phonation and perceived emotional stress. *Journal of the Acoustical Society of America, 101,* 2267–2277.

Prytz, S. (1977). Long-time-average-spectra (LTAS) analyses of normal and pathological voices, *Proceedings of the 17th International Congress of Logopedics and Phoniatrics* (Vol. 1, pp. 457). Copenhagen.

Ptacek, P. H., & Sander, E. K. (1966). Phonatory and related changes with advanced age. *Journal of Speech and Hearing Research, 9,* 353–360.

Qi, Y. (1992). Time normalization in voice analysis. *Journal of the Acoustical Society of America, 92,* 2569–2576.

Qi, Y., HIllman, R., & Milstein, C. (1999). The estimation of signal-to-noise ratio in continuous speech for disordered voices. *Journal of the Accoustical Society of America, 105,* 2532–2535.

Qi, Y., & Shipp, T. (1992). An adaptive method for tracking voicing irregularities. *Journal of the Acoustical Society of America, 91*, 3471–3477.

Qi, Y., Weinberg, B., Bi, N., & Hess, W. J. (1995). Minimizing the effect of period determination on the computation of amplitude perturbation in voice. *Journal of the Acoustical Society of America, 97*, 2525–2532.

Quackenbush, S. R., Barnwell, T. P., & Clements, M. A. (1988). *Objective measures of speech quality*. Englewood Cliffs, NJ: Prentice-Hall.

Rabiner, L. R., & Schafer, R. W. (1978). *Digital processing of speech signals*. Englewood Cliffs: Prentice-Hall.

Rabinov, C. R., Kreiman, J., & Gerratt, B. R. (1994). Comparing reliability of perceptual and acoustic measures of voice. In D. Wong (Ed.), *Proceedings of the Workshop on Acoustic Voice Analysis*. Iowa City, IA: National Center for Voice and Speech.

Rabinov, C. R., Kreiman, J., Gerratt, B. R., & Bielamowicz, S. (1995). Comparing reliability of perceptual ratings of roughness and acoustic measures of jitter. *Journal of Speech and Hearing Research, 38*, 26–32.

Raes, J. P. F., & Clement, P. A. R. (1996). Comments to the BSGVD: Results from aerodynamic measurements. *Acta Oto-Rhino-Laryngologica Belgica, 50*, 343–344.

Ramig, L. A. (1986). Acoustic analyses of phonation in patients with Huntington's disease. *Annals of Otology, Rhinology & Laryngology, 95*, 288–293.

Ramig, L. A., & Ringel, R. L. (1983). Effects of physiological aging on selected acoustic characteristics of voice. *Journal of Speech and Hearing Research, 26*, 22–30.

Ramig, L. A., Scherer, R. C., Klasner, E. R., Titze, I. R., & Horii, Y. (1990). Acoustic analysis of voice in amyotrophic lateral sclerosis: A longitudinal case study. *Journal of Speech and Hearing Disorders, 55*, 2–14.

Ramig, L. A., Scherer, R. C., Titze, I. R., & Ringel, S. P. (1988). Acoustic analysis of voices of patients with neurologic disease: Rationale and preliminary data. *Annals of Otology, Rhinology & Laryngology, 97*, 164–172.

Ramig, L. A., & Shipp, T. (1987). Comparative measures of vocal tremor and vocal vibrato. *Journal of Voice, 1*, 162–167.

Raphael, B. N., & Scherer, R. C. (1987). Voice modifications of stage actors: Acoustic analyses. *Journal of Voice, 1*, 83–87.

Rasch, R. A. (1983). Jitter in the singing voice, *Proceedings of the 10th International Congress of Phonetic Sciences* (pp. 288–292). Dordrecht: Foris Publications.

Ray, G. B. (1986). Vocally cued personality prototypes: An implicit personality theory approach. *Communication Monographs, 53*, 266–276.

Redenbaugh, M., & Reich, A. (1985). Correspondance between an accelerometric nasal/voice amplitude ratio and listeners' direct magnitude estimations of hypernasality. *Journal of Speech and Hearing Research, 28*, 273–281.

Reich, A., Frederickson, R., Mason, J., & Schlauch, R. (1990). Methodological variables affecting phonational frequency range in adults. *Journal of Speech and Hearing Disorders, 55*, 124–131.

Reuter, R., & Herzel, H. (1998). Quantifying correlations in pitch and amplitude contours. In T. Lehmann, C. Palm, K. Spitzer, & T. Tolxdorff (Eds.), *Advances in quantitative laryngoscopy, voice and speech research* (pp. 45–60). Aachen: University Hospital Benjamin Franklin, Free University Berlin.

Rihkanen, H., Leinonen, L., Hiltunen, T., & Kangas, J. (1994). Spectral pattern recognition of improved voice quality. *Journal of Voice, 8*, 320–326.

Ringel, R. L., & Chodzko-Zajko, W. J. (1987). Vocal indices of biological age. *Journal of Voice, 1*, 31–37.

Risberg, A. (1962). Statistical studies of fundamental frequency range and rate of change. *Speech Transmission Laboratory Quarterly Progress and Status Report*, 7–8.

Robbins, J. (1982). *A comparative acoustic study of laryngeal speech, esophageal speech, and speech production after tracheoesophageal puncture*. Unpublished doctoral dissertation, Northwestern University, Evanston, IL.

Roessler, R., & Lester, J. W. (1979). Vocal patterns in anxiety. In W. E. Farm, I. Karacan, & A. P. Porkony (Eds.), *Phenomenology and treatment of anxiety* (pp. 225–235): Spectrum Publications.

Rontal, E., Rontal, M., & Rolnick, M. (1975). Objective evaluation of vocal pathology using voice spectrography. *Annals of Otology, Rhinology & Laryngology, 84*, 662–671.

Rosenberg, A. E. (1971). Effect of glottal pulse shape on the quality of natural vowels. *Journal of the Acoustical Society of America, 49*, 583–590.

Rosenfield, D. B., Viswanath, N., Herbrich, K. E., & Nudelman, H. B. (1991). Evaluation of the speech motor control system in amyotrophic lateral sclerosis. *Journal of Voice, 5*, 224–230.

Rossiter, D., & Howard, D. M. (1996). ALBERT: A real-time visual feedback computer tool for professional vocal development. *Journal of Voice, 10*, 321–336.

Rothenberg, M. (1973). A new inverse-filtering technique for deriving the glottal air flow waveform during voicing. *Journal of the Acoustical Society of America, 53,* 1632–1645. (Reprinted in Kent, R. D., Atal, B. S., & Miller, J. L. [Eds.], [1991]. *Papers in speech communication: Speech production* [pp. 219–232]. Woodbury, NY: Acoustical Society of America.)

Rothman, H. B., & Arroyo, A. A. (1987). Acoustic variability in vibrato and its perceptual significance. *Journal of Voice, 1,* 123–141.

Rothman, H. B., Rullman, J. F., & Arroyo, A. A. (1990). Inter- and intrasubject changes in vibrato: Perceptual and acoustic aspects. *Journal of Voice, 4,* 309–316.

Roy, N., Tasko, S. M., Callan, D., & Bless, D. M. (1997, November). *Documenting outcomes of voice treatment: Which acoustic measures matter?* Poster presented at the annual convention of the American Speech-Language-Hearing Association, Boston, MA.

Rozsypal, A. J., & Millar, B. F. (1979). Perception of jitter and shimmer in synthetic vowels. *Journal of Phonetics, 7,* 343–355.

Ruiz, R., Absil, E., Gramatica, B., Harmegnies, B., Legros, C., & Poch, D. (1995). Spectrum-related variabilities in stressed speech under laboratory and real conditions. In I. Trancoso & R. Moore (Eds.), *ESCA–NATO tutorial and research workshop on speech under stress* (pp. 49–52). Lisbon, Portugal: ESCA.

Ruiz, R., Absil, E., Harmegnies, B., Legros, C., & Poch, D. (1996). Time- and spectrum-related variabilities in stressed speech under laboratory and real conditions. *Speech Communic-ation, 20,* 111–129.

Sansone, F. E., Jr., & Emanuel, F. W. (1970). Spectral noise levels and roughness severity ratings for normal and simulated rough vowels produced by adult males. *Journal of Speech and Hearing Research, 13,* 489–502.

Sapienza, C. M., Murry, T., & Brown, W. S., Jr. (1998). Variations in adductor spasmodic dysphonia: Acoustic evidence. *Journal of Voice, 12,* 214–222.

Sapienza, C. M., & Stathopoulos, E. T. (1994). Comparison of maximum flow declination rate: Children versus adults. *Journal of Voice, 8,* 240–247.

Sasaki, Y., Okamura, H., & Yumoto, E. (1991). Quantitative analysis of hoarseness using a digital sound spectrograph. *Journal of Voice, 5,* 36–40.

Scherer, K. R. (1981). Vocal indicators of stress. In J. K. Darby (Ed.), *Speech evaluation in psychiatry* (pp. 171–187). New York: Grune & Stratton.

Scherer, K. R. (1986a). Vocal affect expression: A review and a model for future research. *Psychological Bulletin, 99,* 143–165.

Scherer, K. R. (1986b). Voice, stress, and emotion. In M. H. Appley & R. Trumbull (Eds.), *Dynamics of stress: Physiological, psychological, and social perspectives* (pp. 157–179). New York: Plenum Press.

Scherer, R. C., Gould, W. J., Titze, I. R., Meyers, A. D., & Sataloff, R. T. (1988). Preliminary evaluation of selected acoustic and glottographic measures for clinical phonatory function analysis. *Journal of Voice, 2,* 230–244.

Scherer, R. C., Titze, I. R., Raphael, B. N., Wood, R. P., Ramig, L. A., & Blager, R. F. (1987). Vocal fatigue in a trained and an untrained voice user. In T. Baer, C. Sasaki, & K. Harris (Eds.), *Laryngeal function in phonation and respiration* (pp. 533–555). Boston: College Hill Press.

Schoentgen, J. (1982). Quantitative evaluation of the discrimination performance of acoustic features in detecting laryngeal pathology. *Speech Communication, 1,* 269–282.

Schoentgen, J. (1985). An acoustic feature related to vocal efficiency in normal and pathological speakers. *Speech Communication, 4,* 277–287.

Schoentgen, J. (1988). Presentation of problem: Performance of jitter in discriminating between normal and dysphonic speakers. *Applied Stochastic Models and Data Analysis, 4,* 127–135.

Schoentgen, J. (1989). Jitter in sustained vowels and isolated sentences produced by dysphonic speakers. *Speech Communication, 8,* 61–79.

Schoentgen, J., & Bucella, F. (1997). Acoustic analysis of dysphonic voices: Descriptors and methods, *Larynx 97* (pp. 37–46). Aix en Provence, France: Universite de Provence.

Schoentgen, J., & De Guchteneere, R. (1991). An algorithm for the measurement of jitter. *Speech Communication, 10,* 533–538.

Schoentgen, J., & De Guchteneere, R. (1995). Time series analysis of jitter. *Journal of Phonetics, 23,* 189–201.

Schoentgen, J., & De Guchteneere, R. (1996). Searching for nonlinear relations in whitened jitter time series, *Proceedings of the International Conference on Spoken Language Processing* (pp. 753–756). Newark, DE: University of Delaware.

Schoentgen, J., & De Guchteneere, R. (1997). Predictable and random components of jitter. *Speech Communication, 21,* 255–272.

Schönhärl, E. (1960). *Die stroboskopie in der praktischen laryngologie*. Stuttgart: Thieme Verlag.

Schroeder, M. R. (1968). Period histogram and product spectrum: New methods for fundamental frequency measurement. *Journal of the Acoustical Society of America, 43,* 829–834.

Schroeder, M. R., & David, E. E., Jr. (1960). A vocoder for transmitting 10 kc/s speech over a 3.5 kc/s channel. *Acustica, 10,* 31–40.

Schultz-Coulon, H. J., Battmer, R. D., & Fedders, B. (1979). Zur quantitativen bewertung der tonhöhenschwankungen im rahmen der stimmfunktionsprüfung. *Folia Phoniatrica, 31,* 56–69.

Schutte, H. K., & Miller, D. G. (1991). Acoustic details of vibrato cycle in tenor high notes. *Journal of Voice, 5,* 217–223.

Scobbie, J., Gibbon, F., Hardcastle, W., & Fletcher, P. (1998). Covert contrast and the acquisition of phonetics and phonology. In W. Ziegler & K. Deger (Eds.), *Clinical Phonetics and Linguistics* (pp. 147–156). London: Whurr Publishers Ltd.

Scripture, E. W. (1902). *The elements of experimental phonetics.* New York: Scribner's and Sons.

Scripture, E. W. (1906). *Researches in experimental phonetics: The study of speech curves.* Washington, DC: Carnegie Institution of Washington.

Scripture, E. W. (1916). Records of speech in disseminated sclerosis. *Brain, 39,* 455.

Scripture, E. W. (1933). Diagnosis by soundtracks. *Nature, 132,* 821–822.

Seaver, E., Dalston, R., Leeper, H., & Adams, L. (1991). A study of nasometric values for normal nasal resonance. *Journal of Speech and Hearing Research, 34,* 715–721.

Seidner, W., Nawka, T., & Cebulla, M. (1995). Dependence of the vibrato on pitch, musical intensity and vowel in different voice classes. In P. H. Dejonckere, M. Hirano, & J. Sundberg (Eds.), *Vibrato* (pp. 63–82). San Diego: Singular Publishing Group.

Shipp, T., Doherty, E. T., & Haglund, S. (1990). Physiologic factors in vocal vibrato production. *Journal of Voice, 4,* 300–304.

Shipp, T., & Huntington, D. A. (1965). Some acoustic and perceptual factors in acute-laryngitic hoarseness. *Journal of Speech and Hearing Disorders, 30,* 350–359.

Shipp, T., & Izdebski, K. (1981). Current evidence for the existence of laryngeal macrotremor and microtremor. *Journal of Forensic Sciences, 26,* 501–505.

Shipp, T., Leanderson, R., & Sundberg, J. (1980). Vocal vibrato. In V. Lawrence & B. Weinberg (Eds.), *Transcripts of the Eighth Symposium, Care of the Professional Voice. Part I: Physical factors in voice, vibrato, registers* (pp. 46–49). New York: The Voice Foundation.

Shoji, K., Regenbogen, E., Yu, J. D., & Blaugrund, S. M. (1992). High frequency power ratio of breathy voice. *Laryngoscope, 102,* 267–271.

Silbergleit, A., Johnson, A., & Jacobson, B. (1997). Acoustic analysis of voice in individuals with amyotrophic lateral sclerosis and perceptually normal voice quality. *Journal of Voice, 11,* 222--231.

Simon, C. (1927). The variability of consecutive wavelengths in vocal and instrumental sounds. *Psychological Monographs, 36,* 41–83.

Singh, S., & Murry, T. (1978). Multidimensional classification of normal voice qualities. *Journal of the Acoustical Society of America, 64,* 81–87.

Sluijter, A. M. C., & van Heuven, V. J. (1996). Spectral balance as an acoustic correlate of linguistic stress. *Journal of the Acoustical Society of America, 100,* 2471–2484.

Sluijter, A. M. C., van Heuven, V. J., & Pacilly, J. J. A. (1997). Spectral balance as a cue in the perception of linguistic stress. *Journal of the Acoustical Society of America, 101,* 503–513.

Smith, B. E., Weinberg, B., Feth, L. L., & Horii, Y. (1978). Vocal roughness and jitter characteristics of vowels produced by esophageal speakers. *Journal of Speech and Hearing Research, 21,* 240–249.

Södersten, M., & Hammarberg, B. (1993). Effects of voice training in normal-speaking women: Videostroboscopic, perceptual, and acoustic characteristics. *Scandanavian Journal of Logopedics and Phoniatrics, 18,* 33–42.

Södersten, M., Hertegård, S., & Hammarberg, B. (1995). Glottal closure, transglottal airflow, and voice quality in healthy middle-aged women. *Journal of Voice, 9,* 182–197.

Södersten, M., Lindestad, P. A., & Hammarberg, B. (1991). Vocal fold closure, perceived breathiness, and acoustic characteristics in normal adult speakers. In J. Gauffin & B. Hammarberg (Eds.), *Vocal fold physiology: Acoustic, perceptual and physiological aspects of voice mechanisms* (pp. 217–224). San Diego: Singular Publishing Group, Inc.

Sorensen, D., & Horii, Y. (1984a). Directional perturbation factors for jitter and for shimmer. *Journal of Communication Disorders, 17,* 143–151.

Sorensen, D., & Horii, Y. (1984b). Frequency characteristics of male and female speakers in the pulse register. *Journal of Communication Disorders, 17,* 65–73.

Souaid, J. P., Tewfik, T. L., & Pelland-Blais, E. (1998). Use of the computerized speech lab in paediatric dysphonia: A preliminary study. *Journal of Otolaryngology, 27,* 301–306.

Soundswell Music Acoustics. (1999). Swell [Computer Software]. Stockholm: Nyvalla DSP.

Stemple, J. C., Stanley, J., & Lee, L. (1995). Objective measures of voice production in normal subjects following prolonged voice use. *Journal of Voice, 9,* 127–133.

Stevens, K. N. (1977). Physics of laryngeal behavior and larynx modes. *Phonetica, 34,* 264–279.

Stevens, K. N., & Hanson, H. M. (1995). Classification of glottal vibration from acoustic measurements. In O. Fujimura & M. Hirano (Eds.), *Vocal fold physiology: Voice quality control* (pp. 147–170). San Diego: Singular Publishing Group, Inc.

Stevens, K.N, Nickerson, R., Boothroyd, A., & Rollins, A. (1976). Assessment of nasalization in the speech of deaf children. *Journal of Speech and Hearing Research, 19,* 393–416.

Stoicheff, M. (1981). Speaking fundamental frequency characteristics of nonsmoking female adults. *Journal of Speech and Hearing Research, 24,* 437–441.

Strand, E. A., Buder, E. H., Yorkston, K. M., & Ramig, L. O. (1994). Differential phonatory characteristics of four women with amyotrophic lateral sclerosis. *Journal of Voice, 8,* 327–339.

Strik, H., & Boves, L. (1992a). Control of fundamental frequency, intensity, and voice quality in speech. *Journal of Phonetics, 20,* 15–25.

Strik, H., & Boves, L. (1992b). On the relation between voice source parameters and prosodic features in connected speech. *Speech Communication, 11,* 167–174.

Sulter, A. M., & Wit, H. P. (1996). Glottal volume velocity waveform characteristics in subjects with and without vocal training, related to gender, sound intensity, fundamental frequency, and age. *Journal of the Acoustical Society of America, 100,* 3360–3372.

Sundberg, J. (1987). *The science of the singing voice.* Dekalb: Northern Illinois University Press.

Sundberg, J. (1995). Acoustic and psychoacoustic aspects of vocal vibrato. In P. H. Dejonckere, M. Hirano, & J. Sundberg (Eds.), *Vibrato* (pp. 35–62). San Diego: Singular Publishing Group.

Sundberg, J., & Askenfelt, A. (1983). Larynx height and voice source: A relationship? In D. M. Bless & J. H. Abbs (Eds.), *Vocal fold physiology: Contemporary research and clinical issues* (pp. 307–316). San Diego: College-Hill Press.

Sundberg, J., & Nordström, P. E. (1976). Raised and lowered larynx: The effect on vowel formant frequencies. *Speech Transmission Laboratory Quarterly Progress and Status Report, 2-3,* 36–39. (Also in Sundberg, J. [1987] *The science of the singing voice,* [pp. 113–114], Dekalb: Northern Illinois University Press.)

Sundberg, J., Thörnvik, M., & Söderström, A. (1998). Age and voice quality in professional singers. *Logopedics Phoniatrics, Vocology, 23,* 169–176.

Sussman, J. E., & Sapienza, C. (1994). Articulatory, developmental, and gender effects on measures of fundamental frequency and jitter. *Journal of Voice, 8,* 145–156.

Takahashi, H., & Koike, Y. (1975). Some perceptual dimensions and acoustical correlates of pathologic voices. *Acta Otolaryngologica Supplement, 338,* 2–24.

Talkin, D. (1994). Cross correlation and dynamic programming for estimation of fundamental frequency. In D. Wong (Ed.), *Proceedings of the Workshop on Acoustic Voice Analysis.* Iowa City, IA: National Center for Voice and Speech.

Terhardt, E. (1974). On the perception of periodic sound fluctuations (roughness). *Acustica, 30,* 201–213.

Ternström, S., & Friberg, A. (1989). Analysis and simulation of small variations in the fundamental frequency of sustained vowels. *Speech Transmission Laboratory Quarterly Progress and Status Report, 3,* 1–14.

Thompson, C. L. (1962). *Wavelength perturbations in phonation of pathological larynges* (Progress Report, Grant NB-04 398): Bethesda, MD: National Institutes of Health.

Timke, R., von Leden, H., & Moore, P. (1959). Laryngeal vibrations: Measurements of the glottic wave. Part II: Physiological considerations. *A. M. A. Archives of Otolaryngology, 69,* 438–444.

Titze, I. (1993). *Vocal fold physiology: Frontiers in basic science.* San Diego: Singular Publishing Group.

Titze, I. R. (1994a). *Principles of voice production.* Englewood Cliffs, NJ: Prentice Hall.

Titze, I. R. (1994b). Toward standards in acoustic analysis of voice. *Journal of Voice, 8,* 1–7.

Titze, I. R. (1995). *Workshop on acoustic voice analysis: Summary statement.* Iowa City, IA: National Center for Voice and Speech.

Titze, I. R., Baken, R. J., & Herzel, H. (1993). Evidence of chaos in vocal fold vibration. In I. R. Titze (Ed.), *Vocal fold physiology: Frontiers in basic science* (pp. 143–188). San Diego: Singular Publishing Group, Inc.

Titze, I. R., Horii, Y., & Scherer, R. C. (1987). Some technical considerations in voice perturbation measurements. *Journal of Speech and Hearing Research, 30,* 252–260.

Titze, I. R., & Liang, H. (1993). Comparison of f0 extraction methods for high-precision voice perturbation measurements. *Journal of Speech and Hearing Research, 36,* 1120–1133.

Titze, I. R., & Winholtz, W. S. (1993). Effect of microphone type and placement on voice perturbation measurements. *Journal of Speech and Hearing Research, 36,* 1177–1190.

Toner, M. A., Emanuel, F. W., & Parker, D. (1990). Relationship of spectral noise levels to psychophysical scaling of vowel roughness. *Journal of Speech and Hearing Research, 33,* 238–244.

Traunmüller, H., & Eriksson, A. (1995). The perceptual evaluation of f0 excursions in speech as evidenced in liveliness estimations. *Journal of the Acoustical Society of America, 97,* 1905–1915.

Trittin, P. J., & de Santos y Lleó, A. (1995). Voice quality analysis of male and female Spanish speakers. *Speech Communication, 16,* 359–368.

Van Bezooyen, R. (1984). *The characteristics and recognizability of vocal expressions of emotion.* Dordrecht, The Netherlands: Foris.

Van Bezooyen, R., & Boves, L. (1986). The effects of low-pass filtering and random splicing on the perception of speech. *Journal of Psycholinguistic Research, 15,* 403–417.

van den Berg, J. (1958). Myoelastic-aerodynamic theory of voice production. *Journal of Speech and Hearing Research, 1,* 227–244. (Reprinted in Kent, R. D., Atal, B. S., & Miller, J. L. [Eds.], [1991]. *Papers in speech communication: Speech production* [pp. 121–138]. Woodbury, NY: Acoustical Society of America.)

van den Berg, J., Zantema, J. T., & Doornenbal, J., P. (1957). On the air resistance and the bernoulli effect of the human larynx. *Journal of the Acoustical Society of America, 29,* 626–631. (Reprinted in Kent, R. D., Atal, B. S., & Miller, J. L. [Eds.], [1991]. *Papers in speech communication: Speech production* [pp. 115–120]. Woodbury, NY: Acoustical Society of America.)

Van Lierde, K., Moerman, M., & Van Cauwengerge, P. (1996). Comment on the results of voice analysis. *Acta Oto-Rhino-Laryngologica Belgica, 50,* 345–351.

Verdonck-de Leeuw, I. M., Koopsmans-van Beinum, F. J., Hilgers, F., & Keus, R. (1997). The development of an instrument to analyse voice quality of male patients with early glottic cancer, *Larynx 97* (pp. 29–32). Aix en Provence, France: Universite de Provence.

Walton, J. H., & Orlikoff, R. F. (1994). Speaker race identification from acoustic cues in the vocal signal. *Journal of Speech and Hearing Research, 37,* 738–745.

Wang, S. (1985). Singing voice: Bright timbre, singer's formants and larynx positions. In A. Askenfelt, S. Felicetti, E. Jansson, & J. Sundberg (Eds.), *SMAC 83—Proceedings of the Stockholm Music Acoustics Conference* (pp. 313–322). Stockholm.

Waters, J., Nunn, S., Gillcrist, B., & VonColln, E. (1995). The effect of stress on the glottal pulse. In I. Trancoso & R. Moore (Eds.), *ESCA–NATO tutorial and research workshop on speech under stress* (pp. 9–11). Lisbon, Portugal: ESCA.

Wendahl, R. W. (1963). Laryngeal analog synthesis of harsh voice quality. *Folia Phoniatrica, 14,* 241–250.

Wendahl, R.W. (1966a). Laryngeal analog synthesis of jitter and shimmer: Auditory parameters of harshness. *Folia Phoniatrica, 18,* 98–108.

Wendahl, R. W. (1966b). Some parameters of auditory roughness. *Folia Phoniatrica, 18,* 26–32.

Wendahl, R. W., Moore, G. P., & Hollien, H. (1963). Comments on vocal fry. *Folia Phoniatrica, 15,* 251–255.

Wendler, J., Doherty, E. T., & Hollien, H. (1980). Voice classification by means of long-term speech spectra. *Folia Phoniatrica, 32,* 51–60.

Wendler, J., Fischer, S., Seidner, W., Rauhut, A., & Wendler, U. (1985). Stroboglottometric and acoustic measures of natural vocal registers. In A. Askenfelt, S. Felicetti, E. Jansson, & J. Sundberg (Eds.), *SMAC 83 - Proceedings of the Stockholm Music Acoustics Conference* (pp. 333–340). Stockholm.

Wendler, J., Rauhut, A., & Krüger, H. (1986). Classification of voice qualities. *Journal of Phonetics, 14,* 483–488.

Wendler, J., Wagner, H., Seidner, W., & Stürzebecher, E. (1976). Methodik bei stimmschallanalysen, *Proceedings of the 16th Congress of the International Association of Logopedics and Phoniatrics* (pp. 518–521). Interlaken, 1974.

Whurr, R., Lorch, M., Fontana, H., Brookes, G., Lees, A., & Marsden, C. D. (1993). The use of botulinum toxin in the treatment of adductor spasmodic dysphonia. *Journal of Neurology, Neurosurgery, and Psychiatry, 56,* 526–530.

Wieser, M. (1980). The long-term period measurement, an instrumental method in phoniatry. *Archives of Otorhinolaryngology, 226,* 63–72.

Wilcox, K. A., & Horii, Y. (1980). Age and changes in vocal jitter. *Journal of Gerontology, 35,* 194–198.

Williams, C. E., & Stevens, K. N. (1972). Emotions and speech: Some acoustical correlates. *Journal of the Acoustical Society of America, 52,* 1238–1250.

Williams, C. E., & Stevens, K. N. (1981). Vocal correlates of emotional states. In J. K. Darby (Ed.), *Speech evaluation in psychiatry* (pp. 221–240). New York: Grune & Stratton.

Williams, R. G., Eccles, R., & Hutchings, H. (1990). The relationship between nasalance and nasal resistance to airflow. *Acta Otolaryngologica (Stockholm), 110*, 443–449.

Winckel, F. (1965). Phoniatric acoustics. In R. Luchsinger & G. E. Arnold, *Voice, speech, language—clinical communicology: Its physiology and pathology* (G. E. Arnold & E. R. Finkbeiner, Trans.) (pp. 24–55). Belmont, CA: Wadsworth Publishing Co.

Winckel, F. (1974). Acoustical cues in the voice for detecting laryngeal diseases and individual behaviour. In B. Wyke (Ed.), *Ventilatory and phonatory control systems: An international symposium* (pp. 248–260). London: Oxford University Press.

Winholtz, W. S., & Titze, I. R. (1997). Conversion of a head-mounted microphone signal into calibrated SPL units. *Journal of Voice, 11*, 417–421.

Winholtz, W. S., & Titze, I. R. (1998). Suitability of minidisc (MD) recordings for voice perturbation analysis. *Journal of Voice, 12*, 138–142.

Winholz, W. S., & Ramig, L. O. (1992). Vocal tremor analysis with the Vocal Demodulator. *Journal of Speech and Hearing Research, 35*, 562–573.

Wirz, S., & Mackenzie Beck, J. (1995). Assessment of voice quality: The vocal profiles analysis scheme. In S. Wirz (Ed.), *Perceptual approaches to communication disorders* (pp. 39–55). London: Whurr Publishers.

Wirz, S. L., Subtelny, J. D., & Whitehead, R. L. (1981). Perceptual and spectrographic study of tense voice in normal hearing and deaf subjects. *Folia Phoniatrica, 33*, 23–36.

Wolfe, V., Cornell, R., & Palmer, C. (1991). Acoustic correlates of pathologic voice types. *Journal of Speech and Hearing Research, 34*, 509–516.

Wolfe, V., Fitch, J., & Cornell, R. (1995). Acoustic prediction of severity in commonly occuring voice problems. *Journal of Speech and Hearing Research, 38*, 273–279.

Wolfe, V. I., & Ratusnik, D. L. (1988). Acoustic and perceptual measurements of roughness influencing judgments of pitch. *Journal of Speech and Hearing Disorders, 53*, 15–22.

Wolfe, V. I., & Steinfatt, T. M. (1987). Prediction of vocal severity within and across voice types. *Journal of Speech and Hearing Research, 30*, 230–240.

Wong, D., Ito, M. R., Cox, N. B., & Titze, I. R. (1991). Observation of perturbations in a lumped-element model of the vocal folds with application to some pathological cases. *Journal of the Acoustical Society of America, 89*, 383–394.

Wuyts, F. L., De Bodt, M., Bruckers, L., & Molenberghs, G. (1996). Results. *Acta Oto-Rhino-Laryngologica Belgica, 50*, 331–341.

Yair, E., & Gath, I. (1988). On the use of pitch power spectrum in the evaluation of vocal tremor. *Proceedings IEEE, special issue on Emerging Electromedical Systems, September 1998.*

Yanagihara, N. (1967). Significance of harmonic changes and noise components in hoarseness. *Journal of Speech and Hearing Research, 10*, 531–541.

Yanagisawa, E., Estill, J., Kmucha, T., & Leder, S. B. (1989). The contribution of aryepiglottic constriction to "ringing" voice quality—A videolaryngoscopic study with acoustic analysis. *Journal of Voice, 3*, 342–350.

Yonick, T., Reich, A., Minifie, F., & Fink, B. R. (1990). Acoustical effects of endotracheal intubation. *Journal of Speech and Hearing Disorders, 55*, 427–433.

Yoon, K. M., Kakita, Y., & Hirano, M. (1984). Sound spectrographic analysis of the voice of patients with glottic carcinomas. *Folia Phoniatrica, 36*, 24–30.

Yumoto, E. (1983). The quantitative evaluation of hoarseness: A new harmonics-to-noise ratio method. *Archives of Otolaryngology, 109*, 48–52.

Yumoto, E., Gould, W. J., & Baer, T. (1982). Harmonics-to-noise ratio as an index of the degree of hoarseness. *Journal of the Acoustical Society of America, 71*, 1544–1549.

Yumoto, E., Sasaki, Y., & Okamura, H. (1984). Harmonics-to-noise ratio and psychophysical measurement of the degree of hoarseness. *Journal of Speech and Hearing Research, 27*, 2–6.

Zemlin, W. R. (1962). *A comparison of the periodic function of vocal fold vibration in a multiple sclerosis and a normal population.* Unpublished doctoral dissertation, University of Minnesota.

Zwicker, E., & Fastl, H. (1990). *Psychoacoustics: Facts and models.* Berlin: Springer-Verlag.

Zwirner, P., & Barnes, G. (1992). Vocal tract steadiness: A measure of phonatory and upper airway motor control during phonation in dysarthria. *Journal of Speech and Hearing Research, 35*, 761–768.

Zwirner, P., Murry, T., Swenson, M., & Woodson, G. E. (1991). Acoustic changes in spasmodic dysphonia after botulinum toxin injection. *Journal of Voice, 5*, 78–84.

Zwirner, P., Murry, T., & Woodson, G. E. (1991). Phonatory function of neurologically impaired individuals. *Journal of Communication Disorders, 24*, 287–300.

Zyski, B. J., Bull, G. L., McDonald, W. E., & Johns, M. E. (1984). Perturbation analysis of normal and pathologic larynges. *Folia Phoniatrica, 36*, 190–198.

CHAPTER 10

Aerodynamic Measures of Voice Production

Robert E. Hillman and James B. Kobler

Aerodynamics play a major role in the production of voice. This chapter provides a brief overview of approaches for measuring aerodynamic parameters associated with voice production in humans. There is a special effort at the end of the chapter to describe the state-of-the-art in applying aerodynamic measures to the routine clinical assessment of patients with voice disorders.

Normal phonation is typically preceded by the inhalation of air to lung volumes above the resting expiratory level (REL), with normal phrases in continuous speech typically being initiated above the tidal volume level (Hixon, 1973). The vocal folds are then adducted and appropriately tensed via laryngeal muscle activity. Positive subglottal air pressure is built up below the vocal folds with the onset of exhalation. When subglottal air pressure exceeds the resistance offered by the vocal folds, they are blown into airflow-induced oscillation. As the vocal folds oscillate, pulses of air are emitted from the glottis (glottal volume velocity waveform) to generate the acoustic energy that is perceived as the voice. In normal continuous speech, there is a tendency to pause and inhale when lung volume approximates (decreases to) the REL (Hixon, 1973).

This simplified description of the phonation process illustrates that air volumes, airflows, and air pressures all play a role in voice production. Approaches for measuring each of these parameters are described in the following sections of this chapter.

1. AIR VOLUME

A major part of respiratory research in human communication has entailed the measurement of the air volumes that are typically expended during selected speech and singing tasks and the specification of the ranges of lung inflation levels across which such tasks are normally performed (cf. Hixon, 1973; Hoit & Hixon, 1987; Hoit, Hixon, Watson, & Morgan, 1990; Thomasson & Sundberg, 1997; Watson & Hixon, 1985). Air volumes are measured in common metric units (liters, cubic centimeters, milliliters) and lung inflation levels are usually specified in terms of a percentage of the vital capacity (volume of air that can be displaced from the lungs following maximal inhalation) or total lung volume (the vital capacity plus the residual volume that remains in the lungs following maximal exhalation).

1.1. Direct Measurement of Air Volume

Direct measurement of air volumes can be accomplished to a limited extent via traditional spirometry in which a mouthpiece or facemask is connected to a closed system for collection of orally displaced air volumes during phonatory tasks (Beckett, 1971). Older mechanical types of spirometers have limited response characteristics and there can be a buildup of CO_2 with prolonged use. Orally displaced air volumes can also be measured by integrating the oral airflow signal from a pneumotachograph connected to a mouthpiece or facemask (see following section on average glottal airflow rate measurement). The use of devices placed in or around the mouth to directly collect oral airflow can interfere with normal speech production. This is particularly true of mouthpieces, which are often used in assessing basic respiratory capabilities (vital capacity, tidal volume, etc.), but essentially limit speech production to vocalic sounds (usually sustained vowels). Sustained vowels can be sufficient for assessing selected volumetric-based phonatory parameters. There are also concerns that facemasks can interfere with normal jaw movements and that the oral acoustic signal is degraded so that auditory feedback is reduced/ distorted and simultaneous acoustic analysis is limited.

1.2. Indirect Measurement of Air Volume

The majority of speech breathing research has been carried out using indirect approaches for estimating lung volumes via the monitoring of changes in body dimensions. The basic assumption underlying the indirect approaches is that changes in lung volume are reflected in proportional changes in torso size. One relatively cumbersome but time honored approach has been to place subjects in a sealed chamber called a body plethysmograph to allow estimation of the air volume displaced by the body during respiration (cf. Draper, Ladefoged, & Witteridge, 1959). More often used for speech breathing research are transducers that unobtrusively monitor changes in the dimensions of the rib cage and abdomen (referred to collectively as the *chest wall*), as it has been shown that the majority of changes in torso dimension during respiration are accounted for by changes in the dimensions of these two regions of the body (Mead, Peterson, Grimby, & Mead, 1967). There have been two types of systems that have been used most often to monitor chest wall dimensions: magnetometers (cf. Hixon, 1973) and inductance plethysmographs (cf. Sperry, Hillman, & Perkell, 1994). Figure 10–1 shows a subject wearing the elastic bands of an inductance plethysmograph. Both of these systems require the placement of two sets of noninvasive transducers on the body surface to monitor changes in rib cage and abdominal dimensions, which are then related to lung volume via calibration procedures (Banzett, Mahan, Garner, Brughera, & Loring, 1995; Sperry et al., 1994). These approaches have been primarily employed to study respiratory function during continuous speech and singing tasks that include both voiced and voiceless sound production, as opposed to assessing air volume usage during phonatory tasks that involve only laryngeal production of voice (e.g., sustained vowels).

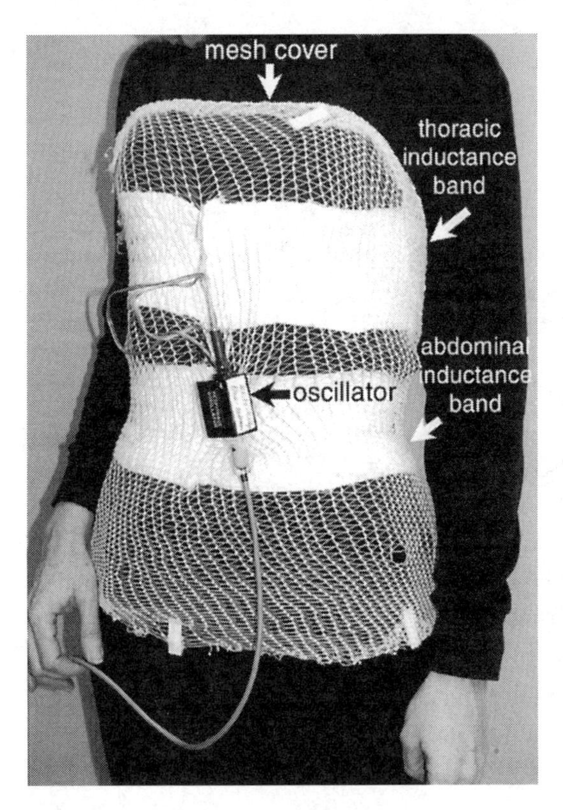

Figure 10–1. Placement of the two elastic inductance bands of the Respitrace™ system for obtaining indirect estimates of lung volume changes via monitoring of changes in body dimensions at the rib cage and abdomen.

There are ongoing efforts to develop more accurate methods for noninvasively monitoring chest wall activity that seek to capture finer details of how the three-dimensional geometry of the body is altered during respiration (cf. Cala et al., 1996).

2. AIRFLOW

Airflow associated with phonation is usually specified in terms of volume velocity (i.e., volume of air displaced per unit of time). Volume velocity airflow rates for voice production are typically reported in metric units of volume displaced (liters or cubic centimeters) per second.

2.1. Average Glottal Airflow Rate Measurement

Estimates of average airflow rates can be obtained by simply dividing air volume estimates (see air volume section) by the duration of the phonatory task. Average glottal airflow rates have usually been estimated during vowel phonation by using a mouthpiece or facemask to channel the oral air stream through a device called a *pneumotachograph* (cf. Isshiki, 1964). Such estimates can be obtained from the oral airflow during vowel production, because the vocal tract is relatively nonconstricted with no major sources of turbulent airflow between the glottis and the lips. The pneumotachograph operates by using a differential pressure transducer to measure the pressure drop (difference) that is created by placing a slight resistance (usually screen material) in the path of the airstream (i.e., there is a buildup of positive back-pressure in front of the resistance). The schematic in Figure 10–2 shows the basic operation of a pneumotachograph. As the goal is to obtain estimates of average flow rates, the signal from the pressure transducer is typically low-pass filtered to remove any fluctuations associated with vocal fold vibration.

There has also been somewhat limited use of hot wire anemometer devices (mounted in a mouthpiece) to estimate average glottal airflow during sustained vowel phonation (cf. Kitajima, Isshiki, & Tanabe, 1978). This approach relies on the relationship between volume velocity flow rate and the amount of current that is needed to maintain constant temperature in a wire that is cooled by being placed in the air stream (i.e., heat dissipation in the wire is linearly related to the square root of the velocity of the gas stream). One limitation of this device is that it cannot differentiate between airflow generated on exhalation versus inhalation.

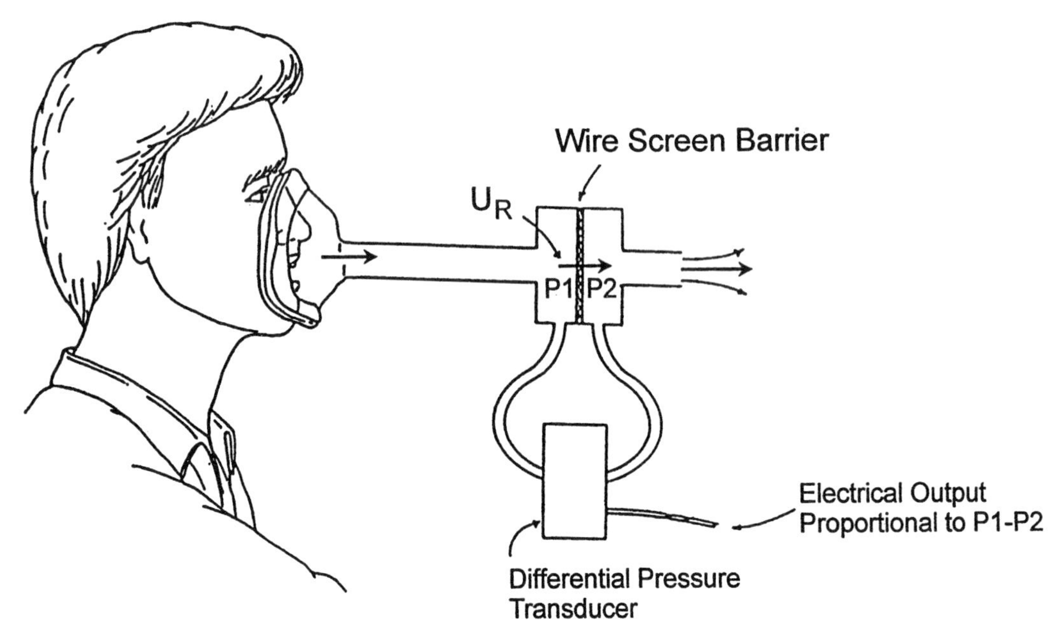

Figure 10–2. Schematic showing the basic operation of a standard pneumotachograph that is mounted in a facemask to measure oral airflow during voice and speech production. (Reprinted with permission from Glottal Enterprises, Inc.)

2.2. Glottal Volume Velocity Waveform Measurement

As indicated previously, the vocal tone is produced by air pulses that are generated as the glottis rapidly opens and closes during flow-induced vibration of the vocal folds. The air pulses comprise a quasiperiodic "glottal volume velocity waveform" (glottal waveform) whose parameters determine most of the salient acoustic characteristics of the voice. Thus, the specification of glottal waveform parameters is of fundamental importance to describing vocal function and/or voice quality.

The glottal volume velocity waveform cannot be directly observed by measuring the oral airflow signal, because the waveform is highly convoluted by the resonance activity (formants) of the vocal tract. Thus, recovery of the glottal volume velocity waveform requires methods that eliminate/correct for the influences of the vocal tract. This has typically been accomplished by a process of inverse filtering in which the major resonances of the vocal tract are estimated and the oral airflow signal is processed (inverse filtered) to eliminate them (Holmberg, Hillman, & Perkell, 1988; Rothenberg, 1973). To do this requires that the oral airflow first be recorded using a fast responding pneumotachograph to allow the capture of as much high frequency-related detail in the airflow waveform as possible. This has been most frequently accomplished with a circumferentially vented facemask that allows faster dissipation of back pressure than standard pneumotachographic-types of devices (Rothenberg, 1977). Figure 10–3 shows a Rothenberg mask, the most frequently used version of a high response-time pneumotachograph. Figure 10–4 depicts examples of parameters that are typically extracted from glottal waveform estimates, which include both volume velocity-based and time-based measures.

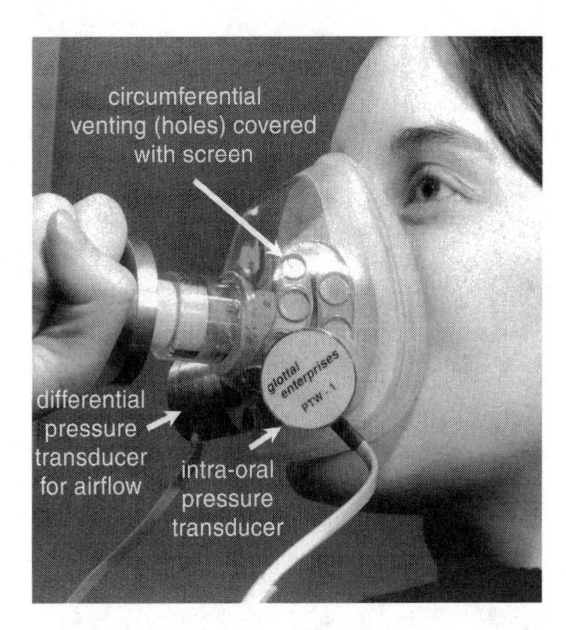

Figure 10–3. Use of a Rothenberg mask to measure oral airflow. The pressure transducer is connected to a thin catheter inside the mask that can be inserted between the lips to obtain simultaneous measures of intraoral pressure (see section 3.2: Indirect Measurement of Subglottal Air Pressure).

Time-based Measures

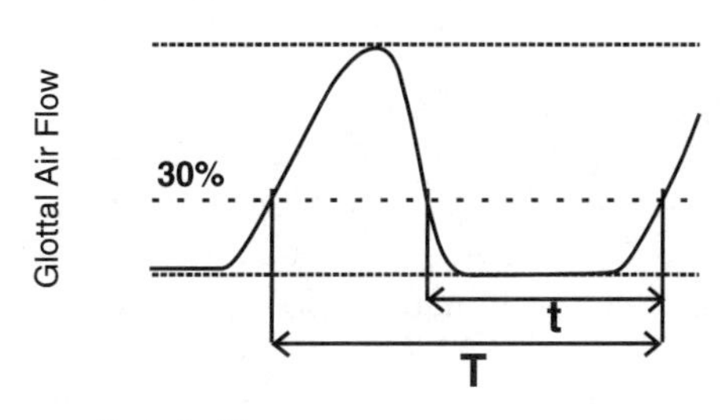

Period = T
Flow Adduction Quotient = t/T

Amplitude-based Measures

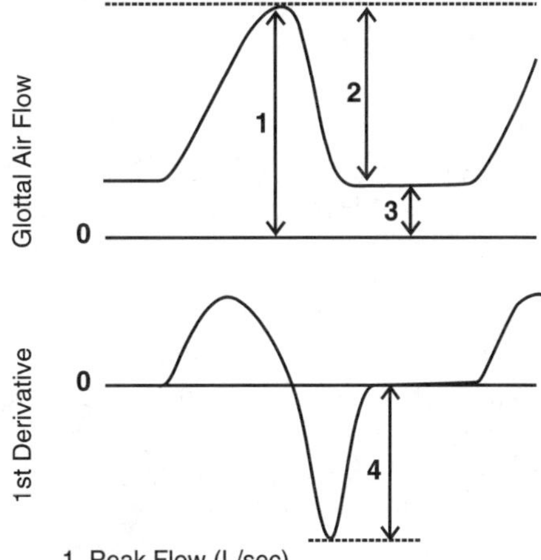

1. Peak Flow (L/sec)
2. AC Flow (L/sec)
3. Minimum Flow (L/sec)
4. Maximum Flow Declination Rate (L/sec/sec)
   AC/DC (RMS about mean of AC portion/mean)

Figure 10–4. Schematic showing idealized glottal volume velocity waveforms with examples of time-based and amplitude-based measures that are typically obtained.

3. AIR PRESSURE

Of primary importance in assessing the aerodynamics of voice production is the measurement of air pressures below (subglottal) and above (supraglottal) the vocal folds. Vocal fold vibration can only be initiated and maintained if there is a transglottal pressure differential, such as during normal exhalatory phonation, where subglottal pressure exceeds supraglottal pressure. Air pressure measurements related specifically to voice production are typically acquired during vowel phonation when there are no vocal tract constrictions of sufficient magnitude to build up positive supraglottal pressures. Under these conditions, it is usually assumed that supraglottal pressure is essentially equal to atmospheric pressure and only subglottal pressure measurements are obtained. Air pressures associated with voice and speech production are usually specified in centimeters of water (cm H_2O).

3.1. Direct Measurement of Subglottal Air Pressure

Subglottal air pressure can be directly measured by inserting a hypodermic needle into the subglottal airway via a puncture in the anterior neck at the cricothyroid space (cf. Isshiki, 1964). The needle is connected to a pressure transducer by tubing. This method is very accurate, but obviously very invasive, requiring that it be done by medically trained personnel in an environment that is well equipped to handle possible complications.

It is also possible to insert a very thin catheter through the posterior cartilaginous glottis (between the arytenoids) to sense subglottal air pressure during phonation. However, this cannot be tolerated by all subjects and it requires heavy topical anesthetization of the larynx, which can affect normal function. A few investigators have also obtained estimates of transglottal air pressure profiles (including subglottal) using an array of miniature transducers positioned directly above and below the glottis (Cranen & Boves, 1985).

3.2. Indirect Measurements of Subglottal Air Pressure

Estimates of tracheal (subglottal) air pressure can be obtained via the placement of an elongated balloon-like device into the esophagus (Kunze, 1964; Lieberman, 1968). The deflated "esophageal balloon" is attached to a catheter that is typically inserted transnasally and then swallowed into the esophagus to be positioned at the midthoracic level. The catheter is connected to a pressure transducer and the balloon is slightly inflated. An esophageal balloon is shown in Figure 10–5. Use of this approach to estimate subglottal pressures associated with phonation requires simultaneous monitoring of lung inflation levels so that the raw esophageal pressure measure can be corrected for the contribution of lung elastic recoil forces. Like subglottal puncture, this is an invasive method that requires the availability of appropriate medical support.

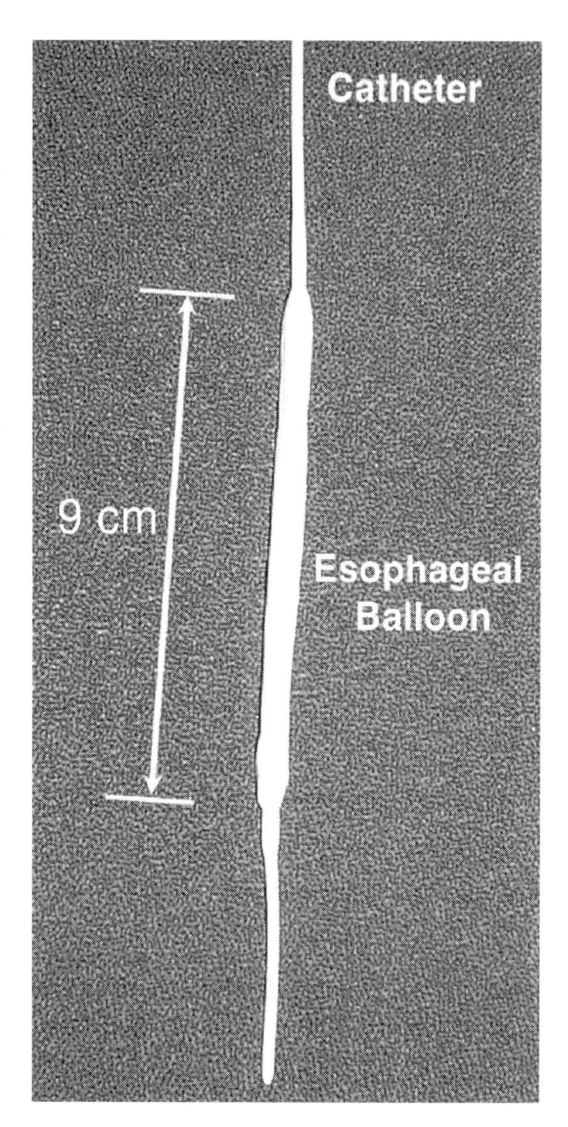

Figure 10–5. The type of esophageal balloon and catheter assembly that can be used to obtain indirect estimates of subglottal air pressure.

Noninvasive estimates of subglottal air pressure can be obtained by measuring intraoral air pressure during specially constrained utterances (Smitheran & Hixon, 1981). This is usually done by sensing air pressure just behind the lips with a translabially placed catheter connected to a pressure transducer. These intraoral pressure measures are obtained as subjects produce strings of alternating bilabial /p/ and vowel syllables (e.g., /pi-pi-pi-pi-pi/) at constant pitch and loudness. This method works because the vocal folds are abducted during /p/ production, thus allowing pressure to equilibrate throughout the airway, making intraoral pressure equal to subglottal pressure. An attempt is usually made to obtain an esti-

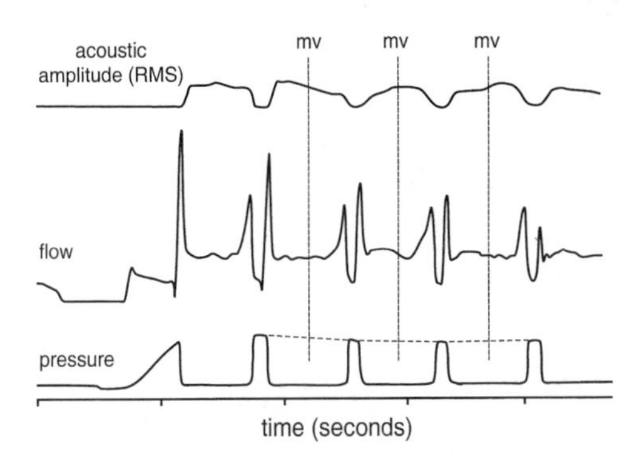

Figure 10–6. Examples of acoustic (top trace), oral airflow (middle trace), and intraoral air pressure (bottom trace) signals obtained during production of a /æ/ syllable string. Vertical dashed lines labeled "mv" (midvowel) indicate the points at which estimates of vocal intensity, average glottal airflow, and average subglottal pressure are obtained.

mate of the subglottal pressure at midvowel (i.e., during phonation) by interpolating between the pressure maximums for the /p/s. The signal measurement technique is illustrated in Figure 10–6. Maximum pressure during lip closure for the /p/ sound should attain some steady-state value to ensure that airway pressure has equilibrated, thus satisfying the major assumption underlying the method.

4. ADDITIONAL DERIVED MEASURES

There have been numerous attempts to extend the utility of the basic aerodynamic measures described by using them in the derivation of additional measures aimed at better elucidating underlying mechanisms of vocal function. One example is maximum flow declination rate (MFDR), which is typically extracted as the maximum amplitude of the negative peak (in L/s^2) in the first derivative of the glottal waveform (see Figure 10–4). This measure is of interest because it relates to vocal fold closure velocity and is highly correlated with the amount of acoustic energy that is generated during phonation (Holmberg et al., 1988; Holmberg, Hillman, Perkell, & Gress, 1994).

Most derived measures usually take the form of ratios that relate aerodynamic parameters to each other, or that relate aerodynamic parameters to simultaneously obtained acoustic measures. A commonly derived measure that interrelates aerodynamic parameters is airway (glottal) resistance, which is simply the ratio between average subglottal air pressure and average glottal airflow rate (cf. Isshiki, 1964; Smitheran & Hixon, 1981). During vowel phonation, this measure has been interpreted as being primarily influenced by the forces that control the resistance of the glottis to airflow, primarily vocal fold adduction and stiffness, although it includes the resistance contributions of the entire airway, which are assumed to be minimal during vowel production.

Measures have also been derived that interrelate glottal volume velocity waveform parameters. For example, AC/DC ratio is a measure that describes the relationship between the magnitude of modulated (AC) versus unmodulated (DC) glottal airflow, as illustrated in Figure 10–4 (Holmberg et al., 1988; Isshiki, 1981).

Vocal efficiency is a measure that compares the aerodynamic power (subglottal pressure × glottal airflow) that is expended to drive vocal fold vibration to the sound power that is produced (Holmberg et al., 1988; Schutte, 1980).

5. NORMATIVE DATA FOR AERODYNAMIC MEASURES

As is the case for most measures of vocal function, there is not currently a set of normative data for aerodynamic measures that is universally accepted and/or applied in research and clinical work. Methods for collecting such data have not been standardized, and study samples have generally not been of sufficient size and/or appropriately stratified in terms of age and sex to ensure unbiased estimates of underlying aerodynamic phonatory parameters in the normal population. However, there

Table 10–1. Examples of normative data for aerodynamic measures, and associated aerodynamically based derived measures from Holmberg et al., 1994. Data are for "comfortable" (normal-habitual) levels of pitch and loudness[1].

	MALES (N = 15)			*FEMALES (N = 15)*		
MEASURES	***Mean***	***SD***	***Range***	***Mean***	***SD***	***Range***
SPL (dB)	77.8	4.4	70.5–85.1	74.0	3.3	60.0–80.5
F_0 (Hz)	112	12	90–132	204	22	181–246
Pressure (cm H_2O)	5.9	1.0	3.8 –7.5	5.5	1.2	3.2–8.7
Average flow (L/s)	.204	.059	.120–.310	.198	.078	.101–.343
Glottal Resistance (cm H_2O/L/sec)	32.6	13.7	16.8–58.2	30.8	9.4	14.2–46.3
Vocal Efficiency (I/ cm $H_2O \times$ L/s)1	15.7	12.7	2.3– 62.0	11.2	9.1	1.4–37.6
Peak flow (L/s)	.41	.087	.276–.552	.286	.100	.152–.476
DC (minimum) flow (L/s)	.08	.045	.021–.155	.130	.063	.049–.256
AC flow (L/s)	.331	.069	.197–.410	.156	.051	.092–.265
AC flow/DC flow	.64	.18	.40–1.00	.30	.08	.18–.44
Adduction quotient (closed t/T)	.52	.06	.38–.61	.43	.04	.37–.52
Max. flow declination rate (L/s^2)	337	127	154–615	184	63	102–288

[1]Vocal efficiency values are from Holmberg et al., 1988 and have been multiplied by 10^5.

are several sources in the literature that provide estimates of normative values for selected aerodynamic measures. One example of such normative data is provided in Table 10–1.

The following publications are examples of additional sources that contain estimates of normative aerodynamic data: (Baken, 1987; Keilmann & Bader, 1995; Kent, 1994; Melcon, Hoit, & Hixon, 1989; Netsell, Lotz, Peters, & Schulte, 1994; Stathopoulos, 1986; Stathopoulos & Weismer, 1985; Tang & Stathopoulos, 1995).

6. CLINICAL USE OF AERODYNAMIC MEASURES TO ASSESS VOCAL FUNCTION

In current clinical practice, aerodynamic assessment of vocal function primarily involves obtaining estimates of average glottal airflow rates and average subglottal air pressures via noninvasive oral measurements during a well controlled utterance (see indirect measurement of subglottal air pressure section). Both measures are easy to obtain, even in young children. One example of a commercially available clinical aerodynamics system is shown in Figure 10–7. It has been shown that average glottal airflow rates can display a relatively high degree of variation across repeated recordings of normal speakers that can not be easily corrected for (Holmberg et al., 1994). There is circumstantial evidence that a likely source of this normal variation is a change in the extent to which the posterior glottis closes across repeated phonations (i.e., variation in posterior glottal chink size). Thus, average airflow rate is most useful and reliable as an indicator of rela-

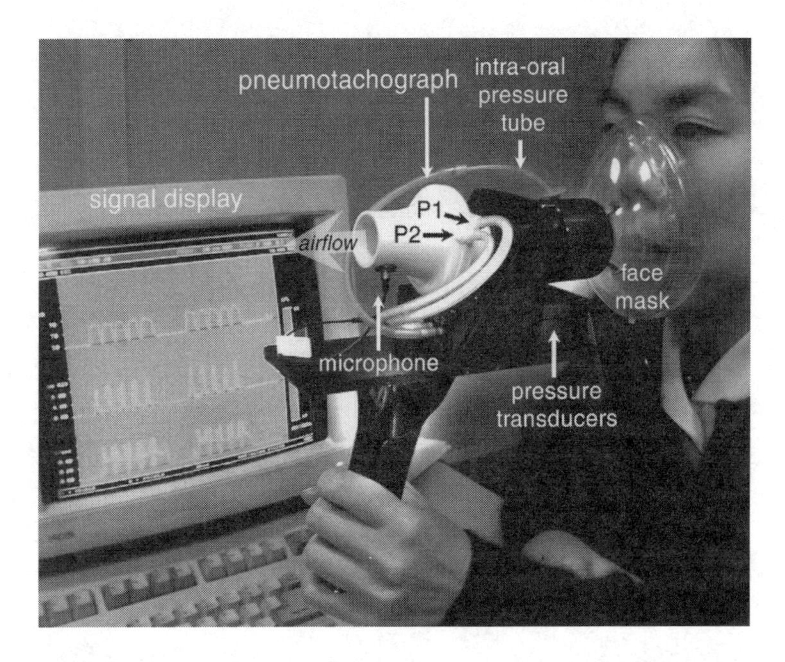

Figure 10–7. An example of a commercially available system (Kay Elemetrics, Inc.) for performing clinical aerodynamic assessment of voice production.

tively large changes in vocal function (e.g., comparing vocal function before and after medialization for vocal fold paralysis).

Subglottal air pressure is highly correlated with the sound pressure level (SPL) of the voice. Thus, the sensitivity and usefulness of subglottal pressure estimates can be greatly increased if simultaneous measures of vocal SPL are obtained (Holmberg et al., 1994). This is accomplished by using age- and gender-specific normative data as a basis for predicting what the appropriate subglottal pressure should be for a patient phonating at a particular SPL. In this way it is possible to determine if a patient is using excessive subglottal driving pressure to produce a given SPL output, even if the absolute pressure value is within normal limits. Such a scenario is often interpreted as evidence of vocal hyperfunction (Hillman, Holmberg, Perkell, Walsh, & Vaughan, 1989). Figure 10–8 shows an example of a clinical report format that includes comparisons of measured pressures with both absolute and predicted (SPL-based) normative values.

The commonly used method of estimating subglottal air pressure from the intraoral air pressure during bilabial stop consonant production assumes that laryngeal conditions (e.g., muscle tension, etc.) do not vary significantly across the test utterance. Although this approach has been validated via tracheal puncture in normals (Lofqvist, Carlborg, & Kitzing, 1982), there is concern that absolute pressure values estimates need to be viewed cautiously when obtained from patients in whom laryngeal conditions can vary significantly across the test utterance, for example, spasmodic dysphonia. However, in such cases, the finding of abnormally high pressures and the monitoring of the relative change in pressure with treatment are still useful and valid.

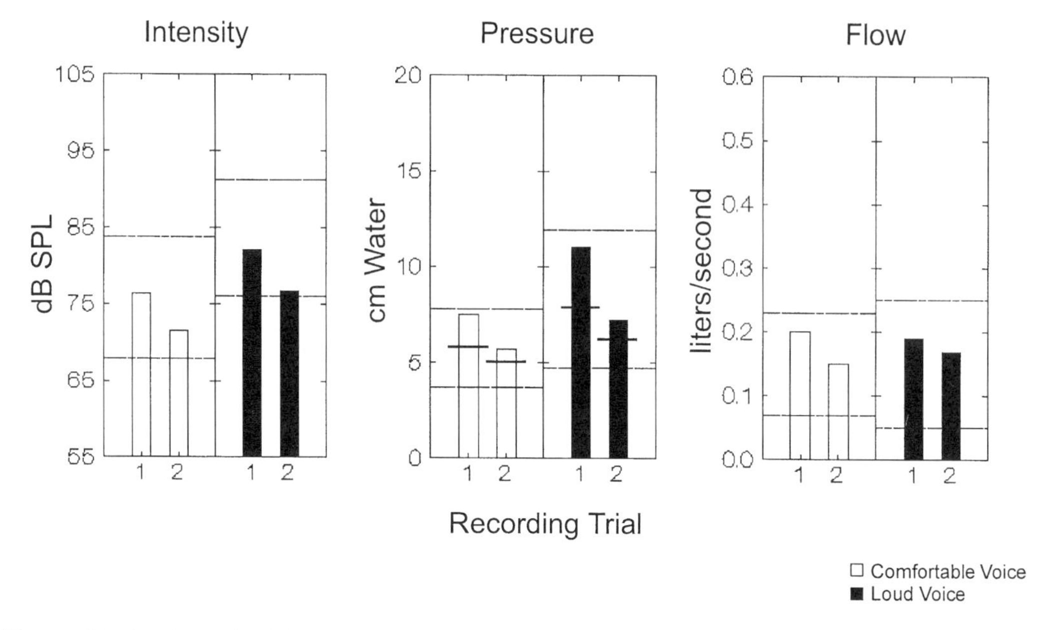

Figure 10–8. Example of format for reporting the results of clinical aerodynamic voice assessments. Shown are measures of vocal intensity in dB_{SPL} (left panel), subglottal pressure in cm H_2O (center panel), and glottal flow rate in L/s (right panel) for phonations produced using comfortable and loud voice across two assessments (Recording Trial), for example, pretreatment versus posttreatment. The horizontal lines in each panel represent estimated normative ranges. The additional small horizontal lines superimposed on the bars in the center panel indicate the predicted subglottal pressure for a normal group phonating at an equivalent intensity (SPL) level.

REFERENCES

Baken, R. J. (1987). *Clinical measurement of speech and voice.* Boston: College-Hill Press.

Banzett, R. B., Mahan, S. T., Garner, D. M., Brughera, A., & Loring, S. H. (1995). A simple and reliable method to calibrate respiratory magnetometers and Respitrace. *Journal of Applied Physiology, 79,* 2169–2176.

Beckett, R. L. (1971). The respirometer as a diagnostic and clinical tool in the speech clinic. *Journal of Speech and Hearing Disorders, 36,* 235–241.

Cala, S. J., Kenyon, C. M., Ferrigno, G., Carnevali, P., Aliverti, A., Pedotti, A., Macklem, P. T., & Rochester, D. F. (1996). Chest wall and lung volume estimation by optical reflectance motion analysis. *Journal of Applied Physiology, 81,* 2680–2689.

Cranen, B., & Boves, L. (1985). Pressure measurements during speech production using semiconductor miniature pressure transducers: Impact on models for speech production. *Journal of the Acoustical Society of America, 77,* 1543–1551.

Draper, M., Ladefoged, P., & Witteridge, D. (1959). Respiratory muscles in speech. *Journal of Speech and Hearing Research, 2,* 16–27.

Hillman, R. E., Holmberg, E. B., Perkell, J. S., Walsh, M., & Vaughan, C. (1989). Objective assessment of vocal hyperfunction: An experimental framework and initial results. *Journal of Speech and Hearing Research, 32,* 373–392.

Hixon, T. J. (1973). Kinematics of the chest wall during speech production: Volume displacements of the rib cage, abdomen, and lung. *Journal of Speech and Hearing Research, 16,* 78–115.

Hoit, J. D., & Hixon, T. J. (1987). Age and speech breathing. *Journal of Speech and Hearing Research, 30,* 351–366.

Hoit, J. D., Hixon, T. J., Watson, P. J., & Morgan, W. J. (1990). Speech breathing in children and adolescents. *Journal of Speech and Hearing Research, 33,* 51–69.

Holmberg, E. B., Hillman, R. E., & Perkell, J. S. (1988). Glottal airflow and transglottal air pressure measurements for male and female speakers in soft, normal, and loud voice. *Journal of the Acoustical Society of America, 84,* 511–529.

Holmberg, E. B., Hillman, R. E., Perkell, J. S., & Gress, C. (1994). Relationships between intra-speaker variation in aerodynamic measures of voice production and variation in SPL across repeated recordings. *Journal of Speech and Hearing Research, 37,* 484–495.

Isshiki, N. (1964). Regulatory mechanisms of vocal intensity variation. *Journal of Speech and Hearing Research, 7,* 17–29.

Isshiki, N. (1981). Vocal efficiency index. In K. N. Stevens & M. Hirano (Eds.), *Vocal fold physiology* (Chap. 15, pp. 195–207), Tokyo: University of Tokyo Press.

Keilmann, A., & Bader, C. A. (1995). Development of aerodynamic aspects in children's voice. *International Journal of Pediatric Otorhinolaryngology, 31,* 183–190.

Kent, R. D. (1994). *Reference manual for communicative sciences and disorders.* Austin, TX: Pro-Ed.

Kitajima, K., Isshiki, N., & Tanabe, M. (1978). Use of hot-wire flow meter in the study of laryngeal function. *Studia Phonologica, 12,* 25–30.

Kunze, L. H. (1964). Evaluation of methods of estimating sub-glottal air pressure. *Journal of Speech and Hearing Research, 7,* 151–164.

Lieberman, P. (1968). Direct comparison of subglottal and esophageal pressure during speech. *Journal of the Acoustical Society of America, 43,* 1157–1164.

Lofqvist, A., Carlborg, B., & Kitzing, P. (1982). Initial validation of an indirect measure of subglottal pressure during vowels. *Journal of the Acoustical Society of America, 72,* 633–635.

Mead, J., Peterson, N., Grimby, G., & Mead J. (1967). Pulmonary ventilation measured from body surface movements. *Science, 156,* 1383–1384.

Melcon, M. C., Hoit, J. D., & Hixon, T. J. (1989). Age and laryngeal airway resistance during vowel production. *Journal of Speech and Hearing Disorders, 54,* 282–286.

Netsell, R., Lotz, W. K., Peters, J. E., & Schulte, L. (1994). Developmental patterns of laryngeal and respiratory function for speech production. *Journal of Voice, 8,* 123–131.

Rothenberg, M. (1973). A new inverse-filtering technique for deriving the glottal air flow waveform during voicing. *Journal of the Acoustical Society of America, 53,* 1632–1645.

Rothenberg, M. (1977). Measurement of airflow in speech. *Journal of Speech and Hearing Research, 20,* 155–176.

Schutte, H. (1980). *The efficiency of voice production.* Groningen, The Netherlands: Kemper.

Smitheran, J. R., & Hixon, T. J. (1981). A clinical method for estimating laryngeal airway resistance during vowel production. *Journal of Speech and Hearing Disorders, 46,* 138–146.

Sperry, E., Hillman, R. E., & Perkell, J. S. (1994). The use of an inductance plethysmograph to assess respiratory function in a patient with nodules. *Journal of Medical Speech-Language Pathology, 2,* 137–145.

Stathopoulos, E. T. (1986). Relationship between intraoral air pressure and vocal intensity in children and adults. *Journal of Speech and Hearing Research, 29,* 71–74.

Stathopoulos, E. T., & Weismer, G. (1985). Oral airflow and air pressure during speech production: A comparative study of children, youths, and adults. *Folia Phoniatrica, 37,* 152–159.

Tang, J., & Stathopoulos, E. T. (1995). Vocal efficiency as a function of vocal intensity: A study of children, women, and men. *Journal of the Acoustical Society of America, 97,* 1885–1892.

Thomasson, M., & Sundberg, J. (1997). Lung volume levels in professional classical singing. *Logopedics, Phoniatrics, and Vocology, 22,* 61–70.

Watson, P. J., & Hixon, T. J. (1985). Respiratory kinematics in classical (opera) singers. *Journal of Speech and Hearing Research, 28,* 104–122.

CHAPTER 11

Laryngostroboscopy

Bert Cranen and F. de Jong

Voice is an indispensible instrument in human communication. Therefore, evaluation of its characteristics is of major importance. Although voice quality has primary significance in the perceptual domain, it is clear that subjective judgments of both speaker and listener are to a large extent determined by the physical and physiological characteristics of the voice apparatus. Therefore, voice evaluation is not complete without a set of objective observations as well. This is particularly true in case a reason must be found why a specific voice does not have desired characteristics. Laryngostroboscopy is a convenient and affordable visualization technique that allows one to obtain that part of the information about the voice that reflects morphological properties and motion of the biomechanical structures involved.

For voiced speech sounds, the primary sound source is located at the vocal folds. Because of the periodic interruption of the airstream by the vibrating vocal folds, the kinetic energy of the airstream is (partly) converted into acoustic energy. If there were no vibrating folds, the stationary airstream from the lungs could escape without any noticeable sound.

The number of times per second the airstream is interrupted by the vocal folds corresponds to the fundamental frequency (F_0) of a sound. For adult males, this is generally around 100 Hz, for adult females around 200 Hz, and for children this may be as high as 400 Hz. The number of glottal closures per second determines the perceived pitch. The other acoustic characteristics, which are more related to voice timbre (like the relative amount of energy contained in the higher frequencies), are directly related to the exact way in which the vocal fold mucosa closes the glottis during each cycle. That large differences between individuals can be observed in the way vocal fold tissue moves, and consequently in the way glottal closure takes place, explains why there are so many different voices. Also the observation that voice characteristics differ with vocal register, frequency, and intensity of phonation and that factors like age, emotional state, and physical health also influence the voice can be understood from this perspective.

Clearly, a true understanding of voice quality requires knowledge of the vibratory behavior of the vocal folds. This knowledge can only be obtained by means of proper observation techniques. Of course, the acoustic product is not the only important aspect of voice production. The voice sound must also be produced without inflicting damage to the vocal folds. Such information can only be obtained by having a direct look at the way in which the vocal folds move.

The vocal fold motions are much too fast (one glottal cycle spanning only 2.5–10 ms) to be studied in detail with the bare eye. Without any extra instrumentation, the moving folds are perceived as a blurred image and special measures are needed to observe the vocal folds in slow motion. One way of achieving this would be to record the vocal fold image on some information carrier (film or other storage device) with several frames per glottal cycle (cf. Chapter 12 on high-speed filming). Playing the recordings afterwards with a reduced speed would give the desired slow-motion version suitable for human eyes to be perceived without blur. A technique that does not need an intermediate information carrier and can be applied in situ is stroboscopy. The principles of this technique and its applicability to voice examination are the subject of this chapter.

Laryngostroboscopy is a method designed to obtain an imaginary picture composed of many snapshots that are taken at cleverly chosen moments in different, subsequent cycles. In doing so, it is assumed that the subsequent cycles look very much alike—so that it makes sense to compose a virtual cycle out of many real ones. Thus, the technique relies rather heavily on the assumption that the vibratory behavior is quasi-steady. Provided this assumption holds (which is approximately true for sustained vowels produced by a healthy voice, but not necessarily for all types of pathological voices), the mucosal wave pattern of the vocal folds and its disturbances can be examined directly. In contrast to most other objective measurement methods such as electroglottography, photoglottography, and oral flow measurement that produce relatively indirect data about the mechanical motions of the vocal folds, laryngostroboscopic examination gives a direct view, and, therefore, is the method of choice to determine morphologic lesions of the vocal folds and their effects on the vocal fold motions. Nowadays, a clinical diagnosis without laryngostroboscopy is hardly conceivable.

1. PRINCIPLES OF LARYNGOSTROBOSCOPY: INSTRUMENTATION

Stroboscopy is a technique in which an object carrying out a periodic motion is illuminated by a pulsed light source. By a clever choice of the timing of the (short) light flashes, an optical illusion may be created that shows the object apparently frozen in its motion during a specific part of the cycle. Figure 11–1 illustrates this process when applied to a white disk with a black dot on it that rotates in a clockwise direction. If the disk is illuminated by a constant light source, the dot will appear as a blurry gray line on the disk. If a flash of light is produced each time the disk has completed 1 revolution, the observer can see the disk brightly lit only when the disk has returned to the same position and gets the impression the disk is standing still.

By constructing a dot detector and feeding its output to a Δf generator the flashing rate could be adjusted according to the rotational speed of the disk. If the disk makes, for instance, F_0 revolutions per second, the detector will yield a pulse train of F_0 Hz. Changing this frequency by means of the Δf generator to a slightly lower value will cause the time between two light flashes to be slightly longer than the time it takes to accomplish one revolution. In other words, the observer "sees" the dot moving slowly in a clockwise direction. The stoboscopic light has "converted" the process, which is actually going on into a slow-motion version, by using many images from subsequent cycles. The smaller the beat frequency (Δf), the slower the observed motion. It is important to realize that the motion observed under strobo-

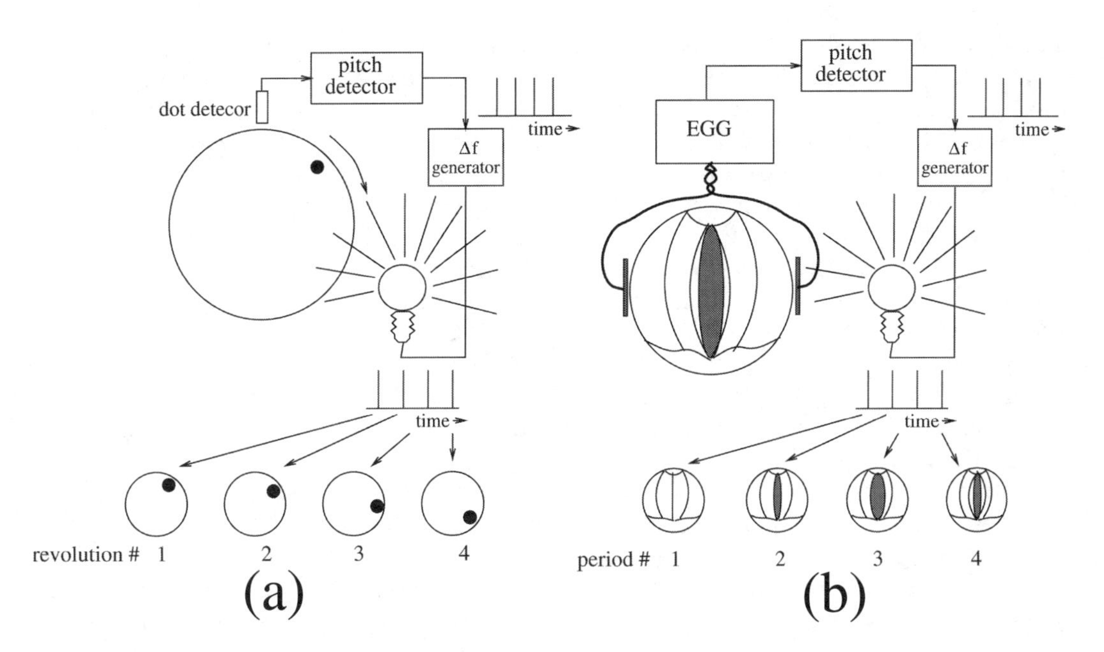

Figure 11–1. A fast periodic motion can be virtually slowed down by illuminating the object with a pulsed light source. The pulses must be generated at a frequency which differs a small amount Δf with that of the periodic motion. Both the slowly varying virtual images of the rotating disk (a) and of the vocal folds (b) are composed of snapshots that are taken from consecutive cycles. The smaller the value of Δf, the slower the virtual motion will be.

scopic light is not always a proper slow-motion version of the real process. For instance, if the light flashes are generated at a frequency slightly higher than F_0, the dot seems to move counter-clockwise.

When applying stroboscopic illumination to study the vibratory behavior of the vocal folds, it is generally referred to as *laryngostroboscopy.* The pulsed light beam can be directed to the vocal folds via a laryngeal mirror or via an endoscope (either rigid or flexible). The use of a mirror has the advantage of stereoscopic viewing the image and, consequently, 3-D perspective is better preserved. When a regular single-fiber endoscope is used, the 3-D perspective is lost, but the pictures can conveniently be stored by attaching a video camera to the eyepiece of the endoscope and recording the images on a videorecorder. Also, by storing the images electronically, further elaboration by digital image processing is possible.

The pictures of a flexible endoscope generally look slightly different from those of a rigid one. This is caused by the different choice of lenses: With a flexible endoscope, with a shorter distance between vocal folds and lens, a wide-angle lens is applied; whereas, with a rigid endoscope, a telescopic lens is preferred. Moreover, because a flexible endoscope cannot be made as thick as a flexible one, the amount of light that can be transported is less and, as a consequence, the colors of a picture taken with a flexible endoscope are generally less natural. Both the optical distortion and the color are properties of the instrumentation, but may easily become a source of misinterpretation if one is not aware of them. In particular, the optical distortion caused by a wide-angle lens makes it often very hard to decide on relative proportions, if the view axis of the endoscope is not exactly in the middle and perpendicular to the transverse plane. However, an important advantage of the flexible endoscope is that phonation during running speech can be properly examined. There is no need for pulling the tongue and possible elicitation of gag reflexes. Also, the flexible endoscope does not prohibit normal motion of the articulatory structures, although recent research seems to indicate that the presence of a flexible endoscope influences the acoustic characteristics of the voice source (Cranen & Norbart, 1997).

Without extra measures, no absolute dimensions can be derived from videostroboscopic images. However, ways can be found to use two endoscopes simultaneously (Fujimura, Baer, & Niimi, 1976; Sawashima et al., 1983). In that case, it is possible to obtain stereo images and to calibrate the equipment such that absolute dimensions can be obtained. In general, however, laryngostroboscopy is primarily used as a clinical tool that allows examination of the mucosal wave pattern of the vocal folds and its disturbances directly and instantaneously in a qualitative sense.

The time resolution obtained with stroboscopy is virtual. The image frames composing the slow-motion glottal cycle perceived by the eye are, in fact, from many different cycles. As a consequence, details of tissue motions within one glottal cycle are lost using laryngostroboscopy. Ultra-high speed photography yields a more accurate view of the vocal fold motions in the sense that it also allows study of individual glottal cycles. For a clinical setting, it will, in general, be too complicated and too expensive (although modern development of fast CCD cameras coupled to endoscopes may become a serious alternative in the future (Honda, Kiritani, Imagawa, & Hirose, 1987; Wittenberg, Moser, Tiggs, & Eysholdt, 1995).

Obviously, stroboscopy is an *event-triggered* observation technique and the quality of the images strongly depends on an accurate detection of the start of a new cycle. In most modern systems for laryngostroboscopy, the fundamental frequency F_0 is derived from either a laryngeal microphone signal or an electroglottogram signal. Both types of signals have in common that they only contain low-frequency components that make pitch detection more easy and reliable. The instantaneous frequency as found by the pitch detector is the primary factor in determining the exact moments at which the snapshots of the folds are taken and also serves as the prime determiner of the quality of the resulting images.

The beat frequency (Δf) between flash rate and fundamental frequency of the periodic motion of the vocal fold mucosa determines the speed with which the observer sees the mucosa move. To obtain a good impression of the vocal fold motion, the Δf is generally chosen in the range 0.5–2 Hz, so that a virtual glottal cycle takes 2–0.5 seconds. By making the frequency difference exactly zero, a static picture can be generated. When Δf is kept equal to zero and the phase angle at which the flash is generated is adjusted, a specific portion of the glottal cycle can be examined.

Assuming the pitch detection circuit works error-free under all circumstances, this feature can in fact be used to show whether irregularities in vibration of the vocal fold mucosa are present. By fixing the flashing rate at the phonation frequency, a completely static picture should result. If certain moving parts are observed anyhow, this points to the fact that these parts show erratic behavior that is not in sync with the light flashes, that is, with the fundamental frequency. Note, however, that if one cannot be sure about the correctness of the pitch markers, there is no way to decide to what extent the observed motion is due to the vocal folds or to the pitch detection circuit. This is a very realistic problem, because the concept of instantaneous F_0 (and thus the concept of instantaneous phase angle at which the snapshot must be taken) may become ill defined when there is too large a random component in the fundamental frequency. In such situations, the interpretation of the lack of stability in the images requires great caution.

In Figure 11–2, an (artificial) example is given of the position of a single point on a vocal fold as a function of time. For illustrative purposes, the excursion of the point is assumed to be an asymmetrical triangle. In the upper trace, 50 periods of a fold that oscillates with 100 Hz can be seen. In all following panels, this real motion is redrawn with a dotted line for reference. The parts of the real curve that coincide with the light flash (which is assumed to last 1 ms) are drawn with a fat line. These "samples" are

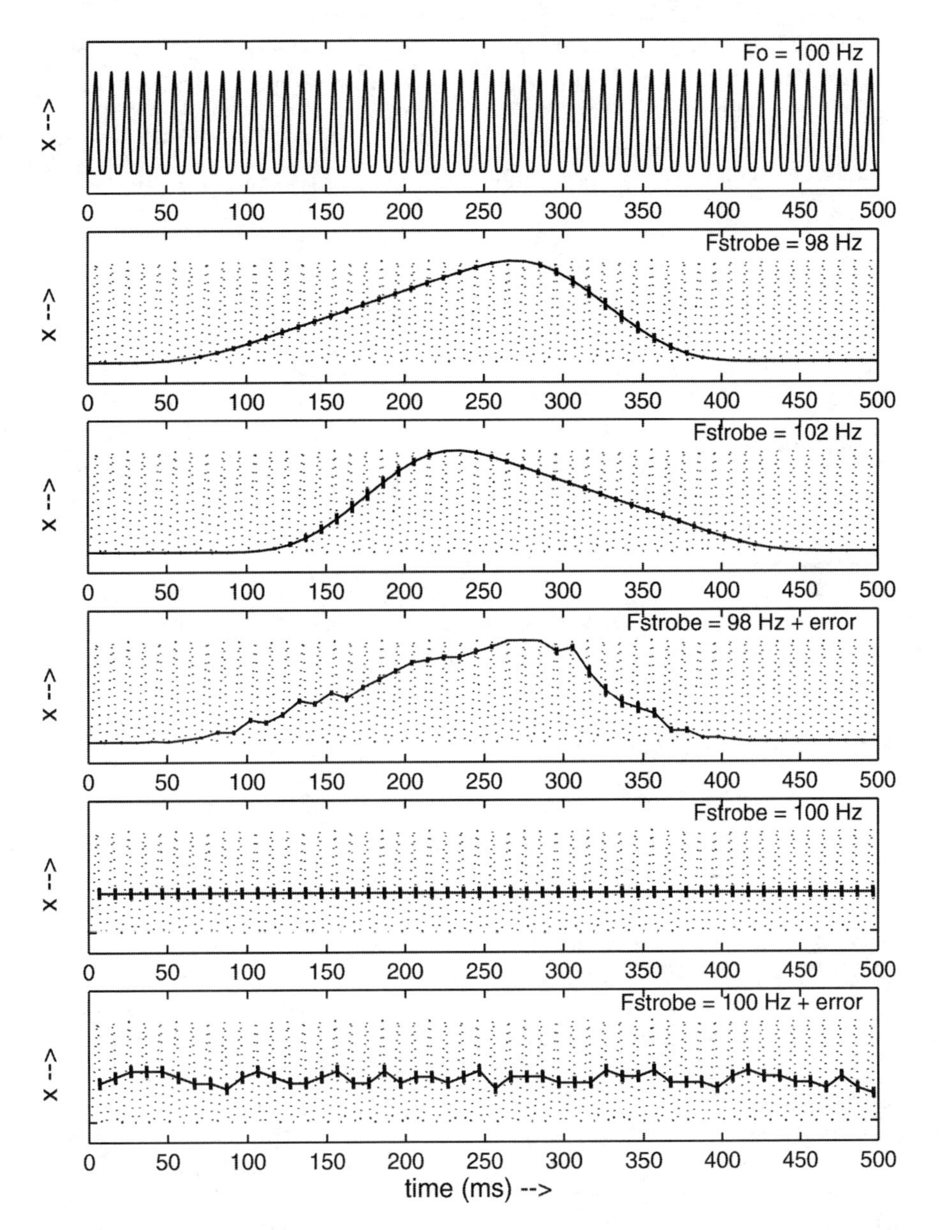

Figure 11–2. The quality of the image one obtains by means of stroboscopy depends strongly on the quality of the event detector (pitch detector) that is used to generate the light flashes. This figure illustrates by means of a computer simulation how the excursion (*x*) of a single point on one of the vocal folds would look like as a function of time, if the real motion has the shape of an asymmetrical triangle. From top to bottom, the panels show (a) the true periodic motion, 0.5 seconds of a purely periodic triangle waveform at a rate of 100 Hz; (b) the slow motion version when the strobe frequency is a constant 98 Hz; (c) the slow motion version when the strobe frequency is a constant 102 Hz; note that the waveform is reversed in time; (d) the slow motion version when the strobe frequency contains a random jitter component; (e) the static picture that results when the strobe frequency exactly matches the F_0, that is, 100 Hz; (f) the unsteady picture resulting from a strobe frequency that matches F_0 but contains an additional random jitter component.

then connected with a normal connected line; this waveform represents the virtual slow motion curve that is obtained by means of stroboscopy. In the second panel, the result when the strobe frequency is 2 Hz lower than the actual phonation frequency can be seen. In the third panel, the direction of time seems to be reversed, because the strobe frequency is 2 Hz higher than the phonation frequency. In the fourth panel, the mean flashing rate is again 2 Hz lower than the phonation frequency, but now the positions in time of the flashes are distributed randomly around the correct point (stdv = 0.25 ms). In the fifth panel, the strobe frequency is chosen exactly equal to the phonation frequency and the timing of the flash is such that it occurs at 6.5 ms after the beginning of the cycle. Finally, in the last panel, the mean strobe frequency is again equal to the phonation frequency, but again the positions of the strobe pulses are distributed randomly around the correct points. What should be a static image (a point which does not move in time) now appears to exhibit a random motion around that point.

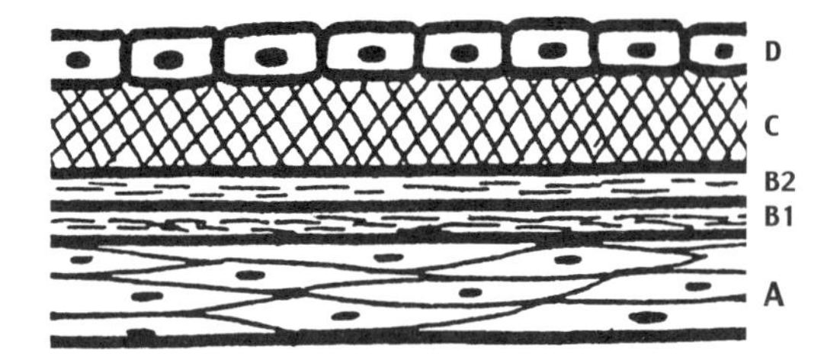

Figure 11–3. The multilayered structure of the membraneous portion of the vocal folds. The thyroarytenoid (vocalis) muscle (A) is covered by a ligamentous structure (vocal ligament) (B) that consists of a relative fibrous deep layer (B1) and a more elastic superficial layer (B2). A loose layer (Reinke's space) (C) separates the epithelial squamous cell layer (D) from the vocal ligament.

2. VOCAL FOLD VIBRATION AND SOUND PRODUCTION

The vocal folds are a multilayered structure (Figure 11–3). Their vibrating membraneous portion consists of five layers. The thyroarytenoid (vocalis) muscle is covered by a ligamentous structure (vocal ligament), which consists of a relative fibrous deep layer and a more elastic superficial layer. A loose layer (Reinke's space) separates the epithelial squamous cell layer from the vocal ligament. The Reinke's space enables easy movement of the epithelial layer, which is of crucial importance for adequate vibration.

Before the start of phonation, the vocal folds move from the respiration (abduction) position to the phonation position (adduction) by a simultaneous three-dimensional motion of the arytenoid cartilages (rotation, sliding, and rocking). At the same time, the vocal folds are appropriately tensioned by the action of the ricothyroid and thyroarytenoid muscles. During phonation, the vocal fold mucosa closes the glottis in a typical cyclic three-dimensional pattern (Figure 11–4). This mucosal wave pattern varies with frequency and intensity of phonation. The mucosal wave can exist by virtue of the loose coupling between epithelial layer and vocal ligament that is described in the body-cover theory of Hirano (1981) (also see Titze, 1994). Because the vibratory pattern of the vocal folds depends on the frequency and intensity of phonation, it is essential that laryngostroboscopic examination be carried out under various conditions of vocal pitch and loudness and that interpretation is being done taking this information into account.

In the transverse plane, the amplitude of the mucosal wave is largest at the mid portion of the vibrating vocal folds. The excursion of the mucosa at the anterior commissure and at the vocal processes is approximately zero. As a consequence, vibration of the vocal fold tissue in combination with a certain degree of abduction will cause closure to take place in a zipper-like fashion and in a ventrodorsal direction. In the coronal plane, the mucosal wave travels in a caudocranial direction: Closure starts at the lower lips of the vocal folds and next the folds make also contact at the midportion, and finally, the upper lips make contact. Depending on the phase difference between upper and lower lip, it may be that the lower lips start their outward movement even before the upper lips have completed their inward movement. Consequently, the folds may or may not be in contact over the entire glottal depth during part of the cycle. During laryngostroboscopy, this will be perceived as a reduced closed portion of the glottal cycle. Opening of the glottis occurs the other way around: It starts with a lateral outward movement of the lower lips, followed by the midportion, and subsequently by the upper lips.

It is important to realize that the motion of the mucosa, being the outer layer of the vocal folds and constituting the boundaries of the glottal air duct, is the primary factor in determining the aerodynamic and acoustic characteristics of the voice. The motion of the mucosal tissue determines how abrupt the airflow is interrupted and how long the glottis effectively remains open. Thus it is responsible for the spectral balance of the harmonics, that is, the specific timbre of the voice sound. This fact, combined with the observation that attachment of the epithelial layer to the vocal ligament, for instance, by fibrotic processes, inevitably results in a decreased voice quality, explains why laryngostroboscopic examinations are focused on visualization of the mucosal wave and on finding possible causes (lesions, muscle [mis]-adjustments, etc.) that might be responsible for preventing such a wave pattern.

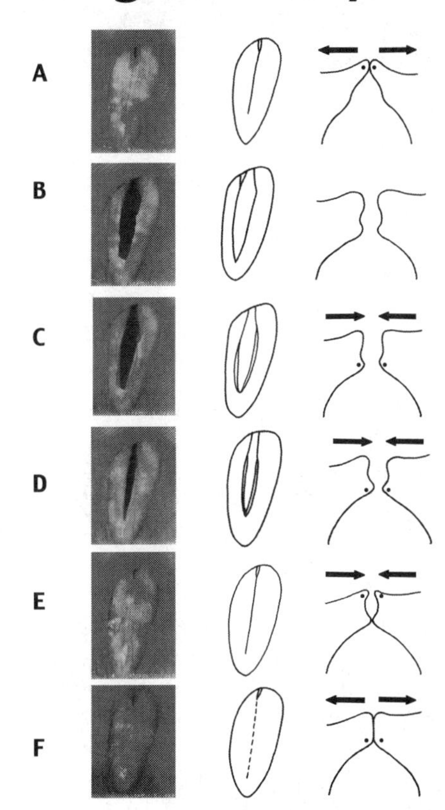

Figure 11–4. One glottal cycle, viewed by laryngostroboscopic examination. From left to right: photographic picture (transverse plane), schematic representation of the photographic picture and schematic view in the coronal plane. The dots indicate the level of the vocal folds at which most of the movement is taking place, with the arrows indicating the direction of movement. In A the end of the *closed phase* is depicted. The cranial edge is still making contact. Subsequently, the cranial vocal fold edges move laterally, initiating the *open phase*: B. In the *open* phase, the *phase of closing* starts with the medial movement of the caudal edge: C. In D the caudal edges almost touch one another. The *closed phase* starts when the caudal edges have made contact. The next stage is a medial movement of the cranial edges: E. In F the vocal folds make maximal contact and the glottis is maximally closed. The glottal cycle continues by lateral movement of the caudal edge, at the beginning of the *phase of opening* after which the situation in A is reached and the glottal cycle starts again.

3. INTERPRETATION OF LARYNGOSTROBOSCOPIC DATA

As may have become clear from the previous sections, drawing conclusions from a laryngostroboscopic examination requires more than just the practical skill to handle a laryngeal mirror or endoscope. First, it is impossible to interpret the images without combining the visual information with other sources of information. To decide which image details deserve special attention and which are irrelevant, one must have at least a basic understanding of the physics of the voice production process. Moreover, sufficient experience is needed to decide what part of all observed morphological and vibratory variation is normal and what is not and under what type of phonatory conditions. Second, insight is needed in the artifacts that may be caused by the instrumentation employed.

As pointed out earlier, the formation of the primary sound at the glottis depends on the specific wave pattern of the vocal fold mucosa that is induced by the passing airstream. A healthy larynx is fairly symmetrical. To obtain a good quality voice sound, the membranous portion of the vocal folds should close completely and vibrate in a periodic fashion, without too many irregularities. One of the tasks during a laryngostroboscopic examination is, taking into account any possible optical distortion caused by the equipment, to estimate the symmetry and degree of glottal closure in both the transverse (horizontal) and coronal (mediolateral vertical) plane. Furthermore, (lack of) periodicity may be assessed by adjusting the beat frequency to zero, mostly a special mode on the laryngostroboscope. In the case of a purely periodic motion, an unblurred, still picture must be expected; in the case of the vocal fold motion being irregular, (part of) the image will be blurred.

Another requirement for a good voice is that the vocal fold tissue does not act as a rigid structure. Rigidity generally causes a decreased and distorted mucosal wave amplitude and mostly results in a voice of bad quality. Especially when the stroboscopic images are recorded on videotape, a slow-motion review of the stroboscopic images allows a more detailed examination of the vibratory pattern of the vocal folds and the impact of vocal fold lesions on the mucosal wave pattern can be determined fairly easy. In the next paragraphs a number of lesions and the way they influence vocal fold motion are discussed. Because lesions of the vocal folds can best be considered from a functional point of view, the elucidation of the nature of voice disorders should preferably also be considered from a functional point of view, that is, by looking at the influence the lesion has on the vocal fold mucosal wave and on glottal closure.

3.1. Vocal Fold Mucosa Amplitude

Different mucosal wave amplitudes are observed in chest and falsetto register. In the chest register, the vocal folds are lax and the mucosal wave amplitude is large. In the falsetto register, the vocal folds are stretched and the anteroposterior distance of the larynx increases. Furthermore, the vocal folds become thinner and the mucosal wave amplitude decreases. As a consequence, the clinical significance of the magnitude of the mucosal wave amplitude is different for different phonation frequencies. A small amplitude is normal in high pitch voicing, but points at a sulcus glottidis, or vocal fold scarring, when occurring during low pitch voicing. Bowing of the vocal fold may be a feature of both vocal fold atrophy and glottal sulcus. A normal mucosal wave amplitude does not necessarily mean that the vocal folds are healthy, although. In case of vocal fold atrophy, the mucosal wave amplitude is normal during low pitch voicing as well.

It should be taken into account that the mucosal wave may be lesser in magnitude when there is insufficient glottal closure. When the folds are separated over a sufficient length, the intraglottal pressure profile will change in such a way that the aerodynamic forces acting on the vocal fold tissue decrease (reduced Bernoulli effect) because the velocities of the air molecules remain relatively low. Smaller excitatory forces may accentuate a possible disturbance of the mucosal wave in, for instance, vocal fold scarring and sulcus and insufficient glottal closure when associated with phonasthenia.

3.2. Vocal Fold Mucosa Irregularities

Vocal fold lesions usually cause a disturbance of the mucosal wave in combination with a smaller or larger glottal closure insufficiency. A different consistency of vocal fold lesion has, in general, a different influence on the mucosal wave. Moreover, it is also dependent on the frequency of phonation. Soft vocal fold nodules may be easily detectable at high frequencies, when the mucosal wave amplitude is small. However, at low phonation frequencies only a minor disturbance of the mucosal wave is visible. In contrast, firm vocal fold lesions influence the mucosal wave and glottal closure also in low-pitched voice to an appreciable degree, although they are more prominent in high-pitched phonation as well.

A global or localized disturbance of the mucosal wave, without distinct morphologic changes may point at a vocal fold cyst, sometimes deeply located. Thus, a disturbed mucosal wave pattern is helpful in establishing the indication for diagnostic cordotomy. Furthermore, laryngostroboscopic examination is very helpful in the diagnosis and follow-up monitoring of premalignant and small malignant lesions with respect to the determination of invasive growth.

3.3. Incomplete Glottal Closure

Incomplete glottal closure may have many different causes. Exophytic and intracordal lesions of the vocal folds can prevent the vocal folds from touching over the entire length and cause a leak at either side of the bulging. If the folds are not completely adducted posteriorly, there will remain a leak that may extend well into the membranous portion of the glottis. Both types of leakage will affect the abruptness with which the glottal airflow is interrupted, and, as a consequence, a negative effect on the acoustic voice quality must be expected. A frame-by-frame analysis of laryngostroboscopic images allows one to obtain a fairly accurate impression of glottal closure. In Södersten (1994), a system is proposed to rate glottal closure. This system is very useful in classifying various types of glottal closure insufficiencies.

However, a warning about this type of descriptive system is appropriate. Not all differences in glottal closure have equal impact on acoustic voice quality. In Cranen and Schroeter (1996) it was argued that a distinction must be made between a glottal opening that affects the abruptness of glottal closure and one that does not. This would mean that, from an acoustic point of view, it is important to adopt a scoring system that treats a glottal leak in the cartilaginous posterior portion of the glottis differently from one in the membranous portion that would require the identification of the vocal processes. Thus, it might appear useful to refine the Södersten system in such a way that the location of the vocal processes is explicitly taken into account.

3.4. Irregular Vibratory Behavior

The mucosal wave picture obtained by stroboscopic examination degrades severely in quality in case of irregular vocal fold vibration. It will be clear that if one chooses to make the (virtual) glottal cycle last 2 seconds, the number of real glottal cycles that are used to compose this virtual picture amounts at least 200. Obviously, the observed motion will only be smooth if the fundamental frequency of the phonation and the maximum excursion of the vocal folds is relatively constant over this entire time interval. If the frequency perturbation (jitter) becomes large or if the excursion of the vocal folds shows an appreciable amount of variation (shimmer), the excursion of the vocal folds in the separate images from which the virtual motion shows a large random component (either because the amplitude is sampled at relatively random phases in the glottal cycle or because the amplitude really showed a large random cycle-to-cycle variation).

Note that a degraded image quality does not necessarily reflect irregular vibratory behavior. It may also result when the stroboscope is not properly fed with information about the phonation frequency. In such a case the light flashes will also occur at more or less random phases within the glottal cycles and a jerky or even completely blurry picture will result (also cf. Figure 11–2). This may easily occur when the microphone/EGG electrodes are not appropriately positioned or when the corresponding signal that is fed to the pitch extractor is not adequately amplified.

4. COMMUNICATING ABOUT LARYNGOSTROBOSCOPIC EXAMINATIONS

To exchange information with other researchers or clinicians about specific findings during laryngoscopic examinations, as well as for the purpose of logging changes in the condition of a patient, it is important that a more or less standardized way of describing observations is agreed on. Extended protocols have been developed to describe the laryngeal morphology and mucosal wave pattern systematically (Hirano, 1981; Hirano & Bless, 1993).

These protocols normally consist of a checklist in which the findings can be noted by means of words, drawings, and numeric scores on a scale. For example, asymmetry of the position and shape of the arytenoid cartilages and vocal folds can be described, along with amplitude of the lateral movement of the vocal folds, and periodicity casu quo regularity of the mucosal wave pattern. Also, local disturbances of the mucosal wave pattern and the degree and shape of glottal closure can be documented in detail. Often these detailed lists contain over a hundred items.

Extended protocols are particularly of value for research purposes and very detailed comparison of the results of different treatments. In the routine clinical setting, however, filling in detailed protocols very often turns out not to be practical, and most of the more experienced practitioners do not really use them in daily practice. As a consequence, uniformity in scoring has not been established until now. In fact, it seems common practice to design a new protocol according to the demands of each new investigation.

5. SUMMARY AND CONCLUSIONS

The generation of the voice sound occurs at the level of the glottis and it is important to realize that the perceived voice quality is very dependent on the exact way in which the glottal geometry changes as a function of time. As this glottal geometry is determined both by the glottal settings at rest and by the mucosal wave pattern that is usually observed during phonation, it is obvious that a technique by means of which visual information can be gathered may be a powerful instrument in detecting problems with a specific voice apparatus. Laryngostroboscopy constitutes such a technique. It is the method par excellence to determine the implications of vocal fold lesions on the mucosal wave and glottal closure. Therefore, it is the most helpful tool in making clinical diagnosis and in decision making for therapy.

Looking for the first time at a pair of vibrating vocal folds makes one realize what an overwhelming amount of information is contained in images. Not all differences between larynges are equally important from an acoustic point of view, although. To pick out and describe the most essential cues, it is important to have a good understanding of the way in which the vocal folds interact with the passing air to generate the final sound that we call voice. Two possibly conflicting demands can be discerned. For efficient sound generation, it is of the utmost importance that the airflow is interrupted abruptly by the vocal folds. This is achieved best by letting the membranous parts of the vocal folds close "instantaneously" over their entire length. However, keeping in mind that at least 100 collisions per second are required during phonation, it is clear that the collisions must take place without exerting too much force on the vocal folds themselves (and certainly no localized forces), because this might lead to tissue damage. Describing laryngostroboscopic images should therefore focus on those aspects that are known to matter from a production point of view. As vibratory behavior may change quite appreciably with phonation condition (pitch, loudness, vocal register, etc.), it is important that a laryngostroboscopic examination includes several phonatory tasks and that a report clearly states which observations were made under what type of conditions.

REFERENCES

Cranen, B., & Norbart, T. (1997, May). *The effect of a flexible endoscope on the acoustics of the voice source.* Paper presented at the First International Conference on Voice Physiology and Biomechanics, Evanston, IL.

Cranen, B., & Schroeter, J. (1996). Physiologically motivated modelling of the voice source in articulatory analysis/synthesis. *Speech Communication, 19,* 1–19.

Fujimura, O., Baer, T., & Niimi, S. (1976). A stereofiberscope with a magnetic interlens bridge for laryngeal observation. *Journal of the Acoustical Society of America,* 65, 478–480.

Hirano, M. (1981). *Clinical examination of the voice.* Berlin: Springer Verlag.

Hirano, M., & Bless, D. M. (1993). *Videostroboscopic examination of the larynx.* San Diego: Singular Publishing Group.

Honda, K., Kiritani, S., Imagawa, H., & Hirose, H. (1987). High-speed digital recording of vocal fold vibrations using a solid-state image sensor. In T. Baer, C. Sasaki, & K. Harris (Eds.), *Laryngeal function in phonation and respiration* (pp. 485–491). Boston: College-Hill Press.

Sawashima, M., Hirose, H., Honda, K., Yoshioka, H., Hibi, S. R., Kawase, N., & Yamada, M. (1983). Stereoendoscopic measurement of the laryngeal structure, In D. M. Bless & J. H. Abbs (Eds.), *Vocal fold physiology: Contemporary research and clinical issues* (pp. 264–276). San Diego: College-Hill Press.

Södersten, M. (1994). *Vocal fold closure during phonation.* (Studies in Logopaedics and Phoniatrics, Vol. 3). Huddinge, Sweden: Huddinge University Hospital.

Titze, I. R. (1994). *Principles of voice production.* Englewood Cliffs, NJ: Prentice Hall.

Wittenberg, T., Moser, M., Tiggs, M., & Eysholdt, U. (1995). Recording, processing, and analysis of digital high-speed sequences in glottography. *Machine Vision and Applications, 8,* 399–404.

CHAPTER 12

High-Speed Digital Image Recording for Observing Vocal Fold Vibration

Shigeru Kiritani

For the study of voice-source characteristics, it is essential to analyze the relationship between the pattern of the vocal fold vibration and the acoustic characteristics of the speech signal. In the past, the observations of vocal fold vibration were generally carried out by means of high-speed motion picture systems (Farnsworth, 1940; Moore, White, & Liden, 1964). However, high-speed motion picture systems were usually massive. To obtain results from a frame-by-frame analysis of exposed film was also time-consuming. Thus, motion picture systems were not suited for flexible data collection covering various phonation types, including pathological cases.

To overcome these difficulties, a method of high-speed digital image recording has been developed (Honda, Kiritani, Imagawa, & Hirose, 1987; Imagawa, Kiritani, & Hirose, 1987). The system employs a solid-state image sensor and a digital image memory. In this system, the output video signal from the image sensor is fed into the image memory through an A/D converter. The stored data are then reproduced as a slow-speed motion picture. Compared to high-speed motion picture systems, a digital image recording system is compact and easy to handle. A simultaneous recording of the speech and other signals, such as EGG, can be performed easily.

In our original pilot system, it was necessary to restrict the number of pixels in the image to achieve a high frame rate. The frame rate was 2,500 frames per second with 126 × 32 pixels. At present, owing to advances in electronic technologies, a system with a higher frame rate and higher resolution is commercially available (Fastcam, Photoron Co. Ltd., Tokyo). The system enables image recording at a rate of 4,500 frames per second with an image size of 256 × 256 pixels. In the following, the performance of the present high-speed digital imaging system will be described, and examples of the images of vocal fold vibration recorded by it, both normal and pathological, will be presented.

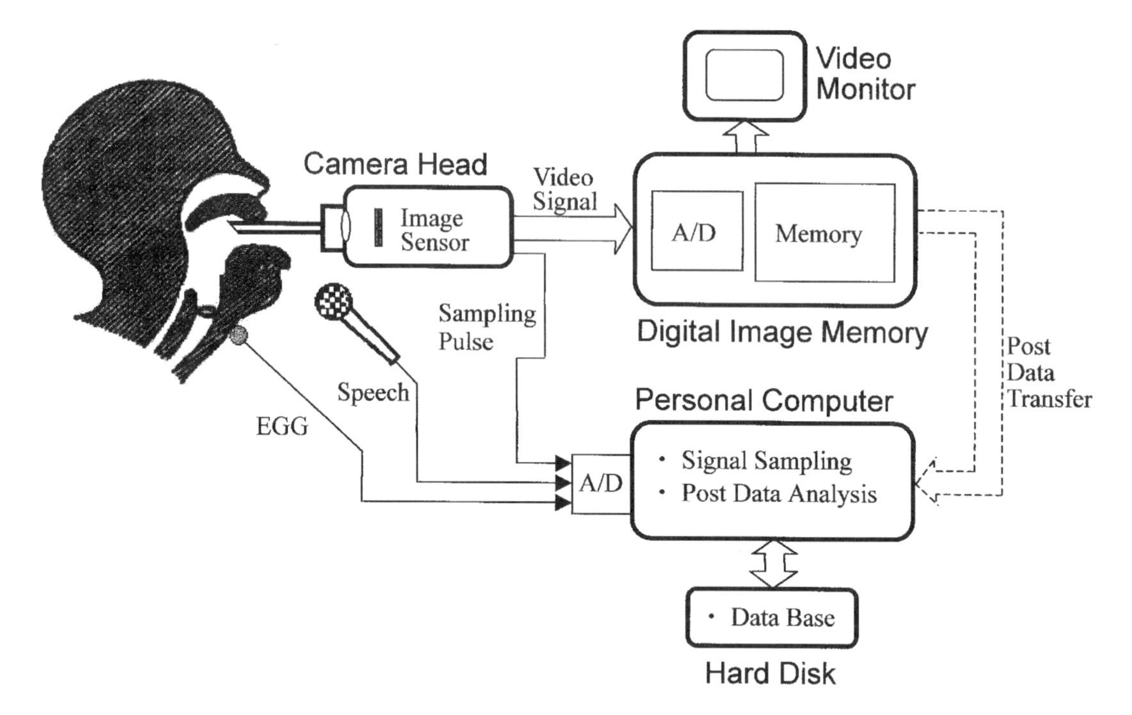

Figure 12–1. Block diagram of our high-speed digital image recording system using a solid endoscope.

1. PERFORMANCE OF THE HIGH-SPEED IMAGING SYSTEM

Figure 12–1 shows a block diagram of our high-speed digital image recording system for observing vocal fold vibration. The system consists of a camera head and a digital image memory. For laryngeal image recording, either an obliquely angled solid endoscope or a flexible fiberscope is attached to the camera head. The output video signals from the image sensor are fed into the digital image memory through A/D converters. The stored data are then reproduced on a video monitor as a slow motion picture.

The camera head contains a special solid-state image sensor specially designed for high-frame rate image recording (Figure 12–2). The sensor contains 256 × 256 picture elements, and, to achieve a high frame rate, the sensor incorporates a parallel read-out of image signals in its pixels (16 parallel channels).

The frame rate of the image recording varies according to the number of pixels used. When the full 256 × 256 pixels are used, the resulting frame rate is 4,500 per second. When the number of pixels is restricted to 256 × 128, the frame rate is 9,000 per second. The video signal is quantized in 8-bit units. The digital image memory can contain a maximum of 192 M Bytes of memory, which can store 3,000 frames of 256 × 256 images (image data from 0.7-second phonation at a frame rate of 4,500 per second).

The digital image memory can be operated as a stand-alone, ordinary video recorder. Data recording is usually done in a pretrigger mode. When the system is set at "READY," the video signal from the camera head is continuously sampled and stored in the image memory, which serves as a cyclic, endless-memory buffer. During this mode, the image on the video monitor is refreshed every 0.1 second. By monitoring this image, the experimenter can adjust the positioning of the scope, and then the subject can start phonation. When the experimenter presses the "RECORD" button, the sampling of the video signal stops and the image data in the memory at that moment is frozen, and the slow-motion display starts.

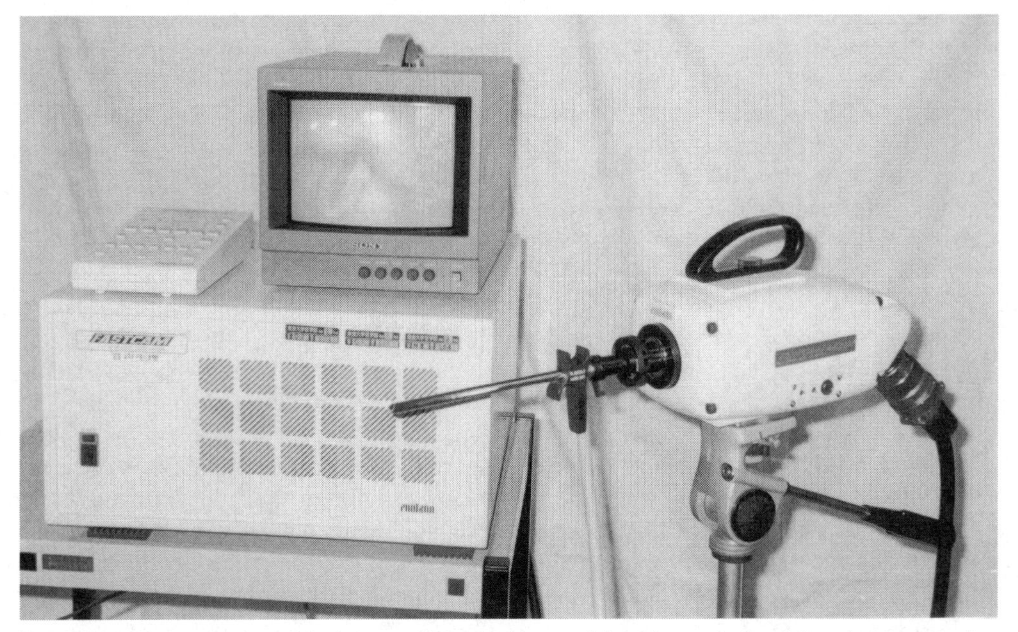

Figure 12–2. A picture of the camera head with an obliquely angled solid endoscope and a digital image memory with a video monitor.

Thus, the image data from a certain time interval just preceding the pressing of the record button is memorized in the digital image memory. The slow motion display can be performed with functions such as PLAY at variable speed, FAST FORWARD, FAST REWIND, STILL, and REPEAT of selected time intervals.

In our system, the speech signal and the electroglottographic signals are recorded simultaneously with the image data using a separate personal computer. To synchronize the sampling of these signals and the image signal, sampling pulses for these signals are generated by down-sampling the master clock pulse in the camera system. When the frame rate is 4,500 per second, four sampling pulses are generated in each image-recording time frame. Consequently, the sampling rate is 18 kHz. For the purpose of later data analysis, the image data stored in the image memory are transferred to the personal computer and stored in its disk memory, together with the digitized data from the speech and EGG signals.

The essential factor that determines image quality in our system is the brightness of the image obtained through the laryngeal scope. At the author's laboratory, an obliquely angled solid endoscope (Type 4450.501, Richard Wolf FMBH, Germany) combined with a 300 W xenon lamp light source (Pentax 3000, Asahi Optical Co. Ltd., Japan) is now being used for the observation of sustained phonation. The outer diameter of the endoscope is 9.7 mm, and the effective diameter of the object lens is ~2.0 mm. This endoscope combined with the present high-speed image sensor has an effective view-angle of 50°, and the vocal folds can usually be imaged at a distance of 3–4 cm, approximately. For most subjects, this system makes it possible to obtain sufficient brightness for image recording at 4,500 frames per second with 256 × 256 pixels.

The use of a flexible fiberscope is indispensable for observing vocal fold vibrations during the production of consonants and/or during running speech. The image obtained through a flexible fiberscope is generally darker than that obtained from a solid endoscope. When a fiberscope is directly connected to the present system, the brightness of the image is not sufficiently high for high-speed image recording. However, the present system can be combined with an image intensifier, and image recording at a rate of 4,500 frames per second is now possible also for fiberscopic observations. The fiberscope used at our lab is an FNL-T15 (Asahi Optical Co. Ltd., Japan) and the light source is the same as that for the endoscope. The diameter of the scope is slightly larger than that for the ordinary clinical use (~4.9 mm); and the object lens is ~1.5 mm. The image intensifier used is of the Channel Plate Type (C6276-01, Hamamatsu Phototonics Ltd., Japan). The effective view angle of the combined system is 60°. The required light intensification factor is about 10. Since it is not so high, the resulting image degradation due to the use of the image intensifier is not significant.

2. EXAMPLES OF NORMAL VOCAL FOLD VIBRATION

2.1. Modal Phonation

Figure 12–3 shows an example of the laryngeal image recorded during modal phonation by a male subject. The image shows the glottis near the moment of its maximum opening. The figure shows that the edges of the vocal folds can be identified through a visual inspection of the image. Thus, the movements of the vocal folds can be measured through a visual inspection of the frame-by-frame display on the computer monitor.

To obtain a simplified measure of the movements of the vocal folds, an effective measure of the glottal width is defined as explained in the figure. Namely, in the glottal image, the area where the brightness is darker than a selected threshold is taken as the area of the glottal opening. A horizontal scan line is selected at an appropriate position on the glottis. By examining the brightness curve along this scan line and comparing it with the threshold value, the points of the right and the left edges of the glottal opening are determined. This measurement is repeated over successive time frames and the temporal course of the effective glottal width is displayed on the computer.

Figure 12–4 shows the speech signal, the EGG signal, the glottal width measure together with the glottal images of one vibratory cycle (A series of pictures displayed in the figure are of 128 × 128 pixels, which show a selected part

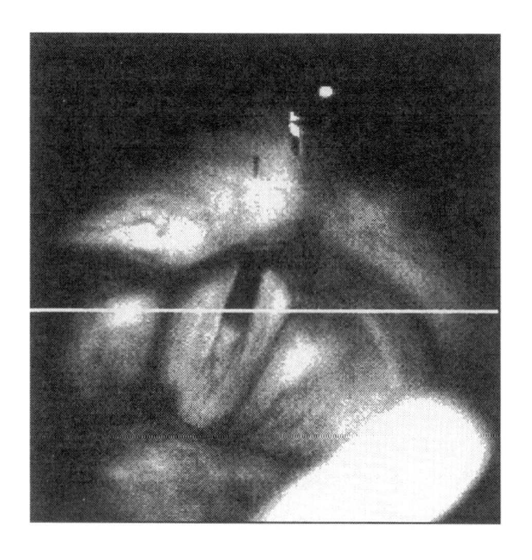

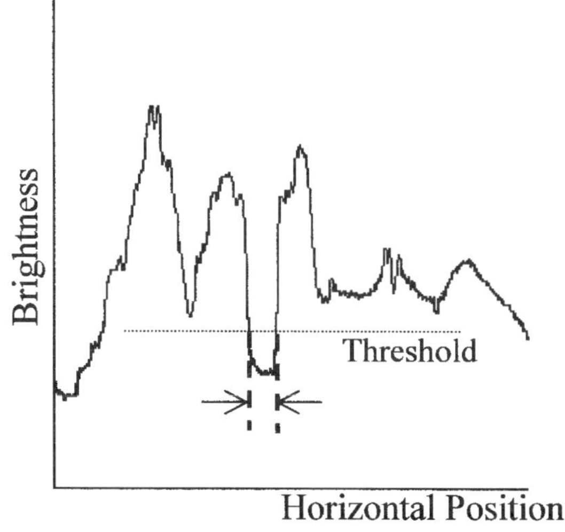

Figure 12–3. An example of the glottal image (256 x 256 pixels; 4,500 frames per second).

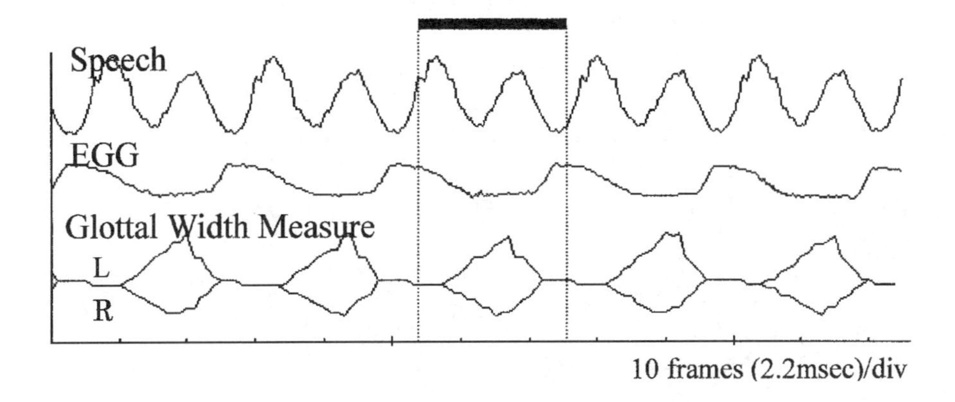

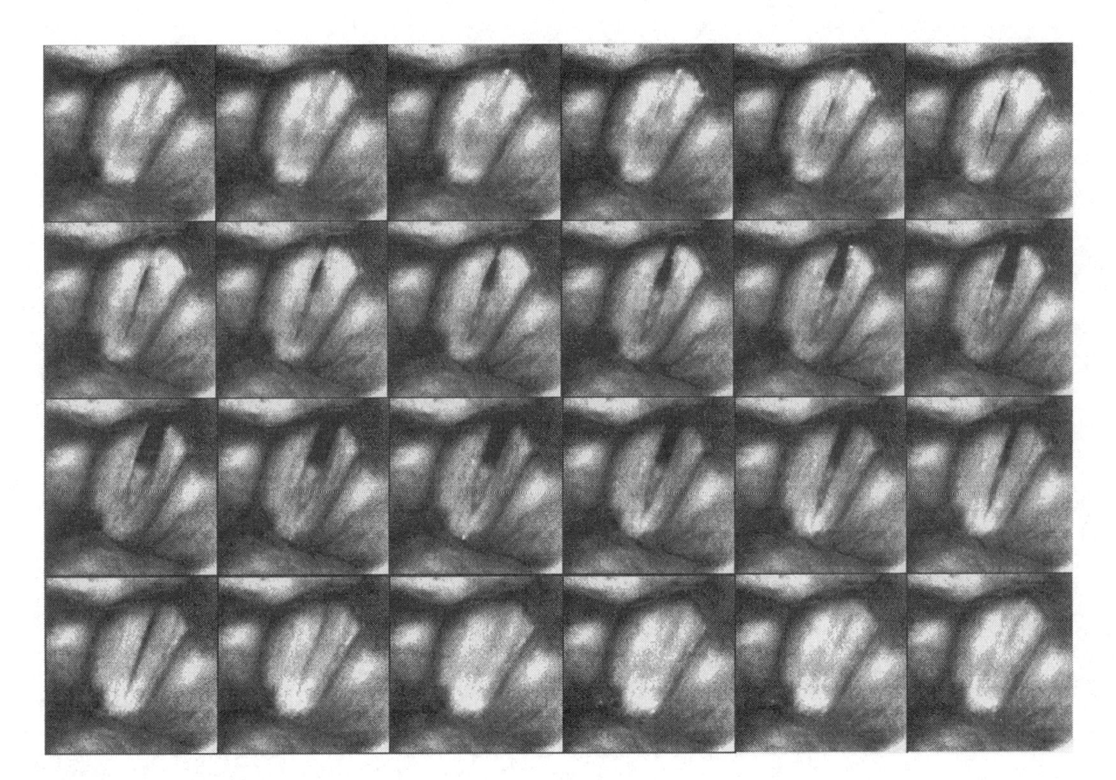

Figure 12–4. Vocal fold vibration for normal modal phonation.

in the original 256 × 256 pixel images. This is also the case for all the subsequent figures). The data shown here conform to the regular pattern of vibration in modal phonation. The vibration shows a relatively long period of closure (the open quotient is relatively small, 0.55 approximately), the moment of the glottal closure coincides with the rise in the EGG signal, which also corresponds to the point of excitation in the speech signal with a delay of approximately 2 ms.

2.2. Hard-, Ordinary-, and H-Attack

Figure 12–5 compares initiation of vocal fold vibration following hard-attack, ordinary-attack, and h-attack. In the case of hard-attack,

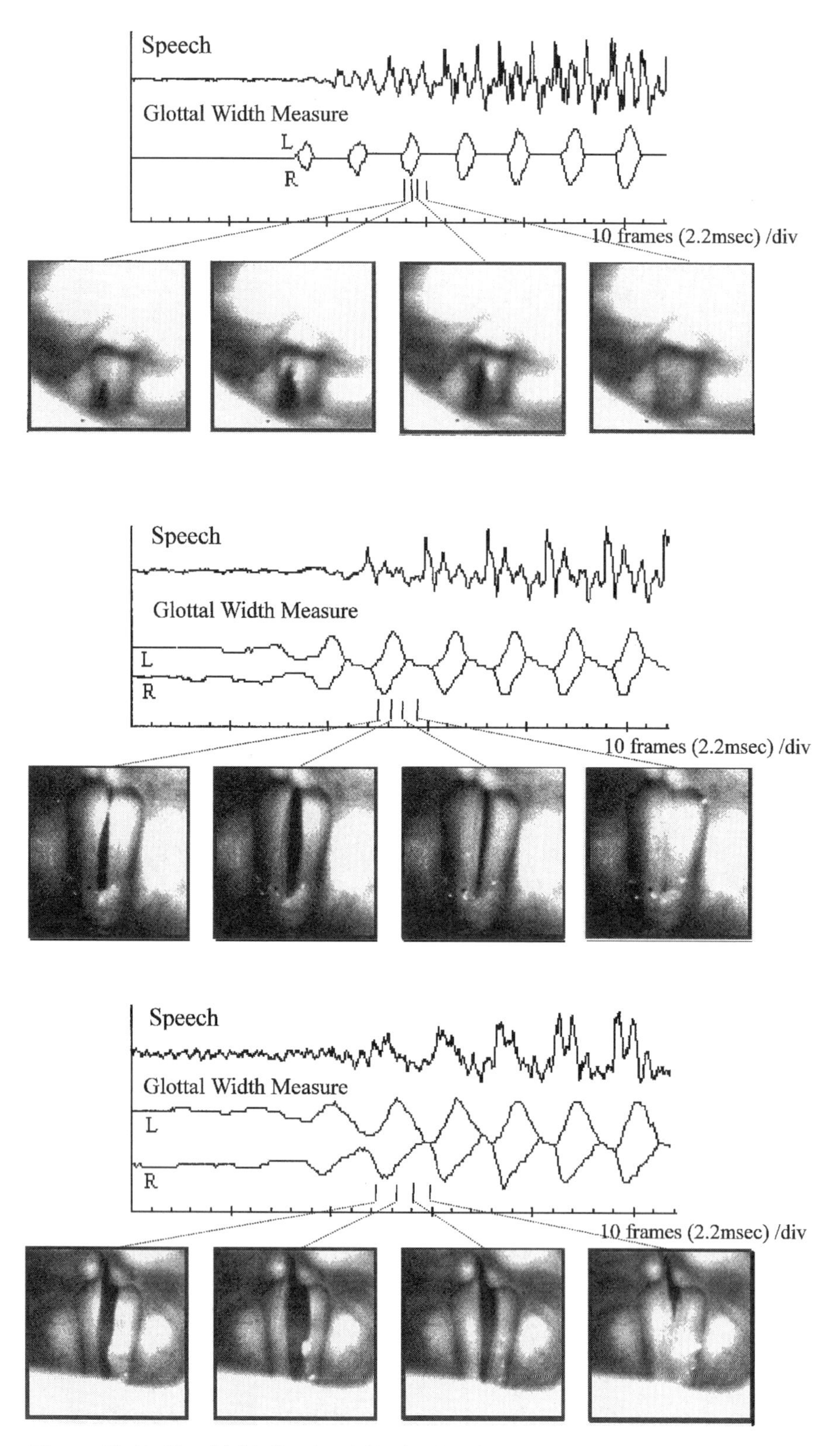

Figure 12–5. Vocal fold vibration following hard-, ordinary-, and h-attack.

the vocal fold vibration starts with the adducted vocal folds. In the first few cycles, the closed phase is long and the open quotient is very small (0.3 approximately). The glottal image shows that in this phonation, the laryngeal frame work is rather constricted. In the case of ordinary-attack, the vocal fold vibration starts with the abducted vocal folds. The first cycle of vibration does not achieve a closure of the glottis and, thus, does not produce a clear excitation in the speech wave. In the case of h-attack, the vibration starts with the vocal folds more widely abducted. In the first two cycles of the vibration, the left and right vocal folds do not make contact. As can be seen in the glottal images, even in the fourth vibration the right and left arytenoid cartilages are clearly separated, although, at the moment of the glottal narrowing, the anterior and middle parts of the left and right vocal folds, respectively, make contact with each other. The opening in the posterior end of the glottis is expected to contribute to the noise component in the speech signal.

2.3. Intervocalic [s] (A Fiberscopic Observation)

Figure 12–6 shows the vocal fold vibration associated with intervocalic [s] in the word [se:se:]. The glottal images in the figure were recorded using a flexible fiberscope.

The temporal course of the glottal width measure shows that during the transition period from the vowel [e] to [s], there are four cycles of vibration in which the vocal folds are not approximated enough to form a glottal closure. These vibrations do not seem to bring about an appreciable excitation in the speech signal.

As for the initiation of voicing after [s], vocal fold vibration resumes complete closure rather quickly. Although the glottal closure is incomplete in the first vibratory cycle, complete closure is generally observed from the second cycle. It should be noted that, in this cycle, the left and the right arytenoid cartilages are approximated and are already in contact with each other. This pattern of glottal activity is distinct from that which occurs during voice onset in the h-attack described above. In the case of h-attack, even when the vibration at the anterior part of the vocal folds becomes large enough to form a partial glottal closure, the left and the right arytenoid cartilages are still separated. This pattern of vocal fold vibration has also been confirmed through fiberscopic observation for the production of intervocalic [h] in Japanese (Kiritani, Hirose, & Imagawa, 1996).

3. ABNORMAL VIBRATION

3.1. Breathy phonation

Figure 12–7 shows the vocal fold vibration associated with breathy voice. The subject had palsy of the left vocalis muscle and his voice gave a perceptual impression of "breathy" and "asthenic" (here and in the following, the terms "breathy," "asthenic," and "rough" are used according to the concept proposed by the Japan Association of Logopedics and Phoniatrics (Hirano, 1979). The glottal images in Figure 12–7 reveal that, during the vibration, the glottal closure is weak and incomplete. Corresponding to this incomplete glottal closure, the speech wave indicates a lack of higher frequency components.

It should be noted that, in this example, the left and right arytenoid cartilages are approximated and the posterior end of the glottis is closed. It has generally been acknowledged that, in some types of breathy phonation, the arytenoid cartilages are separated as in h-attack as described above (Kiritani, Hirose, & Imagawa, 1993). The pattern of vocal fold vibration shown here is different from that following h-attack. It appears that the incomplete glottal closure observed in Figure 12–5 is primarily due to a lack of the tension in the vocal folds.

3.2. Left-Right Imbalance: A Case of Diplophonia

It is well known that many cases of "rough" voice are characterized not by simple random perturbations but by quasi-periodic perturba-

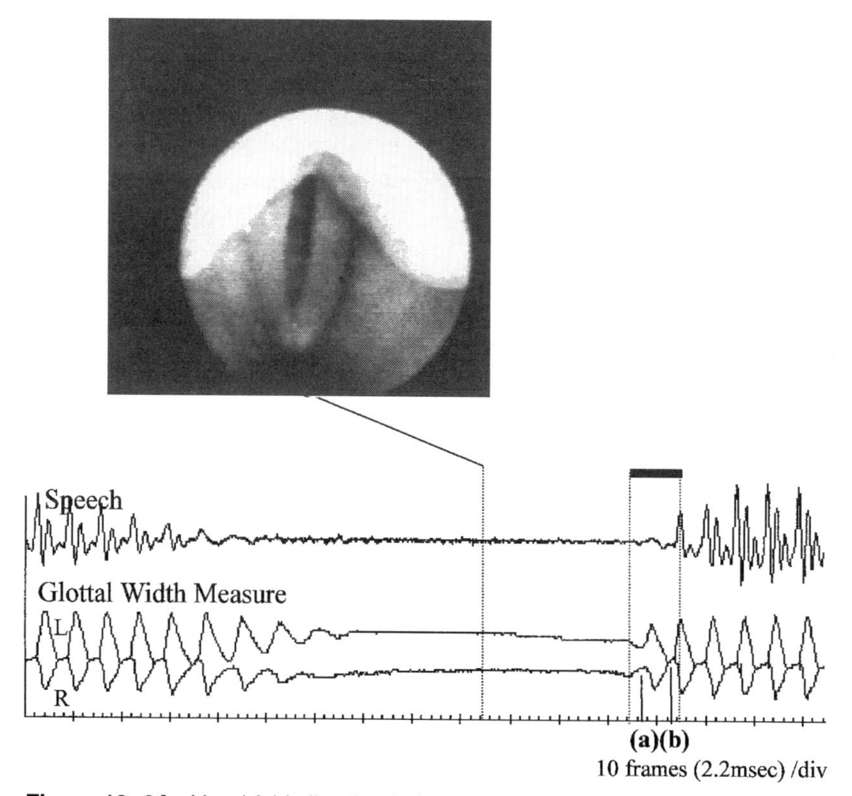

Figure 12–6A. Vocal fold vibration in intervocalic [s] (fiberscopic observation).

tions in vocal fold vibration. In some cases, these voices are perceived as diplophonia. The period of quasi-periodic perturbation is sometimes as long as 5–10 fundamental vibratory periods. Figure 12–8 shows such an example of a subject with a vocal-fold cyst.

The speech signal shows quasi-periodic variations in the amplitude and waveform, which repeat at intervals of about 10 vibratory cycles. The temporal course of the glottal width measure reveals that the left and the right vocal folds vibrate apparently at different frequencies and that the phase difference between the movements of the two vocal folds varies with time. At around A, the movements of the vocal folds are nearly in phase, and the glottis shows a period of complete closure. In the following cycles, the phase difference between the vocal folds become larger, and the glottal closure becomes incomplete. At around B, the phase difference is nearly 180°, and the left and right vocal folds move almost in parallel. Then, for the left vocal fold, one cycle of the outer movement almost disappears. This process cancels and resets the phase difference between the two vocal folds. At this point, the left and right vocal folds resume their synchrony, and the vibration again shows a period of glottal closure. Thus, during this time interval, the right vocal fold has 10 vibratory cycles and the left vocal fold has 9 vibratory cycles.

The temporal change in the pattern of the vocal fold vibration just described explains the pattern of the temporal change in the speech waveform. At around A, where the vocal fold vibration exhibits complete closure, there is a strong excitation pattern in the speech waveform. The amplitude is large, and the formant oscillations are clear. When the glottal closure becomes incomplete, the excitation becomes weaker. The waveform is noisy, and its amplitude becomes smaller.

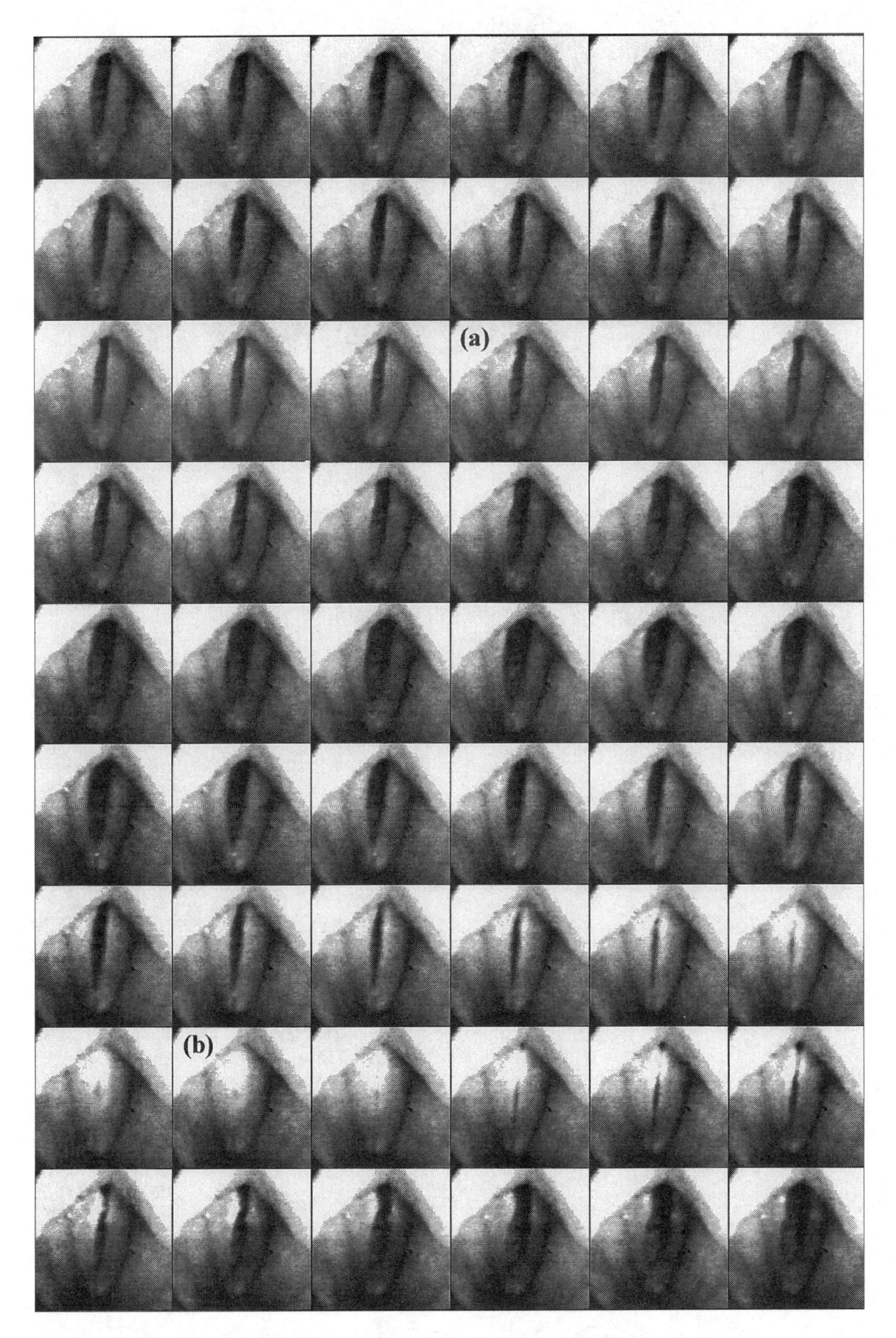

Figure 12–6B. Vocal fold vibration in intervocalic [s] (fiberscopic observation).

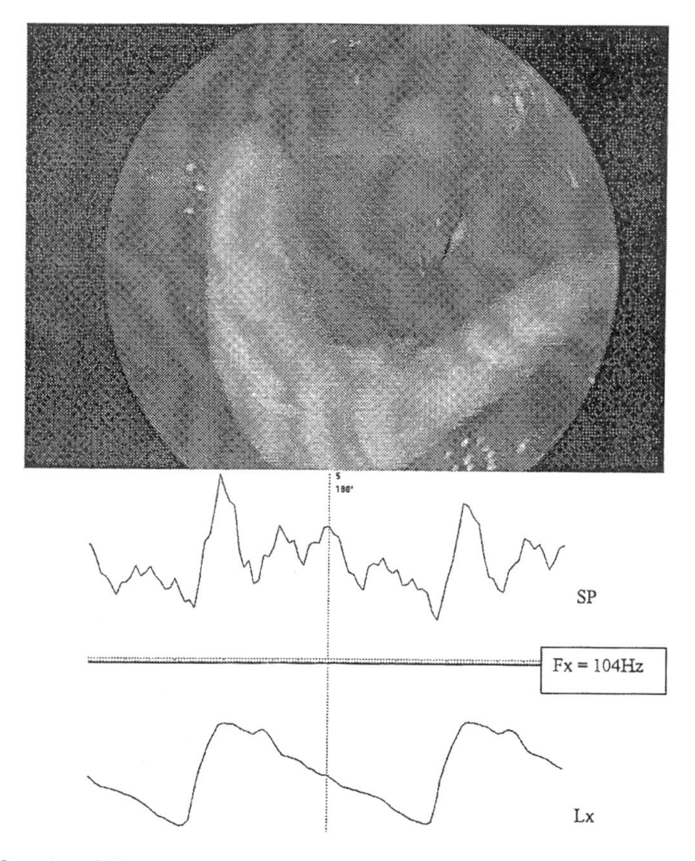

Figure 12–7A. Speaker SK1 Acute Laryngitis. The view has been taken, as shown by the trigger marker, midway between two closures in what would ordinarily be a well defined open phase. The speech and laryngograph waveforms are at the modal frequency.

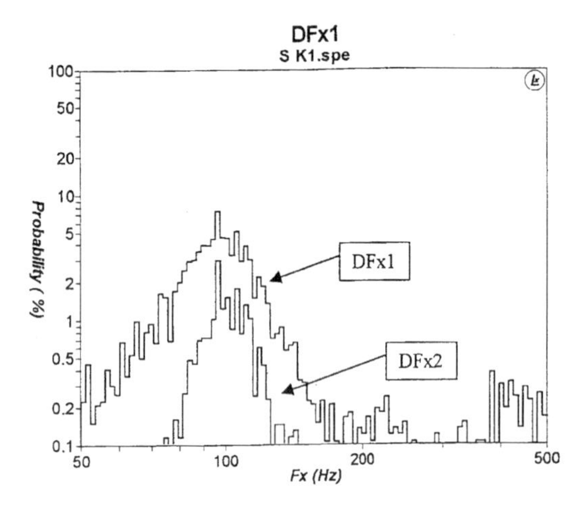

Figure 12–7B. DFx1,2. The basic larynx frequency distribution, DFx1, based on a 2-minute sample of connected speech, is wide and ill-formed. The second order distribution, DFx2 using the same recording, shows by its height and shape that there is a core of well-structured voice of potentially good quality.

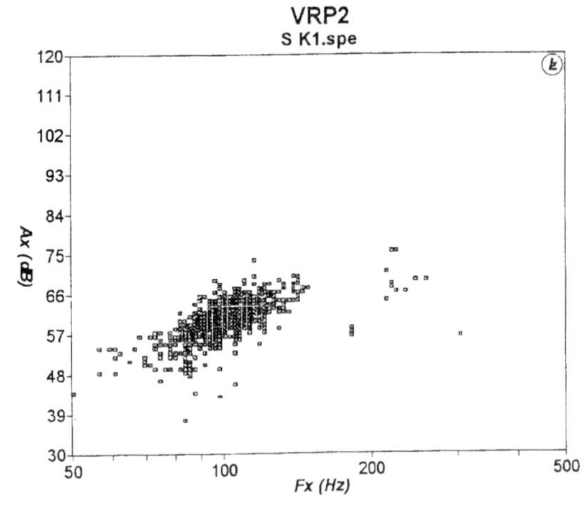

Figure 12–7C. VRP2. The standard first order phonetogram for this speaker is very dispersed in both frequency and intensity. This second order phonetogram, which only shows those pairs of periods falling in the same Ax/Fx bin, indicates the existance of a core of voice regularity now in intensity as well as larynx frequency.

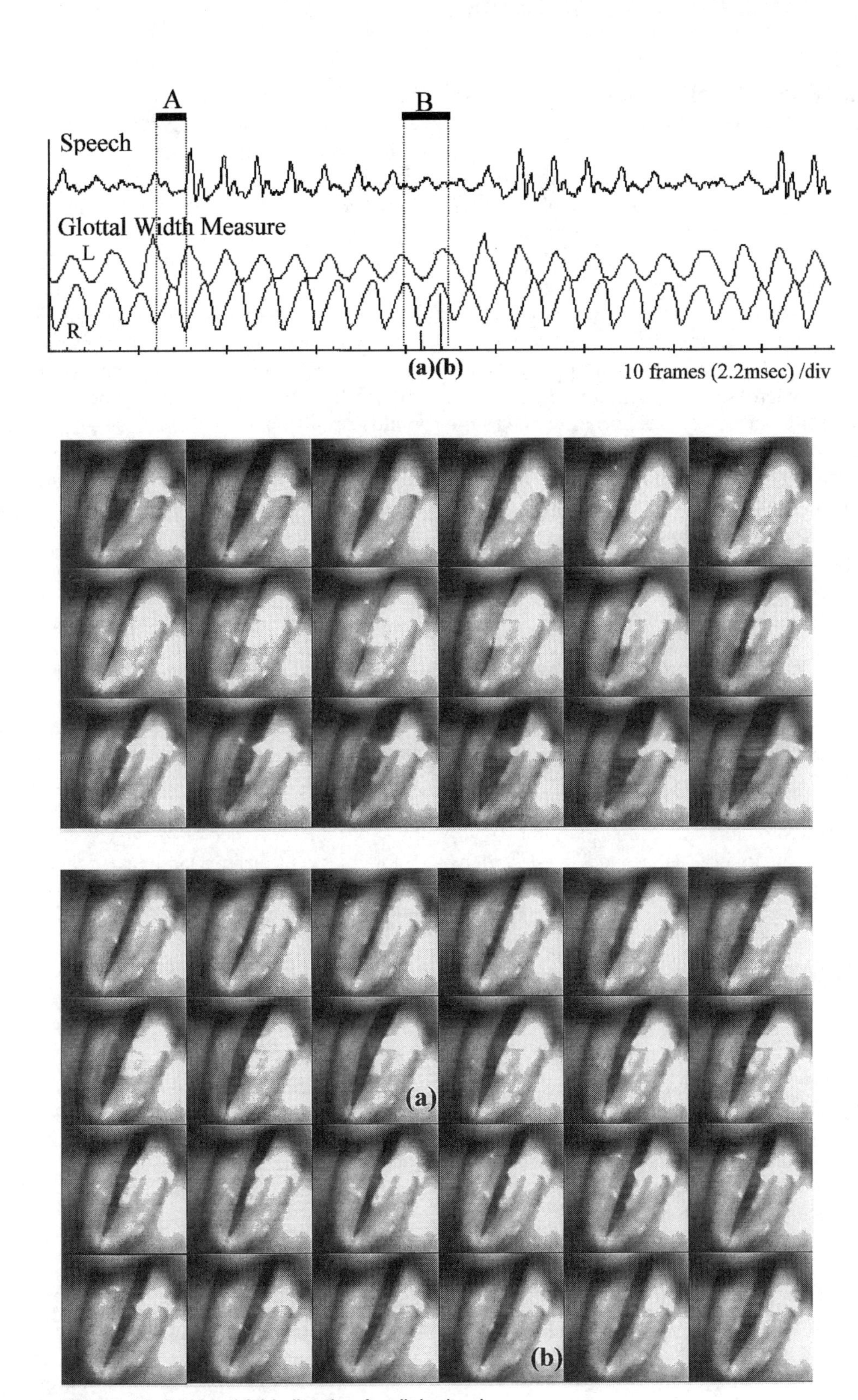

Figure 12–8. Vocal fold vibration for diplophonia.

3.3. Front-Back Imbalance: A Case of Rough Voice

The vocal fold vibration shown in Figure 12–9 displays different characteristics of vibration between the anterior and the posterior part of the glottis. The subject in this case had partial laryngeal palsy. In Figure 12–9, the glottal width measures for the three scan lines at different positions of the glottis are shown. In the anterior portion, the vibration appears nearly regular, whereas in the posterior part, it shows a bifurcate pattern. This is primarily due to the movement pattern of the left vocal fold. The movement of the posterior part of the left vocal fold is smaller at every other cycle, which results in an incomplete closure at every other cycle at the posterior part of the glottis.

This vibration pattern might be conceptualized as follows. If we take the characteristic frequency of the vibration in the anterior portion as F_0, the characteristic frequency in the posterior portion of the left vocal fold seems to be smaller, say $^1/_2\ F_0$. However, through interaction with the other portions of the vocal folds the vibration at F_0 frequency is also partially excited in the posterior portion, resulting in a bifurcate vibration. More quantitative biomechanical analysis is needed to clarify the mechanisms of this kind of vibration.

3.4. Vocal Fry

Figure 12–10 shows the vocal fold vibration associated with vocal fry. They were recorded in two separate sustained phonations. The voices were produced by a normal subject who tended to produce vocal fry when the pitch was lowered during conversational speech. He was also able to produce vocal fry in sustained phonation. Figure 12–10A shows a large fluctuation in the pitch period. However, this fluctuation is mostly due to the variation in the duration of the closure period. From time to time, the closure period becomes very long. It appears that in this phonation the vocal folds tend to stay in a closed position. (Note that in this example, the view of the left vocal fold is partially concealed by the false vocal fold, and the glottal width measure does not give correct information.)

In Figure 12–10B, the vocal fold vibration shows many bifurcate and arifurcate patterns. In these cases, the vibration in the first cycle is weak in that the amplitude of the glottal opening is small and the glottal closure is incomplete. In the following cycles, the vibration is stronger and is followed by a glottal closure. Once a complete glottal closure is formed, the closure period tends to be lengthy. It appears that in this type of phonation, the oscillation builds up in the several successive cycles and when the oscillation becomes sufficiently large the vocal fold vibration shows closure and falls into the lengthy closure period (Whitehead, Metz, & Whitehead, 1984).

4. COMMENTS

The laryngeal images presented in this chapter show that the present high-speed digital image recording system can provide useful information for studying vocal fold vibration in various voice qualities. However, there are a couple of technical points on which further progress can be expected. One is color image recording. For color image recording, laryngeal images with higher brightness and/or an image sensor with higher sensitivity than those presently used are necessary. From the point of view of current CCD technology, it will not be a difficult task to construct an image sensor with higher sensitivity. Another point is the development of a program for the quantitative and automatic measurement of the glottal opening. Such progress will further increase the usefulness of the high-speed digital imaging system in the study of the voice quality (Kiritani et al., 1993).

Acknowledgment

Data collection for the various phonation types was conducted at the author's laboratory in cooperation with Professor Seiji Niimi. Special thanks are due to him for his help in preparing this manuscript.

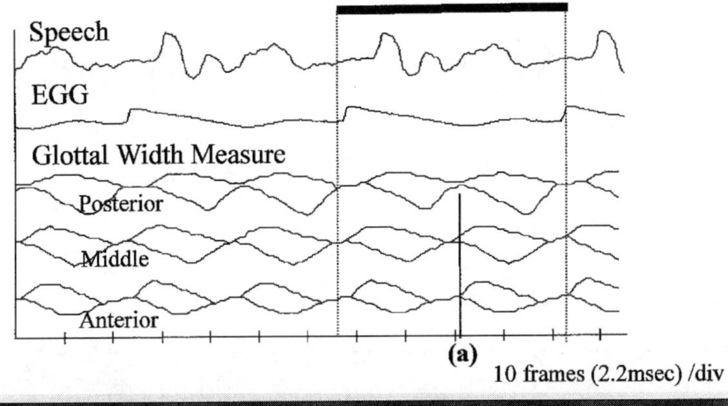

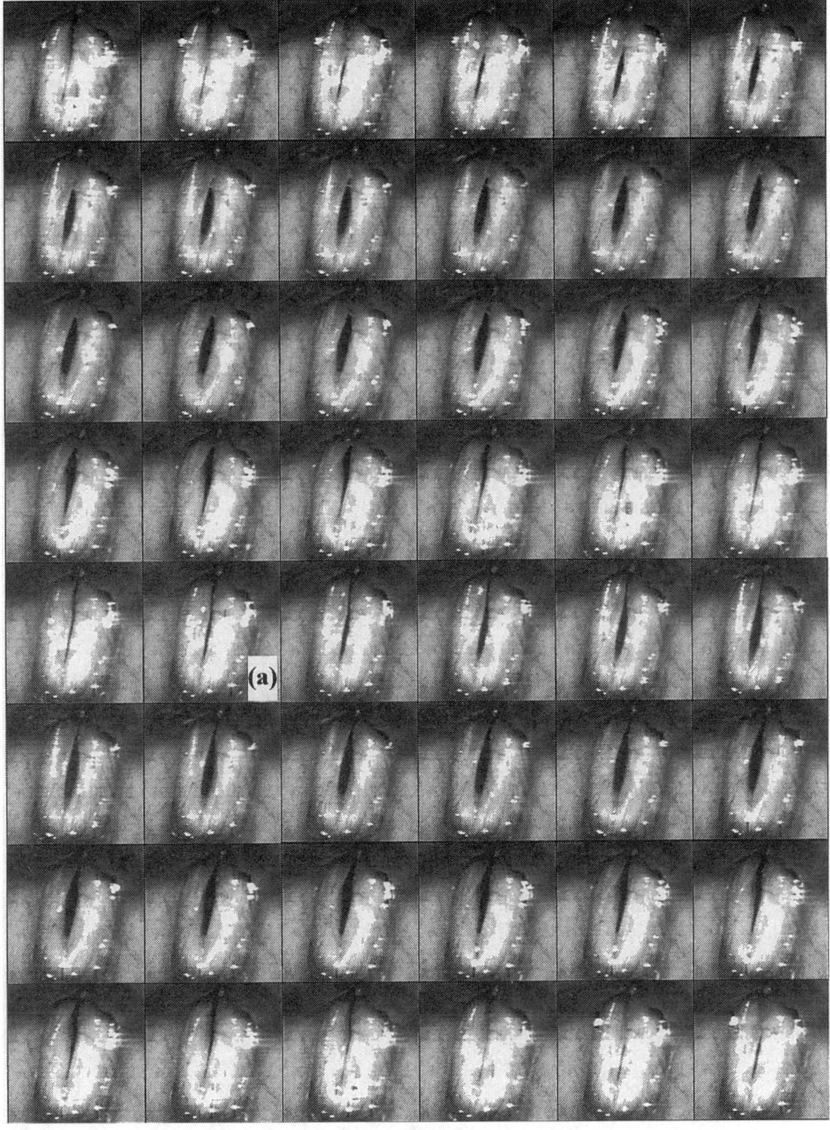

Figure 12–9. Vocal fold vibration for rough voice.

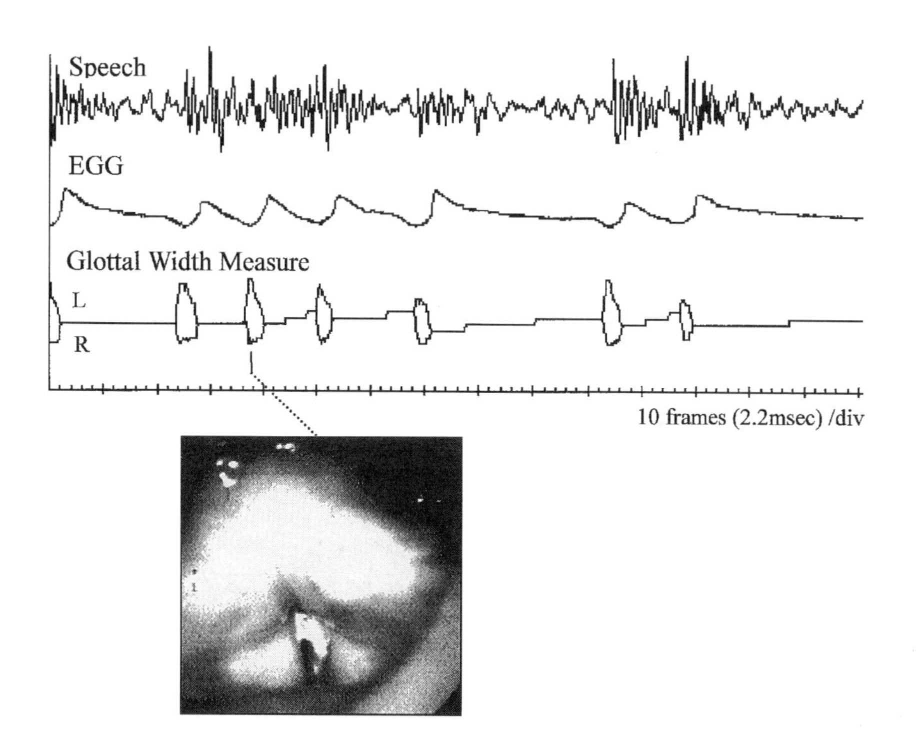

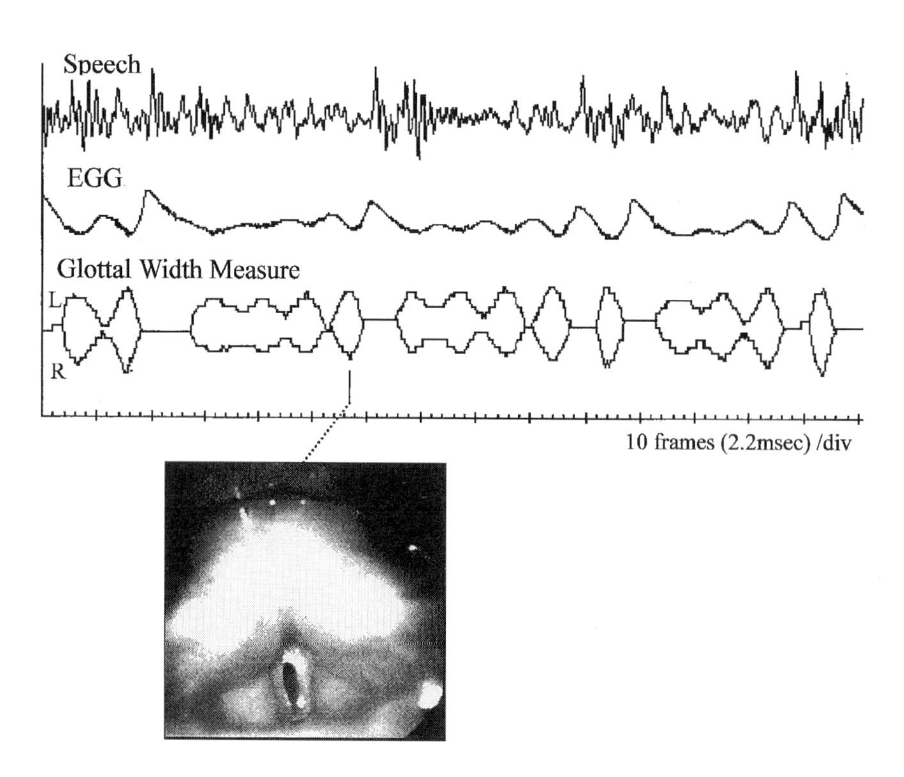

Figure 12–10. Vocal fold vibration for vocal fry.

REFERENCES

Farnsworth, D. W. (1940), High-speed motion pictures of human vocal cords. *Bell Telephone Records, 18,* 203–208.

Hirano, H. (1979). *Clinical examination of voice* (chap. 6). Wien: Springer.

Honda, K., Kiritani, S., Imagawa, H., & Hirose, H. (1987). High-speed digital recording of vocal fold vibration using a solid-state image sensor. In T. Baer, C. Sasaki, & K. S. Harris (Eds.), *Laryngeal function in phonation and respiration* (pp. 485–491). San Diego: Singular Publishing.

Imagawa, H., Kiritani, S., & Hirose, H. (1987). High-speed digital image recording system for observing vocal fold vibration using an image sensor. *Japanese Journal of Medical Electronics and Biological Engineering, 25,* 284–290.

Kiritani, S., Hirose, H., & Imagawa, H. (1993). High-speed digital image analysis of vocal cord vibration in diplophonia. *Speech Communication, 13,* 23–32.

Kiritani, S, Hirose, H., & Imagawa, H. (1996). Vocal cord vibration in the production of consonants—Observation by means of high-speed digital imaging using a fiberscope. *Journal of the Acoustic Society of Japan, 17,* 1–8.

Klatt, D., & Klatt, L. (1990). Analysis, synthesis, and perception of voice quality variations among female and male talkers. *Journal of the Acoustical Society of America, 87,* 820–857.

Moore, G. P., White, F. D., & Leden, H. (1962), Ultra high speed photography in laryngeal physiology. *Journal of Speech and Hearing Disorders, 127,* 165–171.

Whitehead, R. L., Metz, D. E., & Whitehead, B. H. (1984). Vibratory patterns of the vocal folds during pulse register. *Journal of the Acoustical Society of America., 75,* 1293–1297.

CHAPTER 13

Voice Quality and Electrolaryngography

Adrian Fourcin

1. AIM

The aim of this brief overview is to introduce the use of Laryngograph® and EGG voice measurement equipment and to give some examples of the newer methods of voice quality assessment that these techniques are beginning to make available. Special reference is made to the use of these methods in precision stroboscopy, the analysis of connected speech and in regard to their auditory relevance.

2. BACKGROUND

The term "Electroglottograph"—or EGG for short—has become a generic name for a simple electrical method for the noninvasive examination of vocal fold phonatory vibration. The apposition of two electrodes on the alae of the thyroid cartilage provides a circuit element that can be monitored either in terms of its impedance or in regard to its admittance. The technique was first applied to voice work by Fabre (1957) and he used a constant current, impedance-based, method of observation. He also introduced the term *électroglottographie,* considering that the main information derived from the device was in respect of the glottal opening. In fact, however, the real primary information concerns vocal fold contact, and it was for this reason, early on, that the term "laryngograph" was used (Lx is used here as an abbreviation for the resulting signal, now derived via a constant voltage, admittance-based, method). The practical importance of vocal fold contact has since been established in several ways. Direct synchronized cinematic/Lx observation of vocal fold movement with different voice qualities (for example, Lecluse 1977; Donovan, Roach, & Fourcin in Fourcin, 1974) made it feasible reliably to infer the contribution to Lx waveforms made by contact between the opposing faces of the vocal folds. Human experiments in vivo by the interposition of a nonconducting strip within the glottis

(Gilbert, Potter, & Hoodin, 1984) radically established the overriding importance of contact between the folds to the Lx waveform. (Earlier work, based on electrical admittance measurements, had shown that up to 4.5 MHz resistance was potentially the more important electrical contributor to the Lx waveshape than capacitance [Fourcin & Norgate, 1965]). Cadaver experiments have confirmed and extended these results. For instance using an excised single canine vocal fold dynamically abutting a conducting viewing plate (Scherer, Druker, & Titze, 1988), the correspondence between conductance and contact area was shown. Using excised human cadaver larynges the nature of the contact waveform as a function of some of the physical factors influencing vibration has also been investigated (Laukkanen, Vilkman, & Laine, 1992).

Initially, essentially only the Lx signal was presented in the form of a waveform going positive (up) for increasing vocal fold contact area (this was also Fabre's aim, but his actual waveforms were positive for increasing glottal opening). As the result of the work described above, and many other contributions, the near universal practice is now to use both EGG as well as Lx information with positive contact polarity. In normal voice the main acoustic excitation of the vocal tract coincides with vocal fold closure and, since this is a salient aspect (see Baken [1985], pp. 221–227, for an excellent discussion), the Lx signal is widely relied on to provide larynx frequency information. Even though the separate contributions of the two vocal folds cannot be established using Lx, the waveshape is also a potentially rich source of voice quality information. In recent years this has led to the combined use of Lx waveform information together with laryngeal stroboscopy. A first step toward routine clinical use was made by Anastaplo and Karnell (1988) with both synchronization and wave shape now coming from an Lx signal source. A logical extension of this approach is to use a clinical desktop computer to control the stroboscope on the basis of Lx period-to-period closure information. This gives two advantages. First, the instant of illumination of the vibrating vocal folds can be automatically adjusted so that an exact sequence of stroboscopic light pulses can scan through successive periods to provide the basis for the precision storage of vocal fold images in the computer memory for immediate or subsequent animation/examination. Second, a long-standing objection to stroboscopy itself can be, in some measure, avoided by the use of these precisely defined single light flashes, each uniquely linked both to a single image and to a well-defined point on the reference Lx waveform. Pathological voices are often temporally irregular and this variable periodicity makes it impossible with ordinary stroboscopy both to freeze a picture at one point in the vibration cycle and also to adequately interpret a sequence of images. By associating each single image with its corresponding Lx/EGG waveform, these familiar stroboscopic ambiguities are avoidable. This facility has been incorporated in the LxStrobe system.

The following three figures have made use of LxStrobe to exemplify some of the special features of Lx/EGG waveforms for three different normal voice qualities: modal, breathy, and falsetto. Figure 13–1 shows a sequence of eight images uniformly spaced through one vocal fold period during the production of modal voice by a normal speaker. Each of the pictures is linked to the Lx waveform that was responsible for its illumination, and the corresponding trigger instant is shown on that waveform. The images have been automatically acquired to memory in a minimum of phonation time, so, for this normal speaker, there is no observable variation in the Lx waveform across the sequence.

In modal voice, the initial closure of the folds, shown by the sharp rise in the Lx waveform, is well defined. This closure is responsible for the initiation of the very marked acoustic response in the Sp (microphone) waveform shown above the lower Lx signal (typically there is a small air path transmission delay of Sp relative to Lx). Closed phase is also well defined and this interval of contact between the vocal folds isolates the supraglottal resonances from subglottal effects. The mucosal wave which is so important to normal

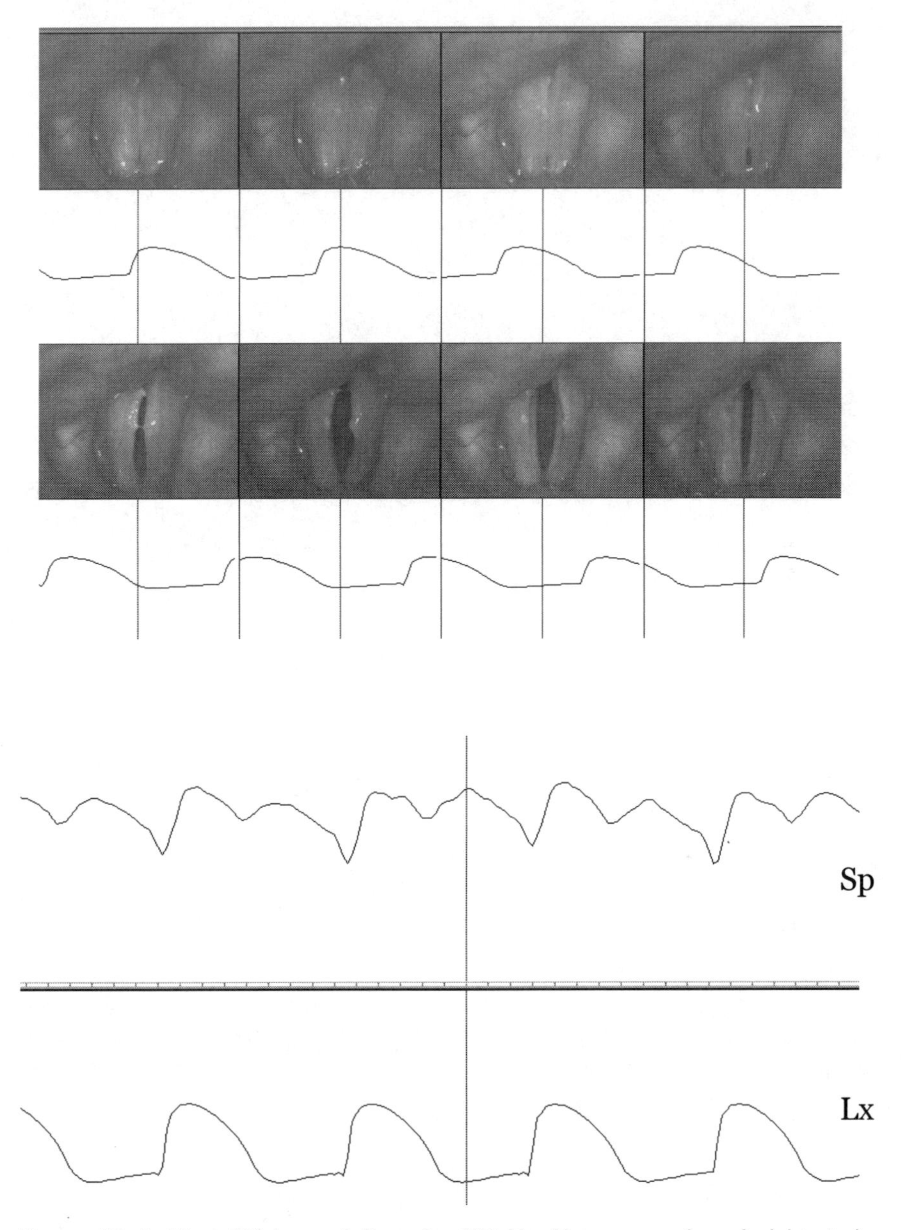

Figure 13–1. Modal Voice: adult male, 120 Hz Above, a series of eight stroboscopically derived images of the vocal folds with the corresponding Lx waveform under each image—together with its trigger instant. Below, the Sp and Lx waveforms for the sixth image.

voice production is clearly seen in the seventh and eighth strobe flash pictures.

The breathy voice phonation quality shown in Figure 13–2 is characterized primarily by its longer open phase. This is especially easy to see both in the Lx waveforms for each of the strobe shots and in the Sp and Lx waveforms at the foot of the figure. During the open phase the supraglottal vocal tract is coupled to the subglottis and, as a consequence, its resonances are more damped than for modal voice. Vocal tract resonances are also less well defined in

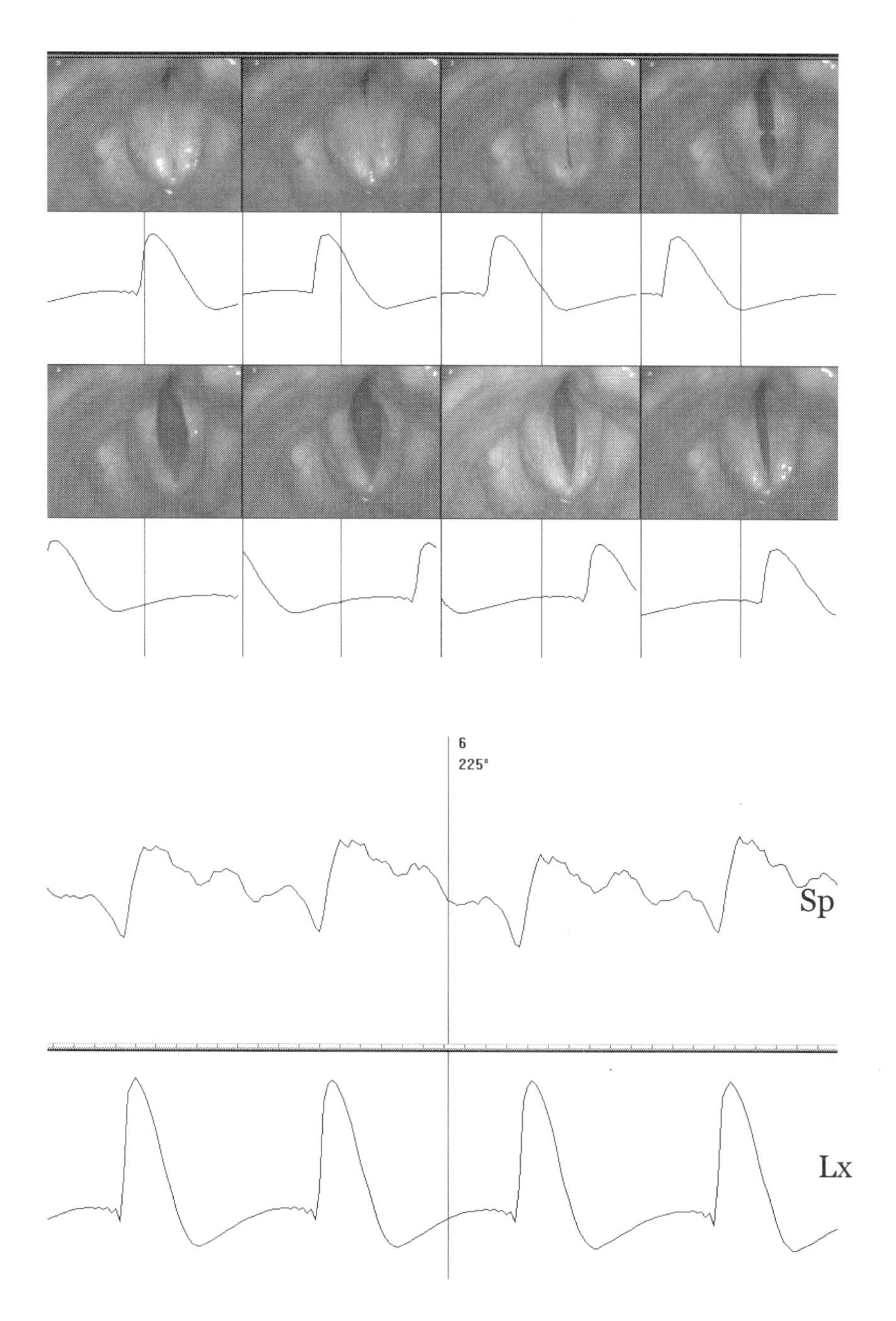

Figure 13–2. Breathy Voice: adult male, 105 Hz Eight stroboscopic images above, each with its triggering instant superimposed on the corresponding Lx waveform. Sp and Lx waveforms below for image 6.

amplitude because this voice quality is often associated with a less rapid closing phase. An additional aspect of breathy voice, as its name implies, is that it is associated with a frictional quality coming from glottal turbulent airflow excitation. Although Lx is periodic, this gives an auditorily perceptible component of irregularity to the Sp waveform from period to

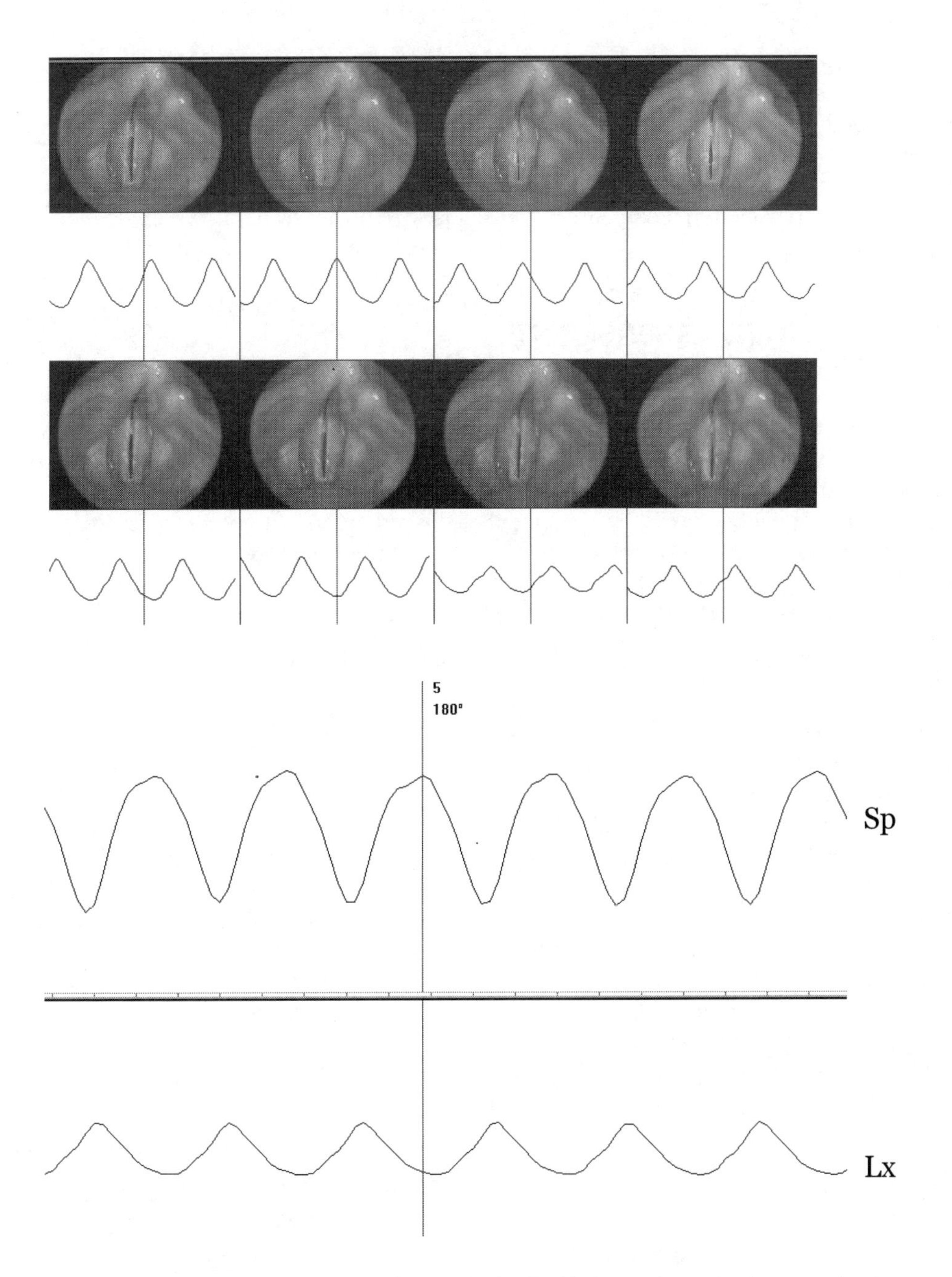

Figure 13–3. Falsetto Voice: adult male, 323 Hz Eight stroboscopic images above, each with its triggering instant superimposed on the corresponding Lx waveform. Sp and Lx waveforms below for image 5.

period that can just be seen in the Sp open phase intervals of the waveform figure.

The falsetto voice quality images and the speech and Lx waveforms displayed in Figure 13–3 show the main features of this phonation type by the length, and extension, of the vibrating vocal folds, the lack of mucosal waves on their surfaces, and the somewhat sinusoidal

Lx waveshape. This phonation type is also characterized by near sinusoidal simplicity of vocal fold motion. The consequently less rapid vocal fold closures give a relative lack of higher spectral components in the vocal tract excitation, and this is reflected in a correspondingly simple Sp waveform.

3. SUBJECTIVE ASSESSMENT AND OBJECTIVE EVALUATION

In many cases the original impetus to seeking a clinical check on voice function comes from the auditory observation that there is a deficiency in voice quality—made by a teacher, family, friends, in the workplace or by the speaker. Normality is partly subjective, it can be culturally determined (e.g., Moore, 1971), phonetically defined as a function of the language environment (e.g., Maddieson, 1984), or simply exist in the ear of the particular listener (e.g., Aronson, 1985). Kent (1996) regards the clinician as the final arbiter and in modern society this must be largely the case, at least administratively, since final outcome measures depend on demonstrable results that can only come from appropriate clinical investigation. Auditory assessment is intrinsically difficult to administer in standard, repeatable fashion and a number of clinical multidimensional scaling approaches have been evolved to objectivize auditory subjective methods. Well known examples are: the GRBAS scale from Japan (Hirano, 1981) and its extended form recently developed and applied in Europe (Dejonckere et al., 1996); in Sweden, Hammarberg and Gauffin (1995) using SVEC have worked on another comprehensive set of clinically relevant voice descriptors with special reference to perception. Laver (1991) has introduced a pseudo-phonetically motivated set of dimensions, which, however, add further to a real dilemma by confounding voice, in the sense of vocal tract excitation, with attributes of the vocal tract setting. All of these approaches suffer from the unresolved problem of providing links between the levels of auditory description used and the levels of objective analysis and measurement that it is convenient and possible to apply clinically.

The auditorily based methods of voice quality assessment aim to provide a basis for quantification with the great advantage of being applicable to connected speech. The main techniques of objective evaluation, however, tend to be directed toward the use of sustained sounds as the foundation for their measurements. Prominent examples are the CSL system (Kay Elemetrics, Computer Speech Laboratory) and the "Dr Speech" system (Tiger Electronics) worked on by Huang and Minifie. A possible reason for this difference in approaches may arise from the obvious need to assess connected "real-life" speech, which motivates subjective work, and the real difficulties that arise in applying rigorous signal analytic techniques to real-life clinical material (mobile telephone networks cannot even cope with some "normal" phonation). The following examples of Lx-based processing of clinically derived pathological material are intended as a modest contribution toward the future solution of some of the problems associated with the development of auditorily significant, rigorous methods of objective speech, and voice quality, analysis.

4. LARYNGOGRAPH DATA AND THE OBJECTIVE ANALYSIS OF CONNECTED PATHOLOGICAL SPEECH[1]

Figure 13–4A gives an open phase view taken from a sequence of eight images uniformly spaced so as to cover, within a sustained utter-

[1] The following four sets of data were derived from Mr. Julian McGlashan's Voice Clinic at Queens Medical Centre Nottingham. The LxStrobe observations were in each case routinely preceded by a speech and laryngograph recording session organized by Beverly Towle. In each case the connected speech sample had a duration of about 2 minutes.

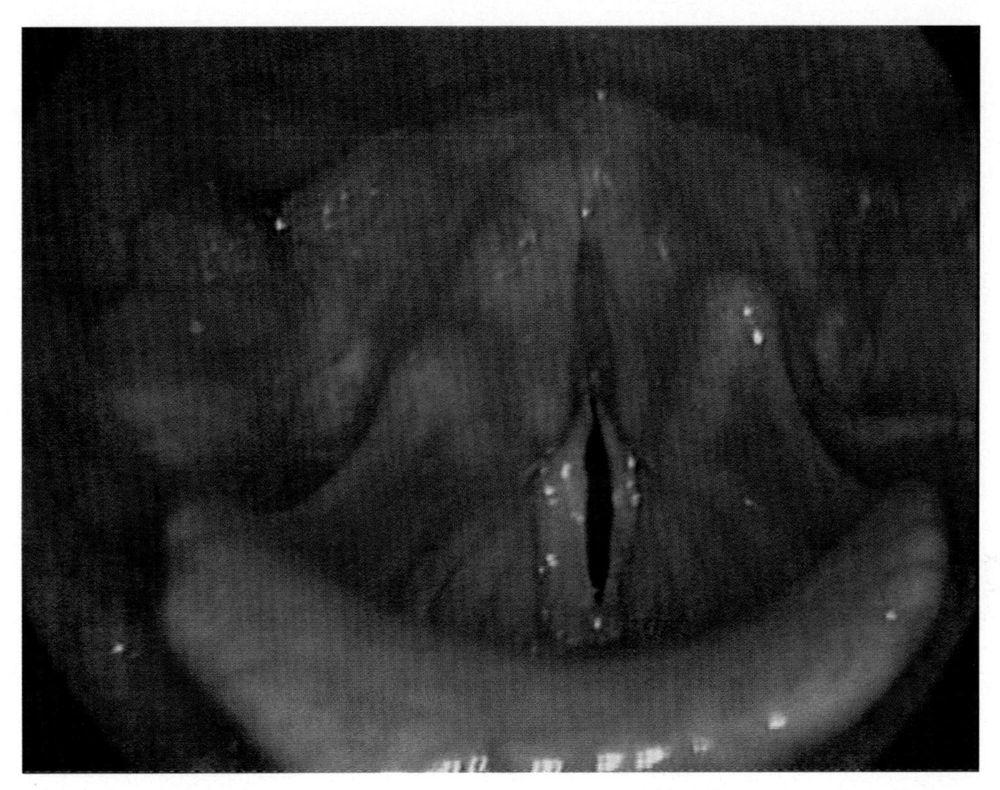

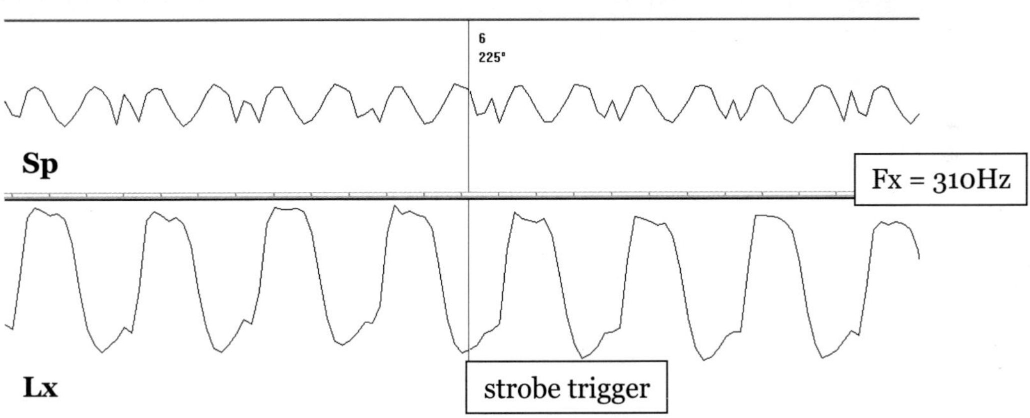

Figure 13–4A. Left vocal fold scarring: speaker CW1 The image shows a single shot, in the middle of the open phase, from a stroboscopic sequence using LxStrobe to cover the interval of one period. The acousic, laryngograph, and strobe trigger (center) signals are below.

ance, one vocal fold period, as for Figures 13–1, 13–2, and 13–3. The speaker is a 35-year-old woman who had previously had a left vocal fold cyst removed. Subsequent to this visual inspection, it was found that her left vocal fold epithelium was very adherent to the underlying ligament. Her preferred "comfortable" frequency of sustained phonation was around 300 Hz, a quite abnormally high value. The use of the laryngograph (Lx) recording makes it

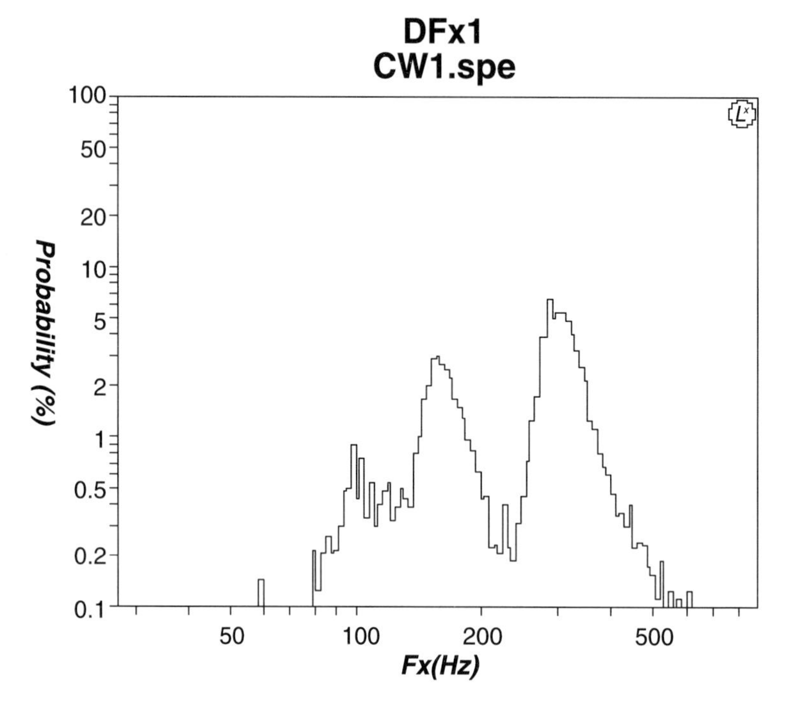

Figure 13–4B. DFx1 Larynx frequency distribution Since the laryngograph signal makes it easy to detect each vocal fold closure on a period by period basis, even very irregular phonatory activity can be measured. The simple larynx period distribution shown here for speaker CW1 has three modal peaks. Only the central mode is appropriate; the others arise from the pathology—but it is the highest which is typically chosen at "comfortable pitch," as in the stroboscopic image.

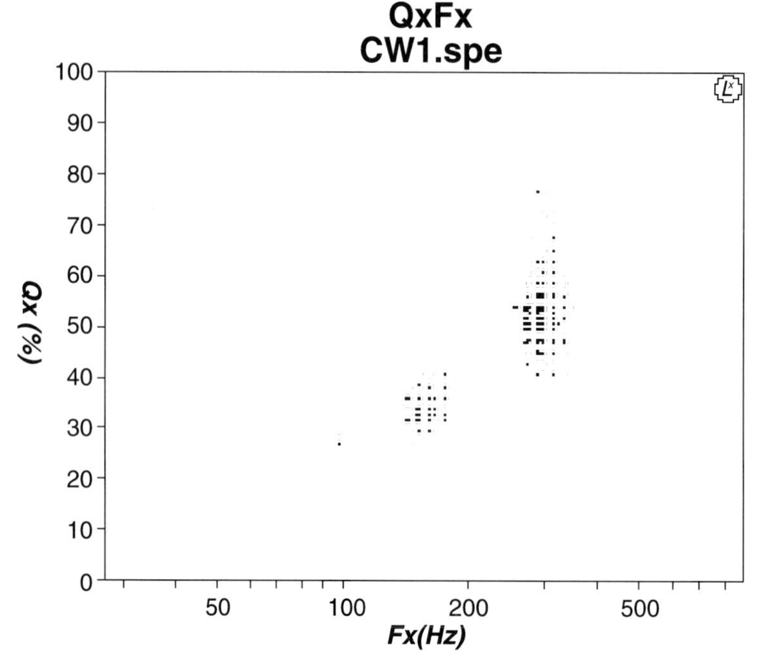

Figure 13–4C. QxFx Quality Index Distribution Contact phase ratio is one of the indices of good quality voice production and the Lx signal can be used to give a useful indication of this parameter, Qx. The distribution on the left shows Qx plotted against Fx. The main concentration of high closed phase ratio voicing is at the abnormal mode, in the vicinity of 300 Hz.

possible to make two, more complete, quantitative checks. The simple larynx frequency distribution of Figure 13–4B (called DFx1) shows that this very high pitch has been chosen because it is at the dominant mode. Although the overall shape of the distribution is grossly abnormal, the sub-mode at 160 Hz is appropriately placed and shaped. It is interesting to note that in the region of 300 Hz the ratio of vocal fold contact duration to period (Qx) in Figure 13–4C, often an indication of good voice quality, is abnormally large. In auditory terms, the two quantitative distributions are related to the subjective impression of a very hoarse, irregular voice (see DFx1) with an unnaturally dominant high pitched component (see both DFx1 and Qx).

These examples of Lx-based processing could not be obtained either as easily or as reliably from the acoustic signal (Sp) alone. The "instantaneous" frequency, Fx, which is measured on a period by period basis from Lx, is especially suitable for the analysis of most pathological voices. And the contact phase ratio within a single period, Qx, can be at least usefully estimated again from the Lx/EGG signal (the values used here are taken from period by period ratio estimates of Lx closure width, 70% down from each positive peak, to the instantaneous period Tx).

Figure 13–5A is from another stroboscopic larynx period-related sequence, here for a 57-year-old man with a voice use problem. Neither this image nor the waveforms indicate any special source of difficulty. Figure 13–5B, however, taken with the folds retracted, shows a granuloma. The distribution of Figure 13–5C, with its marked step down above 200 Hz, also shows an abnormal condition. Using the temporal accuracy of the Lx signal, it is possible to produce larynx frequency distributions that seek out vocal fold vibrational regularity here by only plotting those occasions when two successive periods have essentially the same value (DFx2). A marked reduction in regular vibration is evident from about 120 Hz. Above this vocal fold frequency, the Qx distribution, Figure 13–5D, is also rather broken, indicating poor closure duration control in the upper register. The control of loudness is similarly affected above 120 Hz as shown by the simple connected speech phonetogram in Figure 13–5E (VRP1, in which Fx is, as above, the instantaneous frequency per period, and the intensity is derived from the Lx gated acoustic peak in each Sp period). The three plots relate respectively to important subjective aspects of pitch, projection, and loudness.

The single image shown in Figure 13–6A is taken from a woman of nearly 80 years with previous mild candidiasis. Her sustained voice is of good quality. Her speaking voice is, however, mildly irregular and she complains of its being of low pitch. Both DFx1 and the Qx distributions are not pathological (although the influence of age is shown by the rather ragged shape of DFx1). The third distribution, CFx, in Figure 13–6D gives the clue to the auditory component of her voice complaint. For normal voice (Fourcin, 1979), plotting the frequencies of successive vocal fold vibrations against each other gives a well-defined single diagonal distribution—an indication of regularity of vibration. Different pathologies give different types of deviation from this diagonal. Speaker CW, for instance, has a main diagonal with three distinct parts and two outliers corresponding to the abnormal frequency modes. The present analysis shows a quite distinct type of irregularity. Over a large part of the voice frequency range, there are structured departures from regularity coming from a tendency for a low frequency larynx pulse to be followed by a high—and vice versa. This voice quality characteristic, when it occurs through range of larynx frequencies, leads to the presence of three parallel lines in the CFx distribution. In the low pitch register of the voice this is often referred to as creaky voice (an irregular paired alternation of well and poorly defined vocal fold closures) but here it is spread abnormally into the higher frequencies. This effect would give an impression of roughness even at modal pitches and could account for the speaker's own auditory impression of low voice pitch in spite of the presence of a higher than normal range.

Figure 13–7A is for a male speaker of nearly 50 years with workplace-induced laryngitis. His Lx waveform is abnormal in regard to its opening/open phase shape and his DFx1 (basic voice frequency distribution in Figure 13–7B) is very broad. The second order larynx frequency distribution (DFx2), which picks out regularity in the voice recording, shows a core of well defined voice pitch, which is at the

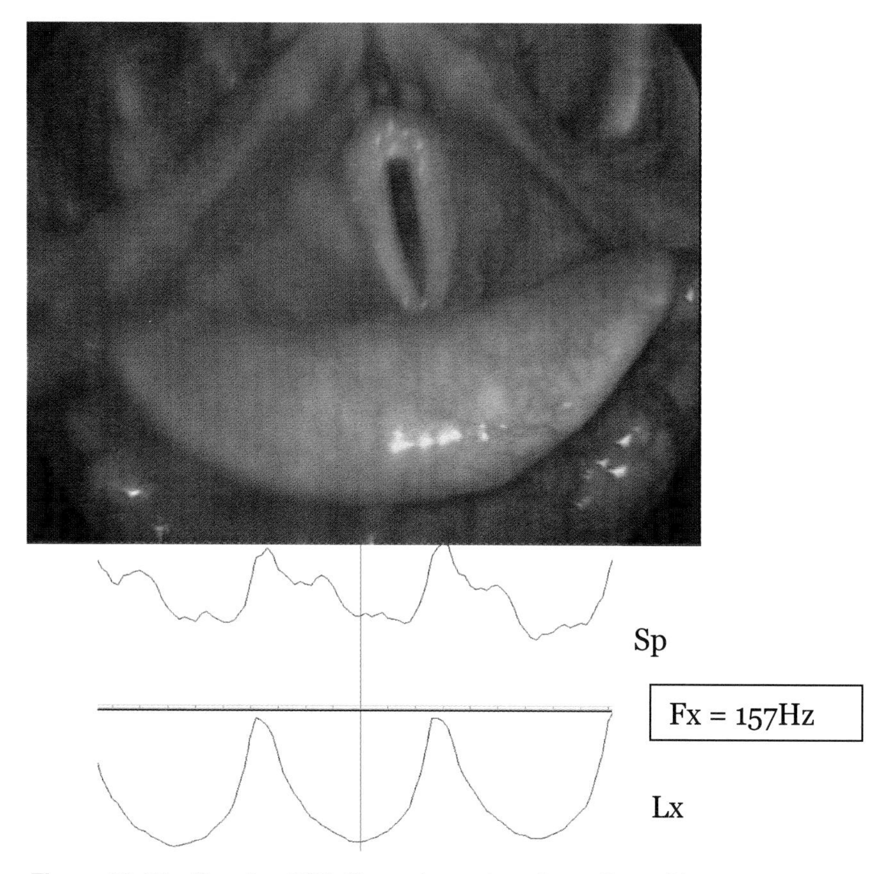

Figure 13–5A. Speaker DC1 Open phase view above; Sp and Lx waveforms and trigger for this view.

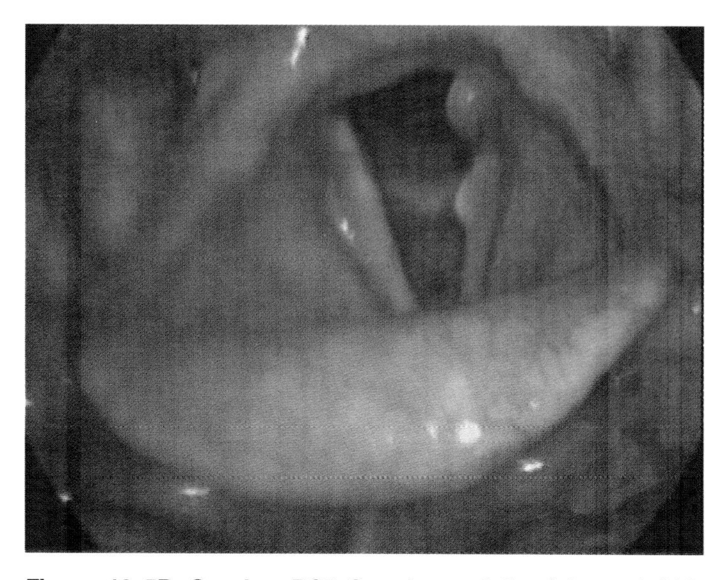

Figure 13–5B. Speaker DC1 Granuloma of the left vocal fold process—visible during abduction (mucus anterior to the granuloma).

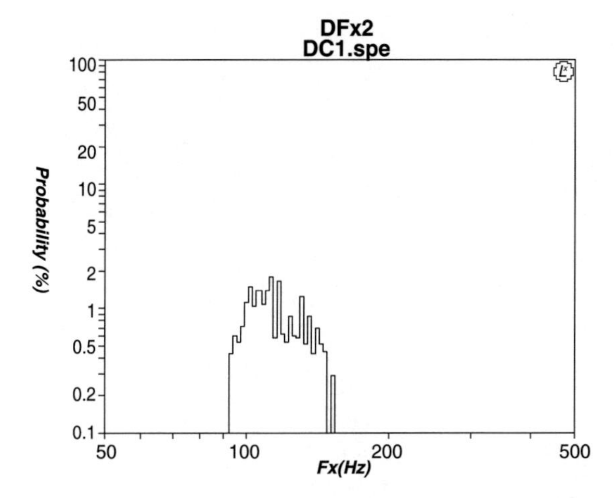

Figure 13–5C. DFx2 The second order larynx frequency distribution on the left is produced by only counting the occasions when two successive vocal fold periods fall into the same Fx frequency bin. This picks up regularity in the speech sample—there is a break around 200 Hz.

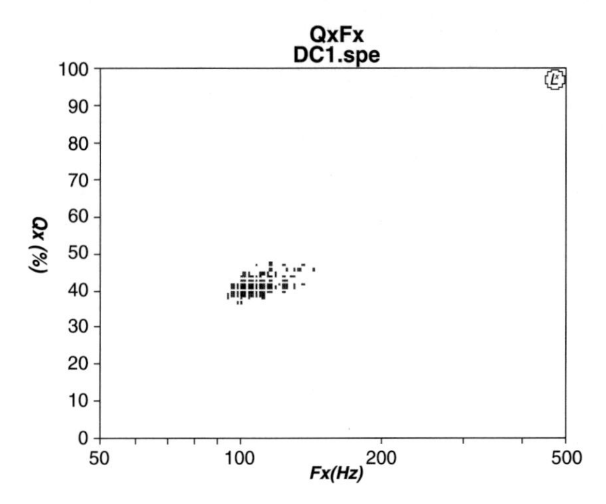

Figure 13–5D. QxFx Qx, the distribution of contact phase ratios is shown here as in figure 13–4C. The speaker has an evident reduction in closed phase ratio for the upper part of his register, and this change in Qx corresponds exactly with the break in the larynx frequency distribution.

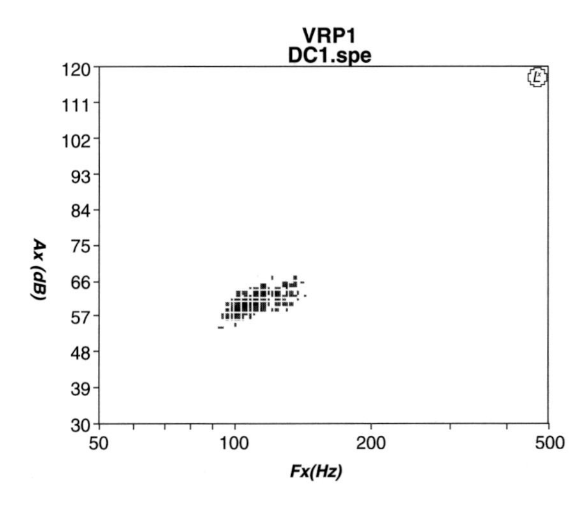

Figure 13–5E. VRP1 This distribution is the familiar phonetogram but applied to connected speech rather than sustained sounds; intensity is plotted against larynx frequency, Fx. There is, however, no smoothing and the same sample of connected speech is used. This plot shows how the intensity is also reduced for the upper part of the register.

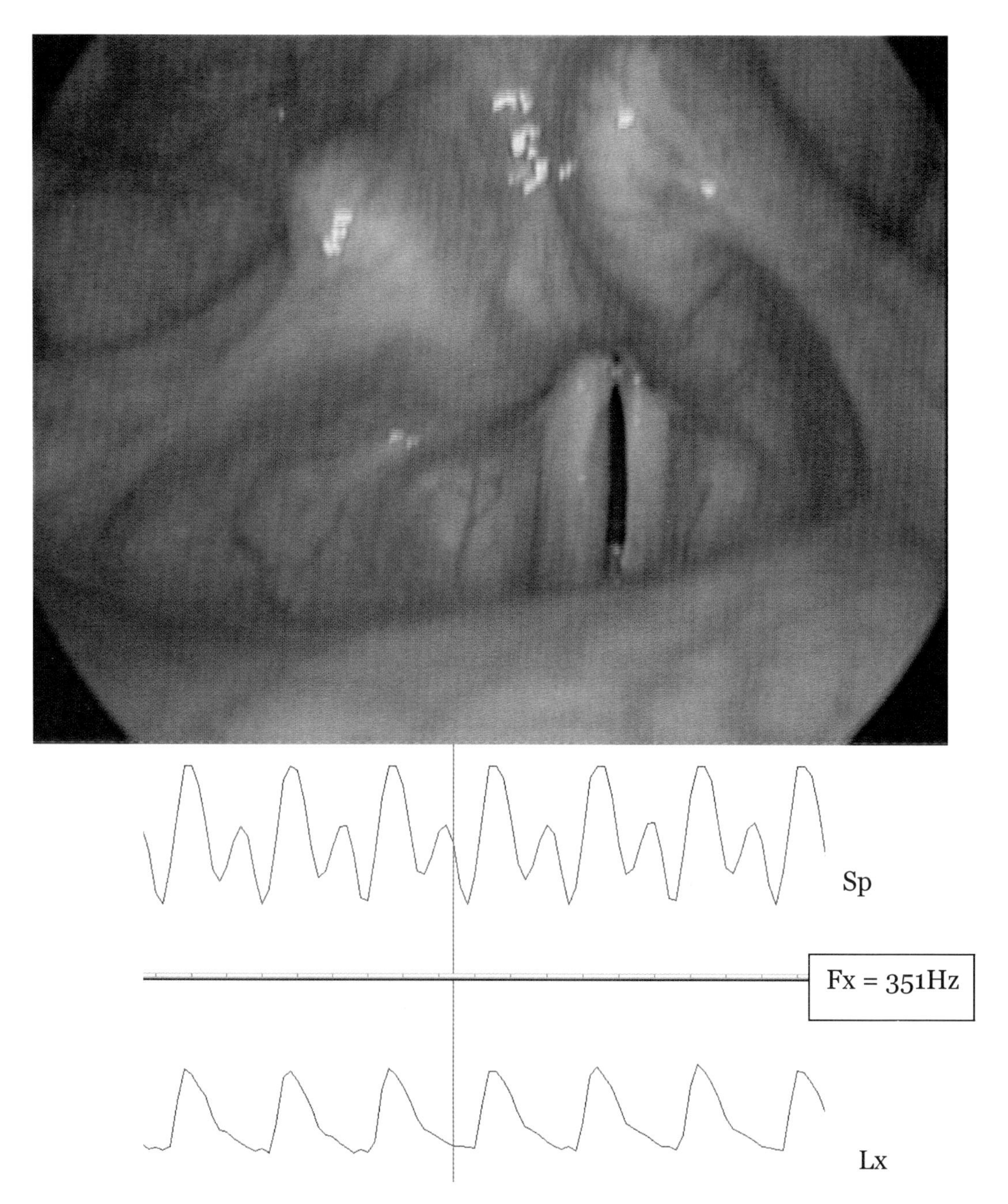

Figure 13–6A. Speaker MF1 An open phase stroboscopic image is shown above together with the speech and laryngograph waveforms that accompanied it and its trigger instant. The images and waveforms show no sign of the irregularity found in connected speech.

heart of his speech. The use of the very simple technique of plotting paired regularities has been applied in Figure 13–7C to the Sp/Lx phonetogram analysis of his 2-minute connected speech sample in regard to both larynx period and speech intensity (on a larynx

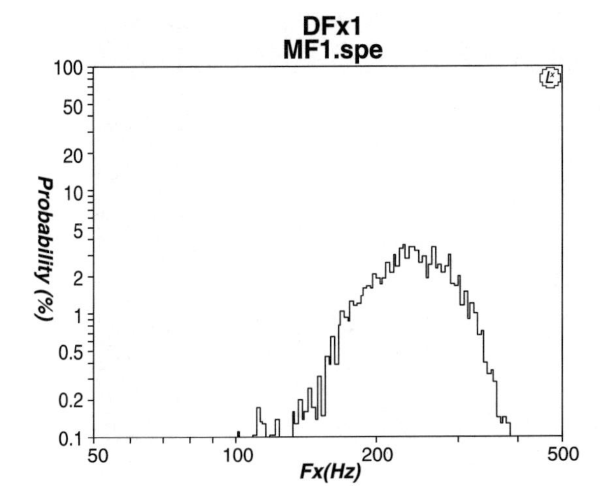

Figure 13–6B. DFx1 The first order Fx distribution is for the female voice of Figure 13–6A. The slight vocal fold asymmetry seen in the figure seems to have given rise to the characteristic broad larynx frequency distribution which is often associated with mild vocal fold vibrational irregularity.

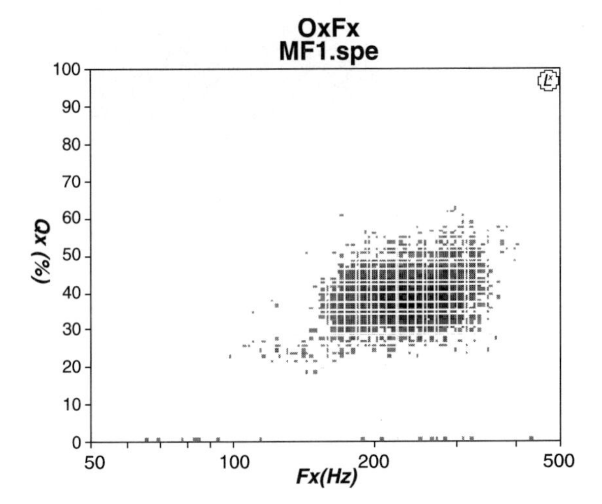

Figure 13–6C. QxFx The heart of the contact phase ratio distribution, of Qx against Fx, is fairly well formed and shows this aspect of the voice to be under appreciable control in the whole of the center register, even though there are outlying irregularities.

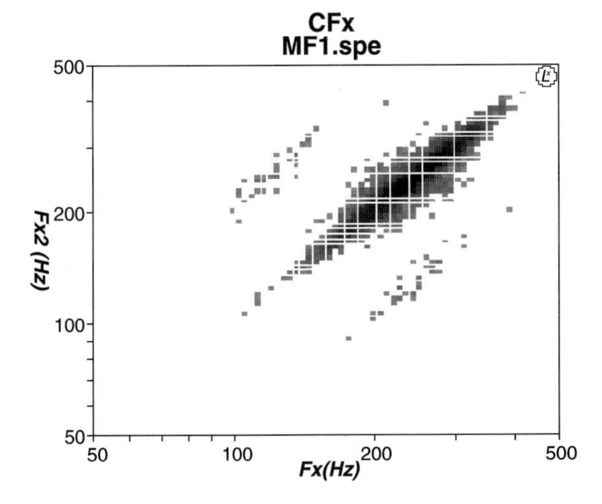

Figure 13–6D. CFx The larynx frequency cross-plot on the left simply indicates the relation between successive pairs of vocal fold periods each of which has been analysed in the sample of connected speech. Normally only a single slim diagonal is found, but here irregularity gives three lines with a broad center.

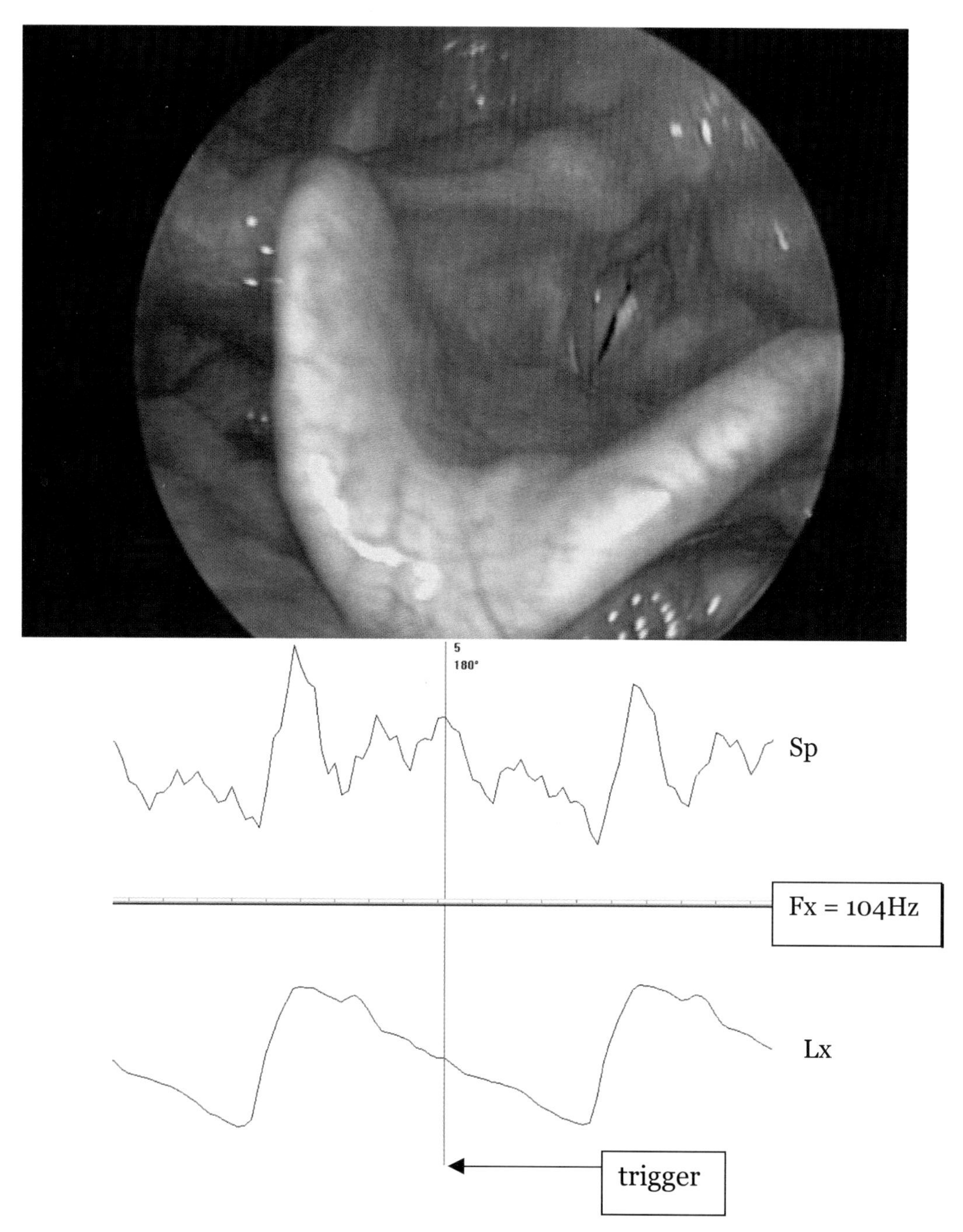

Figure 13–7A. Speaker SK1: Acute Chronic Laryngitis The view has been taken, as shown by the trigger marker, midway between two closures in what would ordinarily be a well defined open phase. The speech and laryngograph waveforms are at the modal frequency.

synchronous basis). This VRP2 plot shows that his speech has a core of both intensity as well as larynx frequency regularity.

In each one of these four pathological voice samples, derived from connected speech, a different aspect of voice quality has been made

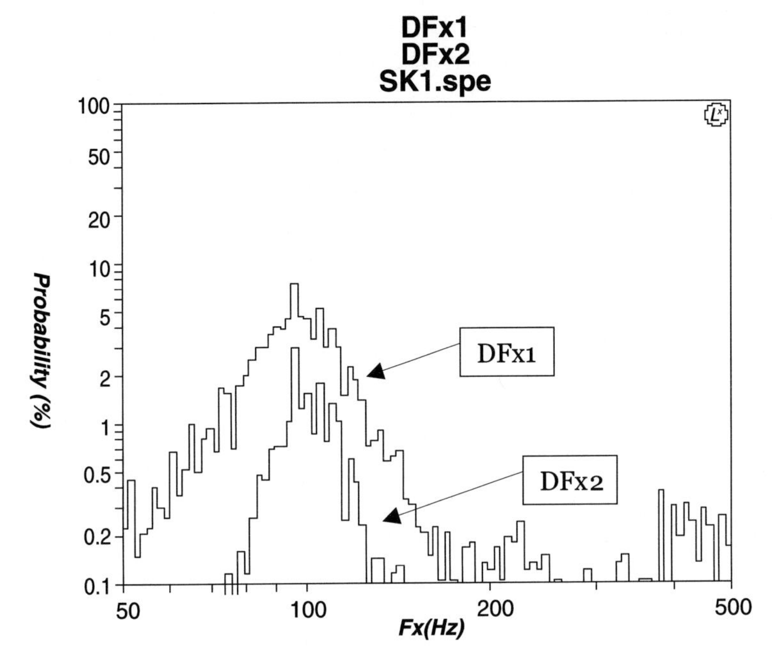

Figure 13–7B. Dfx1,2 The basic larynx frequency distribution Dfx1, based on a 2-minute sample of connected speech, is wide and ill-formed. The second order distribution, DFx2, using the same recording, shows by its height and shape that there is a core of well-structured voice of potentially good quality.

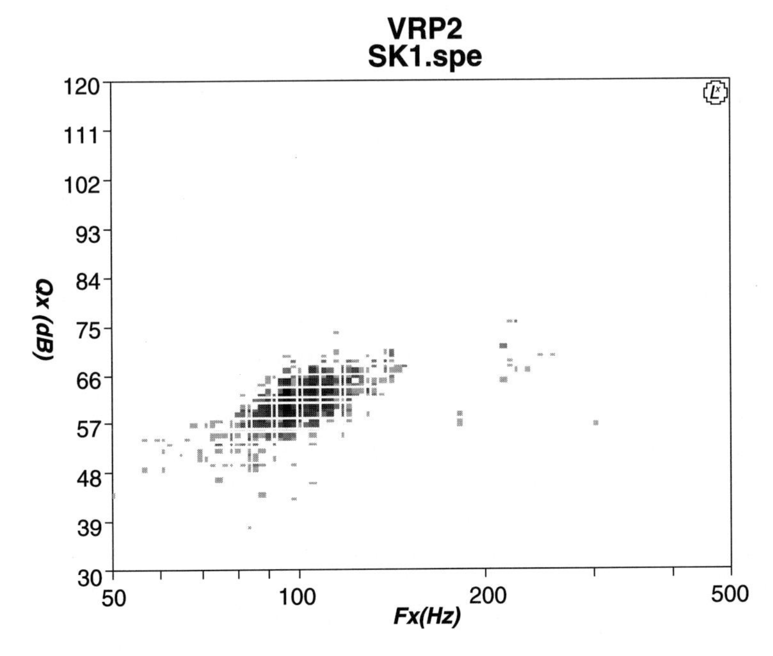

Figure 13–7C. VRP2 The standard first order connected speech phonetogram for this speaker is very dispersed in both frequency and intensity. The second order phonetogram, however, which only shows those pairs of periods falling in the same Ax/Fx bin, indicates the existence of a core of voice regularity now in intensity as well as larynx frequency.

viewable by the use of simple Lx-based processing. But also in each case there is a quantitative analytic aspect of the work that establishes the basis for a rigorous approach to voice quality management that can complement other clinical methods. Speech and laryngograph data files or recordings also provide a basis for comparison over time and contribute to reliable litigation archives.

5. LARYNGOGRAPH DATA AND VOICE QUALITY IN THE SPEECH OF THE DEAF

In a companion chapter, Abberton gives an overview of work concerning the "Voice Quality of Deaf Speakers." Her discussion covers a very wide range of important features and gives instances of the application of EGG/Lx-type approaches not only in respect to analysis but also in regard to assessment, training, and the design of special speech pattern element hearing aids. The quantitative methods discussed here for speech pathology are also, as she has mentioned, applicable to the analysis of the speech of the deaf. Even though the typical deaf speaker has no laryngeal pathology, the lack of appropriate auditory feedback control can give rise to abnormal voice, and Lx information can be of basic assistance in its measurement, understanding, and improvement via interactive training. Abberton refers to the work of Cowie, Douglas-Cowie, and Rahilly (1988) who report work on "timing, intensity range, pitch height and change, and frication" and also to Jones (1967) who uses the descriptors "tense, flat, breathy, harsh, throaty, monotone, lack of rhythm, poor carrying power."

Lx factors can be of very great help in the investigation of many of these factors. In the following very brief discussion, the voices of two speakers are examined by applying methods that follow naturally once the Lx information is available. Both speakers are 10-year-old boys. A is normally hearing, B is congenitally profoundly deaf but has been educated in an intensively oral environment. Figure 13–8 shows particular examples of the voices of these two boys taken from recordings of their connected speech (it is important to note that A has read a standard text while B, who has poor reading ability, has described a familiar set of pictures). In each plot the lower trace is of Fx, the period by period fundamental frequency modulated in width by the amplitude of the acoustic signal, and the upper part of each plot is the wide band spectrum of their fricatives (both voiced and unvoiced). It is not possible to generalize on the basis of such a meager amount of data, but the figures do give a striking indication of what really does happen when, as will be seen below, much longer samples are analyzed. A has well-defined intervals of frication and good control of Fx range and voicing durations. By comparison, B has a tendency to produce very brief intervals of both frication and voicing.

Figure 13–9 shows the results of analyses of intervals of frication in long samples of connected speech for the two boys (>3 minutes, two channel Sp & Lx). The striking differences between the plots of Figure 13–8 are now verified and it is evident that the normally hearing boy has frication segments that do tend to be of greater duration.

Cowie et al.'s reference to timing and frication effects and Jones' comment on lack of rhythm are relevant here. In Figure 13–10 a similar comparison is possible between the distributions of voicing intervals in the same samples of connected speech. Once more there is a quite striking dissimilarity. A has much longer voicing durations than B and this is a quantitative reflection of many of the auditory descriptors given for voicing onset and intonation control in the speech of the deaf. In the two cases, in fact, the Fx ranges are comparable although the patterns of intonation control within the ranges are markedly different.

Finally, the important aspect of voice quality, QxFx, used for example in Figure 13–6C for the examination of pathological speech, is measurable by analyzing the distribution of contact phase intervals in the voicing segments of the two recordings. These Qx distributions, Figures 13–11A and B, once more show that there are striking quantifiable differences between the voices of the two children. The voice of B has a tendency to considerably lower values of Qx—an indicator of breathy voice quality, and a smaller range of control across the span of larynx frequency.

Simple Speech Pattern Displays

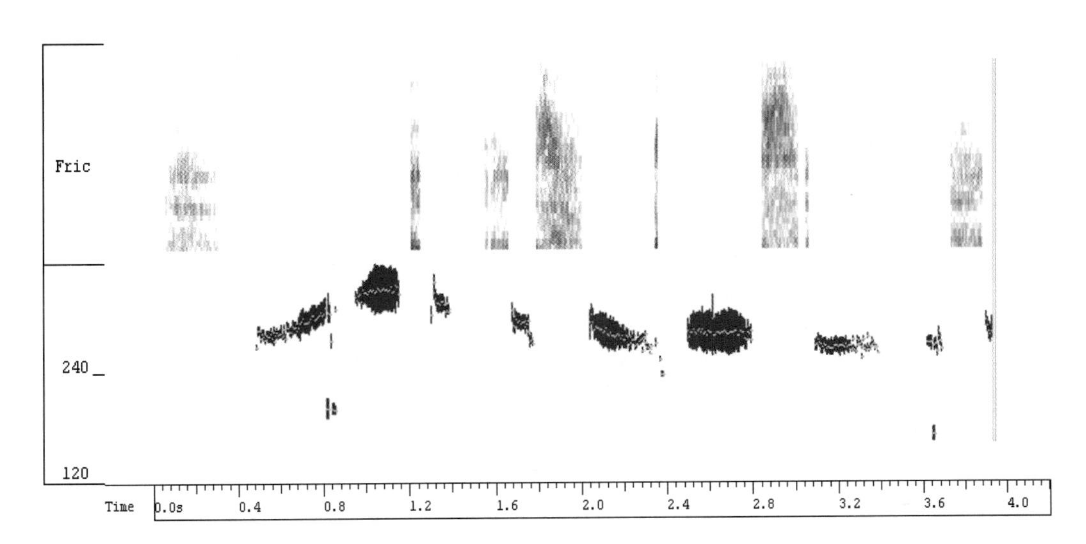

Figure 13–8A. Speaker A: Normally hearing boy—connected speech

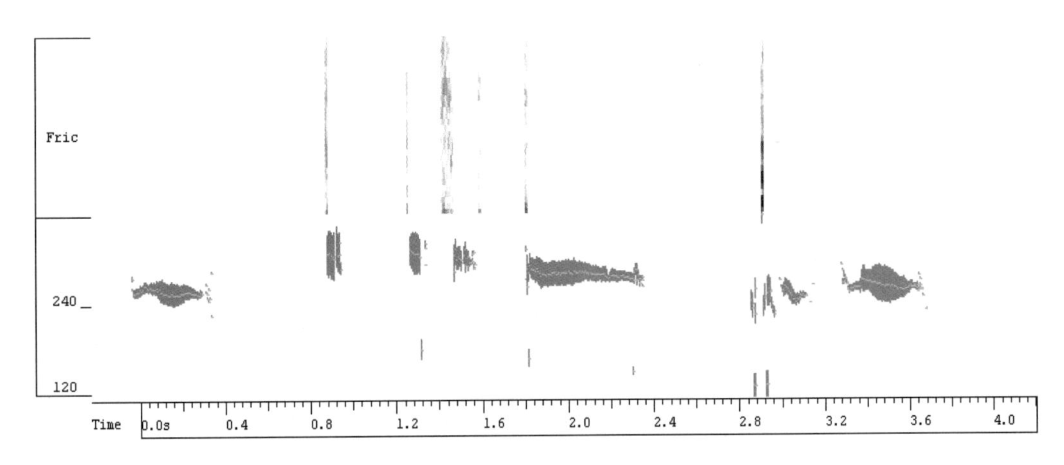

Figure 13–8B. Speaker B: Congenitally deaf boy—connected speech. *Note:* The upper half of each trace is for frication—5 kHz to 10 kHz; the lower half for voiced sounds, two octaves from 120 Hz to 480 Hz and 4 s duration overall, these AxFx traces are controlled in width by the acoustic amplitude for each period. This type of real-time interactive presentation makes it possible to focus attention in therapy on the perceptually salient aspects of production.

On the other hand speaker A is already producing a patterning of Qx control, which tends (by its uniformity across Fx) to be like that of the adult male.

6. NORMATIVE COMPARISONS

Figure 13–12 gives a single overview of the general form of the results that can be

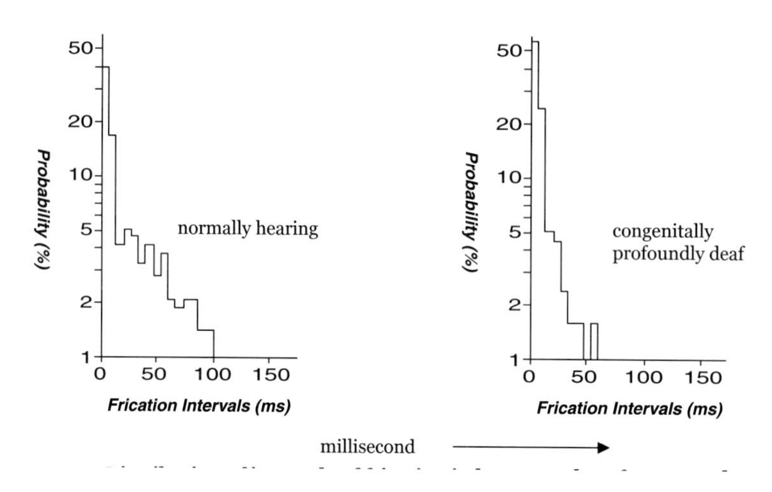

Figure 13–9. Distribution of intervals of frication in long samples of connected speech Speaker **A** on the left; Speaker **B** on the right.

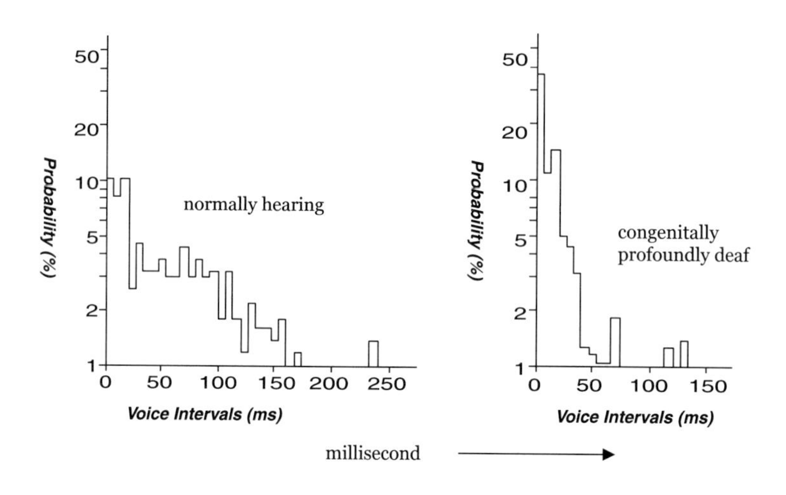

Figure 13–10. Distribution of voicing intervals in long samples of connected speech Speaker **A** on the left; Speaker **B** on the right.

expected from the application to normal speech signals of the analyses used here for the examination of the pathological voice.

- DFx1 and DFx2 are now very similar in shape and do not differ markedly in respect to their relative sizes. This is an immediate indication of the intrinsic regularity that is associated with normal vocal fold vibration.
- CFx, the period by period cross-plot, shows once more that the regularity of vocal fold vibration is high. The complex structures of irregularity and very high irregularity measures are absent in the normal voice.

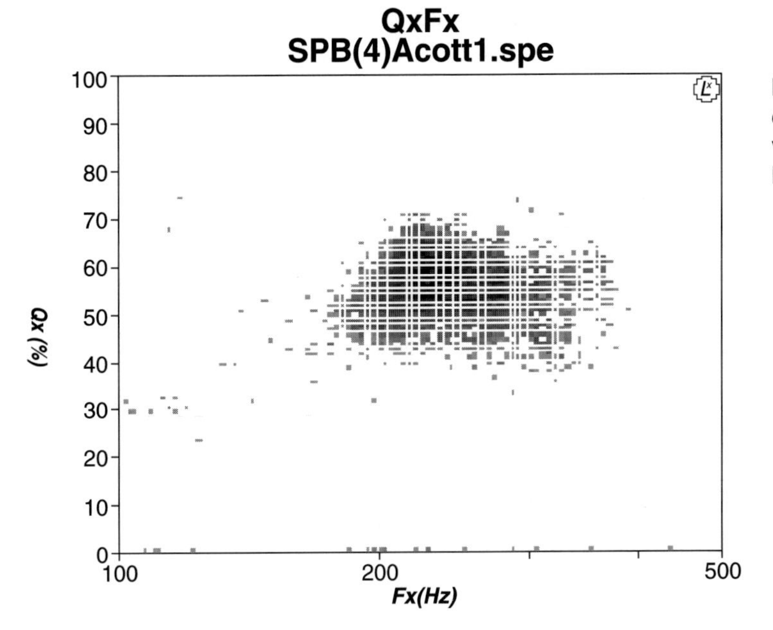

Figure 13–11A. Distribution of vocal fold contact intervals Speaker **A**—normally hearing boy.

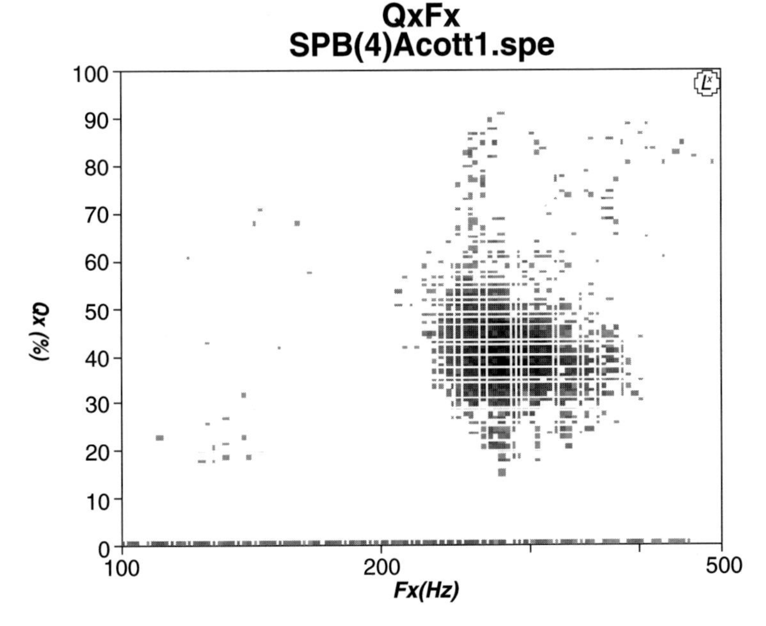

Figure 13–11B. QxFx distribution of vocal fold contact intervals Speaker **B**—congenitally profoundly deaf boy. *Note the lower average value and greater irregularity and spread of Qx for the deaf speech.*

- VRP2 is the second-order connected speech phonetogram. This is a coherent distribution with the well-defined area in amplitude and instantaneous frequency, Fx, which is to be expected from good voice control. The breakdown into separate zones is never found with voices that have a well-defined pitch range.
- QxFx2 is the second order representation of the contact phase ratio as a function of Fx—in which only successive pairs of vocal fold periods that fall in the same analysis bin are plotted. Once more, for the normal voice, this test of regularity still shows a coherence of control that is not ordinarily encountered in pathology.

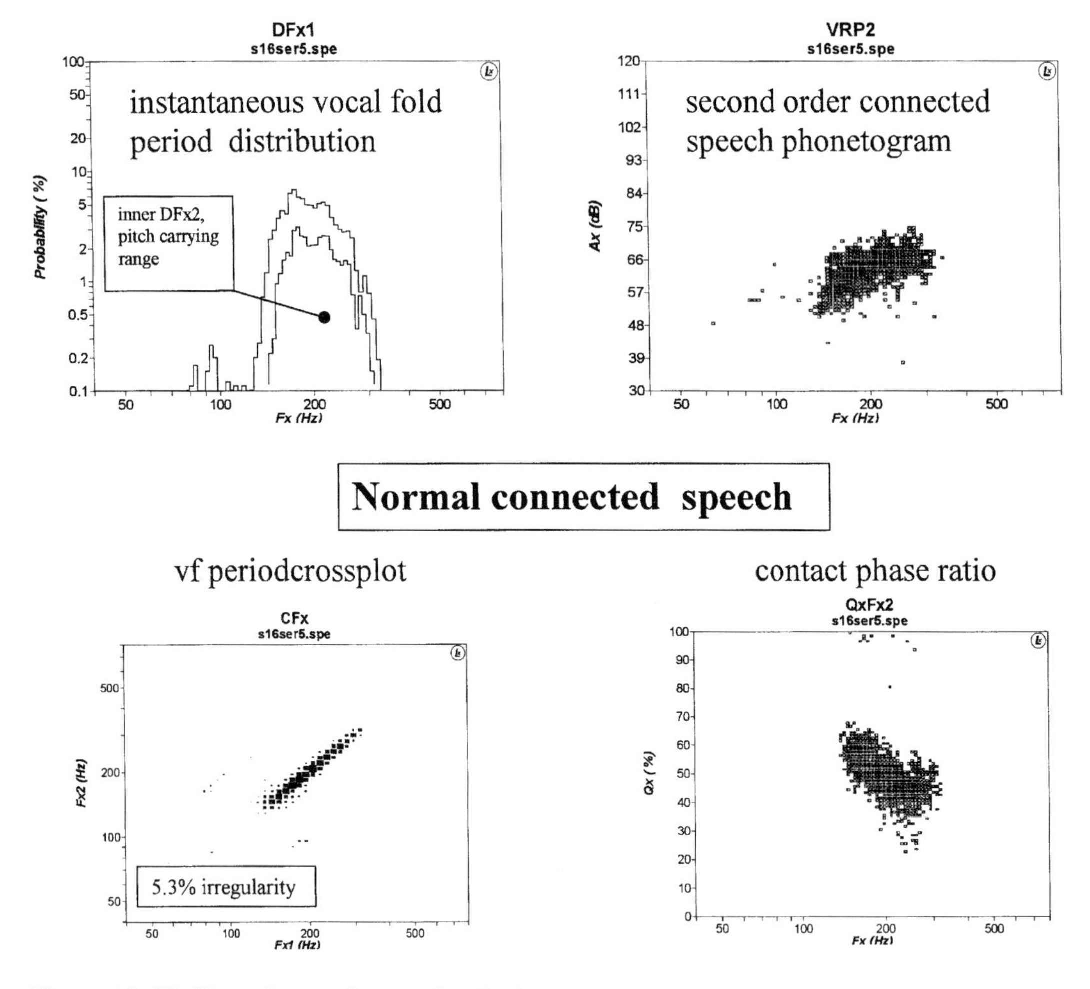

Figure 13–12. Normal speech sample: English woman speaker; analyses based on a 2-minute recording of Sp and Lx derived from a read text.

This very brief discussion of normality and the comparison with voice pathology cannot give a sufficiently full account of a much larger subject. A contribution to more data and information will be found on: http://www.phon.ucl.ac.uk/home/adrian/home.

7. IN CONCLUSION

The main contributions to voice quality analysis which are presently made possible by laryngograph type approaches come from the special physical properties of the equipment and the very close relation between the signals recorded and the processes of voice generation and control.

- Noninvasive sensing gives acceptable access to a wide range of speaker populations
- Response primarily only to vocal fold contact provides an effectively unrivaled accurate basis for larynx frequency measurement.
- Acoustic noise immunity is a special advantage for data gathering in many work environments (including the hospital voice clinic), and, in quiet, this facility gives an extremely useful basis for frication detection.

- The duration of vocal fold contact is represented in the laryngograph waveform with sufficient accuracy to give a basis for closed quotient comparison.

The particular examples discussed in this chapter have tended to concentrate on the links that can be made between objective measurement using Lx-type signals and the use of auditory dimensions of voice quality description. This is an increasingly important area of development. The measurement techniques described are able to provide one way of escaping from the current clinical bias towards the utilization of data (sustained vowels for example) not so much because it is important in real life as because it is convenient in use for the investigator. The 2-minute speech samples (of Sp & Lx) used are easy to obtain and representative of major speech factors such as onset, offset, register change, and vocal tract/larynx interactions which are largely absent from sustained samples.

Acknowledgments

In addition to Mr. Julian McGlashan and Beverly Towle and their colleagues at QMC Nottingham, Mr. John Rubin of the Royal National Throat, Nose, and Ear Hospital, London, and Dr. Elisabeth Fresnel of the Laboratoire de la Voix, Paris, it is a pleasure to acknowledge the laryngograph, stroboscopic, and analytic resources that have been developed by Colin Bootle, Xinghui Hu, and David Miller at Laryngograph Ltd. and used for the figures and discussions of this chapter. Laryngograph® is the registered trademark of Laryngograph Ltd. (www.laryngograph.com).

REFERENCES

Aronson, A. E. (1985) *Clinical voice disorders* (2nd ed.) New York: Thieme Inc.

Anastaplo, S., & Karnell, M. P. (1988). Synchronized videostroboscopic and electroglottographic examination of glottal opening. *Journal of the Acoustical Society of America, 83*, 1883–1890.

Baken, R. J. (1987). *Clinical measurement of speech and voice.* Boston: Little, Brown.

Cowie, R., Douglas-Cowie, E., & Rahilly, J. (1988). The intonation of adults with postlingually acquired deafness: Anomalous frequency and distribution of elements. In B. Ainsworth & J. Holmes (Eds), *Proceedings SPEECH '88, 7th FASE Symposium, Edinburgh, 2*, 481–487.

Dejonckere, Ph., Remacle, M., Fresnel-Elbaz, E., Woisard, V., Crevier-Buchman, L., & Millet, B. (1996). Differentiated perceptual evaluation of pathological voice quality: Reliability and correlations with acoustic measurements. *Revue Laryngologie (Bordeaux), 117*, 219–224.

Fabre, P. (1957). Un procédé électrique percutané d'inscription de l'accolement glottique au cours de la phonation. *Bulletin National Médicine, 141*, 66–99.

Fourcin, A. J. (1974). Laryngographic examination of vocal fold vibration. In B.Wyke (Ed.), *Ventilatory and phonatory control systems* (pp. 315–333). Oxford, UK: Oxford University Press.

Fourcin, A. J. (1981). Laryngographic assessment of phonatory function. *ASHA Reports, 11*, 116–127.

Fourcin, A., & Abberton, E. (1972). First applications of a new laryngograph *Volta Review, 69*, 507–518. [Originally printed in 1971 in *Medical and Biological. Illustration, 21*, 172–182].

Fourcin, A., & Norgate, M. (1965). Measurement of trans-glottal impedance. Progress Report (pp. 34–40). London: Phonetics Laboratory University College.

Gilbert, H. R., Potter, C. R., & Hoodin, R (1984). Laryngograph as a measure of vocal fold contact area. *Journal of Speech and Hearing Research, 27*, 178–182

Hammarberg, B., & Gauffin, J. (1995). Perceptual and acoustic characteristics of quality differences in pathological voices as related to physiological aspects. In O. Fujimura & M. Hirano (Eds.), *Vocal fold physiology* (pp. 283–303). San Diego: Singular Publishing Group.

Hirano, M. (1981). *Clinical examination of voice.* New York: Springer-Verlag.

Jones, C. (1967)."Deaf Voice"—a description derived from a survey of the literature. *Volta Review, 69*, 507–508.

Kent, R. D. (1996). Hearing and believing. *American Journal of Speech-Language Pathology, 5*, 7–23.

Laukkanen, A. -M., & Vilkman, E. (1995). Tremor in the light of sound production with excised human larynges. In P. H. Dejonckere, O. Hirano, & J. Sunberg (Eds.), *Vibrato* (pp. 93–110). San Diego: Singular Publishing Group.

Laver, J. (1991), *The gift of speech.* Edinburgh, Scotland: Edinburgh University Press.

Lecluse, F. L. E., (1977). *Elektroglottografie.* Utrecht, The Netherlands: Drukerijelinkwijk B.V.

Maddieson, I. (1984). *Patterns of sounds.* Cambridge, UK: Cambridge University Press.

Moore, G. P. (1971). *Organic voice disorders.* Englewood Cliffs, NJ: Prentice-Hall.

Scherer, R. C., Druker, D. G., & Titze, I. R. (1988). Electroglottography and direct measurement of vocal fold contact area. In O. Fujimura (Ed.), *Vocal fold physiology* (Vol. 2, pp. 279–291). Philadelphia: Raven Press.

CHAPTER

14

Analysis by Synthesis of Pathological Voices Using the Klatt Synthesizer

Abeer A. Alwan, Philbert Bangayan, Bruce R. Gerratt, Jody Kreiman, and Christopher Long

No accepted standard system exists for describing or measuring pathological voice quality (e.g., Jensen, 1965; Yumoto, Gould, & Baer, 1982; see Kreiman & Gerratt, Chapter 7, for review). Qualities are labeled or rated based on the perceptual judgments of individual clinicians, a procedure plagued by inter- and intrarater inconsistencies and terminological confusions. Synthetic pathological voices could be useful in a standard protocol for quality assessment, because synthesizer parameters quantify vocal quality without the need to decompose quality into individual "qualities" like breathiness and roughness, whose validity is questionable. Further, analysis by synthesis protocols, such as asking a listener to construct a synthetic voice to match a naturally occurring pathological voice, do not require the listener to compare an external stimulus to an unstable internal representation, as occurs in rating scale studies, thus decreasing the error in measures of quality (Gerratt, Kreiman, Antonanzas-Barroso, & Berke, 1993; Kreiman & Gerratt, 1996). This chapter describes a pilot study of the mechanics of synthesizing moderately to severely pathological voices and provides guidelines for synthesizing some kinds of pathological voice qualities.

Speech synthesizers with the ability to model a range of vocal qualities have many applications, including improved vocal prostheses (Qi, Weinberg, & Bi, 1995), analysis and coding of natural-sounding speech (e.g., Karlsson, 1991; Price, 1989), and modeling phonation types in languages with voice quality contrasts (Ladefoged, 1995). Accordingly, source models have received increasing attention in the literature (e.g., Ananthapadmanabha, 1984; Fant, Liljencrants, & Lin, 1985; Fujisaki & Ljungqvist, 1986). Recent studies (Carlson,

Granstrom, & Karlsson, 1991; Gobl, 1988; Gobl & Ní Chasaide, 1992; Imaizumi, Kiritani, & Saito, 1991; Karlsson, 1992; Klatt & Klatt, 1990; Ladefoged, 1995; Löfqvist, Koenig, & McGowan, 1995) have focused on variations in normal quality, rather than on pathology. With the exception of studies by Childers and colleagues (Childers & Ahn, 1995; Childers & Lee, 1991; Lalwani & Childers, 1991), attempts to synthesize pathological voices have not been reported, and synthesis of such voices is not well developed. Childers and colleagues modeled modal, fry, falsetto, and breathy phonation in patients with a variety of diagnoses; other types of pathological voices were not examined. Their work revealed limitations of existing source models and suggested that a turbulent noise component and a pitch perturbation generator were necessary to model breathy voices. These features have proved useful for modeling normal voices as well and have been added to implementations of the popular Liljencrants/Fant (LF) model (Fant et al., 1985) in some laboratories (e.g., Carlson et al., 1991; Karlsson, 1992).

Despite the predominant focus on normal speakers, previous synthesis studies provide some insight into pathologic voices, because many of the qualities examined occur in pathology. Further, modeling continuous speech resembles modeling pathologic voice, in that both tasks require a dynamic source model to mimic changes over the course of an utterance. However, from our perspective, these studies have significant limitations. They typically used small numbers of speakers (often as few as one or two). They examined a limited range of qualities (typically breathiness, creak, hoarseness, harshness, and modal voice, following Laver's classification [1980]), as produced by normal speakers. Finally, formal perceptual evaluation of the resulting synthesis has been very limited or absent in studies of both normal and pathological voice. Most authors determine which LF parameters best sort voices into a priori perceptual categories or merely report whether synthesis quality is "good" or "improved." Lack of detailed perceptual data also makes it difficult to determine the necessary and sufficient parameters to control a synthesizer. Although the LF source model specifies four timing parameters, many different combinations of these parameters can be used to control synthesis. Authors differ considerably in how they define control parameters, largely because perceptual data to guide standardization are lacking. Modeling of voice quality in these studies has not been driven by an interest in acoustic-perceptual relations. Thus, they have generated little insight into the perceptual importance of different features of glottal pulses, or of different synthesizer control parameters (e.g., Ananthapadmanabha, 1984). This information is critical for the development of efficient and standardized synthesis strategies, both for pathological quality and for variations in normal quality.

The present study used the Sensyn 1.1 (Sensimetrics, Cambridge, MA) version of the Klatt formant synthesizer (Klatt & Klatt, 1990) to synthesize a random sample of moderately to severely pathological voices. The Klatt synthesizer was chosen because it is commercially available, widely used, and often referenced. In addition, the synthesizer includes a turbulent noise component, pole and zero pairs that can be used to model tracheal and/or nasal coupling, a provision for time-varying parameters to model unsteady qualities, and a "diplophonia" parameter to model bifurcated phonation. However, the synthesizer was originally designed for synthesizing normal voices, and questions remain about its suitability for producing acceptable pathologic stimuli. In fact, the experiments reported in this study led to a number of suggested modifications to the synthesizer that would facilitate synthesis of pathological voices.

1. ANALYSIS-BY-SYNTHESIS

1.1. Stimuli

Twenty-four samples of the vowel /a/ were selected from a library of voice recordings. Use of vowel stimuli has a number of advantages. First, isolated vowels are often used in clinical practice for evaluation of pathological voice quality. Second, acoustic analysis and synthesis are more straightforward for vowels than for continuous speech. Study of continuous speech is the ultimate goal and an obvious next step. However, valid results based on less complex stimuli are first required.

Signals were recorded with a miniature head-mounted microphone (AKG C410) placed off-axis 4 cm away from the speaker's lips. Signals were low-pass filtered at 8 kHz, digitized at 20 kHz, and then downsampled to 10 kHz, the maximum sampling rate at which all synthesizer parameters could be manipulated. One-second segments were extracted from the middle portion of each natural sample.

Each voice was given an informal severity rating by authors JK and BG, who are experienced in perceptual ratings of pathological voices. Ratings were made on a 6-point equal-appearing interval (EAI) scale, with 1 representing near-normal voice quality and 6 representing extremely severe pathology. Because this study focused on moderately to severely pathological voices, only samples rated 3 or higher were chosen.

1.2. Acoustic Analysis

Time- and frequency-domain analyses of each voice sample were undertaken to guide synthesis efforts. Most of the effort was directed at matching the time-varying spectra of the natural utterances. Most analyses were performed using SpeechStation (version 3.1 for the IBM PC; Sensimetrics, Cambridge, MA), because it is compatible with the Sensimetrics synthesizer and because it can display the natural and synthesized speech files simultaneously. WAVES software (version 5.0 for the Sun SparcStation; Entropic Research Laboratory, Washington, DC) was also used, especially for time-domain analyses.

Time-domain analyses included measuring the amplitude and fundamental frequency (F_0) of the voices. As a first pass, the SpeechStation F_0 tracking algorithm, which consists of center clipping followed by autocorrelation and parabolic interpolation, was used. If the F_0 tracker failed to produce a reasonable F_0 contour, as in the case of voices with high jitter, then F_0 was measured manually from the time waveform.

Frequency-domain analyses included computing 14th-order LPC spectra to measure the formant frequencies and using DFT spectra to determine the overall spectral shape, the strength of the first three harmonics, and the locations of poles and zeros due to nasal and/or tracheal coupling. The analysis window was a Hamming window whose length was varied as necessary to measure variations in quality over the duration of a sample. For example, steady-state segments can be measured with a longer duration window than rapidly varying segments. Spectrograms were used throughout this process to visualize the time course of the waveform.

1.3. Synthesis

Synthetic waveforms were modeled after each of the natural tokens using Sensyn 1.1 implementation of the Klatt synthesizer (Klatt, 1980; Klatt & Klatt, 1990). Synthesis was aimed at matching the spectro-temporal details of the natural waveforms. It was undertaken by authors PB and CL and supervised by author AA who has more than 10 years experience in speech synthesis with the Klatt synthesizer.

The Klatt synthesizer is based on the source-filter theory of speech production and consists of 34 modifiable parameters for the cascade implementation. Default values for these parameters are listed in Appendix 14–A. All samples were synthesized with a sampling rate of 10 kHz, using the cascade branch of the synthesizer and a version of the LF source model (SS = 3).[1] The parameters used to control the glottal pulse shape and timing are the open quotient (OQ), defined as the percentage of time the glottis is open in 1 fundamental period; the speed quotient (SQ), defined as the ratio of the duration of the rising portion of the glottal pulse

[1] **The LF source is implemented as a filtered impulse in this version of the Klatt synthesizer.**

to that of the falling portion; the fundamental frequency (F_0); the tilt of the voicing source spectrum (TL); the amplitude of aspiration noise (AH); the amplitude of voicing (AV); the flutter parameter (FL), which adds a quasirandom component to the nominal F_0 value; and the degree of diplophonic double pulsing (DI).

Synthesis proceeded as follows.

1.3.1. Step 1: Match Parameters in the Frequency Domain

The first step in the synthesis was to match frequency domain parameters, such as F_0, formant frequencies (parameters F_1–F_6), and formant bandwidths (parameters B_1–B_6). Formant frequencies were determined by matching spectrograms of the natural and synthetic utterances. Bandwidths were determined by comparing short-time Fourier spectra. Bandwidths were chosen such that the amplitudes of the natural and synthetic formants matched. The parameter SQ was adjusted if necessary to match the overall spectral slope (also with reference to short-time Fourier spectra). The synthetic sample was then played back to check for vowel quality.

1.3.2. Step 2: Adjust Amplitude of Voicing (AV and GV) and Amplitude of Aspiration Noise (AH and GH)

Next, the parameters AV, GV, AH, and GH were set by matching the intensity of the spectrograms and the energy in the waveforms. The amplitude of voicing was adjusted to match the intensity of the natural waveform as closely as possible. When changing the voicing and noise source amplitudes, it was necessary to alter the formant bandwidths to obtain the correct formant amplitude. This was important because loudness affects the perceived similarity of two voices (Kempster, Kistler, & Hillenbrand, 1991). Likewise, the amplitude of the aspiration noise (AH) was adjusted to match the amount of noise present in the spectrogram of the natural voice. When synthesizing pathological voices, careful manipulation of aspiration noise is as important as that of the amplitude of voicing, because, for example, the degree of aspiration noise can be an important factor in the perception of vocal quality (Kreiman, Gerratt, & Berke, 1994; Kreiman, Gerratt, Precoda, & Berke, 1993). Fine-tuning of GH and GV was guided by perceptual evaluation.

1.3.3. Step 3: Adjust Open Quotient (OQ)

The third step was to alter OQ as necessary to match the natural short-time spectrum and to match the quality of the synthetic and natural voices. Normal voices are characterized by an OQ of about 50%; pathological voices may have OQ either greater or less than 50% (Klatt & Klatt, 1990). In the frequency domain, increasing OQ strengthens the amplitude of the first harmonic.

1.3.4. Step 4: Adjust Low-Frequency Harmonics

It was often difficult to match the amplitudes of harmonics below F_1 in the synthetic vowels to those of the natural samples. This harmonic mismatch resulted in synthetic voices that deviated substantially in quality from the natural voices. The synthesizer provides two pole-zero pairs. One pair (FNP, FNZ) is intended to model a pole and zero that may arise from nasal coupling, with the other pair (FTP, FTZ) modeling a pole-zero pair that may arise from coupling to the trachea. Synthesizer architecture restricts both pairs to frequencies below 3000 Hz.

Adjustments were made with reference to short-time spectra of the natural and synthetic voices. To increase the amplitude of a harmonic, the nasal and/or tracheal pole-zero pairs were placed at that harmonic, keeping the bandwidth of the pole narrower than that of the zero. Similarly, particular frequency regions were attenuated by placing a pole-zero pair in that region with the bandwidth of the zero narrower than that of the pole.

Figure 14–1 illustrates how the amplitude of the first harmonic can be manipulated by

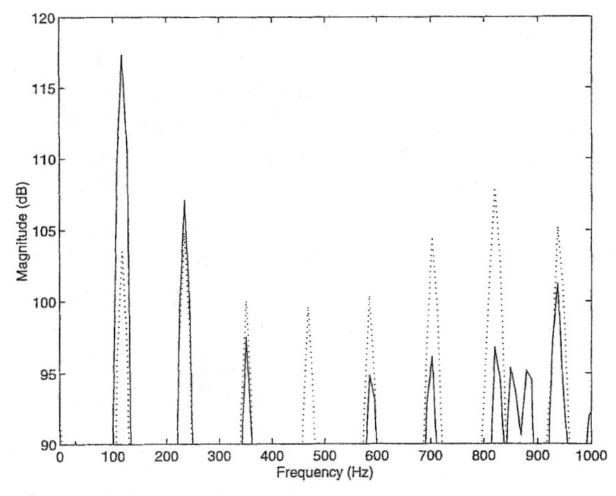

A

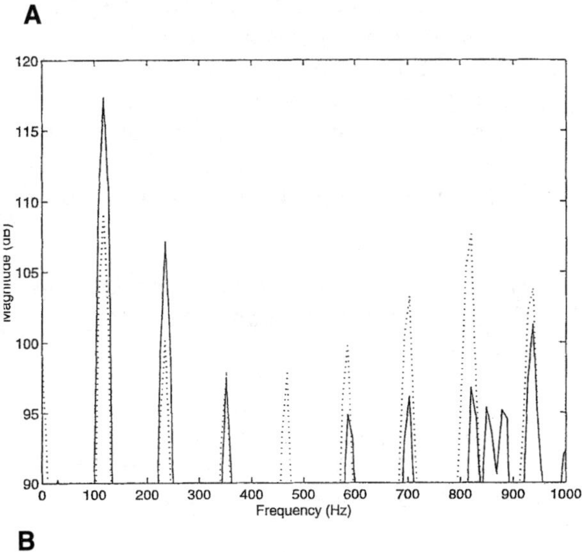

B

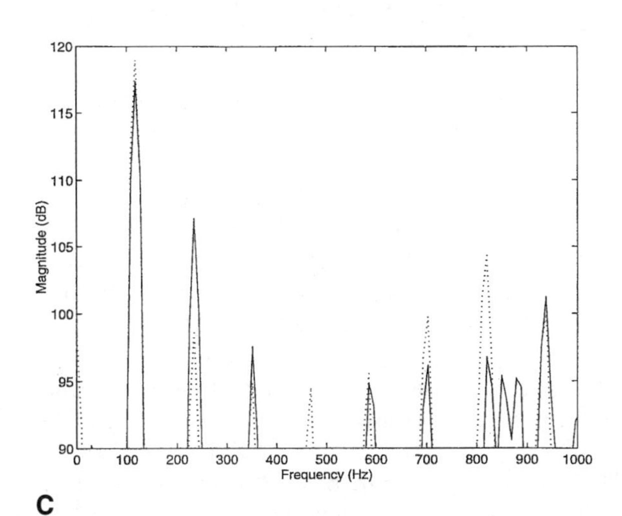

C

Figure 14–1. Discrete Fourier transform (DFT) spectra of a natural (solid line) and synthetic (dashed line) voice. **A.** With OQ = 50%, the first harmonic amplitude for the natural utterance is 14 dB higher than that of the synthesized voice. **B.** Using OQ = 90%, the difference is 8 dB. **C.** Adding a pole/zero pair (FNP, FNZ) at the frequency of the first harmonic and using OQ = 90% yields a better match. The parameters used were FNP = FNZ = 116 Hz, BNP = 40 Hz, BNZ = 180 Hz. Placing a pole-zero pair near any harmonic affects the amplitude of that harmonic.

changing OQ and placing a pole-zero pair at the frequency of the first harmonic. Figure 14–1A shows the energy of the first harmonic when OQ = 50%. In this case, the first harmonic of the synthetic stimulus is 14 dB less than that of the natural stimulus. Increasing OQ to 90% (Figure 14–1B) increases the strength of the first harmonic to 8 dB below that of the natural stimulus. Notice that, in this case, increasing OQ decreases the amplitude of the second harmonic (Klatt & Klatt, 1990). With OQ = 90% and a pole-zero pair placed at the frequency of the first harmonic, the amplitudes of the natural and synthetic first harmonic are about the same (Figure 14–1C). Similarly, the decrease in second harmonic amplitude can be corrected by placing a pole-zero pair at the frequency of that harmonic.

1.3.5. Step 5: Alter Fundamental Frequency (F_0)

Next, F_0 was varied to model the natural utterances. Four approaches were used. In the first, the Klatt parameters FL and DI modulated the F_0 value used in Step 1. FL slowly and regularly varies F_0 as described by:

$$\Delta F_0 = (FL/50)(F_0/100)[\sin(2\pi\, 7.1t) + \sin(2\pi\, 4.7t)] \text{ Hz}$$

DI varies F_0 by delaying every other pulse and decreasing its amplitude. As a result, the pitch period alternates between $T0 - \Delta T0$ and $T0 + \Delta T0$, where $\Delta T0 = DI/100\ T0\ (1 - OQ/100)$. The shorter pitch period is attenuated by $\Delta AV = AV\ (1 - DI/100)$. Figure 14–2 shows the effect of changing DI. Figure 14–2A shows a glottal waveform with DI = 0%; in Figure 14–2B, DI = 50%. This technique improved the naturalness of some voices with relatively steady F_0 values, and of some voices with bifurcated phonation.

The second technique involved importing the F_0 contour calculated with the Speech-Station pitch tracker. This technique worked well for voices with an F_0 that changed slowly enough to be tracked by the pitch tracker, with maximum variations of 20 Hz.

A third technique was to model F_0 as a Gaussian random variable (Hillenbrand, 1987) with mean and variance derived from the natural sample. This worked well for voices with a relatively stable mean F_0 but high cycle-to-cycle fluctuations in period or for which period boundaries were difficult to identify precisely.

When none of the above techniques produced an acceptable sounding F_0 contour, manually calculated F_0 values were used. This technique, although cumbersome, improved the synthesis of some voices with bifurcated phonation.

Special care was taken to set the update interval (UI) equal to the greatest integer (in ms) less than the average period. This is important because F_0 values, unlike some other synthesis parameters, are updated at the beginning of the period rather than at each UI. Thus, with an alternating T0 or a randomly varying F_0, the proper UI must be specified.

1.3.6. Step 6: Alter AV as a Time-Varying Parameter for Amplitude-Modulated Voices

The parameter AV was time-varied to model shimmer (period-to-period variations) and amplitude modulation (longer-term variations) in some voices.

1.3.7. Step 7: Add Additional Pole-Zero Pairs If Necessary

Finally, some voices required pole-zero pairs to model nasal and/or tracheal coupling. This step was performed if the synthesizer's pole-zero pairs were not both used to boost or attenuate the energy in certain frequency regions (Step 4). Adjustments were made with reference to short-time spectra of the natural and synthetic utterances.

These seven steps were repeated and fine-tuned in the following manner, using informal perceptual evaluations and visual comparisons of spectrograms and short-time spectra of the natural and synthetic utterances. As described, visual representations of the voices were critical

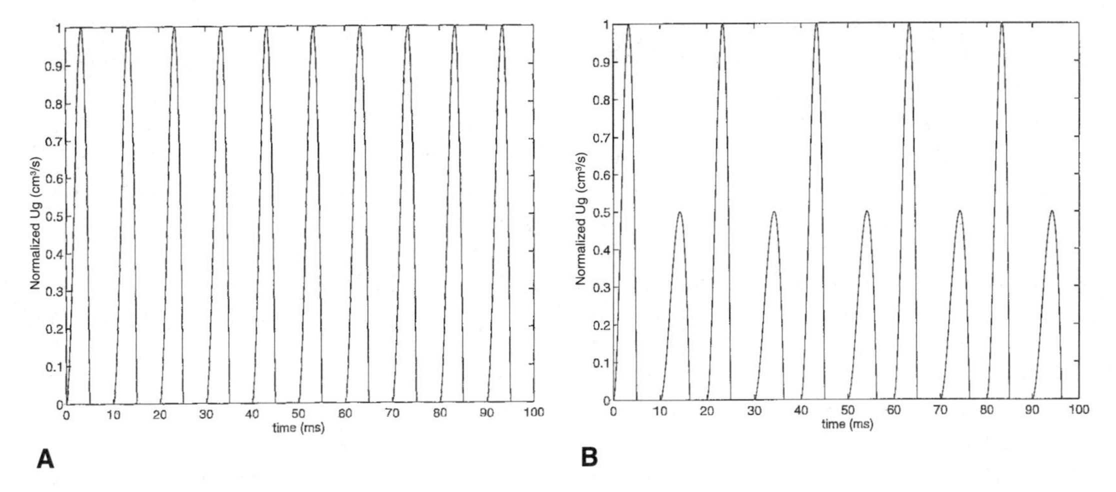

Figure 14–2. Plot of the glottal waveform (volume velocity versus time) with OQ = 50% and **A.** DI = 0%, and **B.** DI=50%.

for five of the seven steps, particularly in the first iteration. Detailed measurements of period-to-period variations (fundamental frequency and amplitude) were also important for guiding adjustment of the time varying parameters F_0 and AV. Once these steps were performed and repeated several times, a reasonably accurate synthetic voice was obtained.

Next, the synthesis was fine-tuned using informal perceptual evaluations. To determine if the fine-tuning improved the synthesis, two synthetic voices were compared to the natural utterance in the pattern: synthetic voice A, natural, synthetic voice B. Synthetic voice A represented the best synthesis thus far, and synthetic voice B differed from A by one or two parameters. When the three voices were played, the better synthetic voice was deemed the new synthetic attempt A. Further alterations were then made to create a new synthetic voice B. This process was repeated until either all attempts to improve the voice resulted in a perceptually worse voice or until these attempts resulted in a synthetic voice B that was perceptually identical to synthetic voice A. At that point, synthetic attempt A was declared the best possible copy of the natural voice sample. Synthesis of a single token took from 1–20 hours, depending on the severity of the vocal pathology.

2. PERCEPTUAL EVALUATION

Some of our attempts to synthesize pathological voices were subjectively more acceptable than others. The following experiment was undertaken to evaluate the overall quality of the synthesis and to determine which voices listeners considered good matches to the original samples.

2.1. Methods

Ten expert listeners (6 speech-language pathologists, 3 otolaryngologists, and 1 phonetician, including authors JK and BG) participated in this experiment. Each had a minimum of 1 year postgraduate experience evaluating voice quality and none reported any speech, language, or hearing difficulties.

The natural and best synthetic versions of the 24 voices described were used as stimuli. Each sample (synthetic and natural) lasted 1 sec. Stimuli were normalized for peak voltage, and onsets and offsets were multiplied by 25 ms ramps to eliminate click artifacts.

All listening tests took place in sound-treated booths. All testing was done in free field. Listeners were seated 3 feet from a high fidelity loudspeaker (Boston Acoustics A40). Stimuli were low-pass filtered at 8 kHz and played through a 16-bit D/A converter at a constant listening level (appx. 80 dB SPL). Responses were recorded and stored by a computer.

Listeners heard each natural sample paired with its synthetic copy and were asked to judge how well the copy matched the original (on a 7-point scale, with 1 indicating a perfect match in quality). Complete listener instructions are given in Appendix 14–B. Voice pairs were always presented in the order natural/synthetic. Three additional pairs consisting of two identical natural stimuli were also included. Tokens within a pair were separated by 500 ms. Each of the 27 voice pairs was presented twice (although listeners were not told this); stimuli were played out, rerandomized, and played out again. Different random orders were used for each listener. Listeners controlled the rate of presentation and were able to replay the voice pairs as often as necessary. The experiment lasted approximately 10 minutes for each listener.

2.2. Results

Test-retest reliability was acceptably high for all listeners. Across listeners, Pearson's r for the first versus second rating of a voice pair was 0.83 (range of individual values = 0.66–0.89); also across listeners, the first and second rating of a voice differed by 0.74 scale value on average. Because most listeners were unfamiliar with synthesized speech, the first set of judgments was treated as practice and discarded.

Performance on trials where voices were identical was also satisfactory. Only 1 listener failed to rate these voices as being identical in quality ("1"). However, that listener used the category "1" much less frequently than other listeners (3/56 trials versus an average of 12.6 trials rated "1" for the other listeners). Given that this listener rated voices consistently (test-retest Pearson's $r = 0.84$; 89.3% of ratings within 1 scale value), we concluded that these ratings probably represent response bias, rather than lapses of attention and data from this subject were retained.

Interrater reliability was also acceptable. Ratings for 8 of the 10 listeners were consistently correlated at $r = 0.7$ or better (mean Pearson's $r = 0.79$, SD = 0.05, range = 0.7–0.88). The remaining two listeners used a limited range of values when making their ratings. One gave 18 of 28 pairs a rating of 1 (identical qualities) and never rated a pair above 4. The second, as described above, rarely used the value 1. Ratings for these listeners were less well correlated with the remainder of the group (average Pearson's $r = 0.59$, SD = 0.14, range = 0.35 to 0.87). However, because they rated voices consistently, their data were retained.

Listeners unanimously reported being pleased by the overall quality of the synthesis. Table 14–1 shows the average rating for each voice, which ranged from 1.3 to 6.3. On the whole, copies of voices with milder pathology were more acceptable than those of more severely disordered voices (Pearson's r comparing mean rating and severity = 0.60, $p < 0.05$). Copies of male voices were more acceptable overall than were copies of female voices (males: mean = 2.99 females: mean = 4.19; $F_{(1,23)} = 5.00$, $p < 0.05$).

3. DISCUSSION

Our efforts to synthesize moderately to severely pathological voices were variably successful. Less severely pathological voices were synthesized best and male voices were synthesized more successfully than female voices: Of the 13 synthetic stimuli rated 3.5 or better, only 3 modeled female voices. This gender difference has been noted previously (e.g., Klatt & Klatt, 1990) and suggests that the synthesizer's glottal source model is better suited to synthesizing male voices than female voices. In addition, efforts to synthesize voices with slow, irregular variations in amplitude of voicing or fundamental frequency (in addition to rapid, period-to-period fluctuations) were often less successful because of the additional complexity of the task.

Although the success of the synthesis is better predicted by severity or gender than by the

Table 14–1. Results of perceptual evaluation.

Token	*Gender*	*Mean Rating*	*SD*	*Voice Severity*
bim2	male	1.3	0.483	4
rm2	male	1.7	0.675	5
bim1	male	1.9	0.994	5
rbrm4	male	1.9	0.738	5
bif1	female	2.0	0.943	4
rbrm1	male	2.3	0.823	3
rf1	female	2.3	0.949	6
rbrm2	male	2.5	0.850	5
rbim	male	2.8	0.789	5
rbrm3	male	2.9	0.994	5
rm1	male	3.0	1.054	4
bim4	male	3.4	1.174	5
bif3	female	3.5	1.269	5
rf2	female	3.8	1.317	6
bif2	female	4.0	1.826	4
bif4	female	4.0	1.700	4
bim3	male	4.3	1.252	5
sbrf1	female	4.5	1.581	6
srf	female	4.6	1.430	6
rbrm5	male	5.4	1.174	6
srm	male	5.5	1.354	6
rbrf1	female	5.8	1.874	6
rbrf2	female	5.9	1.197	6
sbrf2	female	6.3	1.252	6

Note: Mean rating across listeners, for each voice, is shown along with standard deviation, gender of the speaker, and rated severity of vocal pathology. Listeners judged the similarity between natural and synthetic voices on a scale of 1 to 7; 1 implies that the natural and synthetic voice qualities sounded identical, while 7 indicates that the stimuli were heard as differing greatly in quality.

"qualities" a voice might possess, some synthesis procedures and parameters were common to voices with prominent noise and to voices with bifurcated/bicyclic phonation. The following sections describe the analysis-by-synthesis procedures employed for these voices and speculate as to why we were unable to model some tokens adequately.

3.1. Modeling Voices with Prominent Noise

Eleven of the voices were characterized by prominent noise and/or jitter and shimmer. Parameters used to synthesize these voices are listed in Table 14–2. Capturing the variation in F_0 proved critical for successful synthesis of these voices. As shown in Table 14–2, 10 of the 11 voices required some form of F_0 variation; this was achieved by either modeling the F_0 variations with a Gaussian distribution (7 voices), using the flutter parameter (FL) (1 voice), the diplophonia parameter (DI) (1 voice), or by hand-copying the F_0 contour of the natural waveform (1 voice).

Eight of these 11 voices were synthesized with time-varying AV that emulated amplitude modulation. All voices were synthesized with some degree of aspiration noise. In fact, only 1 voice (rbrm1) was synthesized with a greater amplitude of voicing than aspiration (AV + GV

Table 14–2. Voices with prominent noise and/or jitter and shimmer.

	A. Female Voices			
Tokens	***rf1 (6)***	***rf2 (6)***	***rbrf1 (6)***	***rbrf2 (6)***
Time-varying Parameters				
F_0 (Hz)	G	G	G	G
avg	205	185	160	200
min/max	155/248	162/204	75/211	175/220
AV (dB)	G	G	G	
avg	58	67	45	K = 60
min/max	51/64	62/72	42/48	
Constant Parameters				
NF	4	4	5	4
GV (dB)	55	53	63	55
GH (dB)	55	51	60	60
AV	TV	TV	TV	60
OQ (%)	70	90	50	90
SQ (%)	200	200	160	200
AH (dB)	60	73	50	60
F_1 (Hz)	900	780	735	850
B_1 (Hz)	150	130	650	200
F_2 (Hz)	1330	1367	1100	1240
B_2 (Hz)	90	160	250	200
F_3 (Hz)	2700	3000	2400	3470
B_3 (Hz)	300	250	550	300
F_4 (Hz)	3700	3700	3300	3860
B_4 (Hz)	425	450	500	400
F_5 (Hz)	NA	NA	4000	NA
B_5 (Hz)	NA	NA	600	NA
FNP (Hz)	210	180	150	240
BNP (Hz)	40	30	250	40
FNZ (Hz)	210	180	150	240
BNZ (Hz)	100	90	120	120
FTP (Hz)	NA	NA	480	NA
BTP (Hz)	NA	NA	300	NA
FTZ (Hz)	NA	NA	480	NA
BTZ (Hz)	NA	NA	100	NA

	B. Male Voices				
Tokens	***rbrm1 (3)***	***rbrm2 (5)***	***rbrm3 (5)***	***rbrm4 (5)***	***rbrm5 (6)***
Time-varying Parameters					
F_0 (Hz)	G	G	G	G	
avg	119	143	K = 117	71	210
min/max	112/125	105/215		65/78	198/220
AV (dB)				G	G

Tokens	rbrm1 (3)	rbrm2 (5)	rbrm3 (5)	rbrm4 (5)	rbrm5 (6)
Time-varying Parameters					
avg	K = 58	52	K = 60	66	60
min/max		30/57		55/72	58/62
Constant Parameters					
NF	4	4	4	4	4
GV (dB)	61	64	61	53	57
GH (dB)	60	64	60	56	60
Fo (Hz)	TV	TV	117	TV	TV
AV (dB)	58	TV	60	TV	TV
OQ (%)	60	80	90	50	70
SQ (%)	200	150	200	200	200
FL (%)	0	0	5	0	0
AH (dB)	57	59	70	70	57
F_1 (Hz)	680	870	815	595	640
B_1 (Hz)	80	125	180	80	70
F_2 (Hz)	1280	1110	1260	1140	1200
B_2 (Hz)	140	125	200	90	300
F_3 (Hz)	2425	2700	2655	2350	2290
B_3 (Hz)	170	150	180	150	300
F_4 (Hz)	3760	3830	2470	3650	3380
B_4 (Hz)	200	250	300	250	300
FNP (Hz)	NA	NA	116	290	200
BNP (Hz)	NA	NA	40	40	50
FNZ (Hz)	NA	NA	116	290	200
BNZ (Hz)	NA	NA	180	120	150
FTP (Hz)	NA	560	NA	NA	NA
BTP (Hz)	NA	100	NA	NA	NA
FTZ (Hz)	NA	560	NA	NA	NA
BTZ (Hz)	NA	280	NA	NA	NA

C. More Male Voices

Tokens	rm1(4)	rm2 (5)
Time-varying Parameters		
AV (dB)		G
avg	63	65
min/max	61/65	62/68
Constant Parameters		
NF	4	4
GV (dB)	56	57
GH (dB)	56	57
Fo (Hz)	124	88
OQ (%)	90	80
SQ (%)	250	200
DI (%)	20	0
AH (dB)	73	64

Table 14–2. Continued

	C. More Male Voices	
Tokens	***rm1(4)***	***rm2 (5)***
Constant Parameters		
F_1 (Hz)	700	740
B_1 (Hz)	60	130
F_2 (Hz)	1115	1230
B_2 (Hz)	90	120
F_3 (Hz)	2750	2695
B_3 (Hz)	200	175
F_4 (Hz)	3600	3500
B_4 (Hz)	200	350
FNP (Hz)	124	290
BNP (Hz)	35	30
FNZ (Hz)	124	290
BNZ (Hz)	80	100
FTP (Hz)	372	1900
BTP (Hz)	100	200
FTZ (Hz)	372	1900
BTZ (Hz)	280	100

Note: Synthesis parameters for voices characterized by noise, jitter, and shimmer. The parameters are either time-varying (parameter varies throughout the segment) or constant. If a parameter is not specified, it is set to the synthesizer's default value. TV = time varying, K = constant, NA = not activated. The symbol G refers to the use of a Gaussian random variable to model perturbation. The severity rating of the voice is given parenthetically next to the token's label.

> AH + GH), with all the other voices having a greater amplitude of aspiration noise than voicing. To match the increased amplitude of the first harmonic observed in the natural spectra, 9 of the synthetic voices required an OQ > 50%. With the exception of 1 voice (rbrm1), all voices were synthesized with pole-zero pairs placed below F_1 to boost or attenuate the amplitude of the harmonics in that frequency region. When matching the amplitudes of the formant frequencies, formant bandwidths were generally wider for female voices than they were for male voices.

Perceptual ratings for voices in this category ranged from 1.7 (very close match) to 5.9 (poor match). Seven synthesized voices were considered good matches to the natural voices (average ratings of 3.5 or better), with 4 voices having average ratings above 3.5. Spectrograms of the natural and synthetic tokens for the best-rated of these voices (a male, token rm2) are shown in Figure 14–3A. Figure 14–3B shows short-time DFT spectra of the natural stimulus at two places in the time waveform, superimposed on corresponding spectra of the synthetic copy. As can be seen in these figures, the spectral characteristics of the synthetic token provided good matches to those of the natural signal. Using the tracheal and nasal pole-zero pairs (Table 14–2B) was critical in achieving a good copy of this voice. Figure 14–3C shows a portion of the time waveform of the natural token. The shimmer apparent in this figure was mimicked by modeling the AV parameter as a Gaussian random variable.

Figure 14–4A shows spectrograms of the natural and synthetic tokens of female voice (rbrf1) that received a poor rating of 5.8. The spectral match between the natural and synthetic copy is not very good in the mid- and

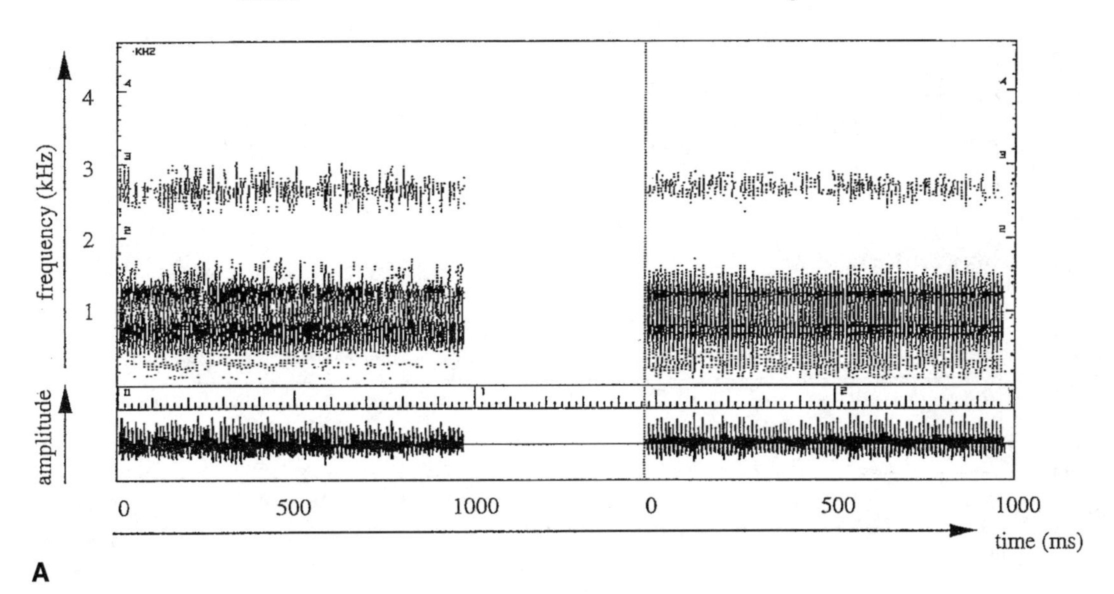

A

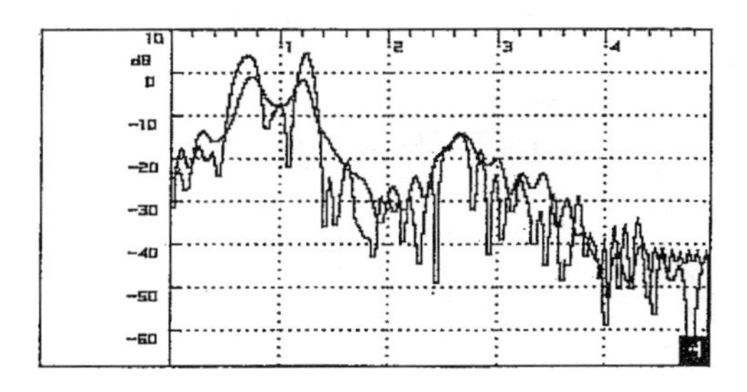

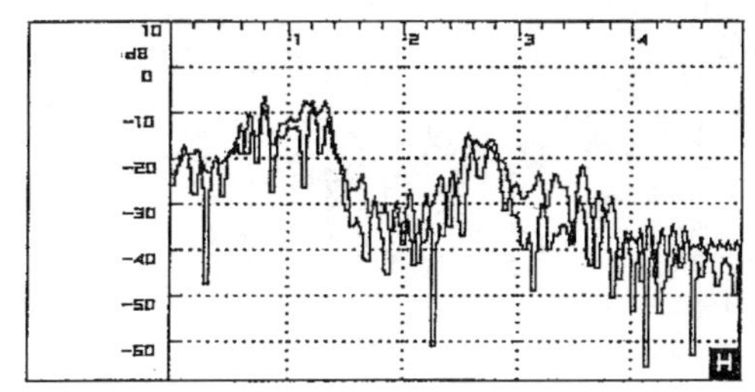

B

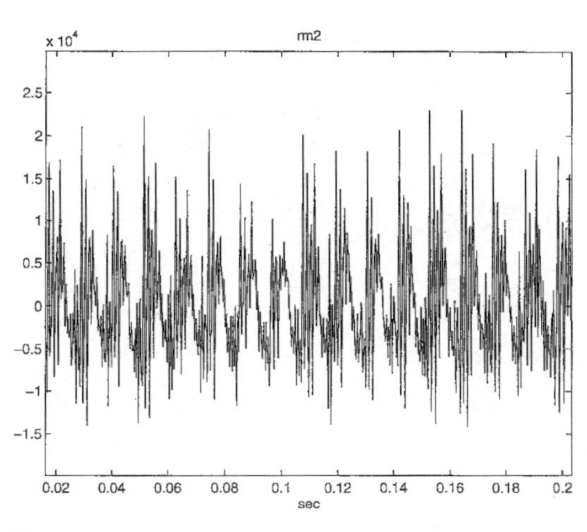

C

Figure 14–3. A. Spectrograms and time waveforms of the natural and synthetic tokens of a male voice (rm2). **B.** DFT spectra (calculated using a 12.8 ms Hamming window) of the natural token superimposed with those of the synthetic token at two different time intervals. **C.** A portion of the time waveform of the natural voice.

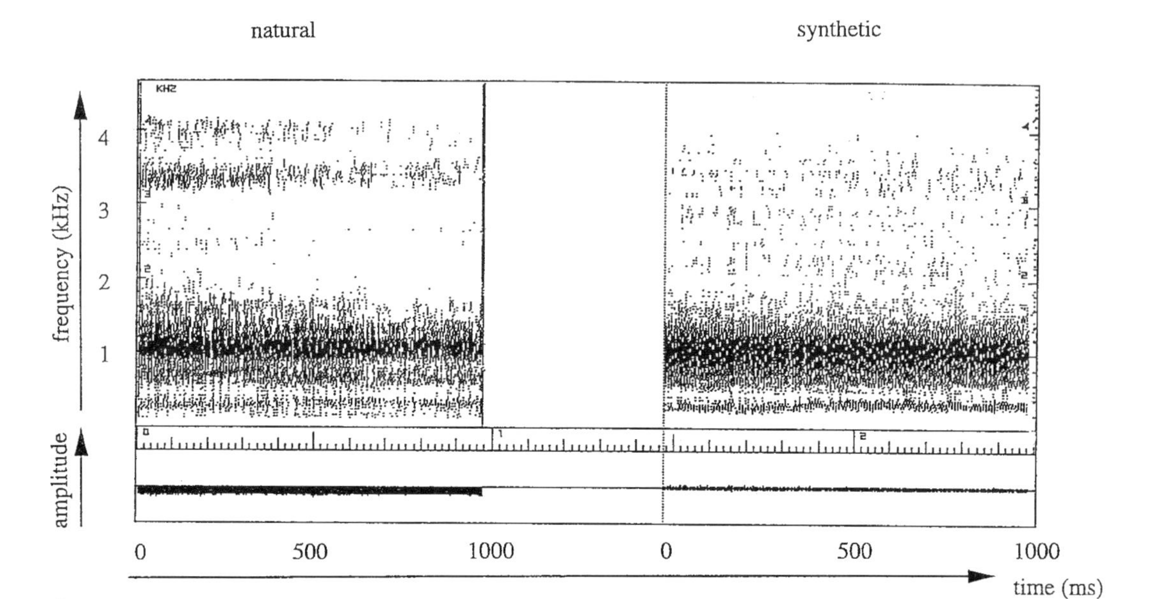

A

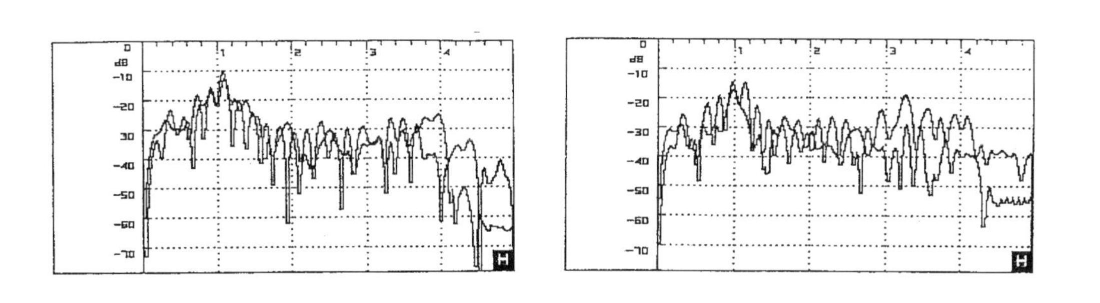

B

rbrf1

-3000
-4000
-5000
-6000
-7000
-8000
-9000

0.4 0.42 0.44 0.46 0.48 0.5 0.52 0.54 0.56

sec

C

Figure 14–4. A. Spectrograms and time waveforms of the natural and synthetic tokens of a female voice (rbrf1). **B.** DFT spectra of the natural token superimposed with those of the synthetic token at 2 different time intervals. **C.** A portion of the time waveform of the natural voice.

high-frequency regions. This can be seen in Figure 14–4B, where DFT spectra of the natural and synthetic copy at two different time intervals are superimposed. The natural voice has significant period-to-period fluctuations (Figure 14–4C). We attempted to mimic these fluctuations by modeling F_0 as a Gaussian random variable and hand-copying AV (Table 14–2C). The mismatch in the spectral domain, combined with large and random temporal variations in the natural voice, may have resulted in the low acceptability of the synthesized copy.

3.2. Modeling Bifurcated Phonation

Bifurcated phonation (e.g., Titze, Baken, & Herzel, 1993; also labeled "diplophonia" [Klatt & Klatt, 1990], "bicyclicity" [Gerratt, Precoda, Hanson, & Berke, 1988], or "dicrotic dysphonia" [Moore & Von Leden, 1958]) is characterized by a pattern of cycles that alternate in fundamental period, amplitude, or both, in a large-small-large-small (AbAb) pattern. Eight bifurcated voices (4 female and 4 male) were analyzed. None showed a perfect pattern of periods alternating in an AbAb fashion. Instead, three patterns emerged: (1) four voices had fundamental frequencies varying randomly between 3 to 9 different F_0 values; (2) three voices had F_0 bimodally distributed; and (3) one voice was increasingly bifurcated with time (see Kreiman et al., 1993, for discussion of the acoustics and perception of such voices).

Synthesis parameters for the 8 bifurcated voices are given in Table 14–3. As this table shows, three methods were used to model F_0. F_0 contours were carefully matched to those of the natural waveforms for three of the eight voices (bif3, bif4, bim4). DI and FL were used with a constant F_0 parameter for three voices (bim1, bim2, bim3), with time-varying F_0 combined with DI for the remaining two voices (bif1, bif2). One voice (bim2) demonstrated considerable shimmer, so time-varying AV was used. In contrast to voices characterized mainly by noise, male and female bifurcated voices differed in OQ values. The male voices had weaker first harmonics than their female counterparts. Hence, OQ was less than 50% for all the male voices, but for only one female voice.

Seven of the 8 voices (4 female and 3 male) required a low-frequency energy boost using the nasal and/or tracheal pole-zero pairs, and in one case (bif4), the tracheal pole-zero pair was used to weaken the second harmonic. Only 1 voice (bif2) was modeled with more aspiration than voicing. All other voices had more voicing than aspiration.

Perceptual ratings for these voices ranged between 1.3 to 4.3. Five synthesized voices were considered good matches to the natural voices (ratings of 3.5 or better), with three voices rated above 3.5. Figure 14–5A shows spectrograms of natural and synthetic tokens for the voice (token bim2) that was the most successfully synthesized in the bifurcated category. The spectral match between the natural and synthetic voice was very good (Figure 14–5B). This voice showed period-to-period fluctuations which were mimicked by hand-copying the amplitude of the waveform, by setting the DI parameter to 8%, and by setting the FL parameter to 5%. F_0 bimodality in the natural and synthetic copies is shown in Figure 14–5C.

Figure 14–6A shows the spectrograms of the natural and synthetic versions of a female voice (bif2) that received a lower rating of 4.0. The fundamental frequency of the natural voice was measured manually; a plot of F_0 for the first 500 ms is shown in Figure 14–6B. F_0 varied randomly between five values in the range 230–250 Hz, and was difficult to mimic properly. In addition, the spectral match in the mid- and high-frequency regions was not perfect, as shown by the DFT spectra of the natural and synthetic voices in Figure 14–6C.

3.3. Other Voices

A number of voices did not fall into traditional categories. Synthesizing these perceptually and acoustically complex stimuli presented particular challenges.

Table 14–3. Bifurcated voices.

	A. Bifurcated Female Voices			
Tokens	***bif1 (4)***	***bif2 (4)***	***bif3 (5)***	***bif4 (4)***
Time-varying Parameters				
F_0 (Hz)				
avg	227	245	182	209
min/max	220/232	237/257	177/187	196/222
DI (%)				
avg	10	K = 7	K = 0	K = 0
min/max	7/14			
Constant Parameters				
NF	4	4	4	4
GV (dB)	57	59	62	59
GH (dB)	57	60	60	58
AV (dB)	62	63	62	65
OQ (%)	70	77	60	40
SQ (%)	200	140	200	150
DI (%)	TV	7	0	0
AH (dB)	60	67	55	60
F_1 (Hz)	930	790	645	990
B_1 (Hz)	200	180	60	200
F_2 (Hz)	1450	1220	1620	1410
B_2 (Hz)	150	90	100	130
F_3 (Hz)	2800	2270	3240	3795
B_3 (Hz)	250	130	250	350
F_4 (Hz)	3740	3150	4200	4245
B_4 (Hz)	150	150	350	450
FNP (Hz)	230	225	194	205
BNP (Hz)	50	40	30	60
FNZ (Hz)	230	225	194	205
BNZ (Hz)	150	100	100	400
FTP (Hz)	460	450	2050	414
BTP (Hz)	50	100	60	150
FTZ (Hz)	460	450	2050	414
BTZ (Hz)	120	200	350	80

	B. Bifurcated Male Voices			
Tokens	***bim1 (5)***	***bim2 (4)***	***bim3 (5)***	***bim4 (5)***
Time-varying Parameters				
F_0 (Hz)				
avg	K = 164	K = 177	K = 140	147
min/max				146/152
AV (dB)				
avg	K = 60	59	K = 63	K = 63
min/max		57/60		

Tokens	*bim1 (5)*	*bim2 (4)*	*bim3 (5)*	*bim4 (5)*
Constant Parameters				
NF	5	5	4	4
GV (dB)	57	62	58	60
GH (dB)	56	60	58	60
Fo (Hz)	164	177	140	TV
AV (dB)	60	TV	63	63
OQ (%)	45	27	30	30
SQ (%)	150	200	200	200
FL (%)	10	5	5	0
DI (%)	23	8	10	0
AH (dB)	60	50	60	55
F_1 (Hz)	755	580	700	790
B_1 (Hz)	60	120	60	150
F_2 (Hz)	1095	1120	1060	1240
B_2 (Hz)	90	30	140	100
F_3 (Hz)	2370	2700	2480	2920
B_3 (Hz)	300	250	90	150
F_4 (Hz)	2980	3330	3000	3760
B_4 (Hz)	200	400	90	150
F_5 (Hz)	3780	3720	NA	NA
B_5 (Hz)	200	500	NA	NA
FNP (Hz)	170	170	NA	280
BNP (Hz)	30	45	NA	60
FNZ (Hz)	170	170	NA	280
BNZ (Hz)	100	90	NA	280
FTP (Hz)	565	340	NA	3760
BTP (Hz)	40	95	NA	60
FTZ (Hz)	565	340	NA	3760
BTZ (Hz)	100	180	NA	300

Note: Abbreviations are defined as in Table 14–2.

One male voice (rbim) was characterized by high levels of jitter and shimmer, noise, and intermittent bifurcations. The fundamental frequency fluctuated between about 100–200 Hz, and aspiration noise was present in the F_3 and F_4 regions. The synthesis parameters for this voice, which received a rating of 2.8, are given in Table 14–4, and spectrograms of the natural and synthetic tokens are shown in Figure 14–7A.

Synthesis involved matching the overall F_0 contour to that of the natural token and using the DI parameter, as for a severely bifurcated voice. Unlike the bifurcated voices, however, this voice was synthesized with 10–14 dB more aspiration than voicing. The spectral details of this voice varied approximately every 100 ms. Figure 14–7B shows DFT spectra of the natural voice superimposed on the spectra of the synthetic copy; the spectral match between the natural and synthetic token was good.

Two female voices (sbrf1, sbrf2) with highly variable vocal qualities were analyzed. Both voices began with strong voicing, but the voicing amplitude decreased in the last 400 ms of the sample. The synthesis parameters for these voices are listed in Table 14–5, and spectrograms of the natural and synthetic utterances for one token (sbrf1) are shown in Figure 14–8A.

These voices were very difficult to synthesize, because of problems matching the widely varying spectral and temporal details of the voices. Figure 14–8B shows DFT spectra at

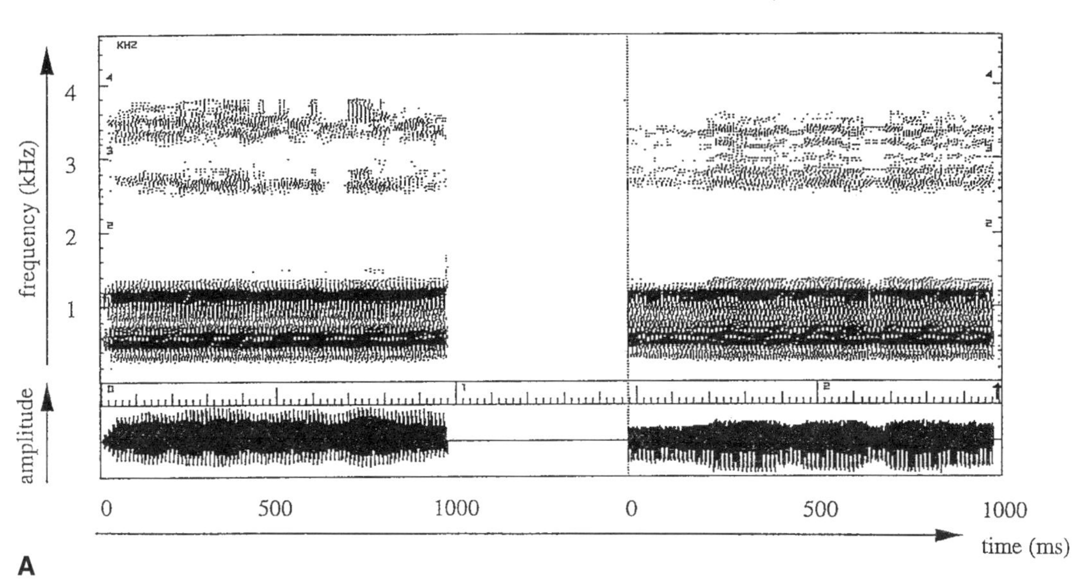

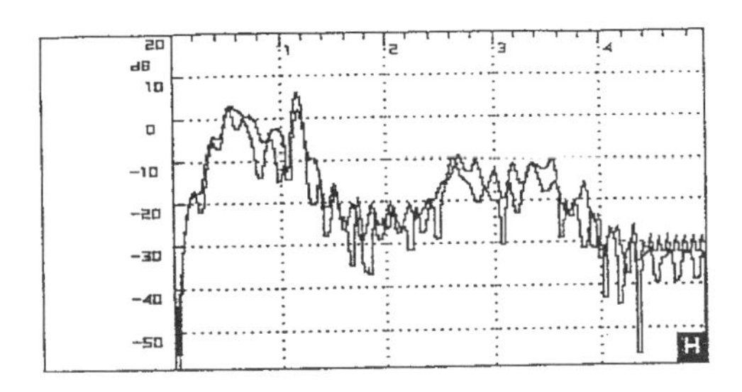
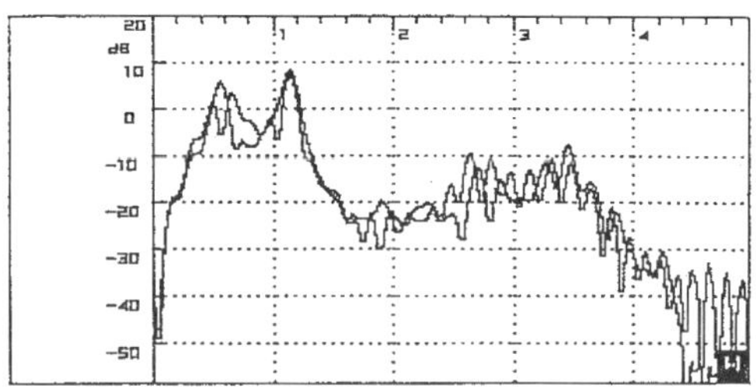

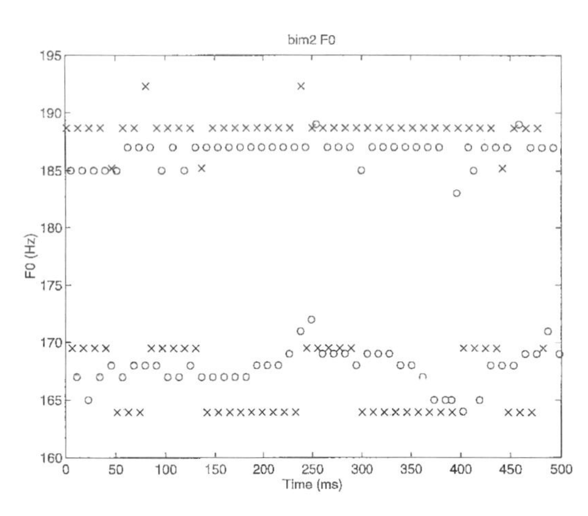

Figure 14–5. A. Spectrograms and time waveforms of the natural and synthetic tokens of a bifurcated male voice (bim2). **B.** DFT spectra of the natural token superimposed with those of the synthetic token at two different time intervals. **C.** Plot of F_0 versus time for the natural (denoted by circles) and synthetic (denoted by the x symbol) tokens.

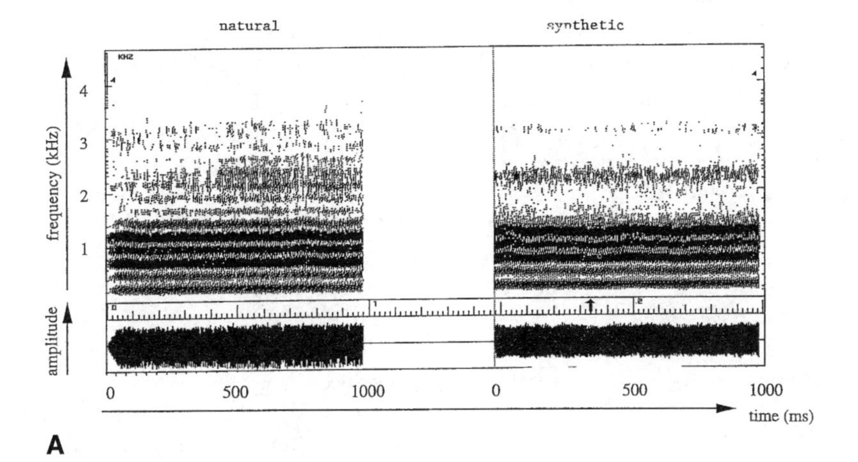

A

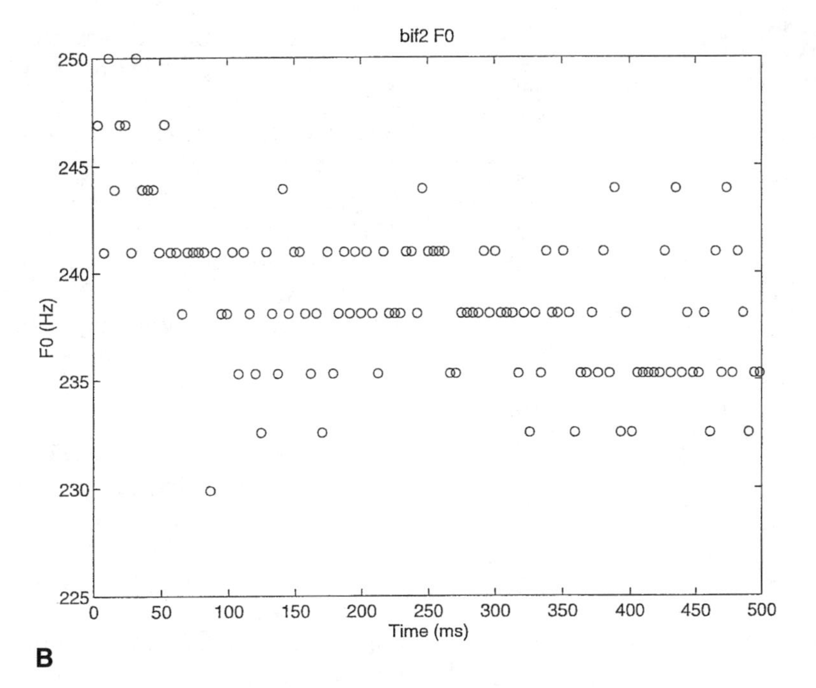

B

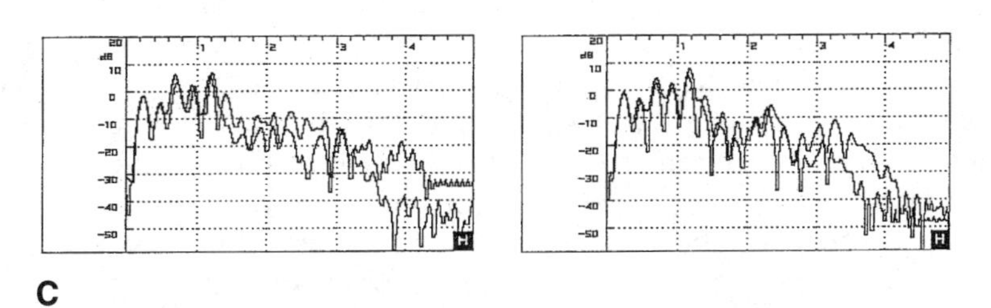

C

Figure 14–6. A. Spectrograms and time waveforms of the natural and synthetic tokens of a bifurcated female voice (bif2). **B.** Plot of F_0 versus time for the natural token. **C.** DFT spectra of the natural token superimposed with those of the synthetic token at two different time intervals.

Table 14–4. Intermittently bifurcated male voice.

Token	*rbim (5)*
Time-varying Parameters	
F0 (Hz)	
avg	152
min/max	80/210
AV (dB)	
avg	61
min/max	58/62
Constant Parameters	
NF	5
GV (dB)	59
GH (dB)	62
OQ (%)	45
SQ (%)	400
DI (%)	2
AH (dB)	69
F_1 (Hz)	450
B_1 (Hz)	60
F_2 (Hz)	1150
B_2 (Hz)	100
F_3 (Hz)	2240
B_3 (Hz)	150
F_4 (Hz)	3000
B_4 (Hz)	350
F_5 (Hz)	3800
B_5 (Hz)	150
FTP (Hz)	1860
BTP (Hz)	140
FTZ (Hz)	1860
BTZ (Hz)	200

Note: See Table 14–2 caption for further details.

three points in the natural waveform; note the significant variation in the spectra. Figure 14–8D shows a portion of the time waveform of this voice, demonstrating significant period-to-period variability.

Techniques used to model the time-varying nature of these voices included sequentially increasing and decreasing OQ to capture variations in quality with time; time-varying AH and AV to model variations in noise; and utilizing FL and time-varying F_0. Perceptual ratings of 4.5 and 6.3 reflect the limited success of our efforts. Figure 14–8C shows DFT spectra of the natural and synthetic copy; note in particular the spectral mismatch at high frequencies.

Finally, two additional voices (1 female, 1 male) with unsteady qualities were analyzed and synthesized. Both voices (srf, srm) were described as "gargly" and both synthetic versions received poor ratings (4.6 and 5.5). The synthesis parameters for these voices are listed in Table 14–6, and spectrograms of the natural and synthetic female token (srf) are shown in Figure 14–9A.

The "gargly" period was limited mainly to the last 400 ms of this voice, and several parameters (F_0, AV, SQ, and FL) were time-varied to capture the unsteadiness in the natural token. Our attempts were not very successful. In particular, it was not possible to significantly attenuate the high-frequency energy in the synthetic copy, especially because both pole-zero pairs (tracheal and nasal) were used to match the spectra below 3 kHz. Figure 14–9B shows DFT spectra of the natural and synthetic copies at two time intervals; in one interval the spectral match was good but in another, there was a clear mismatch at high frequencies.

3.4. Why Exact Matches to Some Voices Could Not Be Achieved

In general, voices with significant amplitude and/or frequency perturbations were difficult to synthesize with the Klatt synthesizer. The flutter parameter (FL), which alters F_0 in a slow time-varying fashion, is available, but does not model jitter appropriately (Klatt & Klatt, 1990). The current implementation of the diplophonia parameter (DI) is also inadequate for modeling jitter, shimmer, or bifurcated phonation. Further, DI produces patterns of amplitude and frequency variation that do not match measurements of natural bifurcated waveforms, for which there is no consistent correlation between amplitude and F_0 (Kreiman et al., 1993). Synthesis would be improved by allowing amplitude to be changed independently of delay and/or by allowing amplitude to be specified for each individual period.

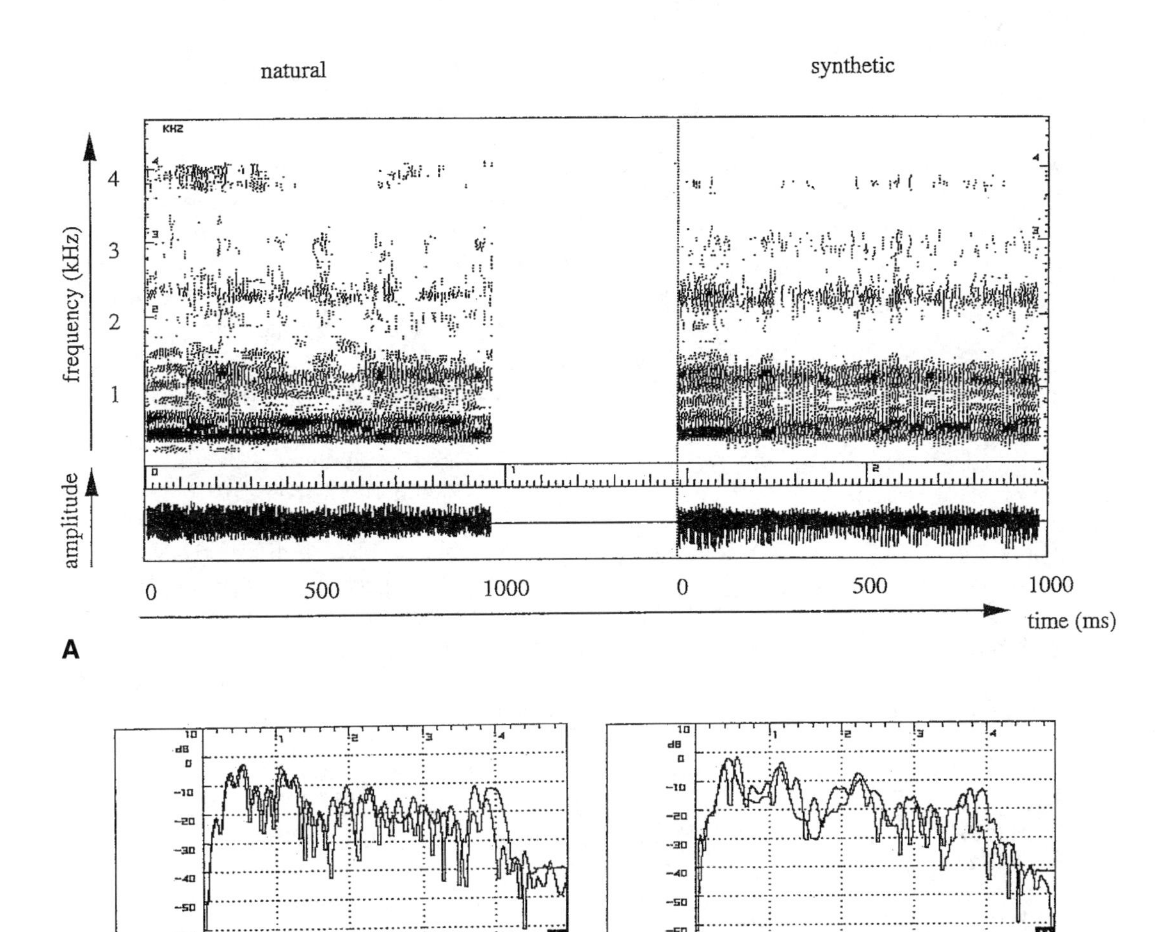

Figure 14–7. A. Spectrograms and time waveforms of the natural and synthetic tokens of a bifurcated male voice (rbim). **B.** DFT spectra of the natural voice superimposed with those of the synthetic voice at two times in the waveform.

One technique that was successful for modeling F_0 in voices with high jitter and shimmer was the use of a Gaussian frequency distribution (Hillenbrand, 1988). This technique involved exiting the synthesizer, generating new random numbers, and importing them back into the synthesizer, which was cumbersome to use. A synthesis parameter that allows F_0 (and possibly AV) to be modeled by a Gaussian random variable with a given mean and variance would greatly facilitate this process.

Most "unacceptable" ratings reflected failures to model unsteady or gargled qualities. Our failure to capture the gargly nature of some voices is due to several factors. First, the synthesizer's update interval (UI) is implemented as a function of time, not period. Some parameters, such as F_0, are updated at the end of each period. However, most time-varying parameters (such as AV) are specified at multiples of UI, and linear interpolation is used to determine time-varying values between update intervals. This poses a problem when one needs to change attributes of one glottal pulse without affecting other pulses. For example, it would be much easier to mimic spikes that

Table 14–5. Strained-noisy female voices.

Tokens	***sbrf1 (6)***	***sbrf2 (6)***
Time-varying Parameters		
F_0 (Hz)		
avg	216	211
min/max	204/250	202/222
AV (dB)		
avg	53	61
min/max	41/57	58/65
OQ (%)		
avg	60	17
min/max	45/70	10/25
FL (%)		
avg	K = 20	13
min/max		10/20
AH (dB)		
avg	77	61
min/max	76/80	58/63
Constant Parameters		
NF	5	
NF	4	4
GV (dB)	58	57
GH (dB)	56	73
Fo (Hz)	TV	202
SQ (%)	180	200
FL (%)	20	TV
DI (%)	6	0
F_1 (Hz)	750	820
B_1 (Hz)	230	400
F_2 (Hz)	1020	1450
B_2 (Hz)	230	200
F_3 (Hz)	2675	2950
B_3 (Hz)	200	300
F_4 (Hz)	3990	3850
B_4 (Hz)	250	600
FNP (Hz)	NA	606
BNP (Hz)	NA	200
FNZ (Hz)	NA	606
BNZ (Hz)	NA	60

Note: See Table 14–2 caption for more details.

occur in the time waveforms of some pathological voices, if it were possible to specify AV at a single period rather than at an update interval. Spikes can usually be modeled adequately if UI = 1 ms, but then we can only synthesize 400 ms because of a limitation imposed by the synthesizer.

It was often difficult to match the low-frequency energy of the natural samples, especially below the first formant. A partial solution is to adjust the open quotient (OQ), which primarily affects the amplitude of the first harmonic. As pointed out earlier, this is often inadequate. Additional pole-zero pairs (nasal and/or tracheal) can be placed at particular frequencies. This solution works well as long as the nasal and tracheal pole-zero pairs are not used elsewhere to model source-tract interactions. Providing more pole-zero pairs, which can be placed at any frequency, would not only alleviate this problem but would also aid in creating better spectral matches between synthetic and natural voices at all frequencies. Alternatively, a new parameter that adjusts the amplitudes of individual harmonics (especially those below F_1) would help.

4. SUMMARY AND CONCLUSIONS

This chapter describes a pilot study into the mechanics of synthesizing moderately to severely pathological voices. Successful synthesis of such voices may ultimately provide a method for evaluating and documenting voice qualities. An analysis-by-synthesis approach using a Klatt formant synthesizer was applied to study 24 tokens of the vowel /a/ spoken by males and females with voice disorders. Both temporal and spectral features of the natural waveforms were analyzed and the results were used to guide synthesis.

Ten expert listeners found that about half the synthetic voices were well-matched to the natural waveforms they modeled. Some modifications to the Klatt synthesizer are necessary to successfully synthesize the remaining pathological voices. Potential modifications include providing a parameter to increase the low frequency energy below F_1; adding more pole-zero pairs; providing jitter and shimmer parameters; changing the update interval parameter to work in periods rather than in

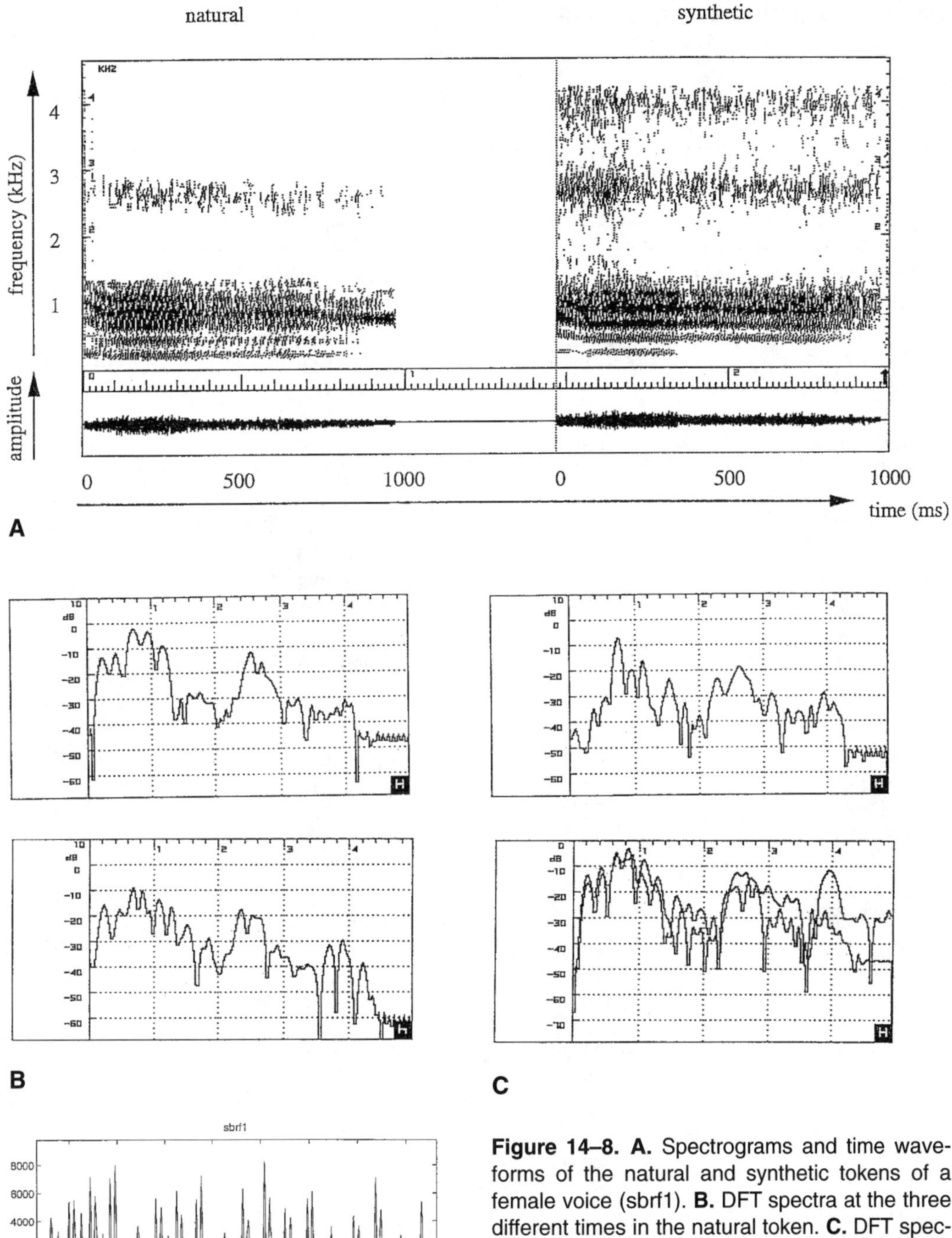

Figure 14–8. A. Spectrograms and time waveforms of the natural and synthetic tokens of a female voice (sbrf1). **B.** DFT spectra at the three different times in the natural token. **C.** DFT spectra of the natural voice superimposed with those of the synthetic voice. **D.** A portion of the time waveform of the natural voice.

Table 14–6. Gargly voices.

A. Female Voice		Male Voice	
Token	***srf (6)***	***Token***	***srm (6)***
Time-varying Parameters		*Time-varying Parameters*	
F0 (Hz)		F_0 (Hz)	
avg	200	avg	170
min/max	195/201	min	160/175
AV (dB)		AV (dB)	
avg	61	avg	56
min/max	58/63	min	53/58
SQ (%)		OQ (%)	
avg	370	avg	50
min/max	300/500	min/max	45/60
FL (%)		SQ (%)	
avg	20	avg	237
min/max	15/30	min/max	200/300
Constant Parameters		*Constant Parameters*	
NF	5	NF	5
GV (dB)	55	NF	4
GH (dB)	60	GV (dB)	60
OQ (%)	35	GH (dB)	60
AH (dB)	52	FL (%)	20
F_1 (Hz)	790	AH (dB)	55
B_1 (Hz)	100	F_1 (Hz)	700
F_2 (Hz)	1200	B_1 (Hz)	60
B_2 (Hz)	130	F_2 (Hz)	1030
F_3 (Hz)	2590	B_2 (Hz)	90
B_3 (Hz)	400	F_3 (Hz)	3100
F_4 (Hz)	3800	B_3 (Hz)	100
B_4 (Hz)	375	F_4 (Hz)	3800
F_5 (Hz)	4200	B_4 (Hz)	100
B_5 (Hz)	375		
FNP (Hz)	402		
BNP (Hz)	60		
FNZ (Hz)	402		
BNZ (Hz)	180		
FTP (Hz)	3000		
BTP (Hz)	180		
FTZ (Hz)	3000		
BTZ (Hz)	120		

Note: See Table 14–2 caption for further details.

absolute time; and modifying the diplophonia parameter so that fundamental frequency and amplitude variations can be independently controlled. Modifying the DI parameter and increasing the number of formants and the pole-zero pairs are straightforward operations. It is less clear how jitter and shimmer parameters should be implemented. One possibility is

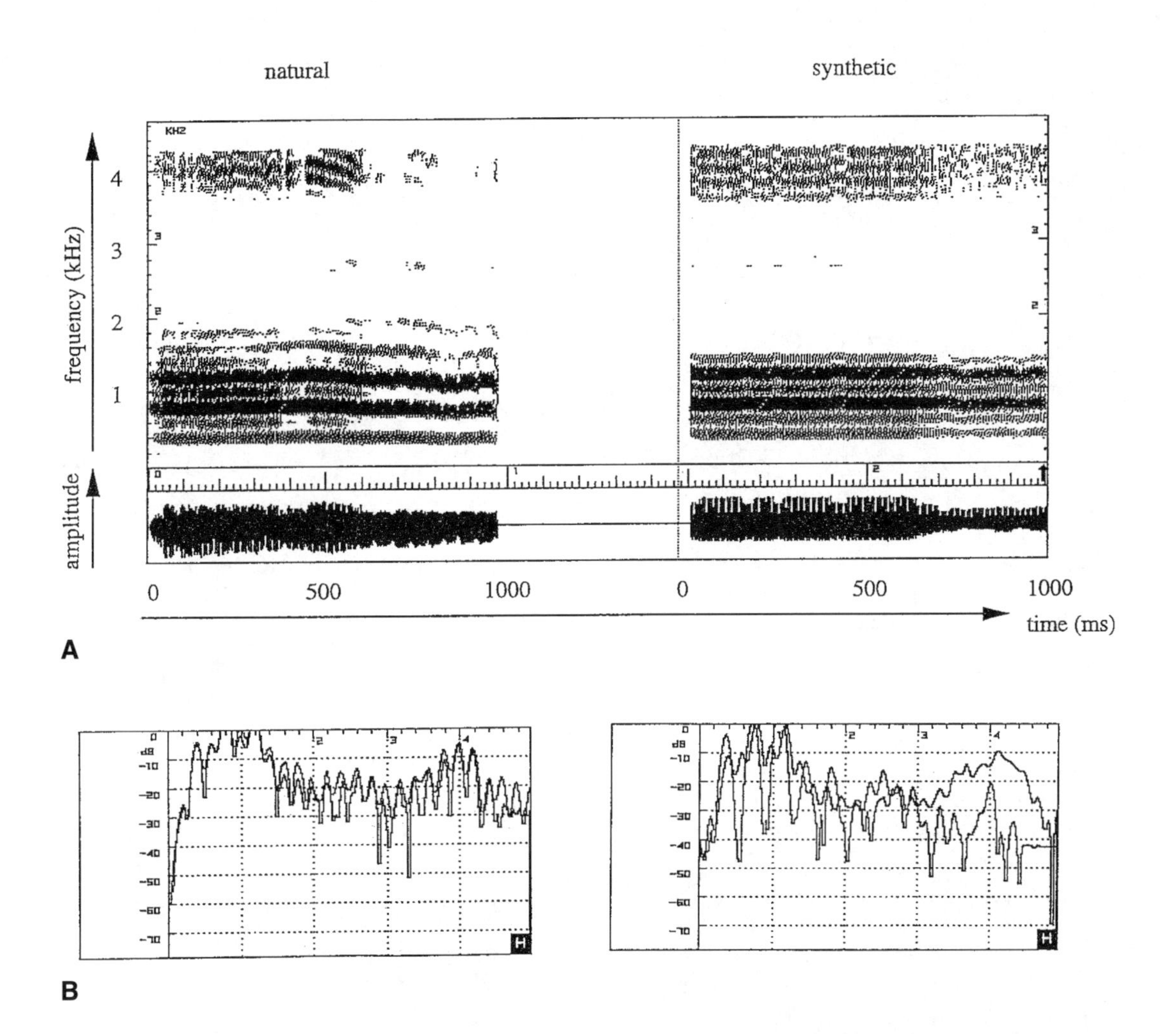

Figure 14–9. A. Spectrograms and time waveforms of the natural and synthetic tokens of a female voice (srf). **B.** DFT spectra of the natural voice superimposed with those of the synthetic voice at two different time intervals in the waveform.

to implement a Gaussian random variable, like the one used in this study.

In this study we were obliged to limit our analysis-by-synthesis to waveforms sampled at 10 kHz because the synthesizer provides only six variable formants, limiting the maximum usable sampling rate to 10–12 kHz. Figure 14–10 shows the high frequency spectral roll-off for a vowel synthesized at sampling rates of 10 kHz and 20 kHz, using the default values for formant frequencies and bandwidths. Figure 14–10A shows a spectrum synthesized with five formants and a sampling rate of 10 kHz, while Figure 14–10B shows a synthetic vowel with eight formants and a sampling rate of 20 kHz. The resulting spectrum for the higher sampling rate slopes downward starting at the fourth formant, due to the lack of formants near the Nyquist frequency (10 kHz in Figure 14–10B). Providing more than six formants with variable frequency and bandwidth would alleviate this difficulty.

This spectral slope has noticeable effects in the resultant synthetic voice quality. For example, Figure 14–11 shows a spectrogram of a natural voice sampled at 20 kHz and of the

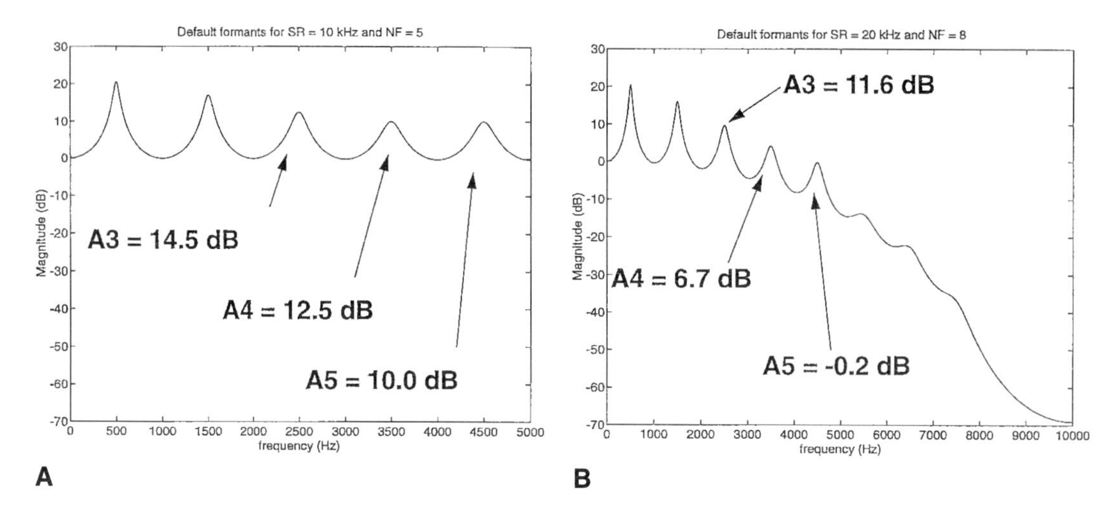

Figure 14–10. Linear predictive coding (LPC) spectra of a central vowel, like "uh," for two different sampling rates. The transfer function is calculated using formants at 500 Hz, 1500 Hz, and so on, plus the synthesizer's default values for the bandwidths. **A.** The vocal tract transfer function for a sampling rate of 10 kHz and 5 formants. **B.** The vocal tract transfer function for a sampling rate of 20 kHz and 8 formants.

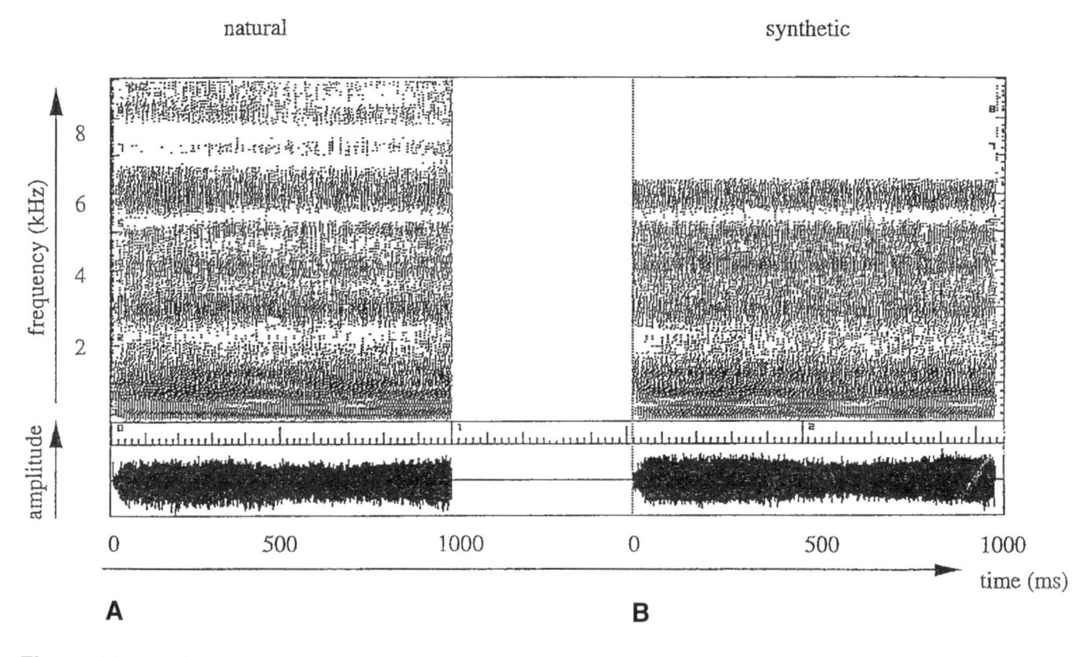

Figure 14–11. Consequences of the limited number of formants when applied to synthesizing a pathological female voice sampled at 20 kHz. **A.** The natural utterance has energy at high frequencies (up to 9 kHz in this example). **B.** The synthetic utterance has most of the energy at frequencies below 6.5 kHz.

synthetic stimulus generated with formant frequencies and amplitudes measured from the original sample. The synthetic stimulus matches the natural one for frequencies below 5 kHz, but not for higher frequencies. Although these high frequencies may not be important for speech perception or intelligibility, they are important aspects of voice quality.

Finally, more acoustic modeling of severe vocal pathology is necessary. As discussed, most models are based on variations in normal speech and do not easily accommodate pathologic cases. Different source models and/or synthesis approaches may ultimately be required to mimic severe pathology adequately. Improved models and synthesizers are essential for improved pathological voice quality evaluation and for the creation of well-matched synthesized voices.

Acknowledgment

This research was supported in part by NIDCD grant DC 01797.

REFERENCES

Ananthapadmanabha, T.V. (1984). Acoustic analysis of voice source dynamics. *Speech Transmission Laboratory Quarterly Status and Progress Report, 2–3,* 1–24.

Carlson, R., Granstrom, B., & Karlsson, I. (1991). Experiments with voice modeling in speech synthesis. *Speech Communication, 10,* 481–489.

Childers, D. G., & Ahn, C. (1995). Modeling the glottal volume–velocity waveform for three voice types. *Journal of the Acoustical Society of America, 97,* 505–519.

Childers, D. G. & Lee, C. K. (1991). Vocal quality factors: analysis, synthesis, and perception. *Journal of the Acoustical Society of America, 90,* 2394–2410.

Fant, G., Liljencrants, J., & Lin, Q. G. (1985). A four parameter model of glottal flow. *Speech Transmission Laboratory Quarterly Status and Progress Report, 4,* 1–13.

Fujisaki, H., & Ljungqvist, M. (1986). Proposal and evaluation of models for the glottal source waveform. *Proceedings of the IEEE International Conference on Acoustics, Speech, and Signal Processing,* vol. 3, 1605–1608.

Gerratt, B. R., Precoda, K., Hanson, D. G., & Berke, G. S. (1988, May). *Source characteristics of diplophonia.* Paper presented at the 115th meeting of the Acoustical Society of America, Seattle, WA.

Gerratt, B. R., Kreiman, J., Antonanzas-Barroso, N., & Berke, G. S. (1993). Comparing internal and external standards in voice quality judgments. *Journal of Speech and Hearing Research, 36,* 14–20.

Gobl, C. (1988). Voice source dynamics in connected speech. *Speech Transmission Laboratory Quarterly Status and Progress Report, 1,* 123–159.

Gobl, C., & Ní Chasaide, A. (1992). Acoustic characteristics of voice quality. *Speech Communication, 11,* 481–490.

Hillenbrand, J. (1987). A methodological study of perturbation and additive noise in synthetically generated voice signals. *Journal of Speech and Hearing Research, 30,* 448–461.

Hillenbrand, J. (1988). Perception of aperiodicities in synthetically generated voices. *Journal of the Acoustical Society of America, 83,* 2361–2371.

Imaizumi, S., Kiritani, S., & Saito, S. (1991). Perceptual evaluation of a glottal source model for voice quality control. In J. Gauffin & B. Hammarberg (Eds.), *Vocal fold physiology: Acoustic, perceptual, and physiological aspects of voice mechanisms* (pp. 225–232). San Diego: Singular Publishing Group.

Jensen, P. J. (1965). Adequacy of terminology for clinical judgment of voice quality deviation. *The Eye, Ear, Nose and Throat Monthly, 44,* 77–82.

Karlsson, I. (1991). Female voices in speech synthesis. *Journal of Phonetics, 19,* 111–120.

Karlsson, I. (1992). Modelling voice variations in female speech synthesis. *Speech Communication, 11,* 491–495.

Kempster, G. B., Kistler, D. J., & Hillenbrand, J. (1991). Multidimensional scaling analysis of dysphonia in two speaker groups. *Journal of Speech and Hearing Research, 34,* 534–543.

Klatt, D. H. (1980). Software for a cascade/parallel formant synthesizer. *Journal of the Acoustical Society of America, 67,* 971–995.

Klatt, D. H., & Klatt, L. C. (1990). Analysis, synthesis and perception of voice quality variations among female and male talkers. *Journal of the Acoustical Society of America, 87,* 820–857.

Kreiman, J., & Gerratt, B. R. (1996). The perceptual structure of pathologic voice quality. *Journal of the Acoustical Society of America, 100,* 1787–1795.

Kreiman, J., Gerratt, B. R., & Berke, G. S. (1994). The multidimensional nature of pathologic vocal quality. *Journal of the Acoustical Society of America, 96,* 1291–1302.

Kreiman, J., Gerratt, B. R., Precoda, K., & Berke, G. S. (1993, May). *Perception of supraperiodic voices.* Paper presented at the 125th meeting of the Acoustical Society of America, Ottawa, Canada.

Ladefoged, P. (1995). A phonation-type synthesizer for use in the field. In O. Fujimura & M. Hirano (Eds.), *Vocal fold physiology: Voice quality control* (pp. 61–76). San Diego: Singular Publishing Group.

Lalwani, A. L., & Childers, D. G. (1991). Modeling vocal disorders via formant synthesis. *Proceedings of the IEEE International Conference on Acoustics, Speech, and Signal Processing, 1,* 505–508.

Laver, J. (1980). *The phonetic description of voice quality*. Cambridge, UK: Cambridge University Press.

Löfqvist, A., Koenig, L., & McGowan, R. (1995). Voice source variations in running speech: A study of Mandarin Chinese tones. In O. Fujimura & M. Hirano (Eds.), *Vocal fold physiology: Voice quality control* (pp. 3–22). San Diego: Singular Publishing Group.

Moore, P., & Von Leden, H. (1958). Dynamic variations of the vibratory pattern in the normal larynx. *Folia Phoniatrica,* 10, 205–238.

Price, P. J. (1989). Male and female voice source characteristics: Inverse filtering results. *Speech Communication, 8,* 261–277.

Qi, Y., Weinberg, B., & Bi, N. (1995). Enhancement of female esophageal and tracheo-esophageal speech. *Journal of the Acoustical Society of America, 98,* 2461–2465.

Titze, I. R., Baken, R. J., & Herzel, H. (1993). Evidence of chaos in vocal fold vibration. In I. R. Titze (Ed.), *Vocal fold physiology: Frontiers in basic science* (pp. 143–188). San Diego: Singular Publishing Group.

Yumoto, E., Gould, W. J., & Baer, T. (1982). Harmonics-to-noise ratio as an index of the degree of hoarseness. *Journal of the Acoustical Society of America, 71,* 1544–1550.

APPENDIX 14–A
PARAMETERS FOR THE CASCADE BRANCH OF THE SYNTHESIZER

Unless otherwise noted, the parameters in the table below were set to these default values.

Symbol	*Default*	*Description*
DU	1000	Duration of the utterance, in ms
SR	10000	Output sampling rate, in samples / sec
NF	5	Number of formants in cascade branch
SS	3	Source switch (1 = impluse, 2 = natural, 3 = LF model)
GV	60	Overall gain scale factor for AV, in dB
GH	60	Overall gain scale factor for AH, in dB
F0	100	Fundamental frequency, in Hz
AV	60	Amplitude of voicing, in dB
OQ	50	Open quotient (voicing open-time/period), in %
SQ	200	Speed quotient (rise/fall time of open period, LF model only), in %
TL	0	Extra tilt of voicing spectrum, dB down at 3kHz
FL	0	Flutter (random fluctuation in F0), in % of maximum
DI	0	Diplophonia (pairs of periods migrate together), in % of maximum
AH	0	Amplitude of aspiration, in dB
F_1	500	Frequency of the 1st formant, in Hz
B_1	60	Bandwidth of the 1st formant, in Hz
F_2	1500	Frequency of the 2nd formant, in Hz
B_2	90	Bandwidth of the 2nd formant, in Hz
F_3	2500	Frequency of the 3rd formant, in Hz
B_3	150	Bandwidth of the 3rd formant, in Hz
F_4	3250	Frequency of the 4th formant, in Hz
B_4	200	Bandwidth of the 4th formant, in Hz
F_5	3700	Frequency of the 5th formant, in Hz
B_5	200	Bandwidth of the 5th formant, in Hz

APPENDIX 14–A (Continued)

Symbol	*Default*	*Description*
F_6	4990	Frequency of the 6th formant, in Hz
B_6	500	Bandwidth of the 6th formant, in Hz
F_7	6500	Frequency of the 7th formant, in Hz (not modifiable)
B_7	500	Bandwidth of the 7th formant, in Hz (not modifiable)
F_8	7500	Frequency of the 8th formant, in Hz (not modifiable)
B_8	600	Bandwidth of the 8th formant, in Hz (not modifiable)
FNP	280	Frequency of nasal pole, in Hz
BNP	90	Bandwidth of nasal pole, in Hz
FNZ	280	Frequency of nasal zero, in Hz
BNZ	90	Bandwidth of nasal zero, in Hz
FTP	2150	Frequency of tracheal pole, in Hz
BTP	180	Bandwidth of tracheal pole, in Hz
FTZ	2150	Frequency of tracheal zero, in Hz
BTZ	180	Bandwidth of tracheal zero, in Hz

APPENDIX 14–B
LISTENER INSTRUCTIONS FOR SYNTHESIS OF PATHOLOGICAL VOICES STUDY

You are about to hear a series of voice pairs. The first voice in each pair was recorded from a dysphonic patient. The second voice is a copy of the dysphonic voice, made with a speech synthesizer. Some of the copies are much more successful at capturing the quality of the original voice than others are. We would like you to listen to each pair and tell us just how successful each synthesized copy is. You may listen to each pair as many times as you like. Please rate the goodness of the copy on a 7 point scale, where "1" means the copy is identical to the original, and "7" means it does not sound like the same person. You need not use the entire scale; if all the copies are rated 1 or 7, that is fine. Please try to judge each pair independently of the others. You will hear the entire set of voice pairs before the study starts to give you an idea of how much they vary.

When judging the pairs, try to focus on the overall quality. Please ignore differences in the loudness of the stimuli as much as possible. Thank you for participating in this study.

PART

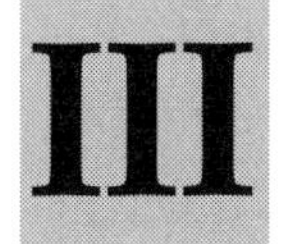

Voice States and Disorders

The chapters in Part III pertain to various voice states and disorders. Whereas the earlier two parts of the book lay the groundwork for perceptual and instrumental assessments of voice quality, Part III addresses vocal quality issues in both normal and pathologic vocal function. The normal versus pathologic constrast is not dichotomous, because the information considered in normal function can be highly relevant to clinical applications, with respect to both establishing normative data and understanding variations in vocal function that occur over the lifespan and in varikous social and personal circumstances. Our vision for Part III was that it would show how voice quality issues pervade speech communication and its disorders.

The opening chapter for Part III, by Gudrun Klasmeyer and Walter F. Sendlmeier, discusses the role of voice quality in emotional expression. They consider how emotion is conveyed by acoustic properties of the voice, and they report on an experiment designed to demonstrate emotion-specific changes in the acoustic parameters of voice quality. Sue Ellen Linville reviews information on the aging voice, including anatomic and physiologic changes, perceptual attributes, and acoustic correlates. This information is essential to an understanding of age-related changes in normal voice and also to effective diagnosis and treatment of voice disorders that arise in aging populations. One common form of vocal pathology is mass lesions. Charles N. Ford and Nadine P. Connor describe the phonatory effects of these lesions, drawing particular attention to the roles of phonatory assessment in the management of individuals with this vocal pathology. Minoru Hirano and Kazunori Mori review the topic of vocal fold paralysis, concluding that the pathology affects the body of the vibrator (the muscle) and that this condition results in specific abnormalities in vocal function. Wolfram Ziegler and Philip Hoole examine the relationship between neurologic diseases and voice, organizing their comments particularly around major etiologies and pathophysiologic states. The spasmodic dysphonias are reviewed in detail by Michael P. Cannito and Gayle E. Woodson. Their review covers a large literature on the nature, diagnosis, and management of this condition. Kim Corbin-Lewis and Thomas Johnson's chapter surveys voice disorders in children, presenting information on the nature and prevalence of these disorders, diagnostic procedures, and treatment alternatives. Evelyn Abberton discusses voice quality issues associated with deafness. She reviews literature that has attempted to describe "deaf voice quality" and shows that a fuller account can be accomplished by considerations of phonological patterning, psychoacoustic abilities, and acoustic analysis. In the final chapter, Nelson Roy and Diane M. Bless review information on personality and emotional adjustment related to voice disorders. They present a theory that identifies personality factors related to the development of voice disorders, including functional dysphonia and vocal nodules.

CHAPTER 15

Voice and Emotional States

Gudrun Klasmeyer and Walter F. Sendlmeier

In natural communication situations, emotional arousal is a quite complex phenomenon. Scherer (1986) proposed a theoretical model of vocal affect expression that is generally accepted. In this model emotion is seen as a process, not as a steady state of the organism. The process includes such components as physiological arousal and expression and feeling as a response to an evaluation of significant events in the environment. The organism's information processing subsystem continously scans external and internal stimulus inputs and performs a series of stimulus evaluation checks that result in the organism's emotional state. This emotional state can be labeled with emotional terms provided by natural languages and referred to as "discrete emotions." In spite of these discrete labels, the emotional arousal, itself, is gradual, can change abruptly, and can also be a mixture of different discrete emotions.

In a vocalization process, the physiological arousal due to an emotion appears to be an involuntary force. A vocalization can further be influenced by voluntary effects in the service of affect control or self-presentation.

Systematic studies of acoustic voice qualities in different emotional states of a speaker have to deal with some problems. Field recordings of emotional utterances usually lack the good quality essential for the analysis of acoustic voice quality parameters; whereas under laboratory conditions, it is quite difficult to sucessfully induce different emotions. A solution to this problem is to record emotional speech produced by actors under laboratory conditions in combination with a perception experiment with naive listeners to evaluate the naturalness and recognizability of the emotions. Drama actors tend to portray emotions in a way that the emotional content can be recognized from a distance, which results in an improper use of the voice source, although the emotional content might be recognizable from the intonation pattern and the speaking rate. Therefore, the actors have to use a special technique: They imagine an emotional situation until they really "feel" the emotional arousal, before the utterances are recorded. The naive listeners have to be instructed to evaluate utterances that sound like "theater clichés" of the emotions as unnatural.

The acoustic analysis of voices is not an easy task, because there is a lot of parallel information in fluent speech. Besides semantic information, spoken language contains evidential information conveyed by signs in speech that act as attributive markers (Laver 1994). These are used by a listener as the basis for attributing personal characteristics to the speaker. The attributes of the speaker fall into three groups:

- Physical markers that indicate characteristics such as sex, age, physique, and state of health;
- Social markers that indicate characteristics such as regional affiliation, social and educational status, occupation, and social role;
- Psychological markers that indicate characteristics of personality and affective state or mood.

The correlation between these attributive markers and acoustic parameters is rather complicated. Laver states that physical characteristics lie in a speaker's voice quality, with social markers including such features as accent and choice of vocabulary. Psychological markers are often taken to reside in a speaker's tone of voice (Laver, 1994). But, given the human vocal apparatus, it is very unlikely that tone of voice should change under emotional arousal without affecting the speaker's general voice quality or type of phonation. It is more realistic to assume that all acoustic parameters that can be used to characterize a speaker's personal voice quality might be influenced by the speaker's mood or affective state.

A listener's attribution of speaker characteristics is usually based on the general impression of the utterance. Attributions based on single acoustic parameters are ambiguous. A high "jitter" value, for example, could be a physical marker for a speaker's personal voice quality or state of health, but it could also be a psychological marker for fear.

This chapter proposes a general approach toward the objective measurement of different voice qualities in fluent speech. Initially, conclusions about typical signal characteristics of the transglottal airflow are drawn from the production strategies of varying types of phonation. The signal characteristics are discussed with regard to the question of how voice quality and type of phonation can be measured in the acoustic speech signal. In natural communication situations, voice quality is often a combination of different types of phonation. This is one reason why several acoustic parameters are required for an adequate description of voice quality. To deal with the fact that some voice qualities can hardly be regarded as quasistationary signals and, hence, are difficult to analyze using common algorithms for stationary signals, some of the introduced parameters are not orthogonal, but represent different approaches to measuring similar phenomena in the frequency and time domains. As mentioned, voice quality can be used by listeners as a basis on which to attribute speaker characteristics.

1. ANATOMY AND CONTROL MECHANISMS OF THE VOICE SOURCE

In human speech production, the breathing organs produce an airflow that is not audible by itself. In the laryngeal system, this airflow is modified into an audible sound wave. The sound wave propagates through the supraglottal cavities, where it is subject to further modifications by the articulators before it is radiated from the mouth as an acoustic speech signal. The major results of all laryngeal control mechanisms are changes in the opening section of the glottis as well as the tension and oscillation characteristics of the vocal folds. Three forces are regarded as being most important for the control of voice quality and type of phonation. These forces are (1) the longitudinal tension of the vocal folds, which is achieved by muscular tension in the musculus vocalis and the cricothyroid muscles; (2) the adductive tension of the ligamental and cartilaginous glottis, which is achieved by tension of the interarytenoid muscles; and (3) the medial compression that closes the ligamental glottis as a secondary effect of a force on the arytenoid cartilages, which is caused by tension of the lateral cricoarytenoid muscles in collaboration with tension in the lateral part of the thyroarytenoid muscles. These forces of longitudinal tension, medial compression and adductive tension are illustrated in Figure 15–1, which shows a cross-section of the human larynx.

It is obvious that emotional arousal can have an influence on the control mechanisms and therefore change the audible voice quality.

In phonetic practice the categories breathy phonation, whispery phonation, modal voice, creak (which is also called glottal fry or vocal fry), and falsetto proposed by Laver (in Chapter 4) are used to label voices. In the next section, acoustic characteristics of these types of phonation are discussed with regard to the question of how the voice quality can be measured objectively.

2. SIGNAL CHARACTERISTICS OF ACOUSTIC SPEECH SIGNALS

The distinction between voiced and voiceless sound segments has already been adequately addressed and solved in the research literature. This chapter focuses on the objective description of voiced sounds, such as breathy voice, whispery voice, modal voice, creaky, and falsetto in terms of acoustic parameters. The listed types of phonation can be determined in the acoustic speech signals by analysis of the spectral distribution of harmonic and noise components in the frequency domain and by parameters derived from the time signal. Among these parameters in the time domain, vocal effort, voicing irregularities, and the speed of changes in the fundamental frequency are important criteria by which voice quality in acoustic speech signals can be characterized.

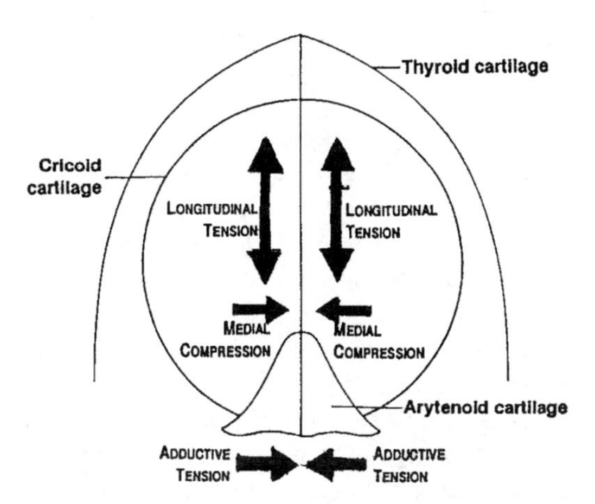

Figure 15–1. Schematic illustration of longitudinal tension, medial compression, and adductive tension.

2.1. Influence of the Supraglottal Cavities

As stated, the source signal that is the object of investigation is modified by the articulators in the supraglottal cavities before it is radiated from the mouth. The modification consists of additional turbulent noise, which has its origin in constrictions of the vocal tract as well as resonances and antiresonances. To investigate the source signal, the modifications caused by supraglottal components and mouth radiation have to be compensated for in the acoustic speech signal. A promising method of extracting the source signal from the acoustic speech signal is to compensate for mouth radiation by an integration filter. Resonances of the vocal tract can be compensated for by inverse filtering with an optimized filter. The filter coefficients are calculated using all-pole linear predictive coding (LPC) during the closed glottis interval of the preemphasized acoustic speech signal (Wong, Markel, & Gray 1979). If antiresonances are also to be compensated for, a pole-zero LPC is required, which is more difficult to handle, because it can lead to unstable filters (Makhoul, 1975). Turbulent noise caused by vocal tract constrictions causes the most difficult problem, because it can only barely be distinguished from turbulent noise originating at the glottis. Therefore the analysis of source characteristics must be restricted to the segments of the acoustic speech signal that are produced with minimal vocal tract constriction. The vowel /a/ is the phoneme spoken with the most open vocal tract and, therefore, seems to be most appropriate for investigations of the voice source in acoustic speech signals.

2.2. Parametric Description of the Source Signal

2.2.1. Modal Voice

In modal voicing, the forces of all laryngeal control mechanisms have to be offset by subglottal pressure to open the vocal folds, which are closed as long as subglottal pressure is absent or small. Therefore, glottal opening is not abrupt but gradual. The transglottal airflow rises from zero to peak flow. At maximum flow, a local pressure drop is created, which allows the vocal folds to return to a closed position. All laryngeal forces support this closing movement, which is much faster than the speed of glottal opening. Both the glottal opening function and the transglottal airflow function re-semble a sawtooth function, with a gradually increasing flank followed by an abrupt but finite time drop and a zero phase. In undistorted speech sounds with modal phonation, the transglottal airflow can be calculated by inverse filtering techniques. The spectral characteristic of an asymetric sawtooth-like triangular function consists of equally spaced spectral peaks at the fundamental frequency and at all higher harmonics, with a spectral damping of about 6 dB per octave toward higher frequencies in normal voices. Obviously, the sawtooth analogy is a very crude approximation of the transglottal flow, because natural signals do not have any sharp edges. However, it serves to illustrate the characteristics of the source signal.

2.2.1.1. Decreased Laryngeal Forces If the muscular forces helping maintain a closed glottis position were decreased, the result would be a steeper opening phase, and the glottal closure would be less abrupt. This skewing of the glottal pulse has been shown to result in decreased loudness and is, therefore, not an effective voicing manner (Sundberg, 1994). In the extreme, the sawtooth shape of the source signal changes into a symmetric triangle, or rather a sinus shape, because there are no sharp edges in physiological signals. In the frequency domain, this signal can be characterized by an increased spectral attenuation of higher harmonics, with a pure sine wave only having one single harmonic at the fundamental frequency. Inverse filtering of an acoustic speech signal produced with minimal laryngeal forces is not possible, because the closed glottis interval is unsuitable for calculation of the filter coefficients for the inverse filter. First, there is no impulse at the beginning of the closed phase, which would be necessary to interpret the acoustic speech signal as an impulse response of the supraglottal cavities during the closed glottis interval, and, second, the closed phase is often too short. But inverse filtering is not necessary, because the spectral damping of the source signal is very high. Higher harmonics that lie in the spectral region of formants have very little energy; therefore the source signal is hardly modified by the supraglottal cavities before it is radiated from the mouth.

2.2.1.2. Increased Laryngeal Forces If the muscular tension at the larynx is increased, the opening of the vocal folds is more difficult. Higher subglottal pressure is required to open the vocal folds. Once the opening starts, the high subglottal pressure will lead to an increased transglottal airflow. In comparison to the sawtooth function discussed previously, the glottal flow signal will have much steeper flanks and, therefore, resemble an impulse rather than a sawtooth function. A periodic train of pulses in the time domain leads to an equally spaced pulse train in the frequency domain. Therefore, it can be concluded that increased laryngeal forces result in a source signal with less spectral damping of its harmonics. Inverse filtering of undistorted speech signals with high muscular forces at the larynx and high vocal effort is possible, as long as the closed glottis interval is long enough to calculate the filter coefficients. It should be emphasized that this is only valid for modal voicing, in which the vocal folds vibrate completely. Falsetto, which is marked by extreme tension of the vocal folds and only partial vibration only, needs to be discussed separately.

2.2.1.3. Increased Fundamental Frequency and Increased Vocal Effort Modal voice is characterized by very little turbulent noise and by regular, periodic components. The fundamental frequency can be varied from lower to higher values. Vocal effort can change from soft to loud. An increase of the fundamental frequency, as well as an increase of vocal effort, leads to steeper glottal pulses and, therefore, to less spectral damping of the harmonics. It might make sense to split the category modal voice into two subcategories: one in which both fundamental frequency and vocal effort are low or moderate and a second category in which both are high, because these voice qualities are perceptibly quite different. Extremely high vocal effort would be shouted voice. Physiologically, the increase of vocal effort can be achieved by an increase of subglottal pressure, which also causes an increase of the fundamental frequency. This secondary effect could theoretically be offset by a relaxation of laryngeal forces, especially by a relaxation of the longitudinal tension of the vocal folds, but in practice this is seldom the case. In human speech production, an increase of subglottal pressure, which is achieved by increased tension of the breathing muscles, is accompanied somewhat by an increase of laryngeal tension, adding to the total fundamental frequency increase.

2.2.1.4. Irregular Glottal Cycles and Abrupt Changes of Fundamental Frequency In the previous schematic discussion, it proved relatively easy to differentiate between voice qualities with high or low laryngeal forces using inverse filtered signals or fast fourier transform (FFT) spectrograms. Problems arise if either the glottal cycles are irregular or the fundamental frequency changes abruptly, as is the case in fluent speech with marked prosody. In both cases, spectral lines at the harmonics will be smeared in the spectrum, which makes the determination of harmonic components more difficult. A parameter designed to deal with this problem is introduced in section 3.2. The Hilbert envelope of separate frequency bands is used to determine the composition of harmonic and noisy components within these bands.

2.2.2. Falsetto

In falsetto, only the thin edges of the vocal folds vibrate, causing the glottal pulses to take on a sinus-like shape rather than an impulse-like shape. Therefore, the spectral damping of higher harmonics can be strong. Inverse filtering is usually impossible because the closed glottis interval is too short. An unambiguous sign of falsetto is the extremely high fundamental frequency.

2.2.3. Creak (Glottal Fry, Vocal Fry)

Creak is characterized by irregular durations of glottal cycles or by a fundamental frequency of about half a speaker's normal fundamental frequency. In this way, creak can easily be determined in the acoustic time signal.

2.2.4. Whispery Phonation

So far, only the spectral distribution of harmonic signal components has been discussed in detail. Turbulent signal components appear if the glottis is neither completely closed nor widely open. The amplitude of the turbulent components can be so dominant that harmonic components are masked in the acoustic signal, at least in some frequency regions. Whispery phonation is characterized by relatively loud turbulent noise, which predominates over the harmonic components. Analysis of spectral damping characteristics of the harmonic components, as well as inverse filtering, is therefore difficult or impossible. But the strong turbulent noise can easily be detected in the acoustic time signal.

2.2.5. Breathy Phonation

Breathy voices are characterized by soft to no turbulent noise, because the glottis is fairly wide open at all times. The difference between minimal and peak transglottal flow is relatively small, which means that the alternating signal components that could be heard as tonal sound quality are also quite soft, although the absolute air flow is registered at comparably high values. The sound production is ineffective. As stated, laryngeal forces are minimal in breathy phonation, which leads to high spectral damping of higher harmonics. Analysis of spectral peaks would result in high bandwidth of the formants. Fundamental frequency is rather low. Typical signal characteristics for phonatory settings are shown in Figure 15–2.

3. ACOUSTIC PARAMETERS

In this section a brief definition is given of the derived acoustic parameters that can be used to determine the type of phonation in fluent speech signals. The parameters were selected according to the previously mentioned typical signal characteristics of the transglottal airflow. Only the combination of several acoustic parameters guarantees a reliable characterization of voice quality.

3.1. Glottal Pulses via Synchronous Inverse Filtering

Inverse filtering techniques to calculate glottal pulses from the acoustic speech signal can only be used in undistorted signals without any frequency-dependent damping or phase shifting. Theoretically, the process of glottal closure resembles an impulse. So in the subsequent closed-glottis interval, the acoustic speech signal can be interpreted as an impulse response of the vocal tract, because the subglottal volume is decoupled from the upper tract during that time. The filter coefficients for inverse filtering are calculated during the closed-glottis interval. The actual point of glottal closure can be determined by inverse filtering, with filter coefficients derived from a time interval that tends to be three to four times longer than one period duration of the acoustic signal. In general, it is more difficult to determine the exact point where the opening begins. In the present study, an 18th order covariance LPC and rectangular data windows were used. The filter coefficients for inverse filtering are calculated during the closed-glottis interval of the middle period of each realization of the German phoneme /a/. Because of different durations of the closed glottis interval in different glottis cycles, the length of the data window has to be adapted to allow for reasonable spectral shaping of the inverse filter. One hundred ms of the speech signal are filtered. Only the middle period within which the LPC coefficients were calculated was examined more closely. An example for an inverse filtered time signal from an utterance spoken with modal voice is given in Figure 15–3. (Transglottal airflow is presented in a negative direction, because this is often the case in electroglottogram displays.) Also discussed in Klasmeyer and Sendlmeier (1995), the glottal cycles may deviate considerably from the normal sawtooth shape. The inverse filtered signal should, therefore, be interpreted as a glottal pulse signal with great care, because some of the conditions for this theory may not be met. For example, pulses filtered from lax speech show hardly any obvious closed-glottis interval and (or because) the closure is not abrupt.

3.2. Spectral Distribution of Energy in Separate Frequency Bands and Detection of Harmonic Components Versus Turbulent Noise Within Separate Frequency Bands

The advantage of analysis techniques in the frequency domain is the ability to interpret

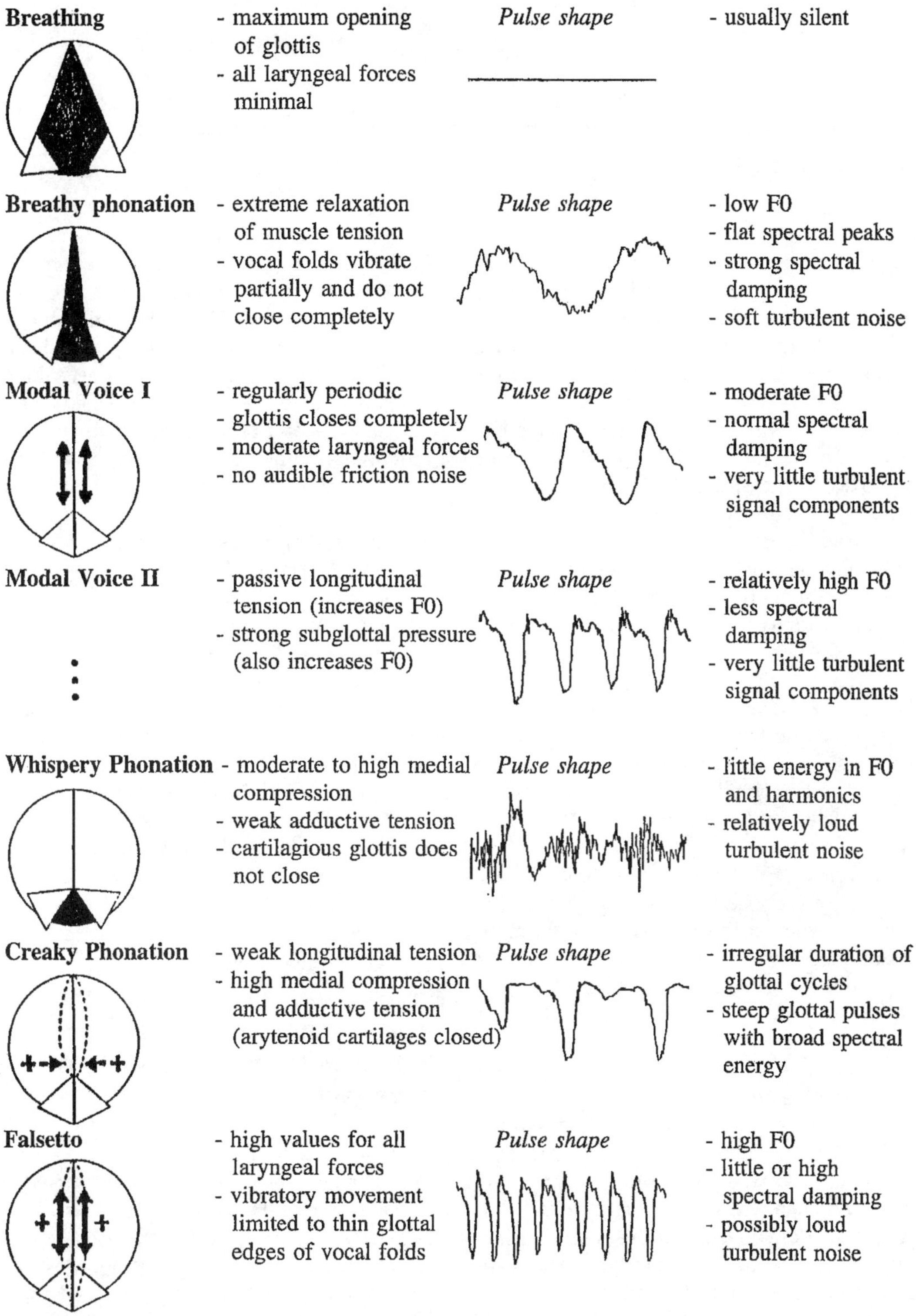

Breathing	- maximum opening of glottis - all laryngeal forces minimal	*Pulse shape*	- usually silent
Breathy phonation	- extreme relaxation of muscle tension - vocal folds vibrate partially and do not close completely	*Pulse shape*	- low F0 - flat spectral peaks - strong spectral damping - soft turbulent noise
Modal Voice I	- regularly periodic - glottis closes completely - moderate laryngeal forces - no audible friction noise	*Pulse shape*	- moderate F0 - normal spectral damping - very little turbulent signal components
Modal Voice II	- passive longitudinal tension (increases F0) - strong subglottal pressure (also increases F0)	*Pulse shape*	- relatively high F0 - less spectral damping - very little turbulent signal components
Whispery Phonation	- moderate to high medial compression - weak adductive tension - cartilagious glottis does not close	*Pulse shape*	- little energy in F0 and harmonics - relatively loud turbulent noise
Creaky Phonation	- weak longitudinal tension - high medial compression and adductive tension (arytenoid cartilages closed)	*Pulse shape*	- irregular duration of glottal cycles - steep glottal pulses with broad spectral energy
Falsetto	- high values for all laryngeal forces - vibratory movement limited to thin glottal edges of vocal folds	*Pulse shape*	- high F0 - little or high spectral damping - possibly loud turbulent noise

Figure 15–2. Typical signal characteristics for phonatory settings.

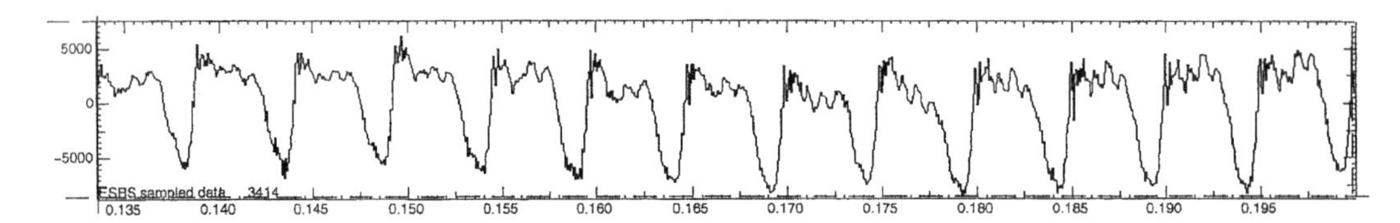

Figure 15–3. Inverse filtered time signal.

slightly phase-distorted signals. Although the inverse filtering technique described in the previous section requires signals without any phase distortion, which can only be recorded in anechoic rooms with special measuring microphones, the spectral parameters are more resilient to phase distortion. Frequency-dependent amplitude distortions will cause mistakes in measuring the time domain, as well as in the frequency domain.

To estimate spectral energy distribution, a quasistationary vowel segment without formant movements is chosen (phoneme /a/) using a wideband spectrogram as shown in Figure 15–4. Four different frequency bands are filtered from the segment: the very low band, which only contains the fundamental frequency; the low-band (0–1 kHz); the mid band (2.5–3.5 kHz); and the high band (4–5 kHz). The energy within the frequency bands is calculated and divided by the entire segment's energy.

A normal FFT of a quasistationary segment of the acoustic speech signal is appropriate for deciding whether the band contains harmonics of the fundamental frequency or turbulent noise only, if there are no voicing irregularities or steep fundamental frequency changes. Otherwise an unsynchronously inverse filtered time signal as shown in Figure 15–5 (residual signal) can be calculated.

The edges of this residual signal are multiplied with a Hanning window in the time domain before it is transformed to the frequency domain using an FFT algorithm. In the frequency domain, separate bands are calculated using spectral Hanning windows at the low band (0–1 kHz), the mid band (2.5–3.5 kHz), and the high band (4–5 kHz). All negative frequencies are set to zero. The analytical signals with frequencies above 0 Hz are transformed to the time domain using a complex inverse FFT algorithm. The Hilbert envelope of the separate frequency bands is calculated from the complex time signal by transforming the real and predicted parts into absolute values. The low-band Hilbert envelope is usually primarily harmonic for all voice qualities. An example is shown in Figure 15–6. Therefore a normalized crosscorrelation between the low and mid band and between the low and high band was calculated. Theoretically a high correlation would indicate harmonic mid-band and high-band components, whereas a low correlation would indicate noisy higher bands. Actually correlation was seldom high, even in those signals that had obvious harmonic components in higher bands. Therefore the decision whether a separate band was mainly harmonic or mainly turbulent was made directly from the Hilbert envelope. Figures 15–7 and 15–8 show examples of a harmonic and a turbulent high-band Hilbert envelope.

3.3. Average Gradient of the Fundamental Frequency Within Separate Increase or Decrease Segments (as an Estimation of Laryngeal Muscle Activity)

The fundamental frequency contour can be seen as an acoustic correlate of speech melody and tone of voice. However, the contour is not discussed in detail here. The average gradient of separate increase or decrease segments is only used to estimate the laryngeal muscle activity as one correlate of voice quality. Figure 15–9 provides an explanation: In the algorithm, local

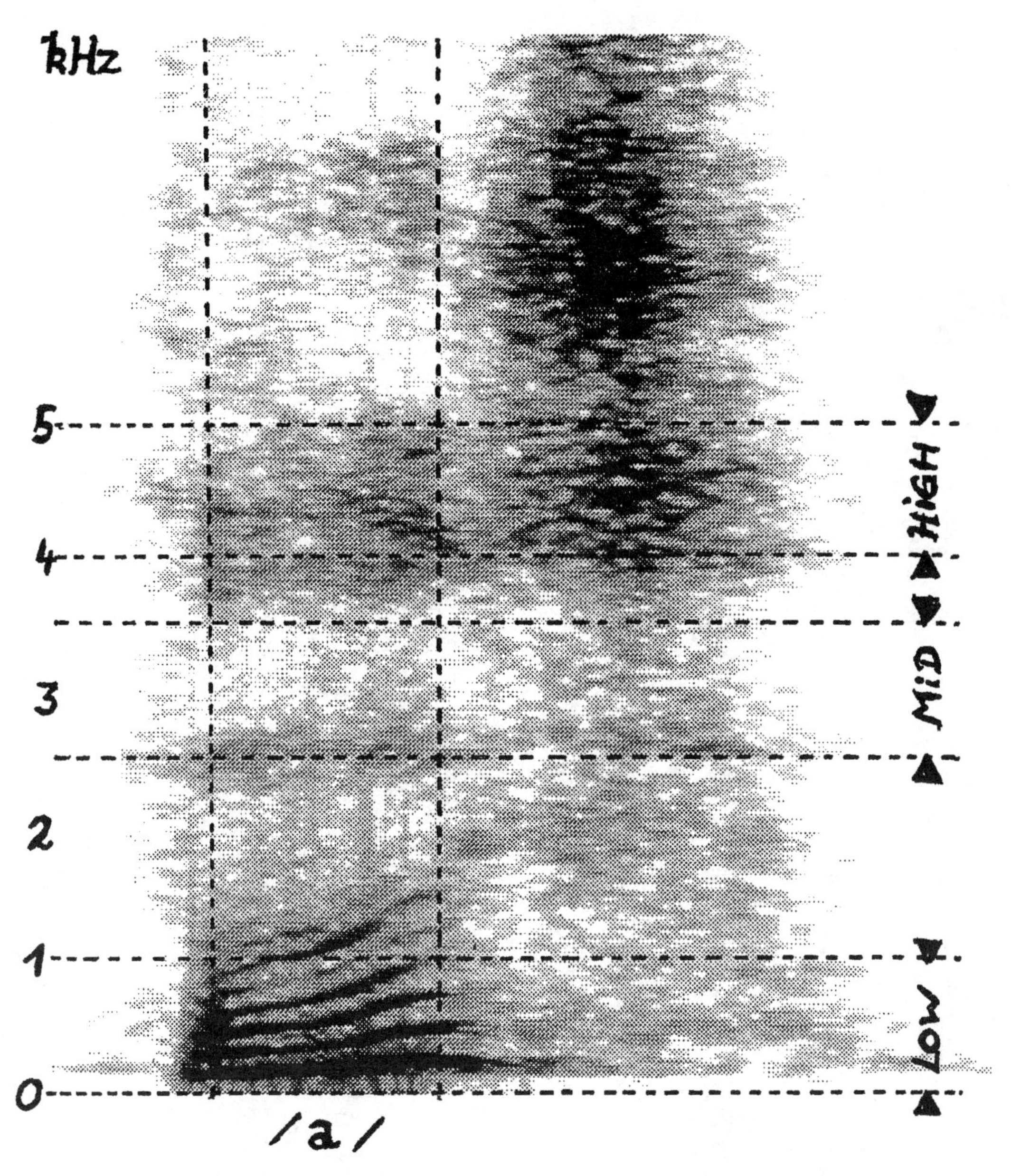

Figure 15–4. Wideband spectrogram, low-band (0–1 kHz), mid-band (2.5–3.5 kHz), and high-band (4–5 kHz).

maxima in the fundamental frequency contour are found. The average gradient is calculated in hertz/s by plotting a straight line through the contour. Rapid changes of the fundamental frequency are achieved by changes in laryngeal forces, especially by the longitudinal tension of the vocal folds.

3.4. Energy Difference of Vowels and Adjacent Fricatives as an Estimation of Vocal Effort

Steep pulses in the source signal are usually a sign of high vocal effort. An additional estimation of vocal effort can be made from an

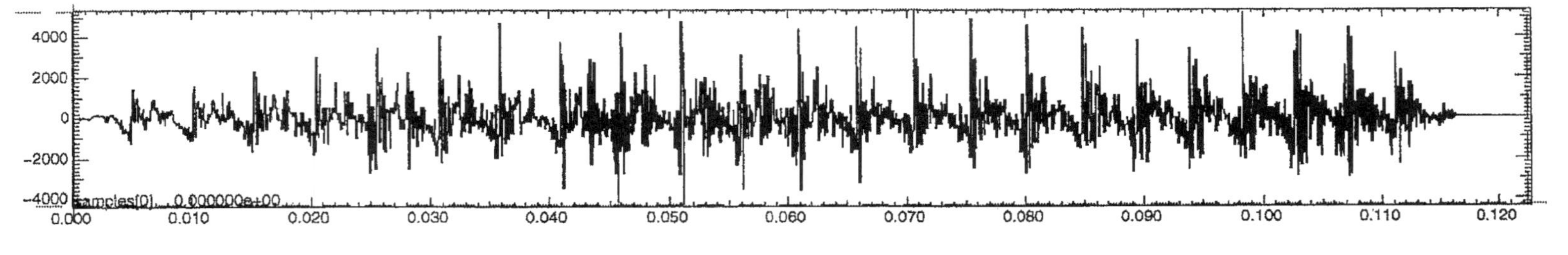

Figure 15–5. Unsynchronously filtered time signal (residual signal).

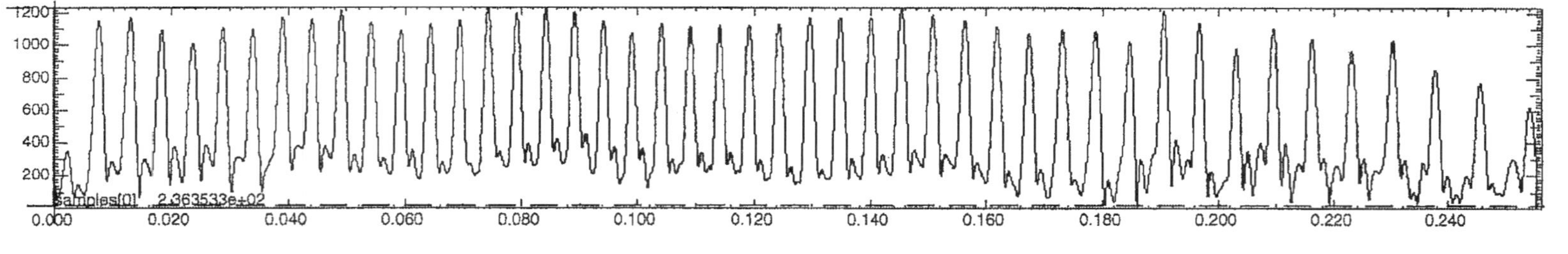

Figure 15–6. Low-band Hilbert envelope (harmonic band).

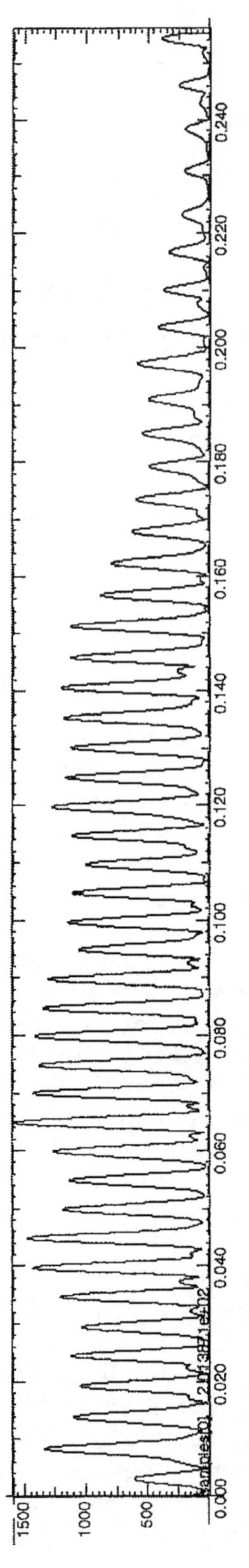

Figure 15–7. High-band Hilbert envelope (harmonic band).

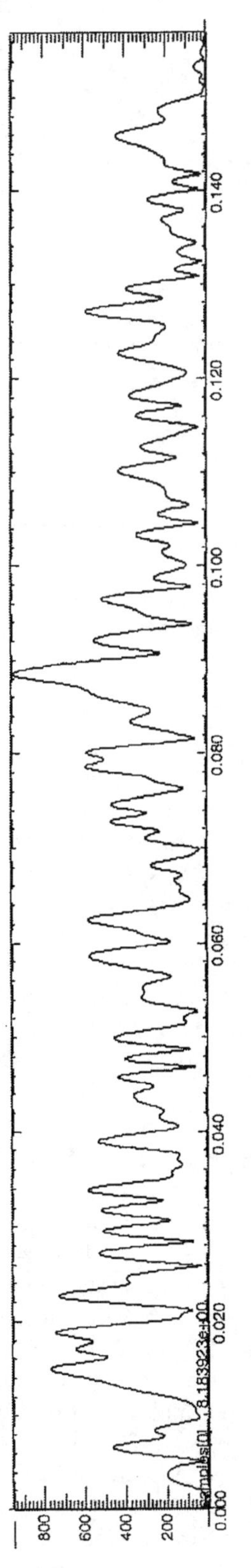

Figure 15–8. High-band Hilbert envelope (turbulent band).

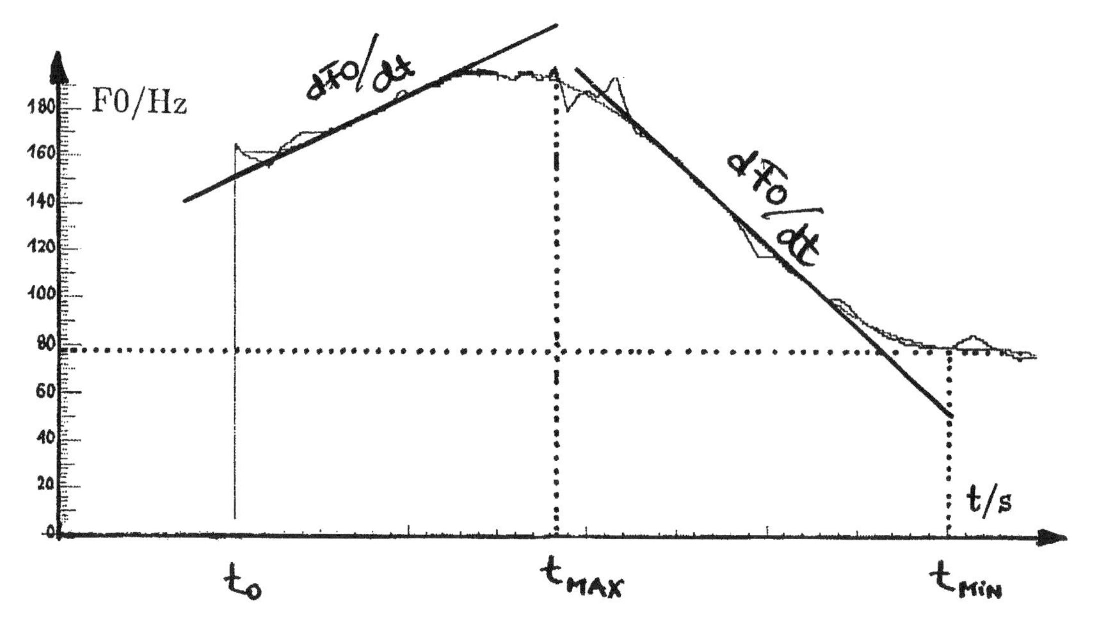

Figure 15–9. Fundamental frequency contour.

energy measurement in a vowel and an adjacent voiceless fricative. The possible loudness range of voiceless fricatives is more limited than the possible loudness range of vowels; therefore the fricative energy can be used as (a rough) reference. The energy difference is measured in decibels. Figure 15–10 shows the energy contour of the phoneme /a/ followed by the phoneme /s/ in an utterance spoken with high vocal effort (above) and with low vocal effort (below).

3.5. Voicing Irregularities (Jitter)

It should be stated that a very reliable fundamental frequency detection algorithm is required to measure voicing irregularities. In clinical voice measurement, a patient produces isolated vowels with flat fundamental frequency contours, whereas in fluent speech there is a continuous rise and fall corresponding to the intonation pattern. This means the parameter jitter has to be measured taking linguistic variation of the fundamental frequency into account. This is done by calculating a polynomial approximation of the fundamental frequency contour as is shown in Figure 15–11 and subtracting this approximation from the measured values. The difference values are used to calculate the absolute jitter, which is divided by the absolute period duration to calculate a relative jitter value (Rosken & Klasmeyer, 1995). This jitter algorithm is also used in forensic speaker identification (Wagner, 1995). In emotional speech, period durations vary; so the relative jitter should be calculated for short segments only. In such regions with short period durations, the measuring error due to low sampling rates or any kind of noise is much higher, therefore, the relative jitter values for high fundamental frequency segments are less reliable.

4. EXPERIMENT

As mentioned at the chapter opening, voice quality can be interpreted as a physical marker that characterizes a speaker's personal vocal equipment or state of health; it can also be interpreted as a psychological marker influenced by the speaker's mood or affective state.

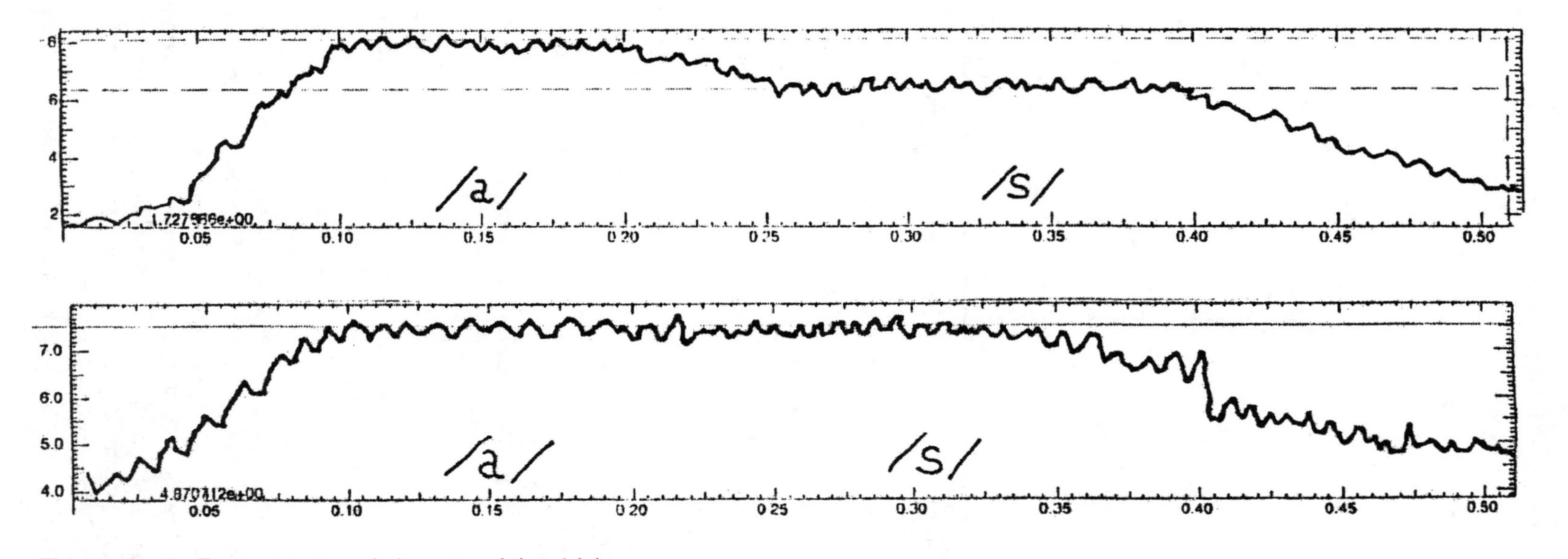

Figure 15–10. Energy contour of phonemes /a/ and /s/.

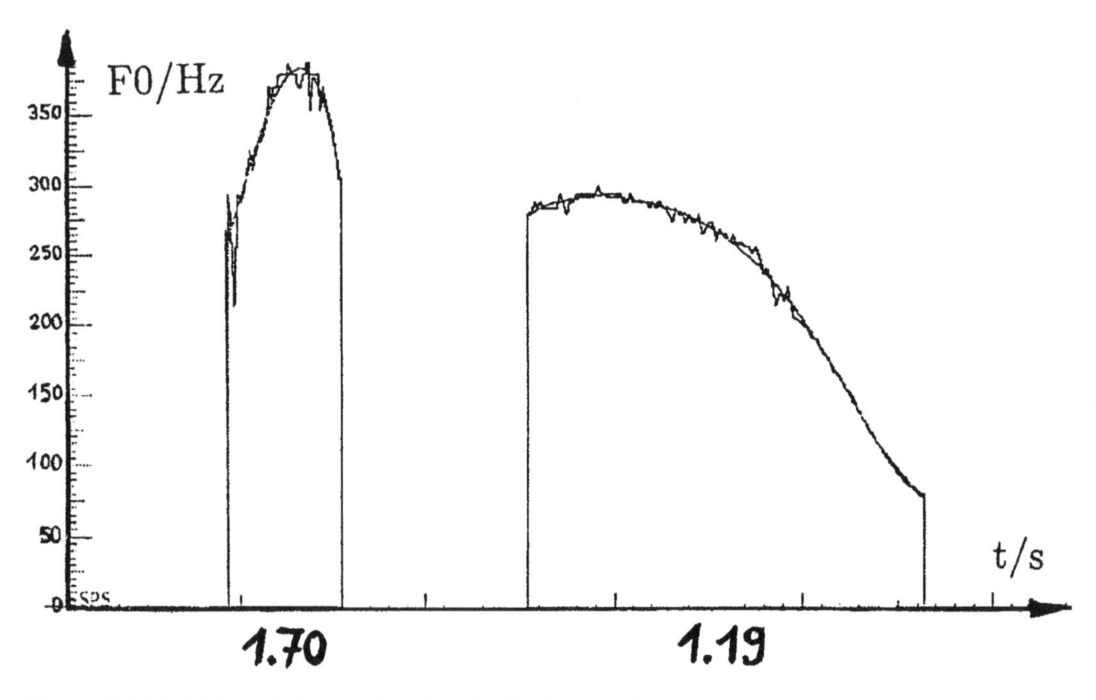

Figure 15–11. Polynomial approximation of a fundamental frequency contour.

The following experiment focuses on emotion-specific changes in the acoustic voice quality parameters introduced in section 3, "Acoustic Parameters."

4.1. Recording of the Database and Recognition Test

Seventy short sentences frequently used in everyday communication, which could appear in all emotional contexts without semantical inconsistency, were recorded under laboratory conditions. The speakers were one female and two male drama students, who did not show any voice pathologies or abnormalities. The sentences were DAT-recorded in separate sessions in an anechoic room using a Bruel and Kiger measuring microphone. Each utterance was spoken several times in a neutral voice and several times with the feigned emotions of: happiness, sadness, anger, fear, boredom, and disgust. To achieve realistic portrayals of emotion, the actors were asked to imagine a situational context in which the sentence could appear. The most appropriate realization was selected by the authors and each actor to be used in a recognition test with naive listeners. The recognition test is important not only to evaluate the recognizability of the emotional content, but also to evaluate the naturalness of the utterances. For each actor, the selected 70 sentences were randomized. Every sentence was repeated three times with 3-second pauses and with a 1-second 1 kHz tone between different emotions. The sentences from each actor were played to 20 naive listeners in separate sessions. The listeners were instructed to mark any utterances that sounded acted or overemphasized as unnatural. The emotional content was evaluated using 8 categories: neutral, happiness, sadness, anger, fear, boredom, disgust, or unnatural or not recognizable emotional content. Only sentences recognized by at least 80% of all listeners were used for the parameter analysis. This recognition threshold is extremely high. In a psychological study, Scherer found a mean recognition rate of 48% for acoustic emotion portrayals. The highest recognition rate was found for anger (78%) and the lowest rate was found for disgust (15%) (Banse & Scherer, 1996).

The utterances used for parameter analysis in the present study were evaluated as natural and the emotional content was deemed unambiguous. For speaker T, 44 out of 70 sentences were used in the analysis. These were 10 neutral sentences, 7 happy sentences, 3 sad sentences, 10 angry sentences, 6 bored sentences, and 8 sentences spoken with fear. None of the sentences with disgust were recognized above the threshold.

For speaker M, 41 of the 70 sentences reached the recognition threshold of 80%. These were 10 neutral sentences, 7 happy sentences, 3 sad sentences, 8 angry sentences, 5 bored sentences, 4 frightened sentences, and 4 sentences spoken with disgust.

For the female speaker, 37 out of 70 sentences were used in the analysis. These were 10 neutral sentences, only 1 happy sentence (the other happy utterances were judged overemphasized), 4 sad sentences, 10 angry sentences, 2 bored sentences, and 10 sentences spoken with fear. None of the sentences with disgust were recognized above the threshold.

The utterances were preselected by the authors and the actors; so high recognition rates were generally expected in the listening test. The relatively low recognition rates for disgust can be explained by the fact that vocal expression of disgust consists of brief affect bursts rather than of a long sentence spoken with a disgust-specific voice quality (Scherer, 1994). In the utterances spoken with disgust that were recognized above the threshold, the last syllable ended in a retching sound. Therefore, the sentences spoken with disgust were not analyzed any further. The relatively low recognition rates for sadness and boredom can be explained by the vocal expressions of sadness and boredom being quite similar; so sad and bored utterances were confused by the listeners.

4.2. Acoustic Parameters

The acoustic parameters previously outlined were used to analyze the emotional utterances. The shape of glottal pulses, as well as spectral distribution of energy and the detection of harmonics versus turbulent noise within different frequency bands, were measured in the vowel /a/ in all sentences. The reason why measurement was restricted to the vowel /a/ is that in the articulation of this vowel, the supraglottal cavities are not expected to cause additional friction noise. The results reflect the type of phonation that is a suprasegmental quality.

The energy difference between vowel and adjacent fricative was measured in the whole sentence. This parameter was used to check the plausibility of the parameters mentioned before. A high energy difference is a sign of great vocal effort that also correlates with steep pulses and little spectral damping of the harmonics.

The average gradient of separate increase or decrease segments of the fundamental frequency contour and the relative perturbation of period durations (jitter) were measured in all voiced segments.

4.3. Results

The experiment focuses on emotion-specific changes in voice quality. The speakers were not selected to represent a wide variety of personal voice qualities. All speakers had completed professional speech training in the same school of acting; they were of the same age and did not show any voice abnormalities. The interindividual differences between the speakers do not stand out from the intraindividual differences within one emotion and, hence, are not discussed any further.

4.3.1. Neutral

In the neutral reference utterances, the vowel energy is 1.2 dB higher than the fricative energy. The glottal pulses are similar to a sawtooth function. Most signal energy is concentrated in the low band below 1 kHz. Energy in all bands is mostly harmonic. Jitter is below 1%. (See Figure 15–12). The type of phonation can therefore be classified as normal modal voicing.

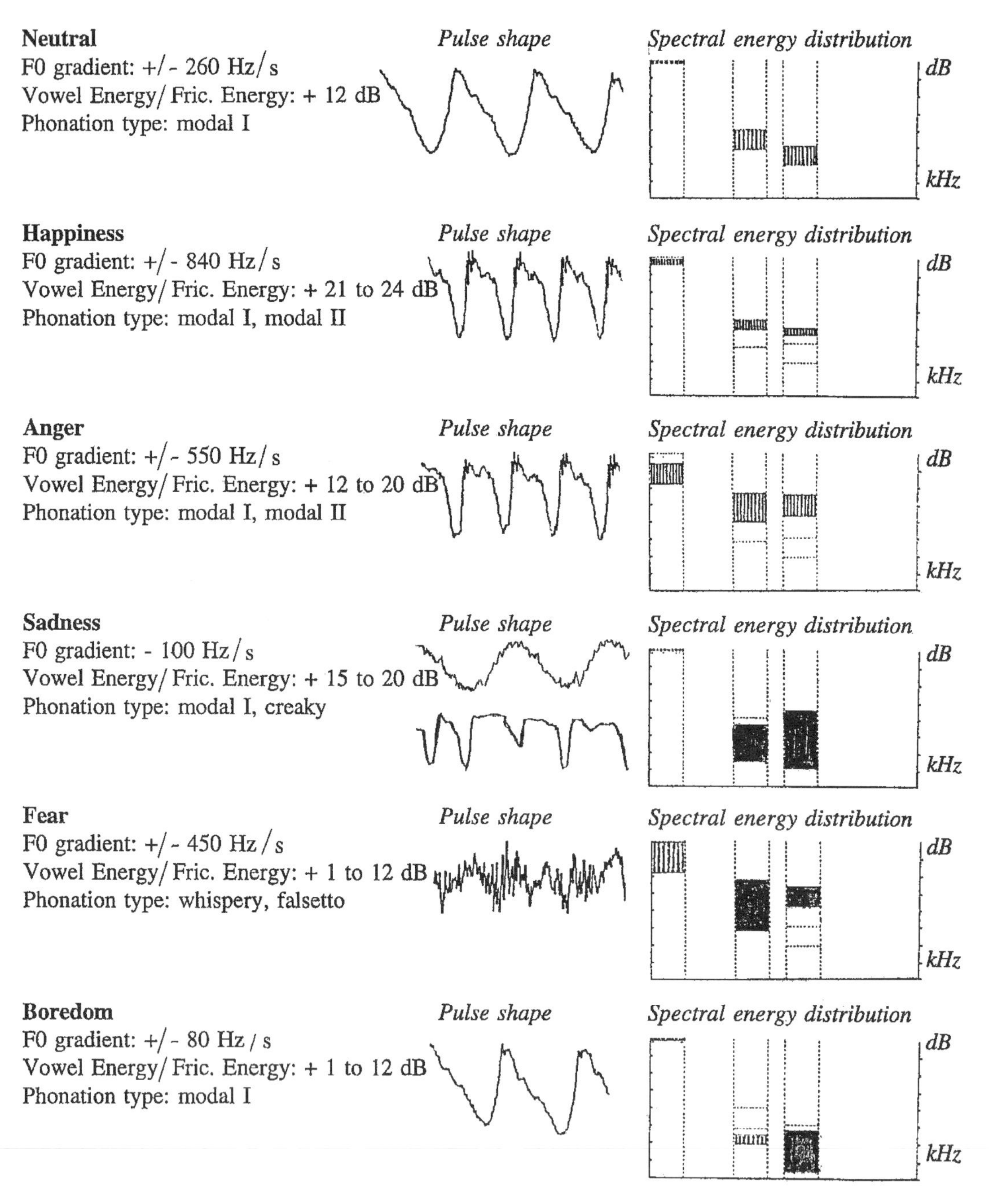

Figure 15–12. Results: Fundamental frequency and amplitude changes, type of phonation, pulse shapes, and spectral distribution of energy for emotional voices.

4.3.2. Happiness

In happy utterances, the vowel energy is 2.1 to 2.4 dB higher than the fricative energy, which also implies a greater loudness than in the neutral utterances. The glottal pulses are steeper than the neutral reference templates. Voiced segments contain largely harmonic energy in all frequency bands. Spectral damping of the harmonics is less than in neutral utterances. The average relative jitter value is slightly above 1%, but as the fundamental frequency reaches extremely high values at localized peaks, this also means that the systematic measuring error is high, as the speech signals were sampled at 16 kHz. The type of phonation can be classified as loud modal voicing with extremely fast changes in the fundamental frequency contour.

4.3.3. Anger

The vowel energy is 1.5 to 2 dB higher than the fricative energy, which also implies a greater loudness than in the neutral reference material. The glottal pulses are very steep with long closed-glottis intervals. As in happy utterances, voiced segments contain mainly harmonic energy in all frequency bands. Spectral damping of the harmonics is less than in neutral utterances. The physical energy in the mid and high band is not as high as in the low band, but considering the frequency-dependent loudness, the mid and high bands in angry speech signals are perceptibly important for the sound impression. As in happy utterances, the average relative jitter is slightly higher than in the neutral reference utterances. But, as was shown for happy utterances, the higher values might be caused by systematic errors at local fundamental frequency peaks. This type of phonation can be classified as shouted modal voicing with strongly marked prosody.

4.3.4. Sadness

The maximum difference between vowel and fricative energy is 1dB. This also means that the speech is not very loud. The inverse filtered signal looks very similar to a pure sine wave with obvious noise components. (The speech signal itself does not differ very much from that either.) This is consistent with the energy measurement, which shows marked spectral damping. Unlike the female speaker, for male speakers, the mid and high bands contain no harmonic, but only turbulent components. The sound impression of voiced segments is determined by the low frequency components, because there is not much energy in higher frequency regions. Most utterances show creak, which often appears at the beginning of voiced segments within a sentence. Creak is equal to a relative jitter value of 40% or 50%. The type of phonation in segments without voicing irregularities can be classified as breathy phonation.

4.3.5. Fear

The difference between vowel and fricative energy varies between 0.1 and 1.2 dB. This indicates a limited loudness. The inverse filtered signal looks very similar to the sad pulse shapes. The spectral distribution shows different values. In contrast to sad utterances, which have strong spectral damping in voiced segments, the utterances spoken with fear have very little spectral damping. This means that the turbulent noise components in the mid and high band are very important for the perceived sound quality. Not even the low band contains pure harmonic components. The fundamental frequency shows irregularities that result in high relative jitter values of between 2% and 8%. It should be mentioned that the utterances under investigation do not represent panic fear. They rather express whispery, suspicious fear. The fundamental frequency is high with little variation in the sense of increases or decreases for linguistic purposes. This type of phonation can be classified as breathy or whispery falsetto. But this conclusion might be wrong, because the turbulent noise components could also originate in an imprecise articulation with fricative constrictions during vowel articulation. The marked elongation of fricatives in the utterances could indicate that fear induces narrow fricative articulation in contrast to the usually more open vowel articulation.

4.3.6. Boredom

The difference between vowel and fricative energy is about 1.2 dB, which indicates a moderate loudness. The pulses are very similar to a sawtooth function, as is the neutral material, although the spectral damping in the mid and high band is stronger than in the neutral utterances. Unlike the female speaker, the male speakers do have turbulent noise in the higher frequency bands, but owing to the relatively low energy, these higher frequencies seem less important for the perceived sound quality. In contrast to sad utterances, bored speech does not show voicing irregularities or creaky phonation. This type of phonation can be classified as normal modal voicing with little dynamics in the fundamental frequency contour, that is, relatively monotonous speech.

5. SUMMARY

In the initial part of this chapter signal characteristics of the transglottal airflow were discussed with regard to the question of how different voice qualities can be measured in the acoustic speech signal. Several acoustic parameters were discussed. To deal with the fact that some voice qualities can hardly be regarded as quasistationary signals and hence difficult to analyze using common algorithms for stationary signals, some of the discussed parameters are not orthogonal, but represent varying approaches to measuring similar phenomena in the frequency and time domains. The combination of these acoustic parameters allows plausibility checks, so that the process can be trusted as a reliable method for the characterization of voice quality. The experiment presented focused on emotion-specific changes in the acoustic voice quality parameters. The speakers were not selected to represent a wide variety of different personal voice qualities. The interindividual differences were not more marked than of the intraindividual differences within one emotion.

Voice quality in neutral utterances could be classified as normal modal voicing for all speakers. In happy utterances, voice quality could be classified as loud modal voicing with extremely rapid changes in the fundamental frequency contour. In angry utterances the speakers used shouted phonation with strongly marked prosody. Sad utterances were spoken with breathy phonation. The type of phonation often changed within the sad utterances. Creak appears at the beginning of voiced segments. In frightened utterances the average fundamental frequency is high with little variation for linguistic purposes. Voice quality in sentences spoken with fear is (presumably) breathy or whispery falsetto. The fundamental frequency shows irregularities that result in high relative jitter values of about between 2% and 8%. Bored speech often resembles sad speech. Voice quality in those utterances that were unambiguously recognized as bored speech, do not show voicing irregularities or creaky phonation as the sad utterances do. This type of phonation can be classified as normal modal voicing with little dynamics in the fundamental frequency contour.

REFERENCES

Banse, R., & Scherer, K. R. (1996). Acoustic profiles in vocal emotion expression. *Journal of Personality and Social Psychology, 70,* 614.

Klasmeyer, G., & Sendlmeier W. F. (1995). Objective voice parameters to characterize the emotional content in speech. *Proceedings of the International Conference of Phonetic Sciences (Stockholm), 1,* 181–185.

Laver, J. (1994). *Principles of phonetics.* Cambridge, UK: Cambridge University Press.

Makhoul, J. (1975). Linear prediction: A tutorial review. *Proceedings IEEE, 63,* 561–580.

Rosken, W., & Klasmeyer, G. (1995). Erfassung von F0-Irregularitäten in gesprochener Sprache als messbarer Parameter zur Beschreibung von Stimmqualitäten. *Fortschritte der Akustik, DAGA 95,* 1047–1050.

Scherer, K. R. (1986). Vocal affect expression: A review and a model for future research, *Psychological Bulletin, 1986, 99,* 143–165.

Scherer, K. R. (1994). Affect bursts. In S. M. H. van Goozen, N. E. van de Poll, & J. A. Sergeant (Eds.), *Emotions: Essays on emotion theory* (pp. 161–196). Hillsdale, NJ: Erlbaum.

Sundberg, J. (1994). Vocal fold vibration patterns and phonatory modes. *Speech Transmission Lab* (Quarterly Progress Status Report 2–3/94). Stockholm: Royal Institute of Technology.

Wagner, I. (1995). A new jitter-algorithm to quantify hoarseness: An exploratory study, *Forensic Linguistics, 2*(1), 18–21.

Wong, D. J., Markel, J. D., & Gray, A. H. (1979). Least squares glottal inverse filtering from the acoustic speech waveform. *IEEE Transactions on Acoustics,*

CHAPTER 16

The Aging Voice

Sue Ellen Linville

It has been recognized for some time that the aging process alters an individual's voice. Changes in voice with aging are of interest to researchers as they work to identify and understand normal age-related changes in any number of health areas. By understanding normal aspects of the aged voice, such alterations can be distinguished from pathological conditions that affect voice.

In this chapter, normal age-related changes that occur in voices are reviewed along with anatomic and physiologic changes in the larynx. In addition, perceptual aspects of aged voice will be discussed. That is, those acoustic cues which result in a voice "sounding old" will be identified and related to acoustic aspects of actual age.

1. AGE RECOGNITION FROM VOICE

A number of studies have indicated that listeners are quite accurate in estimating speaker age from tape recordings of voice samples. When listeners were asked to determine if speakers were young versus old, Ptacek and Sander (1966) reported accuracy rates of 99% from reading passages played forward, 87% from reading passages played backward, and 78% from phonated vowel productions. When listeners were asked to divide female speakers into three perceived age groups (young, middle-aged, old), Linville and Fisher (1985) found that listeners were 51% accurate from phonated vowels and 43% accurate from whispered vowels. When asked to judge age directly from reading passages, correlations of perceived age and actual age ranged from 0.88 to 0.93 (Hartman, 1979; Ryan & Capadano, 1978; Shipp & Hollien, 1969). In each of these studies, listeners were able to accurately judge age at better-than-chance levels. However, as less acoustic information was available in the signal and the task became more difficult for listeners, accuracy rates dropped. This result is to be expected. It is significant, however, that listeners do not appear to be reduced to random guessing even when judging age even from samples devoid of voicing information, such as whispered vowels. Of course, listener accuracy under such conditions is not particularly good, suggesting that a number of individual speakers might be misperceived from whispered vowel samples, even if overall accuracy rates for a large sample of speakers surpasses random guessing levels.

A number of factors have been reported to affect listener accuracy in perceiving age from voice. Young listeners have been reported to be more accurate in their age perceptions than elderly listeners (Huntley, Hollien, & Shipp, 1987; Jacques & Rastatter, 1990; Linville & Korabic, 1986). Female listeners have been reported to be more accurate than male listeners (Hartman, 1979). In addition, young speakers might be identified more accurately than elderly speakers, even if listeners are elderly (Hollien & Tolhurst, 1978; Jacques & Rastatter, 1990; Neiman & Applegate, 1990). It even has been suggested that white male speakers may be identified more accurately with respect to age than black male speakers, regardless of listener race (McCloskey & Moran, 1988).

Occasionally listeners have been asked to describe the vocal characteristics that are displayed by individuals unambiguously judged as old (Hartman, 1979; Hartman & Danhauer, 1976; Ryan & Burk, 1974). Voice characteristics considered characteristic of "old" voices are listed in Table 16–1. It is significant that these features do not always correspond to actual acoustic changes in voice with aging. Similarly, differences exist between these identified features and data from correlational studies in which acoustic parameters of voice were measured and correlated with perceived age estimates (Shipp & Hollien, 1969; Shipp, Qi, Huntley & Hollien, 1992). These inconsistencies are pointed out as the chapter progresses.

2. AGE-RELATED VOICE CHANGES RELATED TO RESPIRATORY/PHONATORY FUNCTION

2.1. Anatomic and Physiologic Changes

The respiratory and phonatory systems undergo significant anatomic and physiologic changes with aging. Anatomic changes in the respiratory system include stiffening of the thorax (Kahane, 1983), decreased force and rate of respiratory muscle contraction (Dhar, Shastri, & Lenora, 1976; McKeown, 1965), and loss of elasticity of the pleural membranes (Pierce & Ebert, 1965). Such anatomic changes in the lungs and thorax with aging affect the functioning of the respiratory system (Rochet, 1991). Specifically, elderly speakers demonstrate increased residual volume (Bode, Dosman, Martin, Ghezzo, & Macklem, 1976) and decreased elastic recoil (Sperry & Klich, 1992). In addition, decreases in vital capacity (Sperry & Klich, 1992), expiratory and inspiratory reserve volume (Chebotarev, Korkushuko & Ivanov, 1974; Hoit & Hixon, 1987; Hoit, Hixon, Altman, & Morgan, 1989) and forced expiratory volume and airflow rate (Chodzko-Zajko & Ringel, 1987) have been reported. However, airflow rate during oral reading in women appears to be unaffected by age (Sperry & Klich, 1992).

Anatomic changes in the larynx include ossification and calcification of cartilages (Kahane, 1980), atrophy of muscle tissue (Segre, 1971), erosion of joint surfaces (Kahane, 1988), and thinning of the lamina propria accompanied by breakdown of subepithelial connective tissue (Hirano, Kurita, & Sakaguchi, 1989; Kahane, 1987). With the possible exception of muscle atrophy, these changes have been reported to be more significant in men than in women (Kahane, 1988; Kahane & Beckford, 1991). Vocal fold edema has been identified as a significant laryngeal change in elderly women (Ferreri, 1959; Honjo & Isshiki, 1980).

2.2. Acoustic Changes

2.2.1. Speaking Fundamental Frequency (SF_0)

In both men and women, speaking fundamental frequency (SF_0) has been documented to change from young adulthood to old age. Different patterns of change with aging can be observed in men and women, however. In

Table 16–1. Vocal characteristics considered by listeners as typical of "old" voices.

Lower vocal pitch (regardless of speaker gender)
Increased strain
Higher incidence of voice breaks
Vocal tremor
Increased breathiness
Reduced loudness
Slower speech rate
Greater hesitancy
Less precise articulation

Note: Compiled from Hartman (1979); Hartman and Danhauer (1976); Ryan and Burk (1974).

Figure 16–1, data are compiled from a number of different studies which suggest that, in men, SF_0 undergoes dramatic lifespan changes (Brown, Morris, Hollien & Howell, 1991; Hollien & Jackson, 1973; Hollien & Shipp, 1972; Mysak, 1959; Pegoraro Krook, 1988). Specifically, SF_0 lowers from young adulthood into middle age and then rises again with the passage into old age. Presumably, by age 85, a man's SF_0 would reach the highest level of his adult life. It has been speculated that the cause of the F_0 drop from young adulthood into middle age in men may be subclinical trauma associated with normal vocal use, although a definitive cause has yet to be determined (Hollien & Shipp, 1972). A rise in SF_0 from middle age into old age might be expected given the muscle atrophy and/or increased stiffness of vocal fold tissue observed in male speakers with advanced age.

The pattern of SF_0 change across adulthood in women is less dramatic than for men, as illustrated in Figure 16–2. In this figure data including both smokers and nonsmokers (Brown et al., 1991; Honjo & Isshiki, 1980; Pegoraro Krook, 1988; Saxman & Burk, 1967) are plotted separately from data including only nonsmokers (Stoicheff, 1981). Speaking fundamental frequency in women remains fairly constant from age 20 until approximately age 50, when a drop occurs. Presumably, the drop in SF_0 in middle age in women follows hormonal changes during menopause that result in vocal fold edema (Kahane, 1983). It is important to note that longitudinal studies have suggested that drops in SF_0 following menopause in women may be of greater magnitude than what is indicated by these cross-sectional data (de Pinto & Hollien, 1982; Russell, Penny, & Pemberton, 1995). As women move from middle age into old age SF_0 appears to change very little. Although some re-searchers have reported a tendency for SF_0 to rise slightly with very advanced age in women (Mueller, Sweeney & Baribeau, 1984; Pegoraro Krook, 1988), such SF_0 changes have been statistically insignificant and must therefore be considered negligible. In addition, other researchers have suggested that SF_0 in centenarian females actually may be lower than previously reported for "younger" elderly women, although variability of SF_0 among the sample of centenarian females examined was quite large (Awan & Mueller, 1992). Smokers and nonsmokers demonstrate the same pattern of SF_0 change during adulthood. That is, smoking appears to simply lower SF_0 for speakers across age levels.

It has been suggested recently that professional singers may display higher SF_0 levels than nonsingers (Brown et al., 1991). However, smoking histories of subjects are unreported in that study. It is premature to conclude that a history of professional singing results in higher

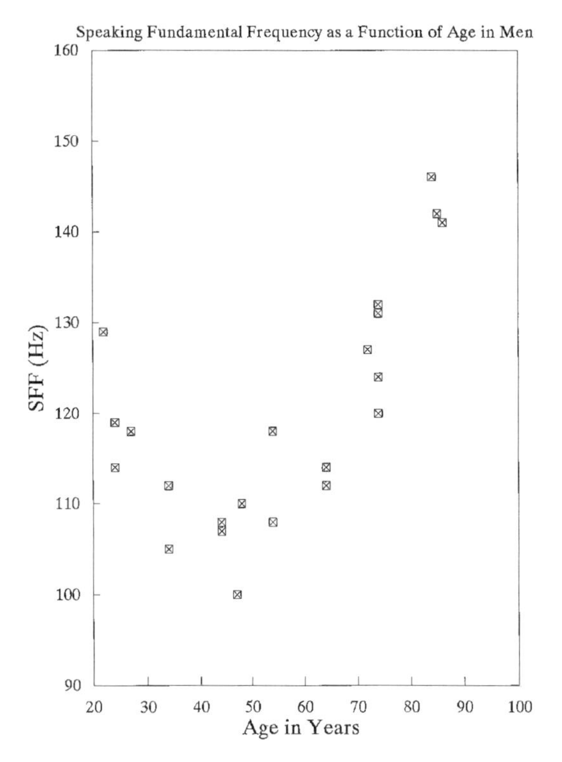

Figure 16–1. Speaking fundamental frequency as a function of age in men. (From "The Sound of Senescence," by S. E. Linville, 1996, *Journal of Voice, 10,* p. 191. Copyright 1996 by Lippincott-Raven Publishers. Reprinted with permission.)

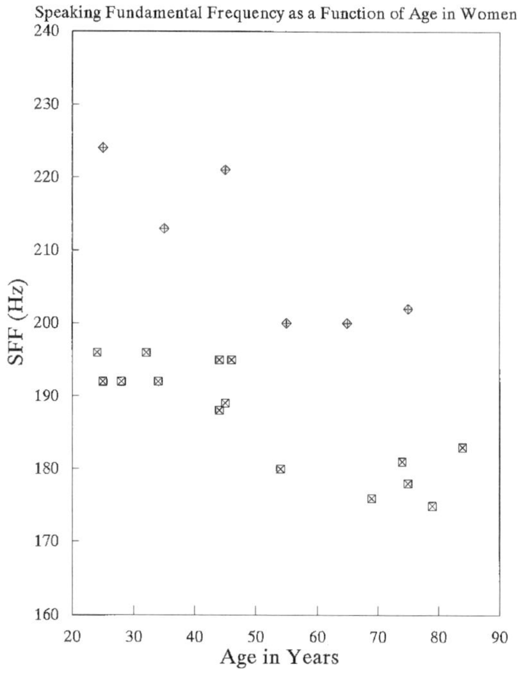

Figure 16–2. Speaking fundamental frequency as a function of age in women. (From "The Sound of Senescence" by S. E. Linville, 1996, *Journal of Voice, 10,* p. 192. Copyright 1996 by Lippincott-Raven Publishers. Reprinted with permission.)

SF_0 levels without first determining that smoking was not a factor affecting SF_0 levels.

It appears that SF_0 strongly influences listeners' judgments of perceived age. Evidence pointing to the power of SF_0 includes: (a) significantly higher accuracy rates in judging age from phonated vowels in comparison with whispered vowels (Linville & Fisher, 1985), (b) similar listener performance in judging age from a tape of unaltered phonated vowels and an altered tape in which resonance features of voice were low-pass filtered from the acoustic signal (Jacques & Rastatter, 1990), and (c) correlation of mean F_0 with listeners' judgments of age from phonated vowels in the absence of correlation of formant information. These findings suggest that SF_0 dominates resonance information in judging age from voice. However, resonance information has been found to correlate with age estimates if F_0 information is unavailable in the signal, as in the case of whispered vowels (Linville & Fisher, 1985).

Correlations of SF_0 with perceived age agree with changes in SF_0 with actual age, at least when sustained vowel productions are used as stimuli. That is, women tend to be perceived as older if their SF_0 is lower, whereas men tend to be perceived as older if their SF_0 is higher (Linville & Fisher, 1985; Shipp et al., 1992). It is interesting, however, that correlations of SF_0 with perceived age do not agree with listeners' reports of reactions to SF_0 when judging age, at least with male speakers. Listeners have reported responding to lower pitch in male speakers as an indicator of advanced age. This finding suggests that listeners may harbor stereotypes of acoustic features that typlify an "elderly" male voice.

2.2.2. Maximum Phonational Frequency Range (MPFR)

MPFR has been defined as the complete range of frequencies that an individual can produce from the lowest sustainable tone (without vocal fry) to the highest falsetto tone (Hollien, Dew, & Philips, 1971). It appears that changes occur at both ends of the MPFR in women with aging, although such changes do not occur during the same time period.

Changes at the low end of the MPFR appear to occur at menopause, with middle-aged, postmenopausal women displaying an ability to produce lower frequencies than both young adult women and elderly women (Linville, 1987). This expanded low frequency capability is probably the result of hormonal changes that increase vocal fold mass. Interestingly, expansion of low frequency capability has not been shown to extend to musically acceptable low pitches (Bohme & Hecker, 1970).

The increased capacity for low frequency production in middle-aged women is not great enough to significantly expand total MPFR capabilities (Linville, 1987). Changes in frequency production capability that have the greatest impact on total MPFR in women are those occurring at the high end of the range later in life (Linville, 1987; Ptacek, Sander, Maloney, & Jackson, 1966). Restriction of the upper end of the MPFR appears to be a biologically determined phenomenon and, as such, occurs even in individuals with professional voice training (Brown, Morris, Hicks, & Howell, 1993). Several factors may account for restriction of high frequency capability in elderly women, including intrinsic muscle weakening, ossification and calcification of laryngeal cartilages, and changes in vocal fold mass.

Elderly women tend to revert back to the low frequency capabilities of young women, losing the expanded low frequency production observed during middle age (Linville, 1987). Similarly, restriction of musically acceptable low pitches occurs after age 65 (Bohme & Hecker, 1970). The passage of time between middle age and old age in women appears to be critical both for reversing a drop in the floor of the frequency range that occurred during middle age as well as restricting the upper end of the MPFR.

In men, findings concerning MPFR have been somewhat contradictory. Ptacek et al. (1966) reported that elderly men display the same restriction of the upper end of the MPFR observed in elderly women. On the other hand, Ramig and Ringel (1983) found that young and elderly men do not differ in MPFR capabilities unless physical condition is taken into account. Ramig and Ringel (1983) acknowledged, however, that factors such as large within-group physiological variation in their subject sample may have obscured significant chronological age effects.

2.2.3. Stability of F_0 and Amplitude

Measures pertaining to stability of vocal fold vibration have been examined as a function of vocal age because such measures are felt to relate to the regulation and control of voice. Researchers have assumed that some subtle loss of function related to anatomic and physiologic changes in the larynx and respiratory system may well accompany the aging process. They reasoned that such an age-related decline might manifest as increased instability of vocal fold vibration.

Similarly, some of the vocal cues that listeners identified as typical of "old" voices suggest increased instability of vocal fold vibration in elderly speakers. Specifically, reports of increased harshness and hoarseness, vocal tremor, and pitch breaks might be related to higher levels of jitter, shimmer, F_0 standard deviation (F_0 SD) or amplitude standard deviation (amp SD) in elderly speakers.

2.2.3.1. Jitter and Shimmer Jitter and shimmer are measures of vocal fold stability reflecting small, cycle-to-cycle fluctuations in vocal fold vibration. Jitter is a measure of cycle-to-cycle fluctuations in the fundamental period of vocal fold vibration. Shimmer relates to cycle-to-cycle variation in waveform amplitude.

At this time, a definitive statement as to jitter and shimmer changes with aging is not possible. Numerous factors have been uncovered recently that can interfere with reliable jitter and shimmer measurements. Specifically, factors such as mean sound pressure level (SPL) of phonation (Orlikoff & Kahane, 1991), mean F_0 of phonation (Orlikoff & Baken, 1990), and analysis system differences (Gelfer & Fendel, 1995; Karnell, Scherer, & Fischer, 1991) may confound jitter and shimmer measurements, particularly in female voices. Because of these methodological issues, results of earlier studies in which jitter and shimmer differences with aging were investigated need to be interpreted with caution.

However, some clue as to age-related changes in jitter and shimmer might be gleaned from examination of recent data from male speakers. In Figures 16–3 and 16–4, jitter and shimmer data from young and elderly men are displayed (Orlikoff, 1990). It appears that mean jitter and shimmer values for elderly men are higher than mean values for young men. It also is evident that elderly men are considerably more variable on measures of jitter and shimmer than are young men. Findings of increased variability in elderly speakers in comparison with young speakers are quite common across a number of studies in which age-related differences in acoustic and physiologic measures have been investigated (Deal & Emanuel, 1978; Kahane, 1980; Linville, 1992; Linville & Fisher,1985; Linville, Skarin, & Fornatto, 1989; Orlikoff, 1990; Ramig & Ringel, 1983). Increased variability in elderly individuals appears to be related, at least in part, to individual health and fitness variables. Indeed, differences in jitter with age may tend to disappear once health and fitness variables are taken into consideration (Orlikoff, 1990; Ramig & Ringel, 1983). However, age-related shimmer differences appear to be less affected by health and fitness issues (Orlikoff, 1990).

2.2.3.2. F_0 SD and amp SD Measures of F_0 SD and amp SD are stability measures that reflect more gross fluctuations over time. These measures tend to increase with advancing age in both men (Figure 16–5) and women (Figure 16–6). In men, mean F_0 SD values more than doubled from young adulthood to old age (Orlikoff, 1990). In women, mean F_0 SD values increased by 71% over the adult lifespan (Linville & Fisher, 1985). Variability of F_0 SD values in both men and women increases with advancing age. However, variability increases in F_0 SD are less dramatic than what has been reported with jitter measures, especially in female speakers (Linville & Fisher, 1985). Indeed, current evidence suggests that F_0 SD measures may be a better predictor of vocal age than jitter (Linville & Fisher, 1985; Orlikoff, 1990). Interestingly, older speakers also have been reported to produce a larger number of upward and downward inflections than younger speakers, along with maximum inflections that are of greater magnitude than younger speakers (Benjamin, 1981).

Amplitude SD also appears to increase with advancing age. In male speakers, Orlikoff (1990) reported amp SD increases of 54% from young adulthood (m = .707 dB) to old age (m = 1.087 dB), with variability also increasing in elderly speakers (range = .863 – 1.727 dB) in comparison with young speakers (range = .542 – .956 dB). Amplitude SD in female speakers with aging has yet to be investigated.

2.2.3.3. Relationship of F_0 Stability to Perceived Age There is evidence that jitter is not associated with perceived age in women (Linville & Fisher, 1985). In other words, women in whom jitter levels are high do not tend to be perceived as older by listeners, even if their jitter levels are as high as values considered characteristic of pathologic voices (Lieberman, 1963). Since jitter and shimmer have been found to be acoustic correlates of a voice quality described as rough or hoarse (Deal & Emanuel, 1978; Lieberman, 1963), these results would indicate that vocal roughness is not a particularly meaningful cue to vocal age in women. Shimmer may be a more sensitive indicator of vocal roughness than jitter, however. Also, it has been suggested that the effects of jitter and shimmer are additive

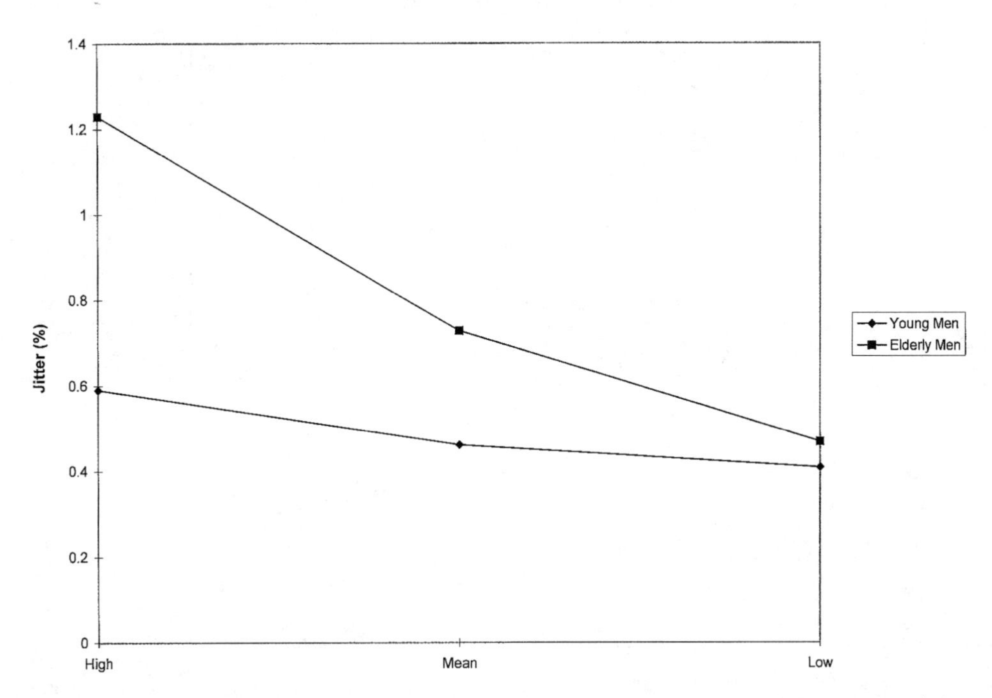

Figure 16–3. Jitter (%) values for two age groups of men during production of sustained /a/ vowels. Abscissa values are the range (high, low) as well as the mean jitter value observed for each age group. (Data are from Orlikoff [1990].)

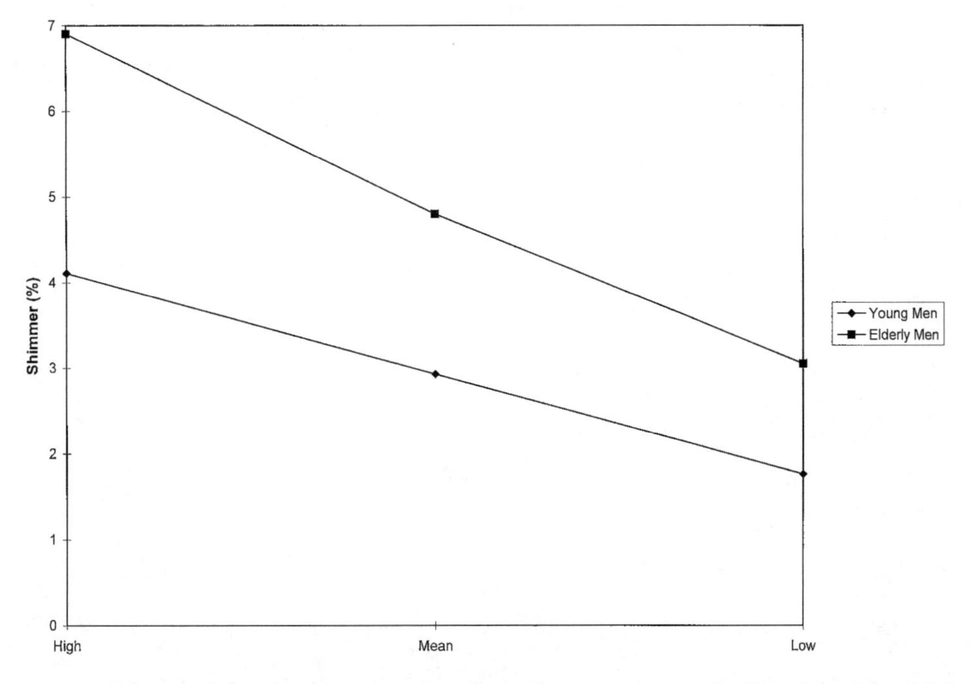

Figure 16–4. Shimmer (%) values for two age groups of men during production of sustained /a/ vowels. Abscissa values are the range (high, low) as well as the mean shimmer value observed for each age group. (Data are from Orlikoff [1990].)

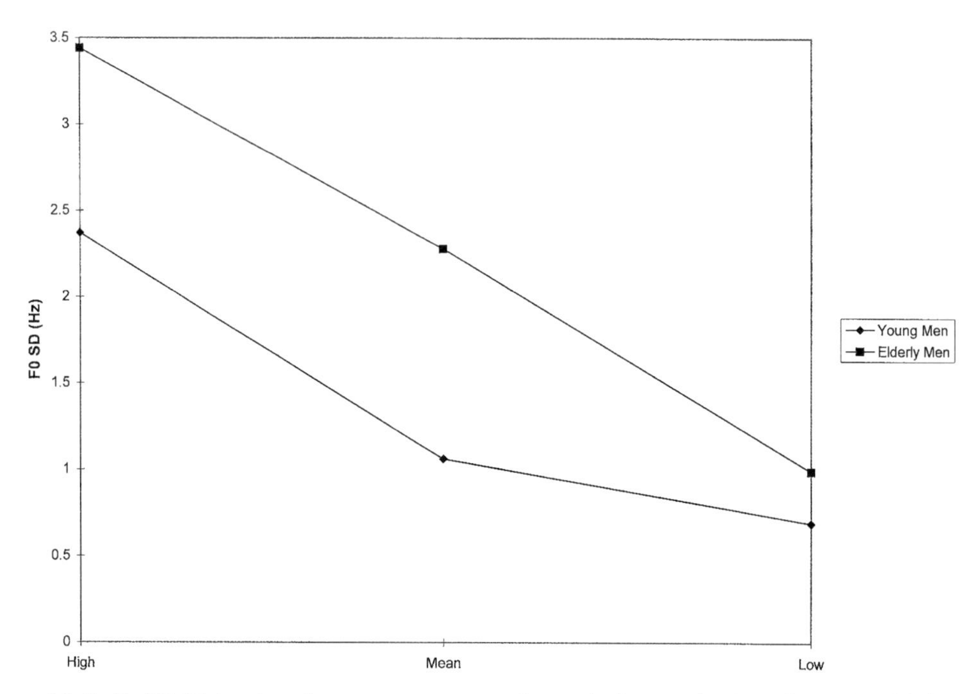

Figure 16–5. F_0 SD (Hz) values for two age groups of men during production of sustained /a/ vowels. Abscissa values are the range (high, low) as well as the mean F_0 SD (Hz) value observed for each age group. (Data are from Orlikoff [1990].)

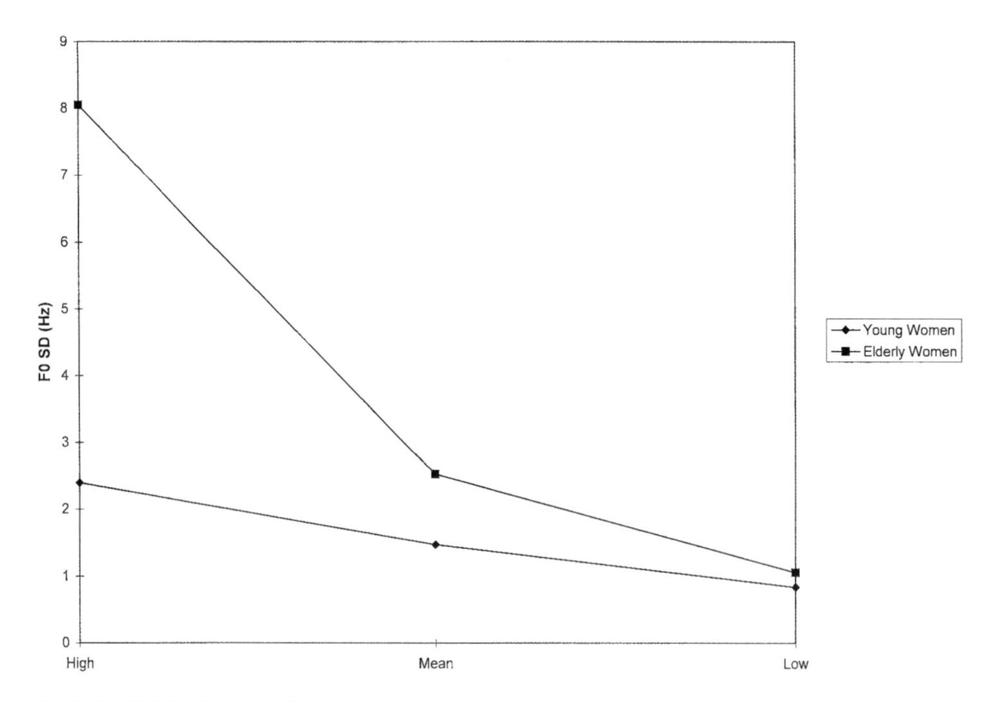

Figure 16–6. F_0 SD (Hz) values for two age groups of women during production of sustained /ae/ vowels. Abscissa values are the range (high, low) as well as the mean F_0 SD (Hz) value observed for each age group. (Data are from Linville and Fisher [1985].)

(Deal & Emanuel, 1978; Hillenbrand, 1988). Further study is indicated to determine definitively the significance of roughness as a perceptual cue to perceived age.

Listeners do appear to respond to F_0 SD in judging vocal age. Higher F_0 SD values have been associated with older age estimates by listeners in judging both men's voices (Shipp et al., 1992) and women's voices (Linville & Fisher, 1985). What is the perceptual phenomenon to which listeners are responding when F_0 SD values are high? Perhaps listeners are sensitive to relatively long-term, systematic variation in F_0, judging voices with such fluctuations as "old." Voices displaying progressive increases in frequency followed by progressive decreases might sound tremulous or "shaky," as opposed to rough or hoarse. Indeed, vocal tremor is one vocal characteristic listeners have labeled as typical of voices judged as old (Hartman, 1979; Ryan & Burk, 1974).

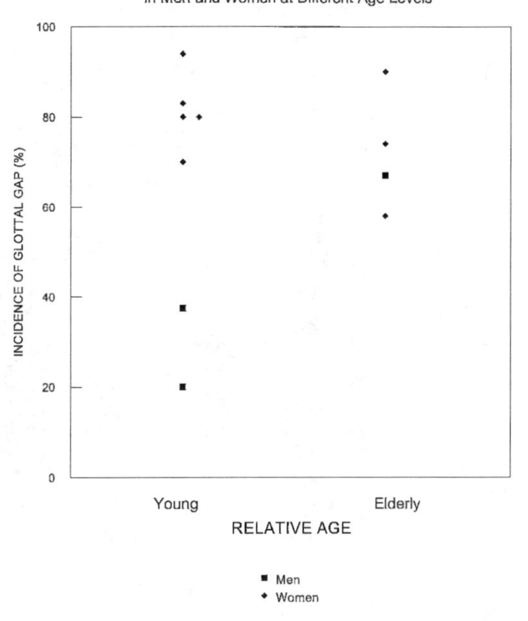

Figure 16–7. Incidence of glottal gap in men and women at different age levels. (From "The Sound of Senescence," by S. E. Linville, 1996, *Journal of Voice, 10*, p. 194. Copyright 1996 by Lippincott-Raven Publishers. Reprinted with permission.)

2.3. Vocal Fold Closure Changes

2.3.1. Assessed From Visual Examination

Age-related changes in the laryngeal mechanism, such as atrophy of the intrinsic laryngeal musculature or atrophy of connective tissue, might be expected to produce glottal gaps. The configuration of any observed glottal gaps would vary as a function of the muscles affected. Whereas weakening to the thyroarytenoid would be expected to result in incomplete closure from the vocal processes to the anterior commissure (a spindle configuration), weakness of the interarytenoids would produce a posterior chink. Incomplete closure along the length of the glottis would be evidenced if generalized weakening of adductor muscles occurred.

In Figure 16–7 glottal gap incidence rates from a number of studies are plotted (Biever & Bless, 1989; Bless, Biever, & Shaik, 1986; Honjo & Isshiki, 1980; Linville, 1992; Peppard, Bless, & Milenkovic, 1988; Sodersten & Lindestad, 1990). In men, advancing age results in an increased incidence of glottal gap. Such an increase in the occurrence of gap might be predicted given reports of atrophy of laryngeal muscles in aged speakers (Bach, Lederer, & Dinolt, 1941; Segre, 1971). Although the cause of muscle atrophy in the elderly larynx has yet to be determined, it is possible that wear and tear factors contribute to muscle weakening.

The data for women are much more interesting. Both elderly and young women demonstrate a high incidence of glottal gaps. Indeed, the overall incidence of glottal gaps for these two groups is not significantly different. Young and elderly women do differ, however, in the configuration of the gaps they exhibit, as well as the phonatory conditions under which gaps occur.

In Figure 16–8, glottal gap configuration data from a study of 10 young and 10 elderly women are displayed (Linville, 1992). Elderly women actually achieved complete closure

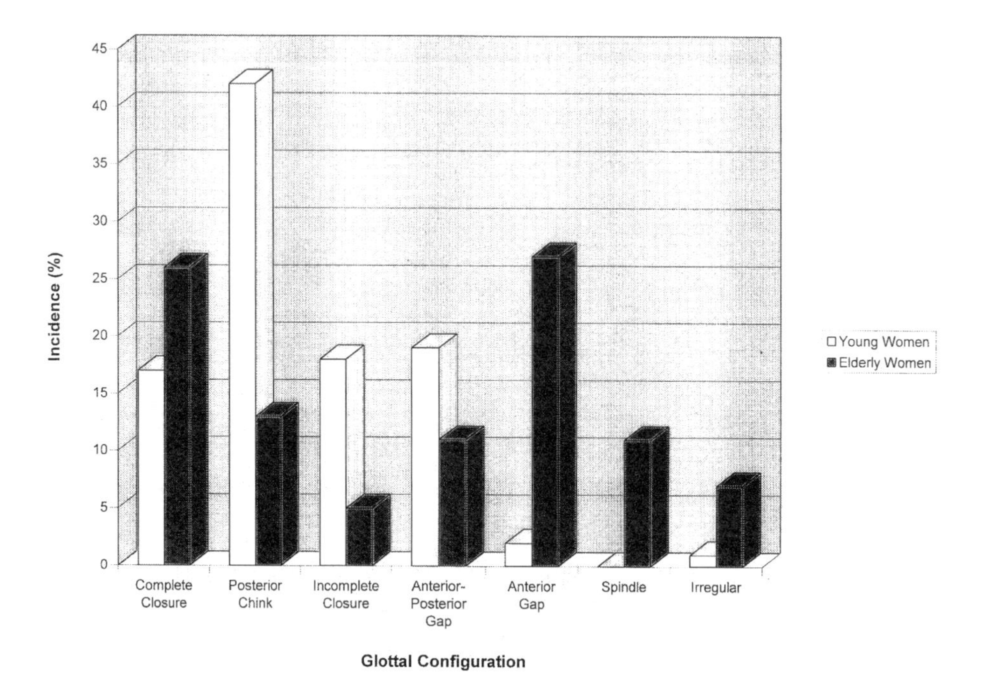

Figure 16–8. Incidence of various glottal configurations (%) for young and elderly women across 9 pitch and loudness conditions. (Data are from Linville [1992].)

more frequently than young women, a finding contradictory to what is expected given anatomical evidence of muscle atrophy in elderly speakers. Elderly women also displayed anterior gap and spindle configuration significantly more frequently than did young women. Young women displayed a particularly high incidence of posterior chink, a finding that supports several earlier studies (Biever & Bless, 1989; Koike & Hirano, 1973; Sodersten & Lindestad, 1990). Incomplete closure also occurred more frequently in young women. Anterior gap and spindle configuration were rarely observed in young women.

Given what is known about age-related changes in the larynx, it is surprising that young women would demonstrate a high incidence of posterior chink in comparison with elderly women. Changes within the larynx such as atrophy of muscle and connective tissue would work against closure of the posterior glottis, not the opposite. Edema, however, would work to increase closure. However, when subjects' videostroboscopic images were examined medically, no edema was reported in any subject. Although a definitive explanation for this finding is not possible, it might be speculated that young women are physiologically capable of achieving vocal fold closure, but fail to do so for functional reasons. That is, opening of the posterior glottis could be an adjustment that is adopted for economy reasons or to achieve a voice quality aim such as slight breathiness. In elderly women this adjustment might be abandoned as gaps begin to develop in the anterior glottis. While this explanation is speculative, there is evidence that young women display a significantly greater degree of perceived breathiness than do young men (Sodersten & Lindestad, 1990). Differences in perceived breathiness in young women and elderly women have yet to be investigated.

A second explanation for higher incidence of posterior chink in young women might be possible. It is conceivable that an age-related alteration in the larynx supraglottally that is as yet undiscovered works to alter the superior view of the posterior larynx. While this explanation also is speculative, there is some evidence that a portion of the posterior glottis remains unclosed normally during vocal fold adduction (Hirano, Kurita, Kiyokawa, & Sato, 1986).

Interestingly, loudness level has proven to be a significant factor in the incidence of posterior chink in young and elderly women (Linville, 1992). While young women demonstrated posterior chink fairly frequently across all loudness levels, elderly women rarely displayed posterior chink during loud phonation. Perhaps elderly women, upon experiencing age-related gaps anteriorly in the glottis, need to close the posterior glottis to phonate loudly. Young women, however, with the advantage of full muscular capability anteriorly, might be able to keep the posterior glottis open and still achieve adequate loudness. There is some support for this hypothesis from a study in which a correlation was found between bowing of the vocal folds and maximum intensity of phonation (Linville et al., 1989).

2.3.2. Inferred From Aerodynamic and Electroglottographic (EGG) Measures

Inverse-filtered airflow waveforms furnish an estimate of the airflow pattern through the glottis during consecutive vocal fold vibrations (Rothenberg, 1973, 1977). Airflow duty cycle, a measure that can be derived from inverse-filtered airflow waveforms, is defined as the ratio of the time above a set baseline divided by the glottal period (Higgins & Saxman, 1991). Likewise, EGG duty cycle can be ascertained from EGG waveforms. EGG duty cycle represents the ratio of the time above a set baseline to the glottal period (Higgins & Saxman, 1991). Duty cycle measurements are associated with less vocal fold contact as well as a shorter period of contact. In other words, as duty cycle increases, a decrease in vocal fold contact and shorter duration of contact is inferred (Childers & Krishnamurthy, 1985). Higgins and Saxman (1991) found interesting age-related patterns when airflow and EGG duty cycle measurements were obtained on speakers, particularly female speakers (Figure 16–9). In men, duty cycle measurements followed the expected age-related pattern. That is, elderly men demonstrated longer duty cycles than did young men, indicating less complete vocal fold closure with aging.

In women, however, lower duty cycle values in elderly women suggest slightly increased vocal fold contact and increased time of contact. This pattern would not be expected if age-related vocal fold atrophy had occurred and produced a higher incidence of laryngeal valving deficits, as had been the case for male speakers. However, this pattern does correspond with findings of stroboscopic studies and provides further evidence that elderly women actually tend to close the glottis more completely than do young women. This age-related pattern in women may be associated with a shift from a larger posterior gap in the young adult years to a smaller anterior gap with advanced age.

Additional support for the notion that vocal aging in women does not increase the incidence of laryngeal valving deficits comes from Sapienza and Dutka (1996). These authors found no significant difference in the magnitude of glottal airflow (peak, alternating, minimum, and minimum to peak) for 70-year-old women in comparison with 20-year-old women, although the older women demonstrated greater variability in peak glottal airflow. Sapienza and Dutka (1996) concured with the hypothesis of Linville (1992) that elderly women may utilize functional adjustments to close the posterior gaps they displayed as young adults when gaps begin to appear more anteriorly in the glottis with advanced age. Of course, all researchers recognize that this explanation is speculative and acknowledge that other factors might be operating to explain age-related glottal closure patterns in women.

2.3.3. Implications of Vocal Fold Closure Changes for Speakers

Elderly men in whom glottal gaps appear may begin to compensate for the closure deficit by use of increased laryngeal adductory forces as a compensatory mechanism (Higgins &

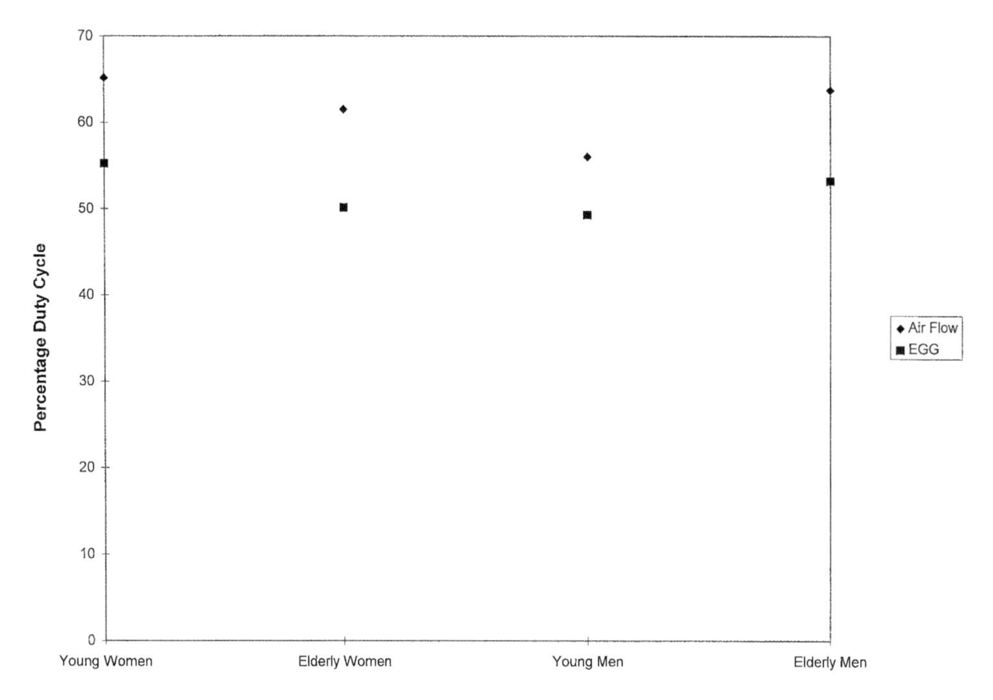

Figure 16–9. Group means for airflow duty cycle and electroglottograph duty cycle obtained during /baep/ and /ae/ productions across four pitch and loudness conditions. (Data are from Higgins and Saxman [1991].)

Saxman, 1991). Such an adjustment might be perceived by listeners as strained vocal quality. Significantly higher estimated subglottal pressure values have been reported for elderly men in comparison with younger men (Higgins & Saxman, 1991). This finding may reflect an increase in vocal fold stiffness (Hillman, Holmberg, Perkell, Walsh & Vaughn, 1989).

Another consequence of glottal closure deficits in the elderly could be a reduction in the number of syllables per breath group. There is evidence that elderly speakers require a greater number of intrasentence breath pauses than do younger individuals (Hoit & Hixon, 1987). Maximum phonation time in both men and women also is reduced with aging (Kruel, 1972; Ptacek et al., 1966). In elderly women, maximum phonation time has been associated with measures of vocal intensity as well as with pitch range measures (Linville et al., 1989). This finding suggests that phonation time reductions in the elderly may be the result of both respiratory control and laryngeal valving factors. Both decreases in vital capacity and maximum expiratory flow rate have been reported for elderly speakers (Gibson, Pride, O'Caine, & Quagliato, 1976; Hoit & Hixon, 1987; Hoit et al., 1989; Lynne-Davies, 1977; Mead, Turner, Macklem, & Little, 1967).

3. AGE-RELATED VOICE CHANGES RELATED TO RESONANCE

3.1. Anatomic and Physiologic Changes

Substantial evidence has been gathered that the supraglottic vocal tract undergoes marked changes with aging (Sonies, 1991). Reported changes include 3%–5% growth of the facial skeleton (Israel, 1968, 1973; Lasker, 1953), atrophy/hypertrophy of the tongue musculature (Balough & Lelkes, 1961; Cohen & Gittman,

1959; Silverman, 1972), tooth loss (Meyerson, 1976), weakening/atrophy of the pharyngeal musculature (Zaino & Benventano, 1977), and restricted movement of the temporomandibular joint (Kahane, 1980). Although no data were reported, it also has been hypothesized that the larynx may lower in the neck with advanced age as a result of stretching of ligaments and atrophy of the strap muscles of the neck (Macklin & Macklin, 1942; Wilder, 1978). Further, Kahane (1980) suggested that weakening of structural support elements in the vertebral column with aging produces a series of changes in the lower respiratory tract, including lowering of both the larynx and the tracheobronchial tree and lungs. Interestingly, Biever and Bless (1989) observed indirect evidence of age-related vocal tract lengthening in women through observation of darker images during stroboscopic examinations on elderly women. Darker images for elderly women suggest greater distance between the camera lens and the vocal folds in comparison with younger women. If of sufficient magnitude, anatomic changes such as these might be predicted to alter vocal resonance in elderly speakers.

3.2. Formant Frequency Changes

A limited number of studies examining vocal resonance changes with aging have been conducted and findings of those studies have been conflicting. Endres, Bombach, and Flosser (1971) studied 4 male and 2 female speakers over periods of up to 29 years and found that the formant frequencies of 7 vowels and 2 diphthongs in content-controlled running speech samples lowered with age. Similarly, Linville and Fisher (1985) found that F_1 frequencies of /æ/ vowels produced by 75 women lowered significantly with aging. F_2 frequencies also lowered significantly in elderly women, although age-related differences in F_2 were less prominent than changes in F_1. Scukanec, Petrosino, and Squibb (1991) also reported lowering of formant frequencies with advancing age in women. Specifically, F_1 frequencies for 3 elderly women lowered in comparison with 6 young women for the vowels /i/, /æ/, /u/ and /a/. Lower F_2 values also were reported for the elderly women, although significant lowering occurred only for /a/ and /u/.

Contradictory findings were reported by Rastatter and Jacques (1990) in a study involving 20 men and 20 women. These authors reported higher F_1 frequencies for front and mid vowels, and lower F_1 frequencies for back vowels, in elderly speakers. The authors concluded that elderly speakers may tend to centralize their tongue position during vowel production.

Studies of resonance changes in speakers with aging have indicated that such changes do occur. However, the precise nature of age-related resonance changes is open to some question. Lowering of formant frequencies across vowels with aging, as reported in three studies, suggests overall lengthening of the vocal tract in the elderly. Variation in formant frequencies as a function of the tongue position of the vowel, however, suggests the possibility of a "sociolect" of age; an elderly speech pattern that corresponds with social expectations for elderly speakers (Ramig, 1986). Additional studies are needed before a definitive conclusion can be drawn regarding the nature and etiology of resonance changes in elderly speakers.

3.3. Relationship of Resonance to Perceived Age Estimates

There is evidence that resonance information provides cues to listeners as to speaker age under limited circumstances. Linville and Fisher (1985) found a correlation between listeners' age estimates and F_1 frequency from women's whispered vowel productions. However, the correlation disappeared when listeners were presented with phonated vowels, suggesting that resonance information is not as meaningful as F_0 cues if both are present in the acoustic signal, at least when sustained vowels are used as stimuli.

It is interesting to speculate as to the significance of resonance information to age estimates from running speech. Judges of speaker age have mentioned "imprecise articulation" as a feature of speech that marked speakers as old (Hartman, 1979; Ryan & Burk, 1974). Since variations in articulatory patterns are reflected in resonance information, perhaps some as yet undiscovered cues to vocal age lie in the resonance patterns of connected speech. Additional research may yield answers to this question.

4. CHANGES IN SPEECH RATE WITH AGING

Elderly speakers demonstrate slower speaking rates than young speakers (Hartman & Danhauer, 1976; Mysak, 1959; Mysak & Hanley, 1959; Ryan, 1972; Ryan & Capadano, 1978). Speculated explanations for slowing of speech rate with aging include neuromuscular slowing (Hartman & Danhauer, 1976; Weismer & Liss, 1991), changes in the respiratory system (Oyer & Deal, 1985; Ramig, 1983), physiological condition (Ramig, 1983), increased cautiousness/expectations of society (Mysak, 1959; Mysak & Hanley, 1959), and fatigue (Hollien & Shipp, 1972). Interestingly, a correlation has been reported between slower reading rates in elderly speakers and reductions in F_0 stability (Linville et al., 1989). Perhaps a generalized loss of physiological control in elderly speakers is reflected both in slower reading rates and greater F_0 instability.

A correlation also has been reported between slower reading rates in elderly speakers and reductions in maximum intensity level (Linville et al., 1989). This finding suggests that changes in the respiratory system or inadequate laryngeal valving with aging may result in slower reading rates. Loss of elastic recoil of lung tissue with aging (Kaltieider, Fray, & Hyde, 1938; Pierce & Ebert, 1965; Turner, Mead, & Wohl, 1968) could produce difficulties in achieving loud phonation as well as producing an increase in the number of pauses during reading. Similarly, inadequate laryngeal valving would necessitate more frequent pauses during speech and also reduce maximum phonation level because of excessive air escape during phonation.

4.1. Relationship of Speech Rate to Age Perception

Speech rate appears to be a factor in listeners' age estimates of male speakers. Specifically, male speakers with slower speech rates tend to be perceived as older than speakers with faster rates (Shipp et al., 1992). In addition, men who utilized a larger number of breaths and longer breath pause durations were judged as older by listeners (Shipp et al., 1992). Studies have not been conducted correlating age estimates to speech rate in female speakers.

5. SUMMARY

The respiratory and phonatory systems, along with the supraglottic vocal tract, undergo significant anatomic and physiologic changes with aging. These changes affect the acoustic properties of voice produced by elderly speakers. Acoustic measures which have been found to vary with aging include speaking F_0, measures of F_0/amplitude stability, temporal aspects of speech, and resonance characteristics of voice. In terms of the performance capabilities of the laryngeal mechanism, aging appears to restrict the high end of the F_0 range in both men and women. Vocal fold closure changes with aging differ in men and women. Whereas elderly men demonstrate a higher incidence of glottal gaps than young men, elderly women may actually tend to close the glottis more completely than young women. Listeners appear to be quite accurate in estimating speaker age from tape recordings of voice samples. Perceived age estimates by listeners appear to be correlated with speaking F_0, F_0 standard deviation, formant frequency measures from whispered vowel productions, and measures related to speaking rate and breath management.

REFERENCES

Awan, S., & Mueller, P. (1992). Speaking fundamental frequency characteristics of centenarian females. *Clinical Linguistics and Phonetics, 6,* 249–254.

Bach, A., Lederer, F., & Dinolt, R. (1941). Senile changes in the laryngeal musculature. *Archives of Otolaryngology, 34,* 47–56.

Balogh, K., & Lelkes, K. (1961). The tongue in old age. *Gerontologica Clinica, 3*(Suppl. ad), 38–54.

Benjamin, B. J. (1981). Frequency variability in the aged voice. *Journal of Gerontology, 36,* 722–726.

Biever, D., & Bless, D. (1989). Vibratory characteristics of the vocal folds in young adult and geriatric women. *Journal of Voice, 3,* 120–131.

Bless, D., Biever, D., & Shaik, A. (1986). Comparisons of vibratory characteristics of young adult males and females. In S. J. Hibi, M. Hirano, & D. Bless (Eds.), *Proceedings of the International Conference on Voice* (pp. 46–54), Kurume, Japan.

Bode, F. R., Dosman, J., Martin, R. R., Ghezzo, H., & Macklem, P. T. (1976). Age and sex differences in lung elasticity and in closing capacity in nonsmokers. *Journal of Applied Physiology, 41,* 129–135.

Bohme, G., & Hecker, G. (1970). Gerontologische Untersuchungen uber Stimmumfang und Sprechstimmlage. *Folia Phoniatrica, 22,* 176–184.

Brown, W. S., Jr., Morris, R. J., Hicks, D. M., & Howell, E. (1993). Phonational profiles of female professional singers and nonsingers. *Journal of Voice, 7,* 219–226.

Brown, W., Morris, R., Hollien, H., & Howell, E. (1991). Speaking fundamental frequency characteristics as a function of age and professional singing. *Journal of Voice, 5,* 310–315.

Chebotarev, D. F., Korkushko, O. V., & Ivanov, L. A. (1974). Mechanics of hypoxemia in the elderly. *Journal of Gerontology, 29,* 393–400.

Childers, D. G., & Krishnamurthy, A. K. (1985). A critical review of electroglottography. *Critical Review of Biomedical Engineering, 12,* 131–161.

Chodzko-Zajko, W., & Ringel, R. (1987). Physiological aspects of aging. *Journal of Voice, 1,* 18–26.

Cohen, J., & Gittman, L. (1959). Oral complaints and taste perception in the aged. *Journal of Gerontology, 14,* 294–298.

Deal, R. E., & Emanuel, F. W. (1978). Some waveform and spectral features of vowel roughness. *Journal of Speech and Hearing Research, 21,* 250–263.

de Pinto, O., & Hollien, H. (1982). Speaking fundamental frequency characteristics of Australian women: Then and now. *Journal of Phonetics, 10,* 367–375.

Dhar, S., Shastri, S. R., & Lenora, R. A. (1976). Aging and the respiratory system. *Medical Clinics of North America, 60,* 1121–1139.

Endres, W., Bambach, W., & Flosser, G. (1971). Voice spectrograms as a function of age, voice disguise, and voice imitation. *Journal of the Acoustical Society of America, 49,* 1842–1848.

Ferreri, G. (1959). Senescence of the larynx. *Italian General Review of Otology-Rhinology-Laryngology, 1,* 640–709.

Gelfer, M. P., & Fendel, D. M. (1995). Comparisons of jitter, shimmer, and signal-to-noise ratio from directly digitized versus taped voice samples. *Journal of Voice, 9,* 378–382.

Gibson, G. J., Pride, N. B., O'Caine, C., & Quagliato, R. (1976). Sex and age differences in pulmonary mechanics in normal nonsmoking subjects. *Journal of Applied Physiology, 41,* 20–25.

Hartman, D. E. (1979). The perceptual identity and characteristics of aging in normal male adult speakers. *Journal of Communication Disorders, 12,* 53–61.

Hartman, D. E.,& Danhauer, J. L. (1976). Perceptual features of speech for males in four perceived age decades. *Journal of the Acoustical Society of America, 59,* 713–715.

Higgins, M. B., & Saxman, J. H. (1991). A comparison of selected phonatory behaviors of healthy aged and young adults. *Journal of Speech and Hearing Research, 34,* 1000–1010.

Hillenbrand, J. (1988). Perception of aperiodicities in synthetically generated voices. *Journal of the Acoustical Society of America, 83,* 2361–2371.

Hillman, R. E., Holmberg, E. B., Perkell, J. S., Walsh, M., & Vaughn, C. (1989). Objective assessment of vocal hyperfunction: An experimental framework and initial results. *Journal of Speech and Hearing Research, 32,* 373–392.

Hirano, M., Kurita, S., Kiyokawa, K., & Sato, K. (1986). Posterior glottis. Morphological study in excised human larynges. *Annals of Otology, Rhinology and Laryngology, 95,* 576–581.

Hirano, M., Kurita, S., & Sakaguchi, S. (1989). Ageing of the vibratory tissue of human vocal folds. *Acta Otolaryngologica (Stockholm), 107,* 428–433.

Hoit, J. D., & Hixon, T. J. (1987). Age and speech breathing. *Journal of Speech and Hearing Research, 30,* 351–366.

Hoit, J. D., Hixon, T. J., Altman, M.E., & Morgan, W. J. (1989). Speech breathing in women. *Journal of Speech and Hearing Research, 32,* 353–365.

Hollien, H., Dew, D., & Philips, P. (1971). Phonational frequency ranges of adults. *Journal of Speech and Hearing Research, 14,* 755–760.

Hollien, H., & Jackson, B. (1973). Normative data on the speaking fundamental frequency characteristics of young adult males. *Journal of Phonetics, 1,* 117–120.

Hollien, H., & Shipp, T. (1972). Speaking fundamental frequency and chronologic age in males. *Journal of Speech and Hearing Research, 15,* 155–159.

Hollien, H., & Tolhurst, G. (1978). The aging voice. In B. Weinberg (Ed.), *Transcripts of the Seventh Symposium Care of the Professional Voice* (pp. 67–73). New York: The Voice Foundation.

Honjo, I., & Isshiki, N. (1980). Laryngoscopic and voice characteristics of aged persons. *Archives of Otolaryngology, 106,* 149–150.

Huntley, R., Hollien, H., & Shipp, T. (1987). Influences of listener characteristics on perceived age estimations. *Journal of Voice, 1,* 49–52.

Israel, H. (1968). Continuing growth in the human cranial skeleton. *Archives of Oral Biology, 13,* 133–137.

Israel, H. (1973). Age factor and the pattern of change in craniofacial structures. *American Journal of Physical Anthropology, 39,* 111–128.

Jacques, R. D., & Rastatter, M. P. (1990). Recognition of speaker age from selected acoustic features as perceived by normal young and older listeners. *Folia Phoniatrica, 42,* 118–124.

Kahane, J. (1980). Age-related histological changes in the human male and female laryngeal cartilages: Biological and functional implications. In V. Lawrence (Ed.), *Transcripts of the ninth symposium care of the professional voice* (pp. 11–20). New York: Voice Foundation.

Kahane, J. (1983). Postnatal development and aging of the human larynx. *Seminars in Speech and Language, 4,* 189–203.

Kahane, J. (1987). Connective tissue changes in the larynx and their effects on voice. *Journal of Voice, 1,* 27–30.

Kahane, J. (1988). Age-related changes in the human cricoarytenoid joint. In O. Fujimura (Ed.), *Vocal physiology: Voice production, mechanisms and functions* (pp. 145–157). New York: Raven Press.

Kahane, J., & Beckford, N. (1991). The aging larynx and voice. In D. Ripich (Ed.), *Handbook of geriatric communication disorders* (pp. 165–186). Austin TX, Pro-Ed.

Kaltieider, N., Fray, W., & Hyde, H. (1938). The effects of age on the total pulmonary capacity and its subdivisions. *American Review of Tuberculosis, 37,* 662–689.

Karnell, M. P., Scherer, R. S., & Fischer, L. B. (1991). Comparison of acoustic perturbation measures among three independent voice laboratories. *Journal of Speech and Hearing Research, 34,* 781–790.

Koike, Y., & Hirano, M. (1973). Glottal-area time function and subglottal-pressure variation. *Journal of the Acoustical Society of America, 54,* 1618–1627.

Kreul, E. J. (1972). Neuromuscular control examination (NMC) for parkinsonism: Vowel prolongations and diadochokinetic and reading rates. *Journal of Speech and Hearing Research, 15,* 72–83.

Lasker, G. (1953). The aging factor in bodily measurements of adult male and female Mexicans. *Human Biology, 25,* 50–63.

Lieberman, P. (1963). Some acoustic measures of the fundamental periodicity of normal and pathologic larynges. *Journal of the Acoustical Society of America, 35,* 344–353.

Linville, S. E. (1987). Maximum phonational frequency range capabilities of women's voices with advancing age. *Folia Phoniatrica, 39,* 297–301.

Linville, S. E. (1992). Glottal gap configurations in two age groups of women. *Journal of Speech and Hearing Research, 35,* 1209–1215.

Linville, S. E., & Fisher, H. B. (1985). Acoustic characteristics of perceived versus actual vocal age in controlled phonation by adult females. *Journal of the Acoustical Society of America, 78,* 40–48.

Linville, S. E., & Korabic, E. W. (1986). Elderly listeners' estimates of vocal age in adult females. *Journal of the Acoustical Society of America, 80,* 692–694.

Linville, S. E., Skarin, B. D., & Fornatto, E. (1989). The interrelationship of measures related to vocal function, speech rate, and laryngeal appearance in elderly women. *Journal of Speech and Hearing Research, 32,* 323–330.

Lynne-Davies, P. (1977). Influence of age on the respiratory system. *Geriatrics, 32,* 57–60.

Macklin, C., & Macklin, M. (1942). Respiratory system. In E.V. Cowdry (Ed.), *Problems of aging* (2nd ed., pp. 185–253). Baltimore: Williams & Wilkins.

McCloskey, L., & Moran, M. (1988). *Socioeconomic and racial effects on the aging male voice.* Paper presented at the annual convention of the American Speech-Language-Hearing Association, Boston.

McKeown, F. (1965). *Pathology of the aged.* London: Butterworths.

Mead, J., Turner, J., Macklem, P. T., & Little, J. B. (1967). Significance of the relationship between lung recoil and maximum expiratory flow. *Journal of Applied Physiology, 22,* 95–108.

Meyerson, M. (1976). The effects of aging on communication. *Journal of Gerontology, 31,* 29–38.

Mueller, P. B., Sweeney, R. J., & Baribeau, L. J. (1984). Acoustic and morphologic study of the senescent voice. *Ear Nose and Throat Journal, 63,* 292–295.

Mysak, E. (1959). Pitch and duration characteristics of older males. *Journal of Speech and Hearing Research, 2,* 46–54.

Mysak, E., & Hanley, T. (1959). Vocal aging. *Geriatrics, 14,* 652–656.

Neiman, G., & Applegate, J. (1990). Accuracy of listener judgments of perceived age relative to chronological age in adults. *Folia Phoniatrica, 42,* 327–330.

Orlikoff, R. F. (1990). The relationship of age and cardiovascular health to certain acoustic characteristics of male voices. *Journal of Speech and Hearing Research, 33,* 450–457.

Orlikoff, R. F., & Baken, R. J. (1990). Consideration of the relationship between the fundamental frequency of phonation and vocal jitter. *Folia Phoniatrica, 42,* 31–40.

Orlikoff, R. F., & Kahane, J. (1991). Influence of mean sound pressure level on jitter and shimmer measures. *Journal of Voice, 5,* 113–119.

Oyer, H. J., & Deal, L. V. (1985). Temporal aspects of speech and the aging process. *Folia Phoniatrica, 37,* 109–112.

Pegoraro Krook, M. I. (1988). Speaking fundamental frequency characteristics of normal Swedish subjects obtained by glottal frequency analysis. *Folia Phoniatrica, 40,* 82–90.

Peppard, R., Bless, D., & Milenkovic, P. (1988). Comparison of young adult singers and non-singers with vocal nodules. *Journal of Voice, 2,* 250–260.

Pierce, J., & Ebert, R. (1965). Fibrous network of the lung and its change with age. *Thorax, 20,* 469–476.

Ptacek, P. H., & Sander, E. K. (1966). Age recognition from voice. *Journal of Speech and Hearing Research, 9,* 272–277.

Ptacek, P., Sander, E., Maloney, W., & Jackson, C. (1966). Phonatory and related changes with advanced age. *Journal of Speech and Hearing Research, 9,* 353–360.

Ramig, L. (1983). Effects of physiological aging on vowel spectral noise. *Journal of Gerontology, 38,* 223–225.

Ramig, L. (1986). Aging speech: Physiological and sociological aspects. *Language and Communication, 6,* 25–34.

Ramig, L., & Ringel, R. L. (1983). Effects of physiological aging on selected acoustic characteristics of voice. *Journal of Speech and Hearing Research, 26,* 22–30.

Rastatter, M. P., & Jacques, R. D. (1990). Formant frequency structure of the aging male and female vocal tract. *Folia Phoniatrica, 42,* 312–319.

Rochet, A. (1991). Aging and the respiratory system. In D. Ripich (Ed.), *Geriatric communication disorders* (pp. 145–163). Austin, TX: Pro-Ed.

Rothenberg, M. (1973). A new inverse-filtering technique for deriving the glottal airflow waveform during voicing. *Journal of the Acoustical Society of America, 53,* 1632–1645.

Rothenberg, M. (1977). Measurement of airflow in speech. *Journal of Speech and Hearing Research, 20,* 155–176.

Russell, A., Penny, L., & Pemberton, C. (1995). Speaking fundamental frequency changes over time in women with age: A longitudinal study. *Journal of Speech and Hearing Research, 38,* 101–109.

Ryan, E. B., & Capadano, H. L. (1978). Age perceptions and evaluative reactions toward adult speakers. *Journal of Gerontology, 33,* 98–102.

Ryan, W. J. (1972). Acoustic aspects of the aging voice. *Journal of Gerontology, 27,* 265–268.

Ryan, W. J., & Burk, K. W. (1974). Perceptual and acoustic correlates in the speech of males. *Journal of Communication Disorders, 7,* 181–192.

Sapienza, C. M., & Dutka, J. (1996). Glottal airflow characteristics of women's voice production along an aging continuum. *Journal of Speech and Hearing Research, 39,* 322–328.

Saxman, J. H., & Burk, K. W. (1967). Speaking fundamental frequency characteristics of middle-aged females. *Folia Phoniatrica, 19,* 167–172.

Scukanec, G. P., Petrosino, L., & Squibb, K. (1991). Formant frequency characteristics of children, young adult, and aged female speakers. *Perceptual and Motor Skills, 73,* 203–208.

Segre, R. (1971). Senescence of the voice. *Eye Ear Nose Throat Monthly, 50,* 223–227.

Shipp, T., & Hollien, H. (1969). Perceptions of the aging male voice. *Journal of Speech and Hearing Research, 12,* 703–710.

Shipp, T., Qi, Y., Huntley, R., & Hollien, H. (1992). Acoustic and temporal correlates of perceived age. *Journal of Voice, 6,* 211–216.

Silverman, S. (1972). Degeneration of dental and orofacial structures. In *Orofacial function: Clinical research in dentistry and speech pathology* (ASHA Reports, No. 7). Washington, DC: American Speech and Hearing Association.

Sodersten, M., & Lindestad, P. A. (1990). Glottal closure and perceived breathiness during phonation in normally speaking subjects. *Journal of Speech and Hearing Research, 33,* 601–611.

Sonies, B. (1991). The aging oropharyngeal system. In D. Ripich (Ed.), *Handbook of geriatric communication disorders* (pp. 187–203). Austin, TX: Pro-Ed.

Sperry, E., & Klich, R. J. (1992). Speech breathing in senescent and younger women during oral reading. *Journal of Speech and Hearing Research, 35,* 1246–1255.

Stoicheff, M. L. (1981). Speaking fundamental frequency characteristics of nonsmoking female adults. *Journal of Speech and Hearing Research, 24,* 437–441.

Turner, J. M., Mead, J., & Wohl, M. E. (1968). Elasticity of human lungs in relation to age. *Journal of Applied Physiology, 25,* 664–671.

Weismer, G., & Liss, J. (1991). Speech motor control and aging. In D. Ripich (Ed.), *Handbook of geriatric communication disorders* (pp. 205–225). Austin, TX: Pro-Ed.

Wilder, C. (1978). Vocal aging. In B. Weinberg (Ed.), *Transcripts of the Seventh Symposium: Care of the Professional Voice. Part II: Life Span Changes in the Human Voice* (pp. 51–59). New York: The Voice Foundation.

Zaino, C., & Benventano, T. C. (1977). Functional involutional and degenerative disorders. In C. Zaino & T. Benventano (Eds.), *Radiologic examination of the oropharynx and esophagus* (pp. 141–176). New York: Springer-Verlag.

CHAPTER 17

Phonatory Effects of Mass Lesions

Charles N. Ford and Nadine P. Connor

Voice production is the result of complex actions and interactions among multiple anatomical, physiological, behavioral, and psychological components. As such, the effect of a vocal fold mass lesion on phonation is greatly influenced by functioning at each level. In other words, vocal fold masses affect the voice differently across individuals, as a pathology is overlaid on a highly idiosyncratic vocal production "platform" (Morrison, 1997). In Morrison's (1997) conceptualization, each individual has a dysphonic platform consisting of four components: (1) posture and muscle usage, or level of vocal skill; (2) behavior, or habits of vocalization; (3) gastroesophageal reflux (GER); and, (4) psychological and emotional factors. These platform components and other factors, including pulmonary function and allergies, must be recognized and addressed in the diagnosis and management of voice disorders.

When multiple platform components are recognized, it becomes apparent that the effect of a mass lesion on the voice goes beyond simple mass loading and may be difficult to predict. For example, identical mass lesions may result in severe, incapacitating dysphonia in one patient, but provoking an imperceptible voice disturbance in another. The vocal abilities of individuals vary to such a degree that some mass lesions may be masked by trained or agile speakers. Conversely, neuromuscular feedback, coordination, and psychological status can augment phonatory effects and result in disruptive hyperfunctional adaptations. Therefore, the challenge to phonosurgeons and voice scientists is to accurately quantify the phonatory effects of mass lesions overlaid on multiple and varied components.

Differential diagnosis of a mass vocal fold lesion is a primary goal for a clinician in determining appropriate management. Unfortunately for the diagnostician, numerous types of mass vocal fold lesions, from focal amyloidosis (Figure 17–1A) to invasive cancer (Figure 17–1B), are capable of influencing phonation. The physical appearance of a lesion, although important in establishing a diagnosis, may not be definitive. As shown in Figures 17–1A and 17–1B, amyloidosis and laryngeal cancer can appear similar, yet the appropriate medical management for each

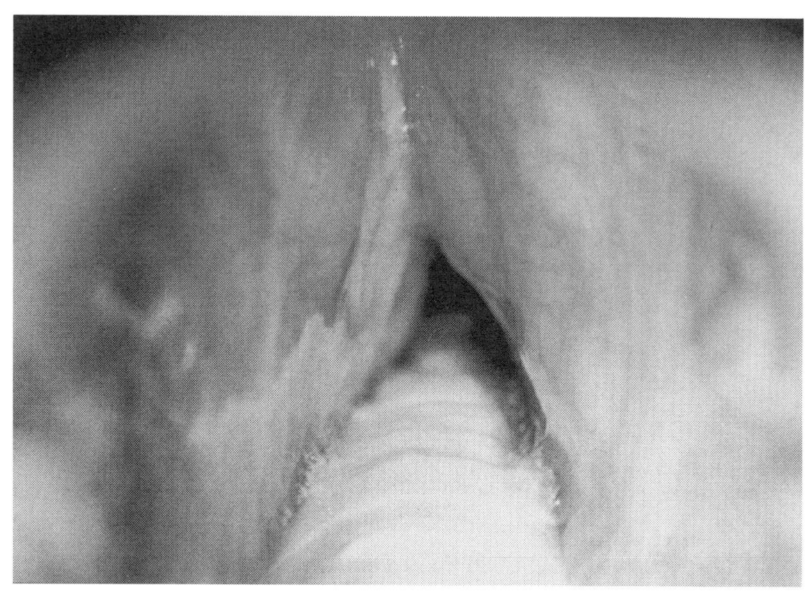

A

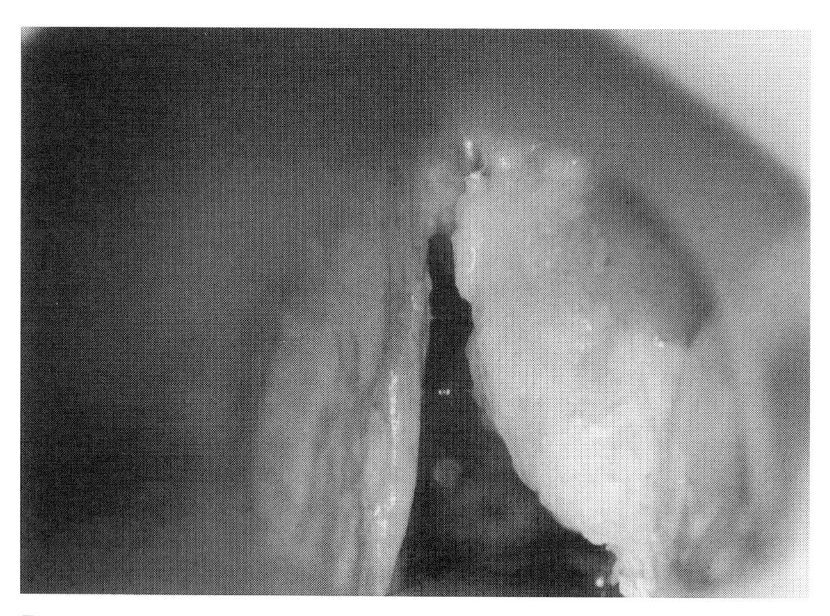

B

Figure 17–1. A. Amyloidosis of the vocal folds and **B.** invasive cancer can be similar in appearance, but appropriate medical management for each disease is very different.

disease is very different. Conversely, as shown for vocal nodules in Figures 17–2A and 17–2B, pathologies of the same type may vary in appearance. Vocal fold nodules, particularly the vascular type shown in Figure 17–2B, may also resemble polyps (cf. Chagnon & Stone, 1966).

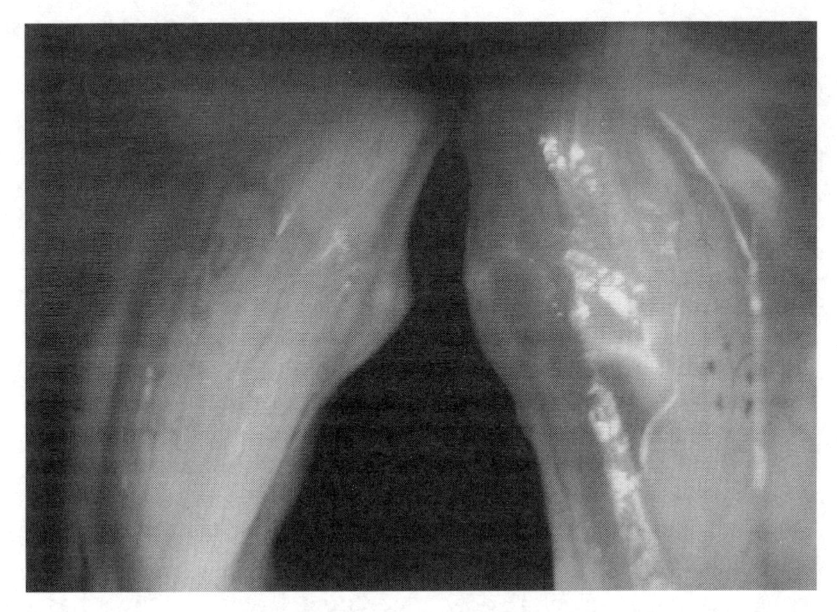

A

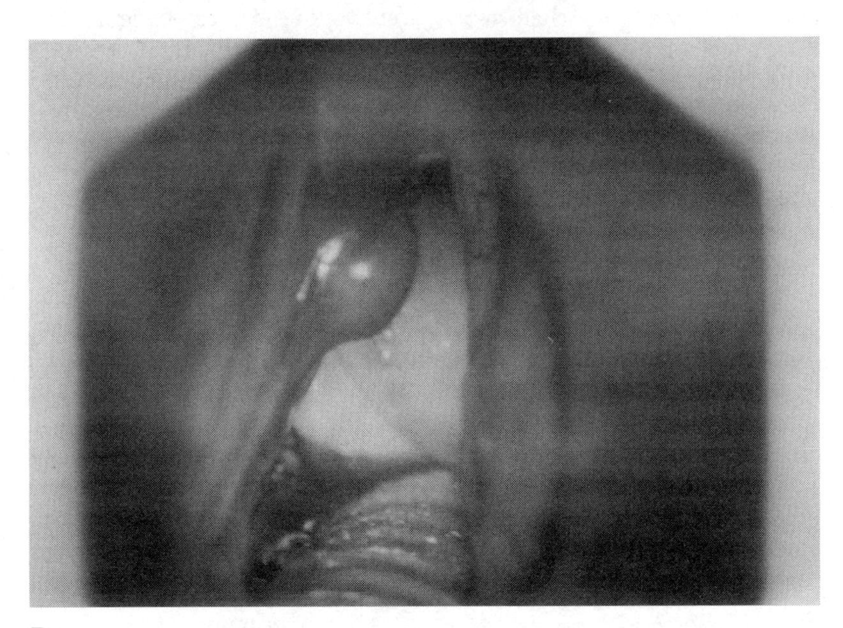

B

Figure 17–2. Vocal fold pathologies of the same type may vary in appearance. Two examples of vocal fold nodules are shown in A and B. In B, the vascular form of vocal nodules may resemble vocal fold polyps.

Further assistance with diagnosis is provided by biopsy results and response to medical and/or behavioral management.

The focus of this chapter is the quantification of the phonatory effects of vocal fold mass lesions. Because the causes of an observed dysphonia may be multifactorial, it is important to first consider the ways in which mass lesions affect phonation. As with most voice disorders, assessment of vocal functioning should be quantified using a profile of multiple parameters, including perceptual measures, acoustic analyses, and aerodynamic or waveform analyses. These particular analysis techniques and their clinical/scientific relevance to the quantification of vocal functioning will be presented.

1. MECHANISM OF PHONATORY EFFECTS

Mass lesions can alter phonation in at least five different ways: (1) increased bulk and/or displacement of the vocal fold, which may produce turbulence, alter vibrational characteristics, promote diplophonia, and/or impede contralateral vocal fold vibratory characteristics via compression; (2) increased stiffness, which results in reduced vocal fold vibratory activity either by direct extension, reactive inflammation, and/or fibrosis; (3) glottic insufficiency due to failure of vocal fold apposition; (4) airway compromise, particularly in the case of large exophytic lesions; and (5) abnormal compensatory mechanisms, such as inappropriate activation of supraglottic muscles. An astute clinician will also recognize that some mass lesions are the result—rather than the cause—of hyperfunctional disorders.

In general, the deeper the level of vocal fold involvement, the more a mass lesion affects the behavior of the adjacent tissues necessary for vocal production. For example, mass lesions that are confined to the epithelium or limited by Reinke's space may have a less profound effect than those involving the underlying vocal ligament or vocal fold musculature. Invasive T3 cancers can produce vocal fold fixation by involvement of the cricoarytenoid joint, laryngeal nerves, or extensive infiltration of the intrinsic laryngeal musculature. Such lesions result in glottic insufficiency, adding yet another component to the dysphonia.

2. PERCEPTUAL MEASURES OF PHONATION

Little guidance in differentiating among types of mass lesions on the basis of vocal function is offered by the research literature, in that most reports of phonatory changes are limited to nodules and polyps (Chagnon & Stone, 1996; Gray, Hammond, & Hanson, 1995; Kitajima & Tanaka, 1993; Koizumi, Taniguchi, & Itakura, 1993; Kotby, Nassar, Seif, Helal, & Saleh, 1988; Shohet, Courey, Scott, & Ossoff, 1996). Understandably, there has been less work concerning the vocal effects of neoplastic disease, as the overriding emphasis must be on survival in laryngeal cancer patients. However, recent interest in organ preservation techniques for advanced laryngeal cancer has provided an interesting opportunity for the study of vocal functioning in these patients (Orlikoff, Kraus, Harrison, Ho, & Gartner, 1997).

It is not surprising that phonatory tests often fail to differentiate among types of mass lesions, given the difficulty of more fine-grained microlaryngoscopic and/or histological quantification (cf. Chagnon & Stone, 1996). Further difficulty in differentiating among mass lesion types on the basis of perceptual measures may be due to: (1) common lesion locations, such as the superficial lamina propria for mucous retention or epithelial cysts; (2) associated inflammatory responses, such as scarring, sulci, and mucosal bridges; and/or (3) the extent of lesion invasion, as in the case of papillomatosis or vocal fold neoplasms.

The patient with a mass lesion of the larynx will typically exhibit an obvious dysphonia, but the perceptual characteristics of the voice are not pathognomonic of specific mass lesion or lesion locations. Lesions may be present supraglottally, in the glottal region, or subglottally. In general, supraglottic lesions will not alter the voice until sufficiently large to partially obstruct the airway or invade the true vocal fold. Typically, hoarseness implies a lesion of the vocal fold proper, which might be most apparent with connected speech or a sustained vowel. Subglottic lesions can produce a brassy timbre due to airway interference or may result in hoarseness if the vocal folds are invaded. Aperiodicity in vocal fold vibration due to the presence of a mass lesion is correlated with perceptions of vocal harshness or roughness, with perception of vocal breathiness related to glottal air leakage and resulting turbulent noise escape (Dejonckere & Lebacq, 1996).

In an attempt to standardize perceptual ratings of vocal functioning, Hirano (1981) introduced the GRBAS scale, a 4-point classification scheme for perceptual ratings of vocal function, which included grade (G), roughness (R), breathiness (B), asthenia (A), and strain (S). With mass lesions, nodules and polyps typically exhibit a 0 rating (i.e., "normal") for asthenia and 1–2 (mild–moderate) for the other parameters. However, as we mentioned previously, trained or agile speakers may not present with predictable perceptual rating profiles. Adaptations in clinical tasks may be required to uncover pathology in professional singers who can mask the phonatory stigmata of these lesions during their normal tasks and performances. For example, a simple approach for the perceptual detection of small focal masses, such as nodules, is to ask the patient to sing softly a staccato on the vowel /i/ and the opening phrase of "Happy birthday to you" at high pitch (Bastian, Keidar, & Verdolini-Marston, 1990; Chagnon & Stone, 1996). In addition, singers with nodules tend to exhibit pitch breaks and diplophonia in the middle, or head, registers (Brodnitz, 1971).

3. ACOUSTIC ANALYSES

Analysis of the acoustic signal provides an indirect measure of vocal fold vibration and status of the vocal tract. As both vibration and vocal tract status are affected by the presence of a mass lesion, alterations of acoustic measures can be anticipated. However, acoustic tests are most useful for monitoring *response* to treatment, rather than in the *diagnosis* of vocal fold mass lesions. Ongoing work with measures such as voice onset time, voice breaks, and modulations of frequency and intensity might prove useful in the future for fine-tuning the diagnostic process.

Unfortunately, there is currently no single measure or battery of acoustic tests with sufficient sensitivity or specificity to be diagnostic. In fact, the maximum performance tasks often used clinically show great intra- and intersubject variability and are also affected by practice, motivation, and instruction (Kent, Kent, & Rosenbek, 1987). Further, although one might expect that decreased fundamental frequency would result from any lesion increasing vocal fold mass, fundamental frequency of the voice may be observed to increase or remain unaffected. Therefore, as with perceptual analyses, normal values do not preclude the presence of lesions because of the varying abilities of speakers. Nevertheless, a number of observations have been made that are commonly associated with mass lesions.

Measures of frequency and intensity range, perturbation measures, or spectrographic analysis, which may reflect a loss of harmonic components and decreased harmonics-to-noise ratios, may have some descriptive value. Patients with nodules typically have a restricted frequency range during connected speech (Blalock, 1992) and reduced intensity range (Bassich & Ludlow, 1986), although habitual loudness levels may be elevated (Hirano, Tanaka, Fujita, & Terasawa, 1991). In children with nodules, two measures of acoustic perturbation, jitter and shimmer, were correlated with severity of dysphonia (Kane & Wellen, 1985).

In monitoring a patient's treatment response, phonosurgeons and speech-language pathologists have found frequency/ intensity profiles, or "phonetograms," to be useful. One recent approach described voice range profiles (e.g., VRPs), which consisted of semitone range, intensity level of the lower contour, locus of the lower frequency values, smoothness of the contours, and presence of intermittencies in the VRP contours (Behrman, Agresti, Blumstein, & Sharma, 1996). Such profiles are useful in that they allow for individualization of outcome measures.

A unique use of acoustic measures was recently used to document the extent of laryngeal impairment in dysphonic patients with laryngeal cancer and to assess the effectiveness of nonsurgical intervention (Orlikoff et al., 1997). The clinical aim was to determine a patient's response to cycled chemotherapy prior to determining the subsequent surgical or radiation treatment pathway. Medically, nonsurgical treatment proved effective when a tumor was reduced in size by more than one-half. In these situations, patients avoided primary extirpation surgery. The important research aim of this work was to document acoustic changes in the voice as a function of reduction in tumor volume. With each patient serving as a self-control, these data are more indicative of the mass effect of the tumor than studies comparing untreated cancer patients to disease-free controls. The findings of this study support the conclusions of Baken (1987) that F_0 variability and range are more indicative of vocal fold pathology than mean F_0, suggesting that this observation applies to large cancer lesions as well as to smaller benign processes. Interestingly, a significant reduction in jitter was reported in patients showing a major tumor reduction and no such trend was found in those patients showing no or minimal response.

4. AERODYNAMIC AND WAVEFORM MEASURES

Aerodynamic measures indirectly assess the efficiency of the laryngeal valve and respiratory support by quantifying airflow, pressure, and volume. These measures are affected by mass lesions that alter the glottal closure pattern and also by supraglottal compensatory behavior. Even small nodules and polyps can produce markedly high and variable airflow rates during sustained phonation, depending on the degree of alteration of glottic closure and supraglottic valving efforts. In general, lesions resulting in poor glottic closure cause decreased vocal efficiency and increased transglottic airflow. Substantial mass lesions that cause vocal fold stiffness result in increased subglottic pressure for phonation. Kitajima and Tanaka (1993) showed that values for the difference in peak pressure between the consonant /p/ and /b/ divided by the estimated subglottal pressure in subjects with vocal fold cancer exhibited different distributions from subjects with polyps.

The Alternating Current/Direct Current (AC/DC) ratio and frequency analysis of the airflow waveform are advocated as reliable measures of vocal efficiency (Woo, Colton, & Shangold, 1987). Kitajima and Fujita (1992) used these techniques to study a group of 361 patients with various laryngeal diseases and compared them to a group of 59 control subjects. The average AC/DC percentage was 55 in the control group, followed by chronic laryngitis (47) and smaller lesions, such as nodules (43), T1 cancers (42), and dysplasias (37). The larger lesions, including polypoid degeneration (38), polyps (34), and more advanced cancers (27) indicated greater impairment in the vibrational capacity of the vocal folds. However, a high degree of variability was suggested by the large standard deviations reported and again suggest that such measures are useful mainly in assessing response to therapy and not in differential diagnosis.

Another approach to the assessment of vocal fold vibration is electroglottography (EGG). As the soft tissues of the neck have relatively good electrical conductance properties, measuring the impedance to a weak alternating current reveals the pattern of vocal fold contact during phonation. This vocal fold closure pattern is altered in the presence of a mass lesion. A distinction in the EGG signal between fibrous and soft edematous mass lesions has been demonstrated (Childers, Alsaka, Hicks, & Moore, 1986). Further, by integrating EGG with videostroboscopy and photoglottography (PGG), three-dimensional representations of glottal vibration have been achieved (Hanson, Jiang, D'Agostino, & Herzon, 1995). Ongoing analysis of this type in patients with a variety of vocal fold pathologies could yield further descriptive information on mass lesions of the glottis.

Altered phonation from mass lesions correlates with vibratory behavior as depicted on laryngeal videostroboscopy (LVS). In addition to visualizing the lesion, LVS gives valuable information on the status of the mucosal wave and the pattern of glottic closure. Nodules and polyps may result in an aperiodicity of vocal fold vibration, but asymmetry of movement is not characteristic. Typically, the mucosal wave is less affected by edematous lesions than by fibrous lesions. The extent of stiffness usually indicates a more extensive lesion with inflammation, fibrosis, or invasion. These manifestations can be valuable in detecting occult cystic lesions and defining the extent of invasive glottic cancers. Shohet and colleagues (1996) found LVS particularly valuable in the preoperative differentiation of vocal fold cysts versus polyps.

5. ROLE OF PHONATORY ASSESSMENT FOR MASS LESIONS

It is clear that phonation is affected by the presence of mass lesions of the vocal fold. Furthermore, mass lesions affect phonation in ways than can be measured using perceptual, acoustic, aerodynamic, and waveform analytical methods. Presently, it is not possible to reliably distinguish lesions using phonatory analysis. This is due, in part, to the tremendous variability of mass lesions, rendering it impossible to generalize across all lesions of a specific type. Furthermore, there is substantial variation in the way individuals are affected by similar lesions. The role of phonatory assessment in the differential diagnosis of mass lesions is currently adjunctive. Ongoing refinement of current techniques of assessment might eventually afford careful discrimination of lesions based on analysis of the phonatory effects. In an intriguing study, Koizumi et al. (1993) devised a noninvasive technique of predicting specific vocal fold polyp characteristics, such as mass and dimensions, by analysis of the hoarse voice. Prediction was accomplished through a series of experiments in which a hoarse voice synthesizer was used to match that produced in patients with polyps of known characteristics. These sorts of advances are promising for future use as diagnostic tools.

6. CONCLUSIONS

In summary, there are three major roles for phonatory assessment in the management of patients with mass lesions of the vocal folds. First, phonatory assessment may assist in describing the lesion. Careful analysis and quantification is essential in establishing a baseline and assisting in the differential diagnosis process. Second, phonatory assessment is useful in tracking the response to therapy. Historically, phonatory assessment has been used to monitor the response of patients to voice therapy. An exciting new application of such techniques in cancer patients suggests a potential value in monitoring the response to chemotherapy and predicting response to definitive cancer therapy. Finally, phonatory function is a major factor in assessing outcomes. As we continue to seek the most effective ways of treating disease, comprehensive outcome evaluation will be increasingly important.

REFERENCES

Baken, R. J. (1987). *Clinical measurement of speech and voice*. Boston: College-Hill Press.

Bassich, C. J., & Ludlow, C. L. (1986). The use of perceptual methods for assessing voice quality. *Journal of Speech & Hearing Disorders, 51*, 125–133.

Bastian, R. W., Keidar, A., & Verdolini-Marston, K. (1990). Simple vocal tasks for detecting vocal fold swelling. *Journal of Voice, 4*, 172–183.

Behrman, A., Agresti, C. J., Blumstein, E., & Sharma, G. (1996). Meaningful features of voice range profiles from patients with organic vocal fold pathology: A preliminary study. *Journal of Voice, 10*, 269–283.

Blalock, P. D. (1992). Management of patients with vocal nodules. *The Visible Voice, 1*, 4–6.

Brodnitz, F. S. (1971). *Vocal rehabilitation*. Rochester,

MN: American Academy of Ophthalmology and Otolaryngology.

Chagnon, F., & Stone, R. E. (Ed.). (1996). Nodules and polyps. In W. S. Brown, B. P. Vinson, and M. A. Crary, *Organic voice disorders* (pp. 219–244). San Diego: Singular Publishing Group, Inc.

Childers, D. G., Alsaka, Y. A., Hicks, D. M., & Moore, G. P. (1986). Vocal fold vibrations in dysphonia: Model versus measurement. *Journal of Phonetics, 14*, 429–434.

Dejonckere, P. H., & Lebacq, J. (1996). Acoustic, perceptual aerodynamic and anatomical correlations in voice pathology. *Journal of Oto-Rhino-Laryngology and Its Related Specialties, 58*, 326–332.

De Foer, B., Hermans, R. Van der Goten, A., Delaere, P. R., & Baert, A. L. (1996). Imaging features in 35 cases of submucosal laryngeal mass lesions. *European Radiology, 6*, 913–919.

Gray, S. D., Hammond, E., & Hanson, D. F. (1995). Benign pathologic responses of the larynx. *Annals of Otology, Rhinology, and Laryngology, 104*, 13–18.

Hanson, D. G., Jiang, J., D'Agostino, M., & Herzon, G. (1995). Clinical measurement of mucosal wave velocity using simultaneous photoglottography and laryngostroboscopy. *Annals of Otology, Rhinology, and Laryngology, 104*, 340–349.

Hirano, M. (1981). Psycho-acoustic evaluation of voice. In *Clinical examination of voice* (pp. 81–84). Wien: Springer-Verlag.

Hirano, M., Tanaka, S., Fujita, M., & Terasawa, R. (1991). Fundamental frequency and sound pressure level of phonation in pathological states. *Journal of Voice, 5*, 120–127.

Kane, M., & Wellen, C. J. (1985). Acoustical measurements and clinical judgments of vocal quality in children with vocal nodules. *Folia Phoniatrica, 37*, 53–57.

Kent, R. D., Kent, J. F., & Rosenbek, J. (1987). Maximum performance tests of speech production. *Journal of Speech & Hearing Research, 52*, 367–387.

Kitajima, K., & Fujita, F. (1992). Airflow study of pathologic larynges using a constant temperature anemometer: Further experience. *Annals of Otology, Rhinology, and Laryngology, 101*, 675–678.

Kitajima K., & Tanaka K. (1993). Intraoral pressure in the evaluation of laryngeal function. *Acta Otolaryngologica, 113*, 553–559.

Kitzing, P. (1990). Clinical applications of electroglottography. *Journal of Voice, 4*, 238–249.

Koizumi T., Taniguchi S., & Itakura F. (1993). An analysis-by-synthesis approach to the estimation of vocal cord polyp features. *Laryngoscope, 103*, 1035–1042.

Kotby, M. N., Nassar, A. M., Seif, E. I., Helal, E. H., & Saleh, M. M. (1988). Ultrastructural features of vocal fold nodules and polyps. *Acta Otolaryngologica, 105*, 477–482.

Morrison, M. (1997). Pattern recognition in muscle misuse voice disorders: How I do it. *Journal of Voice, 11*, 108–114.

Orlikoff, R. F., Kraus, D. H., Harrision, L. B., Ho, M. L., & Gartner, C. J. (1997). Vocal fundamental frequency measures as a reflection of tumor response to chemotherapy in patients with advanced laryngeal cancer. *Journal of Voice, 11*, 33–39.

Shohet, J. A., Courey, M. S., Scott, M. A., & Ossoff, R. H. (1996). Value of videostroboscopic parameters in differentiating true vocal fold cysts from polyps. *Laryngoscope, 106*, 19–26.

Woo, P., Colton, R. H., & Shangold, L. (1987). Phonatory airflow analysis in patients with laryngeal disease. *Annals of Otology, Rhinology and Laryngology, 96*, 549–555.

CHAPTER 18

Vocal Fold Paralysis

Minoru Hirano and Kazunori Mori

Vocal fold paralysis is also known by other terms, including laryngeal paralysis and recurrent laryngeal nerve (RLN) paralysis. Vocal fold paralysis has many different causes, some diseases that are life threatening. In other words, vocal fold paralysis is occasionally the first sign of or alarm for some fatal diseases. Whenever one examines patients with vocal fold paralysis, he or she should recall this possibility and determine and treat, whenever possible, the etiologic disease.

From a neuropathological viewpoint, nerve paralysis is classified into three types: neuropraxia, axonotmesis, and neurotmesis (Figure 18–1). Neuropraxia is a temporary block of conduction of nerve impulses. It occurs, for example, when local anesthesia is injected near the nerve, with the neuromuscular system usually returning to its normal state. In axonotmesis, the axons are cut and, in neurotmesis, the entire nerve fibers are sectioned. Both conditions result in degeneration of the nerve peripheral to the site of lesion and, consequently, denervation of the muscle. Regeneration of the nerve may or may not take place and reinnervation of the muscle may or may not occur accordingly. When the muscle is not reinnervated, it ultimately atrophies.

Unilateral vocal paralysis frequently causes glottic incompetence and subsequent voice disorder, whereas bilateral paralysis often leads to glottic obstruction resulting in dyspnea. Unilateral paralysis is more frequent than bilateral paralysis. The ratio of the number of cases with unilateral paralysis to that with bilateral paralysis varies. It was 7:6 in Tucker's report (1980), whereas it was 9:1 as reported by Tanaka, Tanaka, Fujita, Chijiwa, and Hirano (1993).

1. CLINICAL ANATOMY

The laryngeal muscles, except for the cricothyroid muscle, are innervated by the RLN, which is one of the branches of the vagus nerve. The cricothyroid muscle is innervated by the superior laryngeal nerve (SLN), which is another branch of the vagus nerve. The RLN leaves the vagus nerve in the thorax, below the aortic arch on the left side and below the subclavian artery on the right. As a result, it is longer on the left side than on the right. Paralysis, therefore,

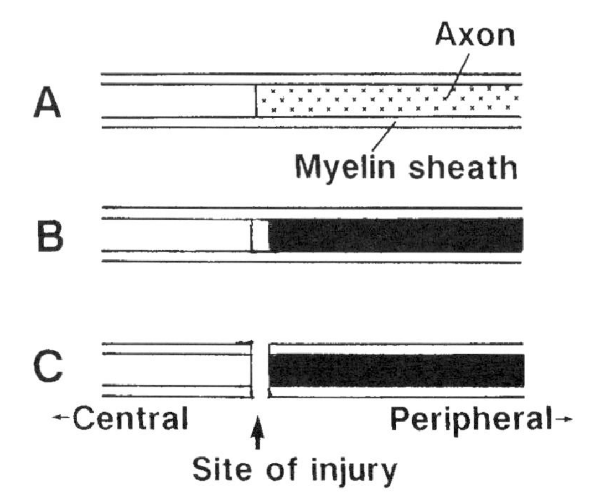

Figure 18–1. Three types of nerve paralysis: **A.** Neuropraxia. **B.** Axonotmesis. **C.** Neurotmesis. Dotted area implies a temporary block of conduction of neural impulses, and solid area depicts degenerating or degenerated axon.

occurs more frequently on the left than on the right.

The motor nuclei of the RLN and SLN are located in the nucleus ambiguus of the medulla oblongata. The laryngeal motor neurons receive innervation from the bilateral cerebral motor cortex. Therefore, unilateral lesions of the cerebral cortex and/or corticobulbar tract do not cause vocal fold paralysis.

Figure 18–2 schematically depicts the laryngeal motor nerves. The upper motor neurons originate from the cerebral cortex and run in the corticobulbar tract to reach the bilateral nucleus ambiguus in the medulla oblongata. The lower motor neurons originating from the nucleus ambiguus leave the cranium through the jugular foramen. They course in the vagus nerve until the laryngeal nerves branch off.

2. ETIOLOGY

Because the motor neurons of the larynx have a long course to reach the muscles, they can be affected by many etiologies at the varying sites shown in Figure 18–1. The overall frequency of a potential etiology varies, depending on the time, place, and age group.

Tables 18–1 and 18–2 show the etiologies for vocal fold paralysis at the Mayo Clinic in two different eras. Before 1932, more than a half of the causes of paralysis were neoplasms, including those of the thyroid gland, hypopharynx, esophagus, mediastinum, and lung. Tuberculosis and syphilis were fairly frequent. There was no paralysis caused by surgery. In the later era, the most frequent cause was thyroid surgery (43.1%). Neoplasms were the second most frequent cause (15.0%). Tucker (1980) pointed out that the frequency of specific etiologies differed between unilateral and bilateral paralysis as shown in Table 18–3. Thyroidectomy was the most frequent etiology for bilateral paralysis, whereas it was rather rare for unilateral lesion. Traumas other than thyroidectomy, including surgeries involving the neck or thorax, were frequent etiologies for both unilateral and bilateral paralysis. Malignant neoplasms were more frequent causes for unilateral than bilateral paralysis .

Table 18–4 demonstrates etiologic diseases in the Kurume University Hospital in three periods: 1960–1970, 1971–1980, and 1981–1990. During the first two periods, the etiology was not verified in approximately 40% of the cases. For many, the cause was suspected to be neuritis. The frequency of undetermined causes reduced in the third era. This may partly have resulted from the use of modern diagnostic tools including the CT scan and MRI. In 1969 and 1970 of the first era, there was epidemic Hong Kong flu associated with vocal fold paralysis. The incidence of neoplasms increased in the second and third eras. The increase of lung cancer was particularly significant. The incidence of surgery markedly increased in the third period. The increase in cases with esophageal cancer surgery was very marked. The incidence of thyroid surgery as the cause of vocal fold paralysis was not as high as that in the reports from the United States.

Table 18–5 shows etiologic factors in the Tokyo University, another Japanese institution. The most frequent etiology was surgery (36.9%). Thyroid surgeries in Tokyo were more frequent than in Kurume. In approximately

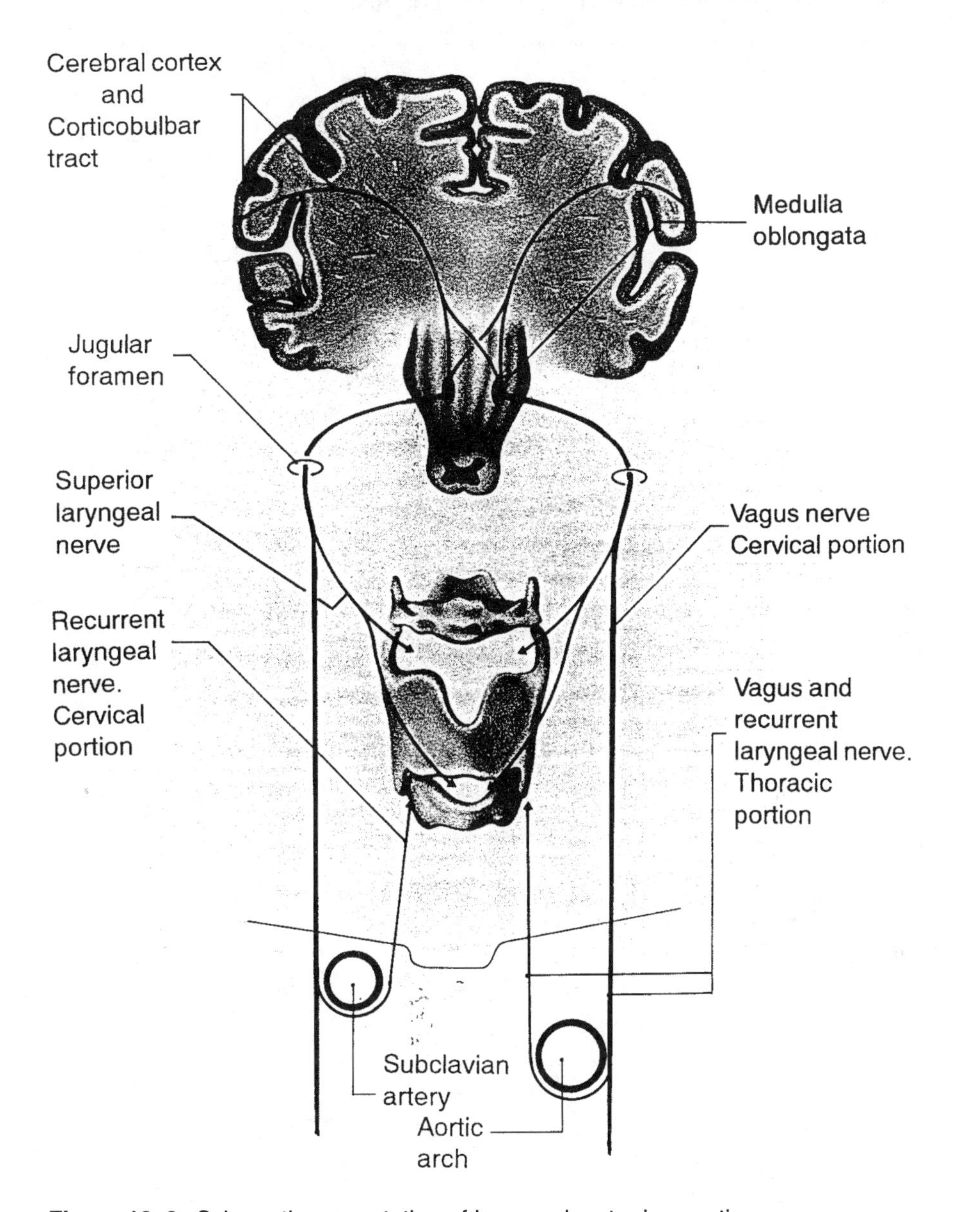

Figure 18–2. Schematic presentation of laryngeal motor innervation.

40% of the cases, the etiology was not determined, the same figure as for the first two eras in the Kurume reports.

In young children, Arnold-Chiari malformation, hydrocephalus, birth trauma, and intubation trauma are frequent causes of vocal fold paralysis (Gentile, Miller, & Woodson, 1986; Rosin, Handler, Potsic, Wetmore, & Tom, 1990; Tucker 1986).

3. ELECTROMYOGRAPHY

Electromyography is useful for three major purposes: to differentiate paralysis from a mechanical fixation, to determine prognosis, and to determine an involvement of the external branch of the SLN.

Mechanical fixations are caused by arthritis of the cricoarytenoid joint, trauma of the joint,

Table 18–1. Vocal fold paralysis etiology (Mayo Clinic N = 217; unilateral 185, bilateral 32, period not specified).

Congenital lesions	3 (1.4%)	
Central origin	24 (11.1%)	
Bulbar lesion		15 (6.9%)
Tabes		9 (4.1%)
Neoplasm	121 (55.8%)	
Nasopharynx		13 (6.0%)
Hypopharynx and esophagus		34 (15.7%)
Thyroid		42 (19.4%)
Neck		4 (1.8%)
Mediastinum, lung, et al.		28 (12.9%)
Trauma, neck	4 (1.8%)	
Syphilis of larynx	10 (4.6%)	
Aneurysm	27 (12.4%)	
Heart disease	10 (4.6%)	
Tuberculosis	11 (5.1%)	
Pneumonia	1 (0.5%)	
Toxic neuritis	6 (2.8%)	

Note: Based on data from New and Childrey, 1932.

Table 18–2. Vocal fold paralysis etiology (Mayo Clinic, N = 633, unilateral 455, bilateral 176, unspecified 2, 1939–1948)

Neurologic (central)	22 (3.5%)	
Cancer	95 (15.0%)	
Breast		19 (3.0%)
Thyroid		15 (2.4%)
Lung		12 (1.9%)
Tongue, mouth, pharynx		11 (1.7%)
Larynx		9 (1.4%)
Lymphoma		9 (1.4%)
Neck		6 (0.9%)
Mediastinum		5 (0.8%)
Esophagus		4 (0.6%)
Miscellaneous		5 (0.8%)
Surgery	287 (45.3%)	
Thyroid		273 (43.1%)
Others		14 (2.2%)
Trauma	13 (2.1%)	
Cardiovascular disease	26 (4.1%)	
Infection	9 (1.4%)	
Undetermined	181 (28.6%)	

Note: Based on data from Huppler, Schmidt, Devine, and R. P. Gage, 1950.

Table 18–3. Vocal fold paralysis etiology (Cleveland Clinic Foundation, N = 390, unilateral 210, bilateral 180, 1975–1978).

	Unilateral (n = 210)	*Bilateral (n = 180)*	*Total*
Thyroidectomy	10 (4.8%)	82 (45.6%)	92 (23.6%)
Other Trauma	77 (36.7%)	54 (30.0%)	131 (33.6%)
Neurologic	5 (2.4%)	10 (5.6%)	15 (3.8%)
Malignancy	46 (21.9%)	14 (7.8%)	60 (15.4%)
Miscellaneous	72 (34.3%)	20 (11.1%)	92 (23.6%)

Note: Based on data from Tucker, 1980.

Table 18–4. Vocal fold paralysis etiology (Kurume University, N = 1,628, 1960–1990).

	1960–70 (n = 400)	*1971–80 (n = 564)*	*1981–90 (n = 664)*
Central	2 (0.5%)	7 (1.2%)	16 (2.4%)
Neoplasm	26 (6.5%)	98 (17.4%)	141 (21.2%)
Thyroid	12 (3.0%)	32 (5.7%)	32 (4.8%)
Esophagus		15 (2.7%)	30 (4.5%)
Lung	28 (7.0%)	31 (5.5%)	64 (9.6%)
Mediastinum		13 (2.3%)	11 (1.7%)
Miscellaneous		7 (1.7%)	4 (0.6%)
Surgery	96 (24.0%)	127 (22.5%)	262 (39.5%)
Thyroid	59 (14.5%)	68 (12.1%)	73 (11.1%)
Esophagus		24 (4.3%)	112 (16.9%)
Lung		8 (1.4%)	34 (5.1%)
Mediastinum		2 (0.4%)	9 (1.9%)
Heart	37 (9.3%)	16 (2.8%)	10 (1.5%)
Aorta		4 (0.7%)	20 (3.0%)
Miscellaneous		5 (0.9%)	4 (0.6%)
Trauma	12 (3.0%)	13 (2.3%)	5 (0.8%)
Endotracheal intubation	18 (5.0%)	63 (11.2%)	80 (12.0%)
Flu	77 (19.3%)		
Miscellaneous	14 (3.5%)	23 (4.1%)	35 (5.3%)
Undetermined	155 (38.8%)	233 (41.3%)	125 (18.8%)
	Unilateral 357	Unilateral 519	Unilateral 584
	Bilateral 42	Bilateral 45	Bilateral 80
	Unspecified 1		

Note: Based on data from Nozoe, Hirano, Shin, and Maeyama, 1972; Yamada, Hirano, and Ohkubu, 1983; Tanaka, Tanaka, Fujita, Chijiwa, and Hirano, 1993.

Table 18–5. Vocal fold paralysis etiology (Tokyo University, $N = 750$, unilateral 663, bilateral 87, 1961–1980).

Central	12 (1.6%)	
Neoplasm	63 (8.4%)	
Thyroid		19 (2.5%)
Esophagus		6 (0.8%)
Lung		27 (3.6%)
Mediastinum		9 (1.2%)
Miscellaneous		2 (0.3%)
Surgery	277 (36.9%)	
Thyroid		160 (21.3%)
Esophagus		14 (1.9%)
Lung		9 (1.2%)
Mediastinum		8 (1.1%)
Heart		42 (5.6%)
Aorta		9 (1.2%)
Miscellaneous		35 (4.7%)
Trauma	17 (2.3%)	
Endotracheal intubation	28 (3.7%)	
Miscellaneous	46 (6.1%)	
Unknown	307 (40.9%)	

Note: Based on data from Hirose, 1978, and Hirose, Sawashima, and Yoshioka, 1981.

scar at the posterior glottis, and scar around the entire glottis. In the first three conditions, normal action potentials are found in the thyroarytenoid muscle. In the latter one, action potentials of the thyroarytenoid muscle are occasionally reduced or absent, as in the case of paralysis. The scar around the entire glottis, however, is usually diagnosed on the basis of history and fiberscopic or telescopic inspection of the larynx.

For the prognostic purpose, electromyography is the most reliable modality. The presence of voluntary action potential indicates a favorable prognosis (Hirano, 1974, 1981a; Parnes & Satya-Murti, 1985). Fibrillation potentials are a sign of denervation and, consequently, they indicate an unfavorable prognosis. Gartlan, Peterson, Luschei, Hoffman, and Smith (1993) reported that electromyography was useful for establishing prognosis in four pediatric cases.

Involvement of the external branch of the SLN is most reliably determined by means of electromyography of the cricothyroid muscle. An absence of or decrease in action potentials of the cricothyroid muscle during a high-pitched phonation is the sign of paralysis of the external branch of the SLN.

4. PERCEPTUAL EVALUATION OF VOICE QUALITY

There is no internationally common or standardized terminology to describe pathological voice qualities.

Hammarberg, Fritzell, and Schiratzki (1984) described pathological voice quality with the use of nine terms; that is, breathy, aphonic, hyperfunctional, hypofunctional, diplophonic, voice breaks, grating, rough, and creaky. The voice quality in patients with vocal fold paralysis tended to be breathy, aphonic, hypofunctional, and/or diplophonic.

The Committee for Phonatory Function Tests of the Japan Society of Logopedics and Phoniatrics proposed the GRBAS scale for describing the degree and nature of hoarse voice. G implies the overall grade; R, rough; B, breathy; A, asthenic; and S, strained (Hirano, 1981a). The voice in the cases with unilateral vocal fold paralysis was often breathy and asthenic. Roughness was audible in about 25% and strained in approximately 15% of the cases (Hirano, 1989).

5. MAXIMUM PHONATION TIME

Maximum Phonation Time (MPT) is a simple but useful parameter to evaluate the vocal function in the cases of vocal fold paralysis, because it reflects, to a certain extent, the degree of glottal incompetence caused by paralysis.

Hirano (1989) investigated 264 consecutive unilateral paralysis patients seen from 1983 to 1987. The logarithmic transformation was applied in statistical analysis. The mean value of MPT was 5.9 s, mean – SD was 2.9 s, and mean + SD was 11.8 s. The MPT value was negatively correlated to the size of glottic gap during phonation. Hirano, Mori, Tanaka, and Fujita (1995) reported MPT values in 228 patients with unilateral paralysis who later underwent intra-fold silicone injection from 1983 to 1993. In general, patients who undergo intrafold injection have more severe dysphonia than those who are treated with voice therapy and those who have no treatments. The MPT value in the 228 patients ranged from 1.4 s to 16.4 s with a mean of 4.3 s (logarithmic transformation again in statistical calculation). In 93.9% of the patients, MPT was shorter than 10 s, the lower borderline of the normal population.

6. AERODYNAMIC MEASUREMENTS

6.1. Mean Airflow Rate During Phonation

Clinically, the mean airflow rate (MFR) is measured during the maximally sustained phonation (MFRm) or during phonation over comfortable duration (MFRc) or both. MFR reflects glottal incompetence caused by vocal fold paralysis.

Hirano (1989) reported that the mean value of MFRm in the 264 consecutive cases with unilateral paralysis was 301 ml/s, mean – SD was 162 ml/s, and mean + SD was 561 ml/s. In the same series, the mean, mean – SD, and mean + SD of MFRc was 340 ml/s, 181 ml/s, and 642 ml/s, respectively. Again, logarithmic transformation was applied in statistical analysis. The MFRm and MFRc values showed a significant positive correlation to the size of glottic gap during phonation. Hirano et al. (1995) reported that, in 228 patients who were subjects of intrafold injection, MFRc ranged from 139 to 1240 ml/s with a mean of 433 ml/s, preoperatively. In 96.5% of the patients, MFRc was greater than 200 ml/s, the upper borderline for normal subjects.

6.2. Subglottic Pressure

Reports on subglottic pressure (P_{SUB}) in patients with vocal fold paralysis are very limited. Hiroto (1966) directly measured P_{SUB} in four patients with unilateral paralysis directly with the tracheal puncture technique and P_{SUB} ranged from 15 to 17 cmH_2O. Kuroki (1969) reported that P_{SUB} measured by means of the tracheal puncture method was 4 to 21 cmH_2O in four cases with unilateral paralysis. Schutte (1980) measured P_{SUB} in three patients with unilateral paralysis by means of an indirect method that consisted of esophageal pressure measurement and abruptly stopping phonation. P_{SUB} in the three patients was 0.98 KPa (9.8 cmH_2O), 0.67 KPa (6.7 cmH_2O), and 1.01 KPa (10.1 cmH_2O), respectively.

7. FUNDAMENTAL FREQUENCY AND SOUND PRESSURE LEVEL OF PHONATION

Hirano (1989) and Hirano, Tanaka, Fujita, and Terasawa (1991) reported results of measurements of the fundamental frequency (F_0) and sound pressure level (SPL) of phonation in 264 consecutive patients with unilateral paralysis. Of the 264, 164 were male and 100 were female. The researchers employed the Nagashima PS-77H for the measurements and determined F_0 for the habitual phonation (habitual F_0), for the lowest pitch (lowest F_0), for the highest pitch (highest F_0), F_0 range, SPL for the habitual phonation (habitual SPL), for the softest phonation (softest SPL), for the loudest phonation (loudest SPL), and SPL range. The values of each parameter were compared with those in normal subjects.

The mean habitual F_0 was A#2 in males and F#3 in females. The former did not significantly differ from that of the normal subjects, but the latter was significantly lower than that in the normal subjects. The mean lowest F_0 was E2 in males and B2 in females. The value in females was significantly lower again. The highest F_0 was B3 in males and F4 in females on the average, both being significantly lower than that of normal control. The mean F_0 range for the entire patients was 18.6 semitones, which was significantly smaller than the mean value of normal subjects. The mean habitual SPL was 74.7 dB and did not differ significantly from that for the normal subjects. The mean softest SPL was 65 dB presenting with no significant difference from that of the normal subjects. The loudest SPL was 87.4 dB on the average and significantly smaller than the mean value of the normal subjects. The mean SPL range was 22.3 dB and it was significantly smaller than that in the normal control.

Hirano et al. (1995) reported F_0 range of phonation examined in 180 patients who later underwent intrafold injection. The F_0 range was 15.3 semitones on the average, ranging from 1.7 to 38.5 semitones. In 69.4% of the patients, F_0 range was smaller than the normal borderline, which was 18.0 semitones. The same authors also measured SPL range of phonation in 209 patients before intrafold injection. The SPL range was from 6 to 47 dB with a mean of 20.7 dB. The SPL range was smaller than the normal minumum borderline (24 dB) in 71.3% of the patients.

8. ACOUSTIC ANALYSIS OF VOICE SIGNAL

Hirano et al. (1995) conducted acoustical analysis of sustained vowels produced by 197 patients with unilateral paralysis who later had intrafold silicone injection. The pitch perturbation quotient (PPQ), amplitude perturbation quotient (APQ), and normalized noise energy for 0–4 KHz (NNEa) were determined by means of the Rion SH10. PPQ ranged from 0.11 to 15.30% with a mean of 0.89%. In 80.2% of the patients, PPQ was greater than the normal upper border, which was 0.43%. APQ was 0.57% at minimum, 34.20% at maximum, and 4.54% on the average. In 83.8% of the patients, APQ was greater than the borderline for normal subjects, which was 1.71%. NNEa was from –30.7 to –0.7 dB and the mean value was –13.36 dB. The NNEa value was greater than the upper borderline of normal subjects (–20.4 dB) in 87.3% of the entire patients.

Hammarberg et al. (1984) made long-term-average-spectrum (LTAS) analysis in 16 patients. The level of the fundamental tone had the highest peak in LTAS.

9. STROBOSCOPY OF VOCAL FOLD VIBRATION

Shönhäri (1960) first conducted systematic studies of vocal fold vibration with the use of a modern laryngo-synchronstroboscope. He investigated 62 patients with vocal fold paralysis, 60 unilateral and 2 bilateral paralysis. Major findings were: (1) vibratory movements of the two folds were asymmetrical in almost all cases, (2) vocal fold vibrations were irregular or aperiodic in the majority of the cases, (3) the amplitude of vibration varied, and (4) the mucosal wave was absent in many cases, and its presence suggested incomplete paralysis or nerve regeneration.

Fex (1969) described that, in cases with vocal fold paralysis, the return of mucosal wave was the first sign of recovery from paralysis. Fex and Elmqvist (1973) confirmed this in 12 patients with vocal fold paralysis associated with Hong Kong flu with the use of stroboscopy and electromyography. Kyttä (1982) also described, on the basis of 32 patients, that a reappearance of mucosal wave was a reliable sign of the recovery from paresis. Hirano (1975) reported that in paralytic immobile vocal folds with normal mucosal wave, 67% of them showed some voluntary action potentials of the thyroarytenoid muscle; in those with reduced mucosal wave, 65% presented with thyroarytenoid voluntary action potentials; and in those with no mucosal wave, 60% had voluntary action potentials.

Hirano, Nozoe, Shin, and Maeyama (1972) and Hirano (1974) reported results of stroboscopy conducted in 113 patients with unilateral paralysis. In 43 patients, stroboscopic examinations were made twice on different clinical stages associated with different stroboscopic findings. Thus, they presented findings of a total of 156 stroboscopic examinations. The vibratory movements of the bilateral vocal folds were asymmetrical in 80%. Irregular or aperiodic vibrations were noted in 41%. The amplitude of vibration of the affected vocal fold was small in 63% and zero in 4%. The mucosal wave on the paralytic vocal fold was small in 42% and absent in 40%. The occurrence of a small amplitude and an absence of mucosal wave was much more frequent in the cases with incomplete glottic closure than those with complete glottic closure.

Sercarz, Berke, Ming, Gerratt, and Natividad (1992) noted that mucosal wave was diminished and delayed in phase on the paralytic vocal fold.

Kokesh, Robinson, Flint, and Cummings (1993) studied the correlation between stroboscopy and electromyography in 20 patients with vocal fold paralysis caused by varying etiologic diseases. Electromyographically, 10 patients had an evidence of reinnervation or partial denervation whereas the other 10 had an evidence of denervation. In the former, 8 presented with mucosal wave but, in the latter, only 3 had mucosal wave. Six patients in the latter group developed mucosal wave after surgical medialization of the paralytic vocal fold.

10. PATHOPHYSIOLOGICAL ASPECTS AND SUMMARY OF VOCAL FUNCTION

When one looks at the vocal fold as a vibrator consisting of a body-cover complex, major pathophysiological issues (Hirano, 1975, 1981b, 1996) in typical unilateral vocal fold paralysis are:

- The pathology is located in the body of the vibrator: the muscle. The cover, consisting of the epithelium and the superficial layer of the lamina propria, and the transition, the vocal ligament, are intact.
- The mass and stiffness of the body are decreased, but those of the cover and transition are normal. Thus, the typical layered structure of the vibrator has deteriorated.
- The mechanical properties of the bilateral vocal folds are asymmetrical.
- There is glottic incompetence along the entire length, causing a decrease in glottic resistance.

These abnormalities are reflected in the vocal function in the following ways:

- The glottic incompetence associated with a decrease in mass and stiffness of the body causes a decrease in MPT, an increase in MFR, a decrease in highest F_0, F_0 range, loudest SPL, and SPL range, a decrease in signal-to-noise ratio (SNR) in acoustic analyses of the voice signal, and an incomplete glottic closure during vibrations. It also contributes to a decrease in vibratory amplitude and mucosal wave.
- Perceptually, the glottic incompetence associated with a flaccid body is reflected in a breathy, asthenic, hypofunctional, and aphonic quality.
- Asymmetrical vocal folds cause asymmetrical vibrations. They also contribute to irregular or aperiodic vibrations, which are manifested by the increase in PPQ and APQ.

REFERENCES

Fex, S. (1970). Judging the movements of vocal cords in larynx paralysis. *Acta Oto-laryngologica, 263,* 82–83.

Fex, S., & Elmqvist, D. (1973). Endemic recurrent laryngeal nerve paresis. *Acta Oto-laryngologica, 75,* 368–369.

Gartlan, M. G., Peterson, K. L., Luschei, E. S., Hoffman, H. T., & Smith, R. J. H. (1993). Bipolar hooked-wire electromyographic technique in the evaluation of pediatric vocal cord paralysis. *Annals of Otology, Rhinology and Laryngology, 102,* 695–700.

Gentile, R. D., Miller, R. H., & Woodson, G. E. (1986). Vocal cord paralysis in children 1 year of age and younger. *Annals of Otology, Rhinology and Laryngology, 95,* 622–625.

Hammarberg, B., Fritzell, B., & Schiratzki, H. (1984). Teflon injection in 16 patients with paralytic dysphonia: Perceptual and acoustic evaluations. *Journal of Speech and Hearing Disorders, 49,* 72–82.

Hirano, M. (1974). Clinical examination for voice disorders in recurrent laryngeal nerve palsy. In E. Loebell (Ed.), *Proceedings of the 16th International Congress of Logopedics and Phoniatrics.* Basel: Karger.

Hirano, M. (1975). Phonosurgery. Basic and clinical investigations. *Otologia (Fukuoka), 21,* 239–422.

Hirano, M. (1981a). *Clinical examination of voice.* Wien: Springer-Verlag.

Hirano, M. (1981b). Structure of the vocal fold in normal and disease states. Anatomical studies. In C. L. Ludlow & M. O. Hart (Eds.), *Proceedings of the Conference on the Assessment of Vocal Pathology.* Rockville, MD: The American Speech-Language-Hearing Association.

Hirano, M. (1989). Objective evaluation of the human voice. Clinical aspects. *Folia Phoniatrica, 41,* 89–144.

Hirano, M. (1996). Laryngeal histopathology. In R. Colton & J. K. Casper (Eds), *Understanding voice problems. A physiological perspective for diagnosis and treatment* (pp. 58–77). Baltimore: Williams and Wilkins.

Hirano, M. , Mori, K., Tanaka, S., & Fujita, M. (1995). Vocal function in patients with unilateral vocal fold paralysis before and after silicone injection. *Acta Oto-laryngologica, 115,* 553– 559.

Hirano, M., Nozoe, I., Shin, T., & Maeyama, T. (1972). Vibration of the vocal cords in recurrent laryngeal nerve paralysis. A stroboscopic investigation. *Practica Otologia (Kyoto), 65,* 1037–1047.

Hirano, M., Tanaka, S., Fujita, M., & Terasawa, R. (1991). Fundamental frequency and sound pressure level of phonation in pathological states. *Journal of Voice, 5,* 120–127.

Hirose, H. (1978). Clinical observations on 600 cases of recurrent laryngeal nerve paralysis. *Auris Nasus Larynx (Tokyo), 5,* 39–48.

Hirose, H., Sawashima, M., & Yoshioka H. (1981). Clinical observations on 750 cases of layngeal palsy. *Annual Bulletin of the Research Institute of Logopedics and Phoniatrics, University of Tokyo, 15,* 173–180.

Hiroto, I. (1966). The mechanism of phonation—Pathophysiological aspects of the larynx. *Practica Otologia (Kyoto), 39,* 229–291.

Huppler, E. G., Schmidt, H. W., Devine, K. D., & Gage, R. P. (1955). Causes of vocal-cord paralysis. *Proceedings of the Mayo Clinic, 30,* 518–521.

Kokesh, J., Robinson, L. R., Flint, P. W., & Cummings, C. W. (1993). Correlation between stroboscopy and electromyography in laryngeal paralysis. *Annals of Otolology, Rhinology and Laryngology, 102,* 852–857.

Kuroki, K. (1969). Subglottic pressure of normal and pathological larynges. *Otologia (Fukuoka), 15,* 54–74.

Kyttä, J. (1982). Prognosis of idiopathic paralysis of the vocal cord in the light of stroboscopy. *Acta Oto-laryngologica, 386*(Suppl.), 193–195.

New, G. B., & Childrey, J. H. (1932). Paralysis of the vocal cords. A study of two hundred and seventeen medical cases. *Archives of Otolaryngology, 16,* 143–159.

Nozoe, I., Hirano, M., Shin, T., & Maeyama, T. (1972). Recurrent laryngeal nerve palsy. A clinical study of 400 cases. *Otologia (Fukuoka), 18,* 411–417.

Parnes, S. M., & Satya-Murlti, S. (1985). Predictive value of laryngeal electromyography in patients with vocal cord paralysis of neurogenic origin. *Laryngoscope, 95,* 1323–1326.

Rosin, D. F., Handler, S. D., Potsic, W. P., Wetmore, R. F., & Tom, L. W. C. (1990). Vocal cord paralysis in children. *Laryngoscope, 100,* 1174–1179.

Schutte, H. K. (1980). *The efficiency of voice production.* Groningen: Kemper.

Sercarz, J. A., Berke, G. S., Ming, Y., Gerratt, B. R., & Natividad, M. (1992). Videostroboscopy of human vocal fold paralysis. *Annals of Otology, Rhinology and Laryngology, 101,* 567–577.

Shönhärl , E. (1960). Die *Stroboscopie in der praktischen Laryngologie.* Stuttgart: Georg Thieme Verlag.

Tanaka, S., Tanaka, Y., Fujita, M., Chijiwa, K., & Hirano, M. (1993). Recurrent laryngeal nerve

paralysis. Clinical study of 1,228 cases for 20 years. *Practica Otologia (Kyoto), 62*(Suppl.), 1–8.
Tucker, H. M. (1980). Vocal cord paralysis—1979: Etiology and management. *Laryngoscope, 90,* 585–590.
Tucker, H. M. (1986). Vocal cord paralysis in small children: Principles in management. *Annals of Otology, Rhinology and Laryngology, 95,* 618–621.
Yamada, M., Hirano, M., & Ohkubo, H. (1983). Recurrent laryngeal nerve paralysis. A 10-year review of 564 patients. *Auris Nasus Larynx (Tokyo), 10*(Suppl.), S1–S15.

CHAPTER 19

Neurologic Disease

Wolfram Ziegler and Philip Hoole

Virtually all neurologic diseases interfering with general motor control can also involve laryngeal motor functions and, as a consequence, lead to voice disorders. Usually, neurogenic dysphonia is part of a more general dysarthric disorder that includes motor problems of the respiratory and the supralaryngeal muscles during speaking as well. The voice problems encountered in these patients may either reflect direct involvement of the laryngeal motor system or a compensatory reaction to respiratory or articulatory dysfunctions.

Unfortunately, most reports about the incidence of speech impairments in neurologic populations fail to distinguish between the disturbances of voice function and those of other speech motor systems, like articulation. In some disorders, such as Parkinson disease, voice problems may appear among the initial symptoms and their recognition may contribute to the early diagnosis of the disorder (Stewart et al., 1995). Depending on its severity, the dysphonia may cause a remarkable communication problem and thereby contribute in a major way to the patient´s overall disability. In particular, neurogenic vocal impairment may interfere with the intelligibility and the naturalness of a subject´s spoken utterances (Ramig, 1992). In the most severe cases, a patient may be completely unable to phonate (aphonia).

This chapter gives an overview of the major etiologies and pathophysiologic states that can cause neurogenic voice disorders and describes the most important diagnostic and therapeutic approaches.

1. NEUROPHYSIOLOGY OF LARYNGEAL MOTOR CONTROL

Compared to other motor systems, very little is known about the neurophysiology of human laryngeal motor control. The major neural systems subserving the motor functions of the larynx are (1) the lower lateral face region of the motor cortex with its descending corticobulbar pathways; (2) the inferior lateral premotor cortex of the dominant cerebral hemisphere, including the anterior insula; (3) medial-frontal cortical areas of the dominant hemisphere; (4) a cortico-striato-pallido-thalamo-cortical loop, often called the extrapyramidal system; (5) the cerebellum, with its afferent and efferent projections; (6) mesencephalic coordinating centers such as the periaqueductal gray; and (7) the nucleus ambiguus in the medulla with its descending Xth cranial nerve (vagus nerve). The latter subdivides into the superior laryngeal nerve (SLN), supplying the cricothyroid muscle and mediating sensory afferents from the larynx, and the recurrent laryngeal nerve (RLN), supplying all other laryngeal muscles except the cricothyroid (Sears, Patten, & Fenstermacher, 1991).

The laryngeal motor system is bilaterally organized in the sense that unilateral stimulation of motor cortical sites results in a contraction of laryngeal muscles of both sides, although the response is probably not entirely symmetric. As in other motor systems, for example the hand, the representation of laryngeal muscles in the motor cortex is based on a many-to-one relation, implying that stimulation of a single cortical neuron may produce complex and functionally significant responses (Zealear, Hast, & Kurago, 1985). The pathway connecting the laryngeal motor cortical area with the nucleus ambiguus is probably indirect (polysynaptic) (Gacek & Malmgren, 1992). It is suspected that the different laryngeal functions, such as in breathing, swallowing, emotional vocalizing, singing, or speaking, are subserved by different neural circuits. Evidence for this comes from various sources: (1) The degree of laryngeal impairment in voluntary or involuntary phonation can be dissociated after brain lesions. After bilateral lesions to the upper motor neuron, for instance, a patient may be unable to phonate voluntarily, but can nevertheless produce voiced phonation during laughing or crying. (2) Animal studies have suggested that the laryngeal motor system subdivides into a limbic vocalization system controlling *emotional* vocal expression and a separate neocortical vocalization system controlling *learned* vocalizations (Jürgens & Zwirner, 1996). (3) Functional imaging studies have revealed differences in the lateralization of prerolandic activation during speaking (predominantly left), syllable singing (predominantly right), or nonverbal articulator movements (bilateral) (Wildgruber, Ackermann, Klose, Kardatzki, & Grodd, 1996).

2. ETIOLOGIES

The various neurologic disorders associated with voice problems are characterized by major differences in brain pathology, prevalence, type of progression, age of onset, prognosis, pattern of accompanying neurologic and neuropsychologic disturbances, and medical management. Thus, characterization of neurogenic dysphonia by its underlying etiology has important clinical implications.

2.1. Cerebrovascular Disease

The major disorders of the vascular system of the brain are ischemic infarction and hemorrhage, that is, intracerebral bleeding as a consequence of hypertension or rupture of arteriovenous malformations (Kase, Fisher, Babikian, & Mohr, 1991). In the Western countries, stroke has an incidence of several hundred new victims per 100,000 people per year and is one of the most frequent causes of death. In the acute phase after stroke, about 35% of survivors are dysarthric, at the chronic stage between 15% and 30% (Arboix & Marti-Vilalta, 1990; Wade, Hewer, David, & Enderby, 1986). Figures describing the frequency of dysphonic signs, specifically, are not available. Speech impairments occur predominantly with particular vascular syndromes, for example basilar artery branch disease, superior cerebellar artery infarction, anterior chorioideal artery infarction, or infarction of the lateral lenticulostriate branches of the middle cerebral artery (Bassetti, Bogousslavsky, Barth, & Regli, 1996); moreover, speech impairments are among the major symptoms of so-called lacunar syndromes (Urban, Hopf, Zorowka, Fleischer, & Andreas, 1996). Because of the bilateral organization of the laryngeal motor system, one-sided infarctions are usually compensated for within several weeks. If pyramidal tract fibers are lesioned on both sides, suprabulbar palsy (or pseudobulbar palsy) results, which is characterized by a bilateral paresis of speech muscles. Voluntary voiced phonation, if possible at all, is characterized by tense voice quality (spastic dysphonia), and there is a marked dissociation between voluntary and involuntary (e.g., emotional, reflexive) motility of the vocal folds (Loeb, Gandolfo, Caponetto, & Del Sette, 1990).

A particular condition associated with stroke is apraxia of speech. This condition occurs predominantly after infarction of the middle cerebral artery of the dominant hemisphere and differs from other unilateral syndromes by its persistent nature and often poor prognosis (cf. section 3.9. following).

A further observation of impaired laryngeal function can be made in patients with lesions to medial frontal cortical areas, the anterior cingulate cortex and the supplementary motor area (SMA). Lesions to the left SMA result in initial complete muteness and subsequent whispery or hypophonic speech, a reduction of spontaneous speech with preserved ability to repeat sentences (transcortical motor aphasia), and an impairment of emotional vocal expression (Jürgens & von Cramon, 1982). Bilateral lesions to the anterior cingulate cortex lead to long-lasting mutism with global akinesia. In both conditions, impaired motility of the vocal folds is not due to paresis or apraxia, but to a loss of motor drive or a disturbance of movement initiation (cf. section 3.4.).

2.2. Closed-Head Injury

In the United States, traumatic brain injury with long-term disability occurs with an incidence of probably more than 100 new cases each year for a population of 100,000 (Willer, Abosch, & Dahmer, 1990). Men are involved twice as often as women, with a marked peak in the age group around 20 years. Brain lesions result from various pathomechanisms, such as contusion, axonal injury, brain hematoma or edema, or secondary hypoxia (Keidel & Miller, 1996). In moderate-to-severe cases, the frequency of motor speech disorders may amount to 50% (Gilchrist & Wilkinson, 1979); in the long run, a quarter of the population of severe closed-head trauma patients has lingering motor speech problems (Schalén, Hansson, Nordström, & Nordström, 1994). Speech motor dysfunctions are only part of an often very complex posttraumatic course, which includes a variety of neurological and neuropsychological deficits (Beukelman & Yorkston, 1991).

The type and severity of voice problems of the closed-head-injured population may vary considerably (Theodoros, Murdoch, & Chenery, 1994). Overall, the prognosis of patients with dysarthric impairments must be considered poor compared to, for example, those with language disturbances (Najenson, Sazbon, Becker, & Schechter, 1978). About 3% of brain-injured patients are completely mute over a substantial period, probably because of a bilateral disruption of corticofugal pathways (Levin et al., 1983). In these patients, a typical pattern of recovery was described by Vogel and von Cramon (1982).

2.3. Degenerative Disorders of the Basal Ganglia

Among the degenerative disorders afflicting the basal ganglia, Parkinson disease and choreatic disorders such as Huntington disease play an important role. A number of other disorders, such as the Steele-Richardson-Olszewski-syndrome, Wilson disease, or the (primary) dyskinesias, are not discussed here (for details see Duvoisin, 1991).

2.3.1. Parkinson Disease

In European countries Parkinson disease has a prevalence of 60–160 per 100,000 in the population more than 40 years old. The disorder results from a depletion of dopamine concentration in the striatum, as a consequence of a loss of neurons in the substantia nigra. In addition to its idiopathic form, Parkinsonism may also occur, for example, after encephalitis, closed-head injury, or as a part of multi-system-degeneration (Duvoisin, 1991). Among the most prominent symptoms of Parkinson disease are tremor, a stooped posture, a slow and short stepped gait, hypomimia, and micrographia. Dysphagia occurs in about half of the overall Parkinson disease population, voice and speech impairments in 50%–80%. Typical vocal problems of Parkinson patients are a soft and breathy voice, monotonous intonation, and voice tremor (Murdoch, Manning, Theodoros, & Thompson, 1997). These symptoms are even named among the early signs of the disease (Stewart et al., 1995). The voice dysfunction of Parkinsonism may be gender-specific, showing predominantly increased pitch and breathiness in males and a quivering voice with a strained quality in females (Hertrich & Ackermann, 1995).

2.3.2. Huntington Disease

Huntington disease (or Huntington chorea) is an autosomal-dominant hereditary disorder characterized by progressive neuronal degeneration in the neostriatum and, in its later course, other subcortical and cortical areas. The disorder has a worldwide prevalence of about 5 per 100,000. Its onset is predominantly in adulthood, and the clinical picture is characterized by, among other things, progressive dementia, emotional lability, behavioral changes, and choreatic movements. The latter include, in more advanced stages, violent flinging movements of the limbs, rapid involuntary movements of other body parts (e.g., the head or the tongue), facial grimacing, lip smacking, and irregular contortions of the trunk (Duvoisin, 1991).

Facial dyskinesias may be marked by almost normal speech; but, during the course of the disease, dysarthria develops in virtually all cases. Voice can be impaired by abrupt involuntary changes of pitch or loudness and by transient changes of voice quality. In the most severe cases, a patient may develop complete mutism (Ramig, 1986).

2.4. Cerebellar Ataxia

The cerebellar ataxias form a group of disorders caused by cerebellar atrophy or by a degeneration of afferent or efferent cerebellar projections. Friedreich ataxia is an autosomal-recessive hereditary disorder associated with a chronic progressive degeneration of spinocerebellar, corticocerebellar, and corticospinal tracts. Its prevalence is estimated by 1–2 per 100,000, with an onset before the age of 25. It is characterized by ataxia, muscle weakness, sensory deficits, and dysarthria (Klockgether & Dichgans, 1996). Speech is scanning, with fluctuating voice disturbances, sometimes a monotonous voice, and hypernasality (Ackermann & Hertrich, 1993). (Pure) cerebellar ataxia can be autosomal-dominant hereditary or sporadic (idiopathic cerebellar ataxia). Both forms may also occur in a variant, including noncerebellar signs, for example, pyramidal or extrapyramidal. These disorders have an estimated overall prevalence of 1 per 100,000 (Klockgether & Dichgans, 1996). In most cases, dysarthric impairments develop during the course of the disease. The dysphonic symptoms may vary depending on the involvement of noncerebellar structures, but usually some ataxic component with rough voice, fluctuating pitch or loudness, or voice tremor is present (Ackermann & Ziegler, 1991, 1994; Kluin, Gilman, Lohman, & Junck, 1996).

2.5. Multiple Sclerosis (MS)

MS is associated with an inflammatory process leading to a demyelination of nerve sheaths in the central nervous system (CNS). The cause of the disease is probably immunologic. In mid-European countries there is an estimated 4–8 new cases per 100,000 per year; the prevalence is between 50 and 60 per 100,000. The disorder usually begins in the third or fourth decade, with women being affected almost twice as often as men. The symptoms of the disorder vary depending on the localization of the "plaques" that develop at the foci of inflammation in the white matter of the brain or in the spinal cord. The most prominent motor signs are paresis or ataxia or a combination of these two. In addition, somatosensory or visual disturbances and cognitive dysfunctions may occur. MS is also highly variable in its course. In many cases, a relapsing-remitting course with slow progression is observed (Martin, Hohlfeld, & McFarland, 1996).

Dysarthria is part of the triad of MS symptoms originally described by Charcot. According to more recent reports, its prevalence in MS is between 40% and 50%. The voice disorder is characterized by spastic or ataxic signs or by a combination thereof. Some patients present with a voice tremor of the cerebellar type, that is, between 2 and 3 Hz (Hartelius, Nord, & Buder, 1995).

2.6. Motor Neuron Disease

Among these disorders, amyotrophic lateral sclerosis (ALS) is most relevant in looking at laryngeal motor control. The disorder has an estimated prevalence of 4–6 per 100,000, with an onset after age 40 and a rapid progression with lethal course within 2–3 years. ALS may involve both the upper and the lower motor neuron as well as the cranial nerve nuclei, which may lead to a coexistence of central and peripheral motor signs. There may also be cortical involvement, with dementia and language impairment. The disorder has a spinal and a bulbar variant, the latter beginning with dysarthria and dysphagia (Borasio, Appel, & Büttner, 1996). Dysphonia may include flaccid as well as spastic signs (see later), depending on the involvement of the lower and upper motor neuron and of the nucleus ambiguus (Langmore & Lehman, 1994).

3. CONDITIONS

Despite the diagnostic value of an etiological classification of neurogenic dysphonias, the nature of the voice problem resulting from many of these disorders is not entirely determined. Multiple sclerosis, closed-head injury, or cerebrovascular disease, for instance, are associated with varying lesion sites and may result in a variety of vocal symptoms. Even in disorders with lesion sites as predictable as Parkinson disease, considerable variation of voice patterns may occur. Part of this variation can be explained by analyzing the different pathomechanisms that may underlie neurogenic dysphonia.

3.1. Flaccid Paralysis

Lesions to the nucleus ambiguus in the brainstem or to its descending Xth cranial nerve or disorders affecting the neuromuscular junction cause flaccid paralysis or weakness of the laryngeal muscles. Since muscle innervation is interrupted on its final path, all motor functions (i.e., reflex activity, emotional vocalizations, and voluntary functions including speech), are involved. Over a longer period, muscle denervation with atrophy and fasciculation occurs.

Bilateral vocal fold paralysis may occur, for example, in motor neuron disease, myasthenia gravis, or after thyroidectomy. Unilateral vocal fold paralysis most commonly results from injury to the recurrent laryngeal nerve, whereas isolated paralysis of the superior laryngeal nerve is a rare condition. Wallenberg syndrome, most often occurring after occlusion of the posterior inferior cerebellar artery, causes unilateral paralysis of laryngeal muscles. As the vagus nerve travels in close proximity to the glossopharyngeal nerve and as both nerves supply the palatal and the pharyngeal musculature as well, vocal fold paralysis is often associated with flaccidity of the soft palate (Sears et al., 1991). Vocal fold paralysis is described in greater detail in Chapter 18.

3.2. Spastic (Supranuclear) Paresis

Spasticity is one of the components of a more complex upper motor neuron syndrome, which is seen after lesions to cortico-nuclear tract fibers descending from the sensorimotor cortex through the interal capsule to the motor nuclei in the brainstem or the spinal cord. Increased excitability of the stretch reflex, resulting in a velocity-dependent resistance of the muscle to passive stretch (spastic hypertonus) is considered one of its underlying pathomechanisms. Spasticity is accompanied by paresis of the involved musculature, increased proprioceptive reflexes, and abolition of fine motor control (Dietz & Young, 1996).

For obvious reasons, the criteria used in the diagnosis of spasticity in the limbs, that is, increased resistance to passive stretching, cannot be employed in the laryngeal motor system. Other clinical features of spasticity, such as a particular affection of antigravity muscles, are not applicable either. However, the mechanoreceptors responsible for the mediation of spastic hypertonus, the muscle spindles, can be found in the laryngeal musculature (Cooper & Lawson, 1992), and specific patterns deemed to be indicative of spastic hypertonicity, for example, hyperadduction and shortening of the vocal folds, have been described repeatedly (Aronson, 1990). The condition of laryngeal spasticity is included within pseudobulbar palsy, but it may also occur in combination with ataxic, hypokinetic, or flaccid signs, such as after closed-head trauma, in multiple sclerosis, in multiple system degeneration, or in ALS. The voice is characterized by a strained-strangled quality, sometimes with increased pitch, reduced pitch range, and reduced loudness. Intonation may be compromised by impoverished fine tuning of vocal fold tension. In severe cases, complete immobility of the vocal folds may result in aphonia. A major criterion for distinguishing between peripheral (flaccid) and central (spastic) paresis is the preservation of reflexive and often emotional motility of the vocal folds and the absence of atrophy and fasciculation in patients with upper motor neuron lesions.

3.3. Rigidity

Rigidity is one of the characteristic symptoms of basal ganglia disorders such as Parkinsonism, Steele-Richardson-Olszewski syndrome, or sometimes Huntington disease. As in spasticity, the affected muscles show increased tone, but muscle tone is increased in both agonist and antagonist muscle groups and the resistance against passive movement is equal in all directions and throughout the whole movement range. The probable pathomechanism underlying muscular rigidity is an increased coactivation of agonists and antagonists (Lee, 1989). Among the muscles relevant for speech, rigidity has been suspected to be present in the intercostal muscles (Solomon & Hixon, 1993) and the perioral muscles (Caligiuri, 1987) of Parkinson patients. Laryngeal rigidity, which has been demonstrated by EMG examinations (Gracco & Marek, 1996), is supposed to result in a bowing of the vocal folds (Hanson, Gerratt, & Ward, 1984). However, the clinical signs of vocal fold rigidity cannot easily be separated from hypokinesia, as both coexist in Parkinson disease (see later).

3.4. Akinesia

Akinesia is defined as the complete loss or the reduction of voluntary motility in the absence of paresis. It is part of the motor symptoms of Parkinson disease and is considered independent of rigidity. Its constituents are bradykinesia, slowing of movements; hypokinesia, reduced movement range; and impaired movement initiation (Marsden, 1989). Among the factors underlying the akinetic condition, insufficient "energizing" of the musculature or a delayed activation of motor cortical neurons have been discussed. Akinesia is considered to result from basal ganglia dysfunction, but mediofrontal connections of the striatum, in particular the anterior cingulate cortex and the supplementary motor area, may also play an important role, as lesions to these structures are known to result in movement initiation problems (Goldberg, 1985).

As regards akinesia of the speech motor system in Parkinsonism, differences from limb motor control are apparent. First, the prolongation of reaction times that characterizes the akinetic condition of Parkinson patients in the extremities cannot be demonstrated for the laryngeal motor system in vocal reaction tasks (Ludlow, Connor, & Bassich, 1987). Second, speech movements of the mandible of Parkinson patients fail to be bradykinetic, although nonspeech mandibular tracking movements are definitely slowed (Connor & Abbs, 1991). It is not known whether bradykinesia of laryngeal speech movements is present in Parkinsonism, but reduced movement amplitude (hypokinesia) can be considered as a potential underlying cause of incomplete vocal fold adduction observed in Parkinson patients. This justifies the use of the term hypokinetic dysarthria, coined by Darley, Aronson, and Brown (1975), although rigid hypokinetic would more appropriately describe the probable presence of muscular rigidity in this patient group.

Akinetic or hypokinetic vocal signs include a weak and breathy, sometimes whispery voice and a monotonous intonation. In severe cases, such as after either bilateral medial-frontal or midbrain lesions, a patient may be completely mute (akinetic mutism; cf. Jürgens & von Cramon, 1982).

3.5. Dyskinetic Conditions

Like rigidity and akinesia, dyskinetic disturbances are also ascribed to a dysfunction at the level of the basal ganglia. Dyskinetic symptoms include chorea, dystonia, athetosis, tardive dyskinesia, and tics, with some authors also including myoclonus (cf. section 3.7.). A distinction can be made between idiopathic (primary) and symptomatic (secondary) forms of dyskinesia (Marsden, 1984).

Choreatic movements are among the core symptoms of Huntington or Sydenham disease (cf. section 2.3.2.), but may also occur after intoxications or infections of the CNS (Duvoisin, 1991). Choreatic impairments at the laryngeal level may lead to abrupt changes in pitch, loudness, or voice quality (cf. section 2.3.2.).

In contrast with choreiform impairments, the dystonias are characterized by slow and persistent muscle contractions that may result in screw-like or repetitive involuntary movements and abnormal posture. Generalized dystonia influences a wide range of body parts, whereas the segmental or focal dystonias only affect circumscribed muscle groups. The cause of primary dystonia is unknown. Secondary dystonia is frequent after focal lesions to the lentiform nucleus and the putamen and is considered to result from increased thalamocortical drive, which may be responsible for the dystonic muscle spasms (Bhatia & Marsden, 1994). Focal dystonia of the larynx, better known as spasmodic dysphonia, will be described in greater detail in Chapter 20.

3.6. Ataxia

Ataxia is characterized by dysmetric (i.e., over- and undershooting) movements, disturbances in the control of movement velocity in aiming or grasping movements or in rapid movement repetitions (dysdiadochokinesia), delayed movement initiation, an inability to maintain a constant motor performance (e.g., a constant force), kinetic tremor with an inability to perform smooth aiming movements, and disturbances in programming multicomponent movements. (Diener & Dichgans, 1992). Among the causes underlying ataxia, disturbances in the processing of time information, of somatosensory information, or problems in the modulation of agonist and antagonist muscle activity have been discussed (Diener & Dichgans, 1992; Ito, 1990).

Ataxia is generally ascribed to dysfunction at the level of the cerebellum or its afferent or efferent projections. With respect to ataxic impairments of motor speech functions, superior paravermal cerebellar areas are considered most important.

Laryngeal ataxia has been investigated by laryngoscopic, electroglottographic, and acoustic methods (for references see Ackermann & Ziegler, 1994). Irregularity of vocal fold adduction gestures and of voice fundamental frequency were among the most prominent symptoms described in these studies. This is in accordance with the observation that pitch fluctuations and vocal harshness are the most salient auditory features of ataxic dysarthria

(Kluin et al., 1988). Voice tremor in the range of cerebellar tremor (2–3 Hz) may occur (Ackermann & Ziegler, 1991). Laryngeal hypotonia has been suspected to be present as well, but Diener and Dichgans (1992) suggest that cerebellar hypotonia is confined to the acute stage of cerebellar dysfunction.

3.7. Tremor and Myoclonus

Tremor is a rhythmical involuntary oscillatory movement of a body part. It may occur in various diseases like Parkinsonism, cerebellar ataxia, multiple sclerosis, head trauma, or dystonia. Tremor is considered to result from abnormal synchronization of motor neurons and is classified according to its frequency (2–12 Hz) or to the particular conditions under which it occurs (resting, postural, action, intention) (Findley & Büttner, 1996). Voice tremor is characterized perceptually by a tremulous, quavering, or wavy voice; sometimes with intermittent complete voice stoppages; and acoustically by rhythmic oscillations of vocal pitch or loudness. It may result from a tremor of respiratory, laryngeal, velopharyngeal, or oral musculature (Brin, Fahn, Blitzer, Ramig, & Stewart, 1992; Tomoda, Shibasaki, Kuroda, & Shin, 1987). Vocal tremor becomes most prominent during sustained vowel prolongation tasks. It may be part of the essential tremor disease (4–12 Hz), of cerebellar ataxia (2–3 Hz) or laryngeal dystonia (irregular frequency), or it may present as an early symptom of Parkinson disease (4–7 Hz) (Findley & Gresty, 1988; Perez, Ramig, Smith, & Dromey, 1996; Stewart et al., 1995).

Myoclonus differs in that it may be less regular than tremor and the movements are mostly brief and shock-like. Myocloni may occur in isolation (essential myoclonus) or with degenerative, infectious or traumatic movement disorders, after intoxication, or with epilepsy. They are considered to be of extrapyramidal origin (Duvoisin, 1991). Some authors classify it among the dyskinesias (Marsden, 1984). Palatal and laryngeal myoclonus can be observed after lesions of the olivopontocerebellar tract, for example, after basilar artery occlusion or closed-head injury. Perceptually, involuntary alterations of pitch or loudness resembling voice tremor can be observed (Brin et al., 1992; Deuschl, Mischke, Schenck, Schulte-Mönting, & Lücking, 1990).

3.8. Stuttering

Contrary to developmental stuttering, acquired neurogenic stuttering in adults is a very rare condition. Disfluency with tonic blocks and iterations may occur in Parkinsonism and other basal ganglia disorders, after stroke or closed-head injury, in combination with spasmodic dysphonia, or in epilepsy (Helm-Estabrooks, 1986; Hertrich, Ackermann, Ziegler, & Kaschel, 1993). Although a clear association of acquired neurogenic stuttering with particular lesion sites has not been established, the medial frontal cortical region and the basal ganglia seem to play some role in fluency control (Ziegler, Kilian, & Deger, 1997). As can be inferred from observations made in developmental stutterers, laryngeal movements and their interaction with other components of the speech motor system play an essential role in the pathogenesis of stuttering (Brin et al., 1992), but the nature of the dysfunction is still unresolved.

3.9. Apraxia

Apraxia is a condition resulting from left hemisphere damage. Apraxic patients are unable to perform gestures on command (Goldenberg & Hagmann, 1997). Their movement disturbances are most often characterized by exclusion, that is, they cannot be explained on the grounds of weakness or paresis, slowness or akinesia, ataxia, or any other elementary motor impairment (Bradshaw & Mattingley, 1995). Quite similarly, apraxia of speech has been described as a motor speech disorder that is not explainable by elementary speech motor deficits, but rather reflects a disruption at some higher level of speech motor control (Darley et al., 1975). A difference from the dysarthrias is that apraxia of speech is a disturbance of the dominant hemisphere, resulting predominantly from left middle cerebral artery infarction. It is characterized by groping and effortful articulation with phonetic and phonemic errors and prosodic problems. Remarkably, in most cases of apraxia of speech there is no major dysphonic component in the sense of poor voice quality or vocal instability. Apart from very severe disorders with complete apraxic mutism (Pineda & Ardila, 1992) or from single cases with a notable disintegration of articulation and phonation (Ruff & Arbit, 1981), apraxic speakers usually present only minor vocal aberrations indicating increased effort or psychological stress (Heeschen, Ryalls, & Hagoort, 1988; but see Ryalls & Scarfone, 1990). Nevertheless, numerous observations point to an involvement of laryngeal motor functions in apraxia of speech, that is reduced F_0 modulation, disturbed tonal coarticulation in tone languages, and a frequent occurrence of voicing errors in articulation (for references see Hoole, Schröter-Morasch, & Ziegler, 1997). Although apraxic speakers are able to perform laryngeal ab- or adductory movements of normal range and rate, there are occurrences of groping, movement delay, undershooting, or aberrant movement shape. In other instances, a required ab- or adduction may be completely absent or a clear laryngeal gesture may occur where none is required (Hoole et al., 1997).

4. ASSESSMENT

Clinical assessment is in the first instance based on perceptual evaluation of a patient´s voice. The most relevant parameters describing voice control in connected speech are related to pitch (decreased or increased), voice quality (breathy, rough/harsh, tense/strained-strangled, glottal fry), vocal stability (pitch breaks, pitch or loudness fluctuations, voice tremor), and pitch or loudness range (increased or decreased variation). Assessment protocols based on auditory features of these kinds were proposed by, among others, Darley et al., (1975), Hartelius, Svensson, and Bubach (1993), or Kluin, Foster, Berent, and Gilman (1993). A less subjective method of evaluating vocal performance in neurologic patients uses speech signal analysis techniques (see Chapter 9). Computations of voice fundamental frequency and F_0 variation provide information about a patient´s average vocal pitch, pitch range, and vocal stability (Ackermann & Ziegler, 1994; Hartelius et al., 1995). Deviant voice quality can be assessed by parameters such as vocal jitter and shimmer as well as by spectral measures such as harmonics-to-noise ratio (Hartmann & Cramon, 1984).

In addition to acoustic and auditory-based evaluations, a physical examination of the larynx is indispensible for the detection of mass lesions (cf. Chapter 18) and for the direct observation of laryngeal motor dysfunctions. This examination includes indirect or telescopic laryngoscopy or transnasal-fiberoptic laryngoscopy, preferably with additional videorecording (Yanagisawa, 1992). A closer examination of the glottal vibratory cycle can be achieved by laryngostroboscopy (see Chapter 11), although this method may fail in cases presenting with poor voice quality. Laryngoscopic observations can be supplemented by photoelectroglottography, which utilizes the light source of the laryngoscope for registration of glottal area changes by means of transillumination (Hoole et. al., 1997).

Electroglottography (EGG) or laryngography is a noninvasive technique for assessing laryngeal dysfunction on the basis of glottal cycle information (cf. Chapter 13). Although the method is clinically applicable and commercial EGG systems are available, there are only few EGG studies of neurogenic dysphonia so far, predominantly for Parkinson disease (Hertrich & Ackermann, 1995; Murdoch et al., 1997).

In certain cases there may be an indication for electromyographic assessment of laryngeal functions in patients with neurogenic disorders. EMG of the larynx can be valuable in the differential diagnosis of peripheral nerve involvement and may be prognostic for the recovery of functions after central vocal fold paralysis (Lovelace, Blitzer, & Ludlow, 1992). A combination of electromyographic techniques with magnetic stimulation of the lower cranial nerves can be used to diagnose upper and lower motor neuron function from cortex to the periphery: Stimulation with a magnetic coil applied at different sites along the corticobulbar tract induces muscle action potentials (MAPs) in the vocalis or posterior cricoarytenoid muscles, the amplitude and latency of which can be measured by bipolar hooked wire electrodes. Lesions to pyramidal tract or peripheral nerve fibers would result in specific alterations of the MAP patterns (Thumfart, Pototschnig, Zorowka, & Eckel, 1992).

5. MANAGEMENT

The clinical management of neurogenic voice disorders is based on speech therapy, pharmacotherapy, and surgery.

Behavioral techniques used by speech therapists to improve insufficient adduction include elicitation of the sphincter function of the larynx or of reflexive phonation, strengthening of respiratory support, digital manipulation of the thyroid cartilage, postural modifications of head and trunk, glottal attack tasks, or maximum phonatory effort tasks. Hyperadduction of the vocal folds can be reduced by relaxation techniques; chewing, humming, or yawn-sigh-exercises; exercises based on utterances with /h/-onset; or modifications of postural and respiratory support. Further specific treatment methods may be focused on stabilizing vocal functions or on improving laryngeal coordination. In some of these approaches, biofeedback techniques can be applied to reinforce laryngeal control functions (Duffy, 1995; Ramig & Scherer, 1992; Vogel, 1998). Controlled treatment studies investigating the efficacy of these methods have only rarely been performed. An exception is the Lee Silverman Voice Treatment (LSVT), which has been shown to improve vocal efficiency and loudness in patients with Parkinson disease (Ramig, Countryman, O'Brien, Hoehn, & Thompson, 1996).

Among the pharmacotherapeutic approaches, botulinum toxin treatment of spasmodic dysphonia has become most prominent (see Chapter 21). Studies of the effects on voice functions of dopamine substitution therapy in Parkinsonism are predominantly negative, and there is no obvious relation of dysphonia to drug cycle fluctuations in this group (Larson, Ramig, & Scherer, 1994; Shea, Drummond, Metzer, & Krueger, 1993). However, modulation of the dopaminergic system may be effective in other populations (Echiverri, Tatum, Merens, & Coker, 1988; Liebson, Walsh, Jankowiak, & Albert, 1994). Voice tremor may be responsive to clonazepam and propanolol (Tomoda et al., 1987).

Injections of Teflon or other substances have been used to reduce glottal insufficiency in various patient groups (Ford, Bless, & Loftus, 1992). RLN surgical section is considered effective in treating spasmodic dysphonia (Dedo & Behlau, 1991), although this approach may in the future be displaced by botulinum toxin injections.

Among the neurosurgical treatments influencing speech and voice, stereotaxic ablation or electrical stimulation of thalamic nuclei have long been used for the relief of severe tremor and rigidity in Parkinson disease, but this method produces dysarthric signs more often than it ameliorates them. A new approach is based on fetal dopamine transplants; but preliminary investigations have revealed that this treatment has no consistent effect on vocal function in Parkinson disease (Baker, Ramig, Johnson, & Freed, 1997).

REFERENCES

Ackermann, H., & Hertrich, I. (1993). Dysarthria in Friedreich's ataxia. *Clinical Linguistics and Phonetics, 7*, 75–91.

Ackermann, H., & Ziegler, W. (1991). Cerebellar voice tremor: An acoustic analysis. *Journal of Neurology, Neurosurgery, and Psychiatry, 54*, 74–76.

Ackermann, H., & Ziegler, W. (1994). Acoustic analysis of vocal instability in cerebellar dysfunctions. *Annals of Otology, Rhinology, and Laryngology, 103*, 98–104.

Arboix, A., & Marti-Vilalta, J. L. (1990). Lacunar infarctions and dysarthria. *Archives of Neurology, 47*, 127

Aronson, A. E. (1990). *Clinical voice disorders*. New York: Thieme-Stratton.

Baker, K. K., Ramig, L. O., Johnson, A. B., & Freed, C. R. (1997). Preliminary voice and speech analysis following fetal dopamine transplants in 5 individuals with Parkinson's disease. *Journal of Speech Language and Hearing Research, 40*, 615–626.

Bassetti, C., Bogousslavsky, J., Barth, A., & Regli, F. (1996). Isolated infarcts of the pons. *Neurology, 46*, 165–175.

Beukelman, D. R., & Yorkston, K. M. (1991). *Communication disorders following traumatic brain injury: Management of cognitive, language, and motor impairments*. Austin, TX: Pro-Ed.

Bhatia, K. P., & Marsden, C. D. (1994). The behavioural and motor consequences of focal lesions of the basal ganglia. *Brain, 117*, 859–876.

Borasio, G. D., Appel, S. H., & Büttner, U. (1996). Upper and lower motor neuron disorders. In T. Brandt, L. R. Caplan, J. Dichgans, H. C. Diener, & C. Kennard (Eds.), *Neurological disorders. Course and treatment* (pp. 811–817). San Diego: Academic Press.

Bradshaw, J. L., & Mattingley, J. B. (1995). *Clinical neuropsychology. Behavioral and brain science*. San Diego: Academic Press.

Brin, M. F., Fahn, S., Blitzer, A., Ramig, L. O., & Stewart, C. (1992). Movement disorders of the larynx. In A. Blitzer, M. Brin, C. T. Sasaki, S. Fahn, & K. S. Harris (Eds.), *Neurologic disorders of the larynx* (pp. 248–278). New York: Thieme Medical Publishers.

Caligiuri, M. P. (1987). Labial kinematics during speech in patients with Parkinsonian rigidity. *Brain, 110*, 1033–1044.

Connor, N. P., & Abbs, J. H. (1991). Task-dependent variations in Parkinsonian motor impairments. *Brain, 114*, 321–332.

Cooper, D. M., & Lawson, W. (1992). Laryngeal sensory receptors. In A. Blitzer, M. Brin, C. T. Sasaki, S. Fahn, & K. S. Harris (Eds.), *Neurologic disorders of the larynx* (pp. 12–28). New York: Thieme Medical Publishers.

Darley, F. L., Aronson, A. E., & Brown, J. R. (1975). *Motor speech disorders*. Philadelphia: W.B. Saunders.

Dedo, H. H., & Behlau, M. S. (1991). Recurrent laryngeal nerve section for spastic dysphonia: 5- to 14-year preliminary results in the first 300 patients. *Annals of Otology, Rhinology and Laryngology, 100*, 274–279.

Deuschl, G., Mischke, G., Schenck, E., Schulte-Mönting, J., & Lücking, C. H. (1990). Symptomatic and essential palatal myoclonus. *Brain, 113*, 1645–1672.

Diener, H.-C., & Dichgans, J. (1992). Pathophysiology of cerebellar ataxia. *Movement Disorders, 7*, 95–109.

Dietz, V., & Young, R. R. (1996). The syndrome of spastic paresis. In T. Brandt, L. R. Caplan, J. Dichgans, H. C. Diener, & C. Kennard (Eds.), *Neurological disorders. Course and treatment* (pp. 861–871). San Diego: Academic Press.

Duffy, J. R. (1995). *Motor speech disorders*. St. Louis, MO: Mosby.

Duvoisin, R. C. (1991). Diseases of the extrapyramidal system. In R. N. Rosenberg (Ed.), *Comprehensive neurology* (pp. 337–364). New York: Raven Press.

Echiverri, H. C., Tatum, W. O., Merens, T. A., & Coker, S. B. (1988). Akinetic mutism: Pharmacologic probe of the dopaminergic mesencephalofrontal activating system. *Pediatric Neurology, 4*, 228–230.

Findley, L. J., & Büttner, U. (1996). Tremor. In T. Brandt, L. R. Caplan, J. Dichgans, H. C. Diener, & C. Kennard (Eds.), *Neurological disorders. Course and treatment* (pp. 853–860). San Diego: Academic Press.

Findley, L. J., & Gresty, M. A. (1988). Head, facial, and voice tremor. In J. Jankovic & E. Tolosa (Eds.), *Advances in neurology. Vol. 49: Facial dyskinesias* (pp. 239–253). New York: Raven Press.

Ford, C. N., Bless, D. M., & Loftus, J.M. (1992). Role of injectable collagen in the treatment of glottic insufficiency: A study of 119 patients. *Annals of Otology, Rhinology and Laryngology, 101*, 237–247.

Gacek, R. R., & Malmgren, L. T. (1992). Laryngeal motor innervation—central. In A. Blitzer, M. Brin, C. T. Sasaki, S. Fahn, & K. S. Harris (Eds.), *Neurologic disorders of the larynx* (pp. 29–35). New York: Thieme Medical Publishers.

Gilchrist, E., & Wilkinson, M. (1979). Some factors determining prognosis in young people with severe head injuries. *Archives of Neurology, 36*, 355–359.

Goldberg, G. (1985). Supplementary motor area structure and function: Review and hypotheses. *The Behavioral and Brain Sciences, 8*, 567–616.

Goldenberg, G., & Hagmann, S. (1997). The meaning of meaningless gestures: A study of visuo-imitative apraxia. *Neuropsychologia, 35*, 333–341.

Gracco, C., & Marek, K. (1996). Laryngeal electromyography findings in Parkinson's disease. *Neurology, 46*, 378

Hanson, D. G., Gerratt, B. R., & Ward, P. H. (1984). Cinegraphic observations of laryngeal function in Parkinson's disease. *Laryngoscope, 94*, 348–353.

Hartelius, L., Nord, L., & Buder, E. H. (1995). Acoustic analysis of dysarthria associated with multiple sclerosis. *Clinical Linguistics and Phonetics, 9*, 95–120.

Hartelius, L., Svensson, P., & Bubach, A. (1993). Clinical assessment of dysarthria: Perform-ance on a dysarthria test by normal adult subjects, and by individuals with Parkinson's disease or with multiple sclerosis. *Scandinavian Journal of Logopedics and Phoniatrics, 18*, 131–141.

Hartmann, E., & von Cramon, D. (1984). Acoustic measurement of voice quality in central dysphonia. *Journal of Communication Disorders, 17*, 425–440.

Heeschen, C., Ryalls, J., & Hagoort, P. (1988). Psychological stress in Broca's versus Wernicke's aphasia. *Clinical Linguistics and Phonetics, 2*, 309–316.

Helm-Estabrooks, N. (1986). Diagnosis and management of neurogenic stuttering in adults. In K. O. St. Louis (Ed.), *The atypical stutterer. Principles and practices of rehabilitation* (pp. 193–217). Orlando, FL: Academic Press.

Hertrich, I., & Ackermann, H. (1995). Gender-specific vocal dysfunctions in Parkinson's disease: electroglottographic and acoustic analyses. *Annals of Otology, Rhinology and Laryngology, 104*, 197–202.

Hertrich, I., Ackermann, H., Ziegler, W., & Kaschel, R. (1993). Speech iterations in Parkinsonism: A case study. *Aphasiology, 7*, 395–406.

Hoole, P., Schröter-Morasch, H., & Ziegler, W. (1997). Patterns of laryngeal apraxia in two patients with Broca's aphasia. *Clinical Linguistics and Phonetics, 11*, 429–442.

Ito, M. (1990). A new physiological concept on cerebellum. *Revue Neurologique (Paris), 146*, 564–569.

Jürgens, U., & von Cramon, D. (1982). On the role of the anterior cingulate cortex in phonation: A case report. *Brain and Language, 15*, 234–248.

Jürgens, U., & Zwirner, P. (1996). The role of the periaqueductal grey in limbic and neocortical vocal fold control. *NeuroReport, 7*, 2921–2923.

Kase, C. S., Fisher, M., Babikian, V. L., & Mohr, J. P. (1991). Cerebrovascular disease. In R. N. Rosenberg (Ed.), *Comprehensive neurology* (pp. 97–156). New York: Raven Press.

Keidel, M., & Miller, J. D. (1996). Head trauma. In T. Brandt, L. R. Caplan, J. Dichgans, H. C. Diener, & C. Kennard (Eds.), *Neurological disorders. Course and treatment* (pp. 531–544). San Diego: Academic Press.

Klockgether, T., & Dichgans, J. (1996). Inherited and noninherited ataxias. In T. Brandt, L. R. Caplan, J. Dichgans, H. C. Diener, & C. Kennard (Eds.), *Neurological disorders. Course and treatment* (pp. 705–713). San Diego: Academic Press.

Kluin, K. J., Foster, N. L., Berent, S., & Gilman, S. (1993). Perceptual analysis of speech disorders in progressive supranuclear palsy. *Neurology, 43*, 563–566.

Kluin, K. J., Gilman, S., Lohman, M., & Junck, L. (1996). Characteristics of the dysarthria of multiple system atrophy. *Archives of Neurology, 53*, 545–548.

Kluin, K. J., Gilman, S., Markel, D. S., Koeppe, R. A., Rosenthal, G., & Junck, L. (1988). Speech disorders in olivopontocerebellar atrophy correlate with positron emission tomography findings. *Annals of Neurology, 23*, 547–554.

Langmore, S. E., & Lehman, M. E. (1994). Physiologic deficits in the orofacial system underlying dysarthria in amyotrophic lateral sclerosis. *Journal of Speech and Hearing Research, 37*, 28–37.

Larson, K. K., Ramig, L. O., & Scherer, R. C. (1994). Acoustic and glottographic voice analysis during drug-related fluctuations in Parkinsons disease. *Journal of Medical Speech-Language Pathology, 2*, 227–239.

Lee, R. G. (1989). Pathophysiology of rigidity and akinesia in Parkinson's disease. *European Neurology, 29*, 13–18.

Levin, H. S., Madison, C. F., Bailey, C. B., Meyers, C. A., Eisenberg, H. M., & Guinto, F. C. (1983). Mutism after closed head injury. *Archives of Neurology, 40*, 601–606.

Liebson, E., Walsh, M. J., Jankowiak, J., & Albert, M. L. (1994). Pharmacotherapy for posttraumatic dysarthria. *Neuropsychiatry, Neuropsychology, and Behavioral Neurology, 7*, 122–124.

Loeb, C., Gandolfo, C., Caponetto, C., & Del Sette, M. (1990). Pseudobulbar palsy: A clinical computed tomography study. *European Neurology, 30*, 42–46.

Lovelace, R. E., Blitzer, A., & Ludlow, C. L. (1992). Clinical laryngeal electromyographyl. In A. Blitzer, M. Brin, C. T. Sasaki, S. Fahn, & K. S. Harris (Eds.), *Neurologic disorders of the larynx* (pp. 66–81). New York: Thieme Medical Publishers.

Ludlow, C. L., Connor, N. P., & Bassich, C. J. (1987). Speech timing in Parkinson's and Huntington's disease. *Brain and Language, 32*, 195–214.

Marsden, C. D. (1984). The pathophysiology of movement disorders. *Neurologic Clinics, 2*, 435–459.

Marsden, C. D. (1989). Slowness of movement in Parkinson's disease. *Movement Disorders, 4*, 26–37.

Martin, R., Hohlfeld, R., & McFarland, H. F. (1996). Multiple sclerosis. In T. Brandt, L. R. Caplan, J. Dichgans, H. C. Diener, & C. Kennard (Eds.), *Neurological disorders. Course and treatment* (pp. 483–505). San Diego: Academic Press.

Murdoch, B. E., Manning, C. Y., Theodoros, D. G., & Thompson, E. C. (1997). Laryngeal and phonatory dysfunction in Parkinson's disease. *Clinical Linguistics and Phonetics, 11,* 245–266.

Najenson, T., Sazbon, L., Becker, E., & Schechter, I. (1978). Recovery of communicative functions after prolonged traumatic coma. *Scandinavian Journal of Rehabilitation Medicine, 10,* 15–21.

Perez, K. S., Ramig, L. O., Smith, M. E., & Dromey, C. (1996). The Parkinson larynx: Tremor and videostroboscopic findings. *Journal of Voice, 10,* 354–361.

Pineda, D., & Ardila, A. (1992). Lasting mutism with buccofacial apraxia. *Aphasiology, 6,* 285–292.

Ramig, L. A. (1986). Acoustic analyses of phonation in patients with Huntington's disease. *Annals of Otology, Rhinology and Laryngology, 95,* 288–293.

Ramig, L. O. (1992). The role of phonation in speech intelligibility. A review and preliminary data from patients with Parkinson's disease. In R. D. Kent (Ed.), *Intelligibility in speech disorders* (pp. 119–155). Amsterdam: John Benjamins Publishing Company.

Ramig, L. O., Countryman, S., O'Brien, C., Hoehn, M., & Thompson, L. (1996). Intensive speech treatment for patients with Parkinson's disease—short-term and long-term comparison of 2 techniques. *Neurology, 47,* 1496–1504.

Ramig, L. O., & Scherer, R. C. (1992). Speech therapy for neurologic disorders of the larynx. In A. Blitzer, M. F. Brin, C. T. Sasaki, S. Fahn, & K. S. Harris (Eds.), *Neurologic disorders of the larynx* (pp. 163–181). New York: Thieme Medical Publishers.

Ruff, R. L., & Arbit, E. (1981). Aphemia resulting from a left frontal hematoma. *Neurology, 31,* 353–356.

Ryalls, J., & Scarfone, D. (1990). Some preliminary observations of voice characteristics in Broca's aphasia. *Journal of Neurolinguistics, 5,* 285–293.

Schalén, W., Hansson, L., Nordström, G., & Nordström, C.-H. (1994). Psychosocial outcome 5–8 years after severe traumatic brain lesions and the impact of rehabilitation services. *Brain Injury, 8,* 49–64.

Sears, E. S., Patten, J. P., & Fenstermacher, M. J. (1991). Diseases of the cranial nerves and brainstem. In R. N. Rosenberg (Ed.), *Comprehensive neurology* (pp. 779–816). New York: Raven Press.

Shea, B. R., Drummond, S. S., Metzer, W. S., & Krueger, K. M. (1993). Effect of selegiline on speech performance in Parkinson's disease. *Folia Phoniatrica et Logopaedica, 45,* 40–46.

Solomon, N. P., & Hixon, T. J. (1993). Speech breathing in Parkinson's disease. *Journal of Speech and Hearing Research, 36,* 294–310.

Stewart, C., Winfield, L., Hunt, A., Bressman, S. B., Fahn, S., Blitzer, A., & Brin, M. F. (1995). Speech dysfunction in early Parkinson's disease. *Movement Disorders, 10,* 562–565.

Theodoros, D. G., Murdoch, B. E., & Chenery, H. J. (1994). Perceptual speech characteristics of dysarthric speakers following severe closed head injury. *Brain Injury, 8,* 101–124.

Thumfart, W. F., Pototschnig, C., Zorowka, P. G., & Eckel, H. E. (1992). Electrophysiologic investigation of lower cranial nerve diseases by means of magnetically stimulated neuromyography of the larynx. *Annals of Otology, Rhinology and Laryngology, 101,* 629–634.

Tomoda, H., Shibasaki, H., Kuroda, Y., & Shin, T. (1987). Voice tremor: Dysregulation of voluntary expiratory muscles. *Neurology, 37,* 117–122.

Urban, P. P., Hopf, H. C., Zorowka, P. G., Fleischer, S., & Andreas, J. (1996). Dysarthria and lacunar stroke. Pathophysiologic aspects. *Neurology, 47,* 1135–1141.

Vogel, M. (1998). Behandlung der Dysarthrien. In W. Ziegler, M. Vogel, B. Gröne, & H. Schröter-Morasch (Eds.), *Dysarthrie. Grundlagen, Diagnostik, Therapie* (pp. 99–132). Stuttgart: Thieme-Verlag.

Vogel, M., & von Cramon, D. (1982). Dysphonia after traumatic midbrain damage: A follow-up study. *Folia Phoniatrica, 34,* 150–159.

Wade, D. T., Hewer, R. L., David, R. M., & Enderby, P. M. (1986). Aphasia after stroke: Natural history and associated deficits. *Journal of Neurology, Neurosurgery, and Psychiatry, 49,* 11–16.

Wildgruber, D., Ackermann, H., Klose, U., Kardatzki, B., & Grodd, W. (1996). Functional lateralization of speech production at primary motor cortex: A fMRI study. *NeuroReport, 7,* 2791–2795.

Willer, B., Abosch, S., & Dahmer, E. (1990). Epidemiology of disability from traumatic brain injury. In R. L. Wood (Ed.), *Neurobehavioural sequelae of traumatic brain injury* (pp. 18–33). New York: Taylor & Francis.

Yanagisawa, E. (1992). Physical examination of the larynx and videolaryngoscopy. In A. Blitzer, M. F. Brin, C. T. Sasaki, S. Fahn, & K. S. Harris (Eds.), *Neurologic disorders of the larynx* (pp. 82–97). New York: Thieme Medical Publishers.

Zealear, D. L., Hast, M. H., & Kurago, Z. (1985). Functional organization of the primary motor cortex controlling the face, tongue, jaw, and larynx in the monkey. In I. R. Titze & R. C. Scherer (Eds.), *Vocal fold physiology* (pp. 57–73). Denver: The Denver Center for the Performing Arts.

Ziegler, W., Kilian, B., & Deger, K. (1997). The role of the left mesial frontal cortex in fluent speech: Evidence from a case of left supplementary motor area hemorrhage. *Neuro-psychologia, 35,* 1197–1208.

CHAPTER 20

The Spasmodic Dysphonias

Michael P. Cannito and Gayle E. Woodson

Intermittent perceptible disruptions of ongoing phonation, or vocal spasms, that manifest as a primary presenting problem in connected speech constitute the core symptomatology of a group of related voice disorders known as the spasmodic dysphonias. Frequently, these events are marked by a brief cessation of phonation, or voice break (Zwirner, Murry, Swenson, & Woodson, 1991). They also are typically attended by a context of laryngealized (e.g., strained-strangled) or aspirate (e.g., breathy) phonatory perturbation (Cannito & Johnson, 1981). Individuals who routinely exhibit such phenomena in the absence of other distinguishable speech or voice disorders are by default diagnosed as having some form of spasmodic dysphonia. A number of additional spasmodic dysphonia characteristics enumerated by Aronson (1978) include "strained strangled voice, hoarseness, harshness, breathiness, excessively high pitch, and excessively low pitch" as well as "staccato or stuttering-like, intermittent, jerky, grunting, squeezed, groaning, and effortful" speech (pp. 553–554). Moreover, spasmodic dysphonia symptoms are reported to be exacerbated by situational stressors or other communicative challenges (e.g., speaking on the telephone) and to improve under specific phonatory conditions, such as speaking at high pitch, whispering, or producing nonspeech vocalizations such as laughing or crying (Aronson, 1990; C. S. Bloch, Hirano, & Gould, 1985). Over the years, spasmodic dysphonia has proven to be notoriously resistant to behavioral interventions (Boone & McFarlane, 1977; Heuer, 1992) and, as a result, a number of more invasive medical treatment options have been explored (Tucker, 1992). The phenomenon known today as spasmodic dysphonia was originally described by Traube in 1871 as a "spastic form of nervous hoarseness" and subsequently by Schnitzler in 1895 as "aphonia spastica" (Schaefer et al., 1985, p. 595). Athough early researchers tended to regard spasmodic dysphonia as a psychogenic phenomenon, in recent years neurological explanations have become more dominant (Schaefer, 1983). In 1968, Aronson and colleagues suggested that the then widely used term "spastic dysphonia" should be replaced by "spasmodic dysphonia" in order to differentiate this intermittent voice disorder from the type of dysphonia observed in association with pyramidal upper motor neuron lesions that typically occurs within a broader context of spastic dysarthria. Over the last 30 years this shift in terminology has been almost complete, reflecting the widely held contemporary view that spasmodic dysphonia is probably a focal hyperkinetic movement disorder of extrapyramidal origin (Cannito, 1991b; Cannito, Kondraske & Johns, 1991; Duffy, 1995). In the present literature review, the terms spastic dysphonia and spasmodic dysphonia are considered interchangeable, providing that the referent is clearly not the dysphonia of spastic dysarthria.

Despite a recent flurry of research interest, stemming largely from the advent of botulinum toxin (Botox) treatment procedures for spasmodic dysphonia, a number of significant clinical questions continue to be unresolved. There remains little consensus even among experts on the proper criteria for its differential diagnosis and clinical subclassification. Debate also persists as to whether spasmodic dysphonia is a unitary disorder or a heterogeneous collection of superficially similar disorders. The etiology of spasmodic dysphonia continues to be poorly understood and no definitive lesion loci or specific pathological process have yet been identified in the majority of cases. Moreover, the primary mode of treatment (i.e., Botox injection of intrinsic laryngeal musculature), although it has clearly benefited many patients with spasmodic dysphonia, may be considered to be largely a Band Aid solution in that it merely masks the symptoms temporarily rather than addressing underlying causation. Apart from these conundrums, or perhaps as a result of them, clinicians and researchers continue to be fascinated by the enigma that is spasmodic dysphonia, because it brings into sharp focus more basic questions regarding the relationship among the nervous system, emotion, and vocal behavior. In the present chapter, in addition to presenting research findings related to the nature, assessment, and treatment of spasmodic dysphonia, the current status of these persistent controversies is considered and important directions needed for future research are set forth.

1. SYMPTOMATOLOGY AND DIAGNOSTIC CRITERIA

There is as yet no bureau of standards for the diagnosis of spasmodic dysphonia. Consequently, even experts sometimes disagree on specific cases that may depart in some way from what is considered the classic symptom complex. Some studies rely solely on consensus of expert opinion for including participants in a spasmodic dysphonia sample, with others descrying the marked extent of heterogeniety found within the diagnosis of spasmodic dysphonia (Freeman, Cannito, & Finitzo-Hieber, 1985a). Building on existing literature, Cannito and Kondraske (1990) proposed the diagnostic criteria listed in Table 20–1, which they found to be useful and that have been employed in a number of subsequent studies (Cannito, 1991a; Cannito et al., 1997; Cannito, Ege, Ahmed, & Wagner, 1994; Cannito et al., 1991; Cannito, Kondraske, & Sussman, 1998). Although rigid adherence to fixed criteria is important for research, it should be recognized that in clinical practice not all of the criteria may apply in every case.

The first criterion, absence of perceptual symptoms of dysarthria, addresses that spasmodic dysphonia presents primarily as a disorder of phonation. Although the presence of movement disorders elsewhere in the body is not uncommon in individuals with spasmodic dysphonia, involvement of supralaryngeal vocal tract musculature resulting in salient motor disturbances of articulation and resonance would suggest a more generalized form of dysarthria rather than a true spasmodic dysphonia. Moreover, when the occurrence of abnormal articulatory movements have been noted in spasmodic dysphonia speech, these have usually been ascribed to incoordination of phonatory function with articulatory activity (Aronson, Brown, Litin, & Pearson, 1968; Free-

Table 20–1. Diagnostic criteria for spasmodic dysphonias.

I.	Absence of perceptual symptoms of the classical dysarthrias[a]
II.	Occasional moments of normal sounding voice
III.	Presence of intermittent breaks in voicing
IV.	Intermittent occurrence of strained-strangled dysphonia or breathy dysphonia
V.	Normal or near normal sounding whispered speech
VI.	Improved voice quality for nonspeech vocalizations
VII.	Improved voice quality for phonation at high pitch levels
VIII.	Reported worsening of dysphonia with increased situational stress

[a]This assumes that otolaryngological exam has ruled out structural pathology of the vocal folds and that neurological exam has ruled out symptomatic neurologic diseases such as Parkinson's or multiple sclerosis.

Note. Based on material in "Rapid Manual Abilities in Spasmodic Dysphonic and Normal Female Subjects," by M. P. Cannito and G. V. Kondraske, 1990. *Journal of Speech and Hearing Research, 33*, 123–133.

man et al., 1985a). Similarly, respiratory abnormalities are not characteristic of spasmodic dysphonia; however, respiratory patterns such as lung volumes employed for speaking or the distribution of inspiratory pauses may be altered secondary to the abnormal laryngeal behaviors (Sapienza, Cannito, & Erickson, 1996). The second criterion, occasional moments of normal sounding voice, refers to the intermittency of symptoms as a hallmark of the disorder. Phonatory spasms may be more or less frequent or more or less sustained in time, but they are not constant. Consequently, over the course of an in-depth interview, a clinician will observe at least a few and perhaps several occasions (however fleeting) of normal or near-normal sounding voice.

Third, the presence of intermittent breaks in voicing is almost definitional to the diagnosis of spasmotic dysphonia. Brief gaps may be demonstrated acoustically within or between syllables in phonetic contexts wherein continuous, modal, quasiperiodic voicing is expected to occur. Exceptions to this rule may be seen at the extremes of the severity continuum. In some very mild or incipient cases, vocal spasms tend to take the form of brief episodes of either fry phonation or breathy phonation without true cessation of voicing during ongoing speech. Conversely, in some profoundly impaired cases, the vocal spasms take the form of long silent intervals between words or phrases during which the speaker struggles at the level of the glottis to "get anything out" and may seem to glottalize, or "swallow," a number of syllables in the process.

The perceptible occurrence of intermittent dysphonia is the fourth criterion. Spasmodic dysphonia is typically characterized by inappropriate glottal configurations resulting from either abnormal adductory gestures of the vocal folds (termed adductor spasmodic dysphonia) or abnormal abductory gestures (termed abductor spasmodic dysphonia) or a combination of the two (termed mixed spasmodic dysphonia). These aberrant gestures may be either fleeting or sustained in time. Abnormal adduction resembles vocal fry, both perceptually and acoustically; however, rather than a true pulse register, in spasmodic dysphonia this phonatory pattern appears to be generated by excessive medial compression (over pressure) of the vocal folds that must be overcome via increased subglottal driving pressure. This abnormal type of laryngealized phonatory perturbation has been described perceptually as strained-strangled voice and is characterized by widely and irregularly spaced vertical striations representing glottal pulses in the acoustic spectrogram. Abnormal abduction results in occurrence of aspiration or glottal frication in inappropriate phonetic contexts (i.e., non /h/ or non [C^{h}V]), which may be generated either by widening of the glottis at times when the vocal folds should be adducted for ongoing phonation or by a delay in vocal fold adduction following an appropriate abductory gesture associated with production of a voiceless obstruent consonant. This abnormal type of aspirate phonatory perturbation is perceived either as intermittent breathiness, evident in the acoustic spectrogram as an inappropriate occurrence of voiced or voiceless /h/ segments within vowel nuclei, or as prolonged voice onset times following initial voiceless stops.

It is also possible for an individual with spasmodic dysphonia to exhibit both types of abnormal features to varying degrees. Although this mixed type of spasmodic dysphonia is considered by many to be less common than either the pure adductor or abductor types, it should be recognized that adductor spasms tend to be more perceptually salient and may mask the presence of cooccurring abductor spasmodic dysphonia. It has also been suggested that some individuals with mixed spasmodic dysphonia may truly exhibit bidirectional adventitious movements of the vocal folds, although in others these episodes may represent attempts to compensate for a primary deficit of the opposing type (Blitzer & Brin, 1992). Other authors have suggested that individuals with spasmodic dysphonia exhibit both adductor and abductor characteristics in differing proportions at different times, consequent to laryngeal dyskinesia and discoordination and that spasmodic dysphonia symptoms generally are distributed along a harshness-breathiness continuum rather than in binary categories (Cannito & Johnson, 1981; Freeman et al., 1985a; Hanson, Logemann, & Hain, 1992). There is currently a need for systematic research focusing specifically on the mixed form of spasmodic dysphonia and its response to treatment.

The fifth, sixth, and seventh criteria cover speaking conditions that ameliorate spasmodic dysphonia symptoms. Various authors have suggested that whispered spasmodic dysphonia speech is perceived clinically to be of normal or near-normal quality. This observation must be tempered, however, by acoustic evidence that whispered spasmodic dysphonia speech, although it does sound better, is frequently produced more slowly than the whispered speech of nondisabled controls (Cannito, Ege et al., 1994; Cannito, McSwain, & Dworkins 1996). The perceived contrast between whispered and phonated speech in spasmodic dysphonia is also helpful clinically for teasing apart the differential effects of spasmodic dysphonia versus supralaryngeal dysarthrias. Similarly, the phonation of individuals with spasmodic dysphonia is typically perceived to be more normal in the context of nonspeech vocalizations, such as laughing, crying, grunting, or sighing or in speech immediately adjacent to such vocalizations (Bloch et al., 1985; Freeman et al., 1985a). The percept of improved phonation at higher pitch levels, in comparison to modal or habitual pitch within a given patient, is also a widely held cornerstone of clinical lore (Aronson, 1990; Izdebski, 1992). However, the extent to which nonspeech vocalization and phonation at high pitch actually do improve or differ from those of nondisabled speakers has not been systematically documented in a significant sample of spasmodic dysphonia speakers.

The last criterion, a reported worsening of spasmodic dysphonia symptoms in association with increased situational stress, has also been noted by a number of clinicians (Rosenfield, 1988; Schaefer, 1983). In a recent study of responses of spasmodic dysphonia patients to the *Shortened Version of the Erickson Scale of Attitudes Toward Communication* (Andrews & Cutler, 1974), Cannito, Murry, and Woodson (1994) demonstrated that spasmodic dysphonia speakers exhibited significantly more negative attitudes than normal controls both before and following Botox intervention. For example, 78% of the spasmodic dysphonia sample were impaired on the item "Even the idea of giving a talk in public makes me afraid" and none improved following treatment. Findings such as these tend to support anecdotal stress-related observations; however, as yet there has been no direct evaluation of spasmodic dysphonia speech produced under conditions of differing degrees of situational stress.

In addition to criteria necessary to establish differential diagnosis and clinical subclassification, a number of additional or cooccurring voice and speech symptoms have been reported in association with spasmodic dysphonia. These include a variety of acoustic and physiological aberrations of phonatory function, the frequent presence of associated voice tremor, as well as abnormalities of speaking rate, prosody, and fluency. Reports of abnormal phonatory function in spasmodic dysphonia have included significantly increased electromyographic activity in various intrinsic laryngeal muscles while speaking, including the thyroarytenoid, posterior cricoarytenoid, interarytenoid, and crichothyroid, for all types of spasmodic dysphonia (Ludlow, Hallet, Sedory, Fujita, & Naunton, 1990; Ludlow, Naunton, Terada, & Anderson, 1991; Roark, Dowling, DeGroat, Watson, & Schaefer, 1995; Shipp, Izdebski, Reed, & Morrisey, 1985; Watson, McIntire, Roark, & Schaefer, 1995; Watson et al.,1991). Phonatory airflow rates are decreased in adductor spasmodic dysphonia but increased in abductor spasmodic dysphonia (Merson & Ginsberg, 1979; Zwirner, Murry, Swenson, & Woodson, 1992).

Acoustic analyses of fundamental frequency and harmonic structure in both adductor and abductor spasmodic dysphonia indicate that a wide variety of parameters are abnormal (Cannito et al., 1996; Ludlow & Conner, 1987; Ludlow et al., 1991; Rontal, Rontal et al., 1991; Zwirner et al., 1992). These include decreased range of vocal intensity, increased shimmer and jitter, increased standard deviation of F_0, increased percentage of aperiodic phonation, and decreased harmonic-to-noise ratio. Mean fundamental frequency, however, has not been found to differ from that of normal controls.

The phenomenon of vocal tremor, most evident on sustained phonation, has been observed repeatedly in association with both adductor and abductor spasmodic dysphonia (Aronson & Hartman, 1981; Hartman & Aronson, 1981; Rosenfield, 1988). These repetitive fluctuations in the acoustic waveform may manifest as amplitude tremor, most prominently demonstrated on an acoustic intensity contour, or frequency tremor, most prominently demonstrated on an acoustic fundamental frequency track or narrow band spectrogram (Freeman, Cannito, & Finitzo-Hieber, 1985a). The dominant tremor frequency tends to occur in a range from 4 to 7 cycles per second and is similar to that generally associated with abnormal postural tremor (Hartman, Abbs, & Vishwanat, 1988). Some investigators have interpreted these low frequency oscillations in the acoustic waveform as benign essential voice tremor being a cause of spasmodic dysphonia, wherein the perceived spasms may represent extreme fluctuations in the depth of the tremor cycles (Aronson et al., 1968). Others have interpreted them as concomitant symptoms of laryngeal dystonia (Cannito, 1991b). It is possible that both tremor variants exist. Moreover, there may be other tremor frequencies of interest in addition to the dominant frequency of oscillation (Hartelius, Buder, & Strand, 1997). Additional systematic research on the nature of tremors associated with spasmodic dysphonia is important because it may be a prognostic factor on response to treatment, although results of recent studies have proven to be equivocal (Ludlow, Bagley, Yin, & Koda, 1992; Whurr et al., 1993).

In addition to voice quality alterations, the occurrence of spasmodic dysphonia may have marked detrimental consequences for the smooth, continuous forward flow of connected speech (Adams, 1982). Temporally based abnormalities affecting the rate and rhythms of speech production have been among the most frequently and consistently reported characteristics of spasmodic dysphonia speech, irrespective of type. Acoustic evidence of temporal prolongation of spasmodic dysphonia speech included increased duration of sentences, words, syllables, intersyllabic intervals, and phonetic segments (Cannito & Johnson, 1981; Cannito et al., 1996; Freeman et al., 1985a; Ludlow, Nauton, Sedory, Schulz, & Hallett, 1988; Ludlow et al., 1991; Merson & Ginsberg, 1979). Wolfe, Ratusnik, and Feldman (1979) reported abnormalities in perceived speaking effort, syllable stress, and rhythm of speech, in addition to the perceived phonatory attributes of extreme pitch change, monotone, hoarseness, harshness, and strained-strangled voice. Moreover, they suggested that these perceptual features were distributed along a severity continuum. These researchers also demonstrated acoustically that there is a neutralization of stressed versus unstressed syllables in spasmodic dysphonia that contributed to perceived dysprosody.

Numerous researchers have suggested that spasmodic dysphonia is a disorder of fluency as well as voice (Adams, 1982; Aronson et al., 1968; Luchsinger, & Arnold, 1965; McCall, 1974; Silverman & Hummer, 1989); however, little direct evidence is available to support this claim. One recent study empirically examined the hypothesis that dysfluency is an integral component of spasmodic dysphonia using a combination of perceptual scaling of dysfluency, frequency counting of dysfluency behavior, and temporal acoustic analysis of the connected speech of 20 speakers with spasmodic dysphonia and matched nondysphonic controls (Cannito et al., 1997). Spasmodic dysphonia speech was found to be significantly more dysfluent than controls on all types of fluency related measures except reading errors. Moreover, more than three-fourths of the variability in perceived dysfluency was explained by a linear combination of objective fluency measures. Lastly, all fluency-related measures were predictive of independent clinical ratings of severity of spasmodic dysphonia. These results were consistent across spasmodic dysphonic subclassifications by type of vocal spasm and voice tremor. Importantly, however, 25% of the spasmodic dysphonia speakers were not found to be dysfluent. These findings suggest that dysfluency is not definitional in the diagnosis of spasmodic dysphonia, but that it is a primary determinant of clinical ratings of severity. Unlike developmental stuttering, abnormal dysfluencies in spasmodic dysphonia typically occurred in close association with episodes of severely aberrant voice quality, which implies a common underlying physiological mechanism.

Temporal and fluency-related aspects of spasmodic dysphonia also may be important treatment variables. Behavioral fluency therapy approaches have been applied to spasmodic dysphonia, with modest success in two case studies (Cannito, 1991b; Meyers & Anderson, 1985). In addition, reports in the literature suggest that Botox treatment enhances speaking rate and fluency in spasmodic dysphonia (Blitzer, Brin, Fahn, & Lovelace, 1988b; Ford, Bless, & Patel, 1992; Ludlow et al., 1988; Ludlow et al., 1991). Cannito, Woodson, Murry, and Newman (1996) have demonstrated that change in temporal acoustic measures accounts for a significant proportion of the variance in perceived improvement of overall speech quality following Botox intervention in adductor spasmodic dysphonia.

2. ETIOLOGICAL CONSIDERATIONS

The precise etiology of spasmodic dysphonia remains unknown. This is true both in terms of immediate causation and the underlying site of neurologic lesion or disease process. Historically, spasmodic dysphonia was regarded as a psychogenic disorder, wherein some psychic conflict becomes somatized to the laryngeal sphincter (Arnold, 1959; P. Bloch, 1965; Brodnitz, 1976; Heaver, 1959). Direct psychological testing, however, failed to differentiate individuals with spasmodic dysphonia from a more general hospital population (Aronson et al., 1968). Although individuals with spasmodic dysphonia, as a group, do appear to be more anxious and depressed than typical (Cannito, 1991a), they probably are not any more so than other individuals who suffer from chronic debilitating illness. Studies of psychological improvement following recurrent laryngeal nerve (RLN) resection and Botox injection of the vocal folds appear to support the exogenous or reactive nature of the affective disturbance in the majority of cases (Cannito et al., 1994; Ginsberg, Wallack, Srain, & Biller, 1988; Murry, Cannito, & Woodson, 1994). It also should be recognized, however, that psychogenic versions of spasmodic dysphonia, perhaps from stress reaction or conversion disorder, do occasionally occur and may remit spontaneously or as a result of psychologically oriented therapy (Aronson, 1990; Chevrie-Muller, Arabia Guidet, & Pfauwadel, 1987; Sapir, 1993). Such cases typically acquire a retrospective diagnosis of psychogenic spasmodic dysphonia. Unfortnately, clear-cut criteria for prospective diagnostic differentiation of these cases from nonpsychogenic forms of spasmodic dysphonia have not been forthcoming in the literature.

In recent years, the notion that spasmodic dysphonia is a laryngeal dystonia has gained widespread clinical acceptance (Blitzer & Brin, 1992). This view has been predicated on physiological documentation of spasmodic laryngeal activity (Blitzer et al., 1988a; Ludlow & Connor, 1987; Ludlow et al., 1990), documentation of abnormal motor functions external to the larynx (Aminoff, Dedo, & Izdebski, 1978; Cannito & Kondraske, 1990; Cannito et al., 1990; Cohen et al., 1989; Rosenfield et al., 1991), other neurophysiological observations such as brain imaging studies (Finitzo & Freeman, 1989), and the favorable response of spasmodic dyphonia to Botox intervention. Along with the dystonia interpretation of spasmodic dysphonia, has come, by implication, a certain amount of intellectual baggage. This includes the interpretation that spasmodic dysphonia must result, like other dystonias, from an impairment of the basal ganglia system. Further, to the extent that some dystonias are inherited, the notion that spasmodic dysphonia may be a genetic disorder has also emerged. However, it must be recognized explicitly that no hard evidence to date has localized the underlying pathology of spasmodic dysphonia to the basal ganglia or any other specific lesion site in a majority of cases—nor is a familial history of spasmodic dysphonia, voice tremor, or movement disorders elsewhere in the body characteristic of the majority of cases. Spasmodic dysphonia has also been described as an action-induced or function-specific dystonia, similar to dystonic writers' cramp (Marsden, 1976); however, some authors report occurrence of abnormal laryngeal motor function during quiet breathing as well as during voice production (Ludlow et al., 1990; Woodson, Zwirner, Murry, & Swenson, 1991).

Clearly, a substantial body of evidence that spasmodic dysphonia is a neuromotor disorder has accumulated over the last few decades. Proposed lesion loci have spanned virtually the entire nervous system from peripheral motor and sensory nerve fibers to the cerebral cortex. Cannito (1991b) carefully reviewed existing literature to support a probable site of neurologic lesion. Any neurological model of spasmodic dysphonia, he posited, must be able to account for its apparent focality, function specificity, heterogeneity, intermittency, and affect sensitivity. It was concluded that spasmodic dysphonia is not a peripheral but a central nervous system disorder—that it is probably supranuclear, involving motor control elements above the level of the hindbrain lower motor neuron pools and that it is probably not of limbic system origin. Beyond that, there is some converging evidence that the locus of abnormality in spasmodic dysphonia may be cerebral (i.e., involving cortical, subcortical white matter, or basal ganglia components). Available evidence, however, does not entirely rule out rostral brain stem elements that participate in sensorimotor control loops with the basal ganglia, cerebellum, and cerebral cortex.

Whether spasmodic dysphonia is, in fact, a classical dystonia remains unclear. Whereas classical definitions of dystonia emphasized that the contractions were sustained in time, often over several seconds, more recent usage includes rapid repetitive contractions of single or adjacent muscle groups that do not flow randomly from one body part to another (Jankovic & Fahn, 1993). Both sustained glottal squeezing and fleeting spasms that alternate with normal voicing may occur in spasmodic dysphonia. Moreover, an extensive amount of heterogeneity in speech and nonspeech symptoms seems to characterize the population (Davis, Boone, Carroll, Darveniza, & Harrison, 1988; Pool et al., 1991). Consequently, some authors have suggested that spasmodic dysphonia is a *symptom complex* rather than a specific disorder and that the underlying etiology may vary across individuals (Aronson et al., 1968). In a reanalysis of Darley, Aronson, and Brown's (1975) perceptual study of the dysarthrias, Cannito (1991b) found the phonatory characteristics of spasmodic dysphonia to be most similar to those of pseudobulbar palsy, dystonia, and Huntington's chorea, but less similar to ALS, Parkinson disease, cerebellar ataxia, and bulbar palsy. Hanson et al. (1992) suggested that spasmodic dysphonia may be associated with functional disorders, dystonia, essential tremor, other forms of tremor, myoclonus, chorea, athetosis, progressive supranuclear diseases, and mixed neurological diseases. Rosenfield et al. (1990) reported a series of 100 consecutive cases in which 71% exhibited an underlying essential tremor, 25% had Meige syndrome, 12% had hypothyroidism, and 27% had either a functional disturbance or focal dystonia. These authors suggest that it would be preferable to address the differing underlying causes of the spasmodic dysphonia symptoms rather than restricting the nomenclature to exclude all but a single and as yet poorly understood etiology (i.e., focal laryngeal dystonia). Until such issues have been sorted out, it seems more prudent to regard neurogenic spasmodic dysphonia as a heterogeneous group of idiopathic focal laryngeal hyperkinesias of probable supranuclear origin.

3. ASSESSMENT OF SPASMODIC DYSPHONIA

The assessment of spasmodic dysphonia is a multidisciplinary endeavor. The collaborative interaction of speech-language pathology and otolaryngology is essential; however, in some cases neurology and psychiatry or psychology also should be actively involved. Swenson, Zwirner, Murry, and Woodson (1992) suggest that neurological consultation is appropriate when there is evidence of movement disorders external to the larynx or when there is suspicion that the laryngeal symptoms may be the presenting manifestation of a symptomatic neurological disorder such as Parkinson's disease or multiple sclerosis. Cannito (1991a) suggests that, for individuals who continue to exhibit high levels of depression and anxiety during treatment, it will be difficult to realize significant lasting gains in behavioral voice therapy. Similarly, if individuals remain clinically anxious and depressed after Botox treatment, the degree or duration of voice improvement may lag (Murry et al., 1994). Moreover, the occurrence of spasmodic dysphonia may harm self-esteem, family relationships, and occupational status of the afflicted individual (Freeman et al., 1985b). For any of these reasons, consultation of an appropriate mental health professional may be warranted. In addition to the clinical interview, the use of standardized psychometric tests such as the *State-Trait Anxiety Inventory* (Spielberger, Gorusch, Luschene, Vagg, & Jacobs, 1983) and the *Self-Rating of Depression Scale* (Zung, 1967) may be useful in determining the need for such referral.

The history and physical examination, typically completed by an otolaryngologist, provide the first line of medical evaluation for most individuals with spasmodic dysphonia. If the physical examination reveals other neurological signs, neurological consultation is indicated and selected laboratory tests can be ordered at that time (Swenson et al., 1992). Flexible videolaryngoscopy is routinely performed, as it permits dynamic visualization of the larynx during sustained vowel phonation, as well as connected speech, singing, and quiet breathing (Woodson, Zwirner, Murry, & Swenson, 1992). Visualization of supralaryngeal structures including the velum may also be accomplished as needed in specific cases (Lundy, Casiano, Lu, & Xue, 1996). Table 20–2 lists major intrinsic and extrinsic laryngeal endoscopic features of interest in spasmodic dysphonia assessment (Woodson et al., 1991). Positive physical signs supporting the diagnosis of spasmodic dysphonia include tremor in the larynx, soft palate, or pharynx, as well as observable spasms of the larynx during speech and/or quiet breathing. Tremor of the soft palate is most easily detected during sustained phonation of the vowel /i/. Although spasms are pathognomic of spasmodic dysphonia, visible tremor is not present in all patients. The status of the thyroarytenoid muscles (TA) also should be assessed, as patients with such muscle atrophy have greater side effects with lower doses of Botox. Abductor spasms are most apparent during speech tasks in which the patient switches from a voiceless plosive or an /h/ to a vowel. The arytenoid cartilages tend to "hang up" laterally just after release of the consonant, delaying onset of the voiced portion of the syllable.

Although sophisticated analysis of EMG signals may be used to document inappropriate levels of EMG activity in the majority of spasmodic dysphonia patients (Blitzer, Loveless,

Brin, Fahn, & Fink, 1985), routine qualitative or quantitative analysis does not reveal any specific patterns that are characteristic of the condition. However, for patients in whom Botox is ineffective or is losing its efficacy, EMG may be helpful in elucidating the problem (Woodson, 1994). Temporary RLN blockade also is not recommended in routine pretreatment evaluation for Botox. Because the effects of focal denervation (Botox injection) may be quite different from complete unilateral paralysis (nerve block), the results may be misleading. RLN blockade may be useful, however, in evaluating patients who do not respond to Botox.

The evaluation of speech and voice characteristics is typically completed by a speech-language pathologist. This should include a thorough speech mechanism examination (Cannito et al., 1991) and a hearing screening. Informal evaluation of speech and language characteristics are completed during a clinical interview to rule out the presence of other potentially confounding communicative disorders. Vocal elicitation procedures should address a wide range of tasks to explore the relative occurrence of spasmodic dysphonia behaviors in a variety of phonatory contexts (Izdebski, 1992). These include sustained vowels /i/ and /a/ at habitual, low, and high pitches, plus at varying intensity levels; glissando /a/, a spontaneous speech sample (e.g., Job Task); a reading passage (e.g., first paragraph of The Rainbow Passage); reading or repeating phonetically controlled sentences (all vocalic, voiced, voiced-voiceless, and /h/ loaded) that are produced both with phonation and while whispering; and production of phonated and whispered diadochokinetic syllable trains (Cannito, 1991a). Because many individuals with spasmodic dysphonia mask their underlying spasms by means of compensatory strategies (e.g., whispering, inspiratory, falsetto, or buccal speech), the clinician must help such individuals to avoid these compensations and allow their natural voice breaks to emerge (Freeman et al., 1985a). In addition, potentially facilitative nonspeech vocalizations including yawning, coughing, laughing, singing, and paralanguage are elicited. Based on perceptual analysis of all of these activities, a judgment is made as to whether the observed disorder is consistent with a diagnosis of spasmodic dysphonia (see Table 20–1). If so, it should be further subclassified on the basis of predominant type of vocal spasms, overall severity, and the presence or absence of vocal tremor (Freeman et al., 1985a). Diagnostic subclassifications are summarized in Table 20–3. Used in conjunction with Tables 20–1, 20–2, and 20–3, the Appendix to this chapter provides a convenient checklist for such an evaluation (Cannito, 1986). A notable effort toward standardization of the perceptual assessment of adductor spasmodic dysphonia was recently reported by Stewart et al. (1997).

The perceptual evaluation of spasmodic dysphonia may be supported with a variety of instrumental assessments of phonatory function (Woodson et al., 1992). These include acoustical

Table 20–2. Laryngeal videoendoscopic features for assessment of spasmodic dysphonia.

I. Excessive phonatory activation of intrinsic laryngeal muscles[a]
    A. Excessive arytenoid adduction
    B. Excessive arytenoid abduction
    C. Vocal fold rigidity
II. Extrinsic muscle hyperfunction[b]
    A. Degree of false vocal fold closure
    B. Extent of anterior posterior compression
III. Tremor with phonation and at rest[c]
IV. Presence of spasmodic movements during respiration[c]

[a] glottal characteristics
[b] supraglottal characteristics
[c] either glottal or supraglottal characteristics

analysis of standard deviation of F_0, harmonic-to-noise ratio, and voice break factor (Zwirner et al., 1992), as well as aerodynamic analysis of phonatory airflow and pressure (Witsell, Weissler, Donovon, Howard, Martinkosky et al., 1994; Woo, Colton, Casper, & Brewer, 1992), during sustained vowel production. Such measures are not used to diagnose the disorder, but to quantify severity, to aid in determining whether an injection should be unilateral or bilateral, and to establish the optimal dose (Woodson, 1994). Because Botox intervention is typically an ongoing process wherein phonatory response to treatment may vary over the long term, ongoing assessment of phonatory function is also recommended as an adjunct to patient self-reports.

4. TREATMENT OF SPASMODIC DYSPHONIA

Behavioral approaches to treatment, including psychotherapy and speech therapy, are rarely effective in patients with moderate to severe spasmodic dysphonia. Some patients achieve success in ameliorating symptoms with speech therapy regimens, but treatment is intensive, requiring strong commitment from both patient and therapist (Cooper, 1980). In the early stages of spasmodic dysphonia, however, voice therapy often serves to reduce the severity of spasms under certain speaking conditions. Voice therapy is also helpful as an adjunct to surgery or pharmacological therapy (Rosenfield, 1991).

Voice therapy for adductor spasmodic dysphonia is directed at reducing the tightness in the laryngeal area. One approach that has been reported to be effective is the use of inverse phonation. In this technique, patients are taught to phonate during inspiration (Freeman et al., 1985a). Spasms are far less likely to occur during this mode of phonation, presumably because it is a profoundly different motor task. Some patients are able to use inverse phonation as the primary means of communication, with others able to generalize the glottic relaxation achieved by this technique to expiratory speech. Other approaches include the use of a whisper voice, continuous airflow, establishing easy voice onset, using /h/ onset, and speaking with an overall higher pitch.

Table 20–3. Diagnostic subclassification of spasmodic dysphonias.

I. Predominant type of phonatory spasm
   A. Adductor type
   B. Abductor type
   C. Mixed (adductor-abductor) type
II. Severity of dysphonia
   A. Normal (clinical rating = 0)[a]
   B. Mild (clincal rating = 1)
   C. Moderate (clinical rating = 2)
   D. Severe (clinical rating = 3)
   E. Profound (clinical rating = 4)
III. Audible voice tremor
   A. Voice tremor absent
   B. Voice tremor present
IV. Putative etiology
   A. Idiopathic
   B. Neurogenic
   C. Psychogenic

[a] This category may be observed following successful treatment in some individuals

Voice therapy for abductor spasmodic dysphonia employs a "continuous voicing" technique. Patients are taught to maintain phonation during normally unvoiced consonants (e.g., /p/ becomes /b/ and /s/ becomes /z/) and to maintain weak vocal fold vibration between syllables (Greene & Mathieson, 1989; Heuer, 1992). This avoids the sudden onsets and offsets of voicing that provoke many of the spasms in abductor spasmodic dysphonia. Rate reduction, particularly syllable prolongation, is sometimes beneficial for both types of spasmodic dysphonia as it allows for additional time for the patient to coordinate phonatory gestures with respiration and articulation.

Dedo reported the dramatic beneficial effects of surgical transection, which paralyzes one side of the larynx (Dedo, 1976). The goal of this procedure for spasmodic dysphonia is to relieve glottic tightness, so that less effort is required to speak. Although speech is more fluent after the surgery, there are variable degrees of breathiness and, in some patients, the voice is quite weak. The initial success rate of RLN section was reported as 92%, but with increasing experience, it became apparent that the failure rate was higher, and that recurrent symptoms were often worse than the original presentation. One series reported a recurrence rate of 64% within 3 years (Aronson & De Santo, 1983). Dedo reported a recurrence rate of 15% and felt that his success rate was related to patient selection criteria (Dedo, 1990; Dedo & Izdebski, 1983). He has also suggested adjunctive procedures to improve results, including Teflon injection for glottal incompetence and vocal fold thinning for recurrent spasticity.

Modifications of RLN section have been suggested in an effort to improve results. Laryngeal nerve crush initially showed some promise, but the sustained success rate was only 13% (Biller, Som, & Lawson, 1983). Transection of only the adductor branch of the RLN has been reported, but only limited data are available regarding the outcome of this procedure (Carpenter, Snyder, & Henley-Cohn, 1981). Netterville studied patients with recurrent spasms after RLN section and found strong evidence that recurrent symptoms resulted from nerve regeneration (Netterville, Stone, Rainey, Zealear, & Ossoff, 1991). To decrease the chance of regeneration, he proposed recurrent nerve avulsion, wherein the nerve is pulled forcefully from the larynx and a large segment of nerve is resected. Using this technique, 13 of 18 patients retained benefit after 3 years, but 6 required vocal fold medialization for breathiness (Weed et al., 1996). Despite its shortcomings, RLN surgery is a viable option for some patients with severe spasm, particularly when frequent Botox injections are required to maintain phonatory control. When, for whatever reason, the patient prefers a permanent surgical solution, RLN avulsion is preferred to RLN section.

Other surgical approaches to the treatment of adductor spasmodic dysphonia have been proposed, but are not widely used. Laryngeal framework surgery has been used to decrease tension in the vocal folds (Tucker, 1989). The anterior thyroid cartilage is incised to create a superiorly based flap containing the anterior commissure. This flap is displaced posteriorly to relax the vocal fold. Despite early encouraging results, the procedure is not widely used. Many patients developed recurrent symptoms and attempts at surgical reversal have been extremely difficult. An implantable RLN stimulator was reported to be effective in 5 patients, but long-term outcome and safety are not known (Friedman, Toriumi, Grybaukas, & Applebaum, 1989). More recently, resection of a portion of the thyroarytenoid muscle has been proposed as a treatment for adductor spasmodic dysphonia (Genack, Woo, Colton, & Goyette, 1993).

Currently, Botox is widely considered to be the treatment of choice for spasmodic dysphonia (Blitzer et al., 1988b; Ludlow et al., 1988; Miller, Woodson, & Jankovic, 1987). Numerous studies have documented significant improvements in spasmodic dysphonia symptoms following injection using a variety of physiological, acoustic, and perceptual measurement techniques (Ford et al., 1992; Ludlow et al., 1990; Ludlow et al., 1991; Rontal et al., 1991; Whurr et al., 1993; Witsell et al., 1994; Woodson et al., 1991; Zwirner et al., 1992). Botox induces focal muscle paralysis by blocking the release of acetylcholine from neuromuscular junction (Simpson, 1992). Recovery of function requires several weeks. This therapy is particularly effective in patients with adductor spasmodic dysphonia. Injections of Botox into the thyroarytenoid muscles reduce the incidence and intensity of adductor spasms. Botox can also be effective in some patients with abductor spasmodic dysphonia, using injections into the posterior cricoarytenoid or cricothyroid muscle (Blitzer, Brin, Stewart, Aviv, & Fahn, 1992; Ludlow et al., 1991; Rontal et al., 1991). However, the success rate of Botox is much lower in patients with the abductor form of spasmodic dysphonia.

Although the voice of a patient with adductor spasmodic dysphonia typically is vastly improved by Botox therapy, the treatment does not completely restore normal function. The voice is often quite breathy for the first 2 weeks after injection and in a few patients may remain weak and breathy for the duration of the therapeutic effect. Even in patients with an optimal response, voice projection is reduced and singing is impaired. Many patients complain of minor alterations in swallowing for the first week or two. Further, the beneficial results are temporary, lasting from 4 to 12 months. Nonetheless, the injections and the side effects are usually very well tolerated, and patients report that the benefits outweigh the minor morbidity. The optimal dose of Botox varies among patients and systematic clinical evaluation is required to identify the proper treatment protocol. Patients with severe and frequent spasm require larger doses than patients with mild or intermittent problems, although patients with vocal fold atrophy have greater side effects with lower doses of Botox.

The earliest technique for injecting Botox into the larynx was percutaneous, using EMG guidance, and this is still widely used. This technique causes minimal patient discomfort and allows for objective confirmation that the injector needle is in active muscle tissue. Alternative approaches include transoral injection using a long, curved needle and visualizing the larynx with a mirror or endoscope, and injecting via the working channel of a fiberoptic endoscope (Ford, Bless, & Lowery, 1989; Rhew, Fiedler, & Ludlow, 1994). Transoral and endoscopic approaches cause more discomfort and require local anesthesia of the mouth, throat, and larynx. The endoscopic injection requires two clinicians, an endoscopist and a person doing the injecting. Further, the injection systems have a considerable volume of dead space, so that dose delivery is less accurate and some toxin is wasted. Irrespective of the injection method employed, Botox treatment is highly effective for adductor spasmodic dysphonia. However, Botox is less successful in patients with abductor spasmodic dysphonia. In patients with mixed spasmodic dysphonia, treatment of adductor spasms can unmask abductor spasms, resulting in unacceptable amount of breathiness. Thus, it is important to evaluate the patient carefully before initiating therapy.

The major clinical question in managing patients with adductor spasmodic dysphonia is not whether or not Botox is likely to work, but how much toxin should be used, and whether injection should be unilateral or bilateral. Both unilateral and bilateral injection can eliminate voice breaks, but there are significant differences. Bilateral injection requires a smaller total dose to achieve the same clinical effect (S. G. Adams, Hung, Charles, & Lang, 1993). Using the American preparation of toxin (Botox, Allergan), injection of 1.25 units into each TA muscle is therapeutically equivalent to a unilateral injection of 10 to 15 units (Woodson, 1994). However, bilateral injection is generally associated with more pronounced side effects of breathiness and swallowing problems, particularly in the first 2 weeks after injection (Zwirner, Murry, & Woodson, 1993; Maloney & Morrison, 1994). As 1.25 units is practically the lowest dose that can be reliably delivered, unilateral injection permits the use of a wider therapeutic range, so that one-side injections of 1.25 to 10–15 units may be used. For mild or intermittent symptoms, unilateral injection of 1.25 to 2.5 units is generally effective. For moderate symptoms, unilateral injection of 5 to 10 units is usually required. Patients with significant or severe spasmodic dysphonia require bilateral treatment of 1.25 to 2.5 units per side.

The optimal treatment effect is a smooth voice with no breaks and normal airflow for at least 16 weeks benefit. If there is excessive breathiness, or if side effects persist for more than 2 weeks, the dose should be reduced for the next injection. Dose increase is indicated if there is only a brief improvement or if voice breaks persist. Treatment should be repeated when symptoms reappear. The duration of effect often increases with sequential injections and voice therapy improves the voice and prolongs the duration of benefits.

Results of Botox therapy for abductor spasmodic dysphonia are disappointing when compared to the results achieved for the adductor type. Slightly more than half of the patients with abductor spasmodic dysphonia respond significantly to Botox. A major problem is that weakening of the posterior cricoarytenoid muscle (PCA) reduces the capacity of the glottis to open during inspiration. Sometimes the amount of weakness required to eliminate spasms results in airway compromise. Many patients are willing to accept some degree of exercise intolerance in exchange for a smoother voice, but stridor during moderate activity is unacceptable. Another issue is that the pathophysiology of abductor spasmodic dysphonia appears to differ from that of the adductor type. Not only do patients have abductor muscle spasm, but there is also diminished TA contraction during phonation. Thus, even when abductor spasms are eliminated, there may still be glottal insufficiency and a breathy voice.

Injection of Botox into the PCA muscles is intended to suppress abductor spasm and decrease phonatory airflow. In almost all abductor spasmodic dysphonia patients, abductor spasms are asymmetric, with a larger amplitude of abductor spasm on one side. This side should be injected with sufficient toxin to abolish the abductor spasms, usually from 5 to 10 units and occasionally as high as 20 units. This will markedly reduce abduction during forced inspiration. Unilateral injection is not often sufficient for controlling symptoms, as small amplitude spasms persist in the nondominant or less spasmodic side, but to avoid airway compromise this dose should be small (i.e., 1.25 units).

The PCA muscle may be injected percutaneously by rotating the larynx. The position of the carotid artery should be carefully monitored during needle insertion. An alternate approach is to pass the needle through the anterior cricothyroid space, across the airway, and through the posterior lamina of the cricoid cartilage. This requires endoscopic guidance. With either technique, the position in the PCA is confirmed by detecting EMG activity when the patient sniffs. When Botox is ineffective for abductor spasmodic dysphonia, then surgical procedures to medialize the vocal fold should be considered, such as Type I thyroplasty or vocal fold injection with fat or collagen. Thyroplasty is more precise and results in a long-term solution. To judge the likelihood of success, a trial of Gelfoam injection is recommended prior to any permanent medialization.

Clinicians have also begun to explore the use of combined treatment modalities. Murry and Woodson (1995) demonstrated that the duration of benefit from Botox may be increased in adductor spasmodic dysphonia by the use of adjunctive voice therapy. The average time between injections exhibited by a Botox only group ($N = 10$) was 15 weeks, in comparison to an average time of 27 weeks in the Botox plus voice therapy group ($N = 17$). Acoustic and aerodynamic analyses demonstrated that although the two groups did not differ from each other prior to treatment, there were statistically significant differences in favor of the Botox plus voice therapy group following treatment. Adjunctive medical therapy with baclofen in addition to Botox injection may also prolong benefits and decrease the amplitude of associated tremor. The use of combined modalities offers a promising direction for future treatment efficacy research. Behavioral treatment in conjunction with orally administered pharmacotherapy has also been reported (Cannito, 1991b; Rosenfield, 1991).

5. CONCLUSIONS AND DIRECTIONS FOR RESEARCH

An extraordinary amount of research has been conducted on the topic of spasmodic dysphonia over the past several decades. Perceptual, acoustic, and physiologic data have been provided to document the phonatory and other clinical characteristics of the disorder. Tentative diagnostic criteria have been developed and some progress has been made toward elaborating the neurological and psychological concomitants. A variety of treatment options have been explored with relative degrees of success, the most current of which is Botox injection of the intrinsic laryngeal muscles, alone or in combination with behavioral voice therapy.

Despite many advances in assessment and treatment, from the foregoing review it must be concluded that there remains much to learn about the underlying nature, evaluation and management of spasmodic dysphonia. Of particular value would be a universally accepted set of diagnostic criteria that clearly differentiates spasmodic dysphonia from other voice disorders and from the dysarthrias. Additional systematic comparisons of the similarities and differences among the putative subcategories of abductor, adductor, and mixed spasmodic dysphonias, versus the alternative continuum hypothesis are also warranted. It is possible that other classification taxonomies may prove to be more clinically relevant. Further research regarding etiologies may eventually elucidate the neural substrates of spasmodic laryngeal activity and the pathophysiology from which it is derived. Recent advances in brain imaging technology that provide an opportunity to examine neural structure and function during on line activation tasks such as speaking (see, for example, Ingham et al., 1996) will be of particular importance.

From a management perspective, the study of prognostic indicators of response to medical treatment as well as functional outcomes research is currently needed. Botox treatment is both costly and ongoing and may not be the most cost-effective strategy in some specific types of cases. Also needed is additional research regarding the differentiation of functional or psychogenic cases, who may benefit from behavioral therapies, from more organically based etiologies requiring direct medical intervention. Moreover, the long-term efficacy of combined therapies that may prolong the effects of Botox and assist patients in adjusting to their ongoing "peaks and valleys" over the long-term course of this form of management remain to be systematically explored. It is hoped that the information synthesized in this chapter will stimulate such activity and lead to an improved outlook for patients afflicted with the spasmodic dysphonias.

Acknowledgments

Preparation of this chapter was supported by a grant from the National Institutes of Health (NIDCD Area Grant 1-R15-DC/OD02299-01A1). The authors gratefully acknowledge University of Memphis doctoral students Brenda Bender and Richard Dressler for their assistance in the development of the reference list.

REFERENCES

Adams, M. (1982). Fluency, non-fluency, and stuttering in children. *Journal of Fluency Disorders, 7,* 171–185.

Adams, S. G., Hung, E. J., Charles, D. A., & Lang, A. E. (1993). Unilateral versus bilateral botulinum toxin injections in spasmodic dysphonia: Acoustic and perceptual results. *Journal of Otolaryngology, 22,* 171–175.

Aminoff, M. J., Dedo, H. H., & Izdebski, K. (1978). Clinical aspects of spasmodic dysphonia. *Journal of Neurology, Neurosurgery, & Psychiatry, 41,* 361–365.

Andrews, G., & Cutler, J. (1974). Stuttering therapy: The relation between changes in symptom level and attitudes. *Journal of Speech and Hearing Disorders, 39,* 312–319.

Arnold, G. E. (1959). Spastic dysphonia: I. Changing interpretations of persistent affliction. *Logos, 2,* 3–14.

Aronson, A. E. (1978). Differential diagnosis of organic and psychogenic voice disorders. In F. L. Darley & D. C. Spriestersbach (Eds.), *Diagnostic methods in speech pathology* (2nd ed., pp. 535–560). New York: Harper & Row.

Aronson, A. E. (1990). *Clinical voice disorders: An interdisciplinary approach.* New York: Thieme, Inc.

Aronson, A. E., Brown, J. R., Litin, E. M., & Pearson, J. S. (1968). Spastic dysphonia: II. Comparison with essential (voice) tremor and other neurologic and psychogenic dysphonias. *Journal of Speech and Hearing Disorders, 33,* 219–231.

Aronson, A. E., & De Santo, L. W. (1983). Adductor spastic dysphonia: Three years after recurrent laryngeal nerve resection. *Laryngoscope, 93,* 1–8.

Aronson, A. E., & Hartman, D. E. (1981). Adductor spastic dysphonia as a sign of essential (voice) tremor. *Journal of Speech and Hearing Disorders, 46,* 52–58.

Biller, H. F., Som, M., & Lawson, W. (1983). Laryngeal nerve crush for spastic dysphonia. *Annals of Otology, Rhinology and Laryngology, 92,* 469.

Blitzer, A., & Brin, M. F. (1992). Treatment of spasmodic dysphonia (laryngeal dystonia) with local injections of botulinum toxin. *Journal of Voice, 6,* 365–369.

Blitzer, A., Brin, M. F., Fahn, S., & Lovelace, R. E. (1988a). Clinical and laboratory characteristics of laryngeal dystonia: A study of 110 cases. *Laryngoscope, 98,* 636–640.

Blitzer, A., Brin, M. F., Fahn, S., & Lovelace, R. E. (1988b). Localized injections of botulinum toxin for the treatment of focal laryngeal dystonia (spastic dysphony). *Laryngoscope, 98,* 193–197.

Blitzer, A., Brin, M. F., Stewart, C., Aviv, J. E., & Fahn S. (1992). Abductor lagyngeal dystonia: A series treated with botulinum toxin. *Laryngoscope, 102,* 163–167.

Blitzer, A., Lovelace, R. E., Brin, M. F., Fahn, S., & Fink, M. E. (1985). Electromyographic findings in focal laryngeal dystonia (spastic dysphonia). *Annals of Otology, Rhinology and Laryngology, 94,* 591–594.

Bloch, P. (1965). Neuro-psychiatric aspects of spastic dysphonia. *Folia Phoniatrica, 17,* 301–364.

Bloch, C. S., Hirano, M., & Gould, W. J. (1985). Symptom improvement of spastic dysphonia in response to phonatory tasks. *Annals of Otology, Rhinology and Laryngology, 94,* 51–54.

Boone, D. R., & McFarlane, S. C. (1977). *The voice and voice therapy.* (2nd ed.). Englewood Cliffs, NJ: Prentice-Hall.

Brodnitz, I. S. (1976). Spastic dysphonia. *Annals of Otology, 85,* 210–214.

Cannito, M. P. (1986). *Extralaryngeal functions in spasmodic dysphonia: Vocal tract and upper extremity control.* Unpublished doctoral dissertation, University of Texas, Dallas.

Cannito, M. P. (1991a). Emotional considerations in spasmodic dysphonia: Psychometric quantification. *Journal of Communication Disorders, 24,* 313–329.

Cannito, M. P. (1991b). Neurobiological interpretations of spasmodic dysphonia. In D. Vogel & M. P. Cannito (Eds.), *Treating disordered speech motor control: For clinicians by clinicians* (pp. 275–317). Austin, TX: Pro-Ed.

Cannito, M. P., Burch, A. R., Watts, C., Rappold, P. W., Hood, S. B., & Sherrard, K. (1997). Disfluency in spasmodic dysphonia: A multivariate analysis. *Journal of Speech, Language, and Hearing Research, 40,* 627–641.

Cannito, M. P., Ege, P., Ahmed, F., & Wagner, S. (1994). Diadochokinesis for complex trisyllables in individuals with spasmodic dysphonia and nondisabled subjects. In J. A. Till, K. M. Yorkston, & D. R. Beukelman (Eds.), *Motor speech disorders: Advances in assessment and treatment* (pp. 91–100). Baltimore: Paul H. Brookes.

Cannito, M. P., & Johnson, J. P. (1981). Spastic dysphonia: A continuum disorder. *Journal of Communication Disorders, 14,* 215–223.

Cannito, M. P., & Kondraske, G. V. (1990). Rapid manual abilities in spasmodic dsyphonic and normal female subjects. *Journal of Speech and Hearing Research, 33,* 123–133.

Cannito, M. P., Kondraske, G. V., & Johns, D. F. (1991). Oral-facial sensorimotor function in spasmodic dysphonia. In C. A. Moore, K. M. Yorkston, & D. R. Beukelman (Eds.), *Dysarthria and apraxia of speech* (pp. 205–225). Baltimore, MD: Paul H. Brookes.

Cannito, M. P., Kondraske, G. V., & Sussman, H. M. (1998). Influence of voicing on verbal/ manual interference in typical speakers and speakers with spasmodic dysphonia. In M. P. Cannito, K. M. Yorkston, & D. R. Beukelman (Eds.), *Neuromotor speech disorders: Nature, assessment, and management* (pp. 293–305). Baltimore: Paul H. Brookes.

Cannito, M. P., McSwain, L. S., & Dworkin, J. P. (1996). Abductor spasmodic dsyphonia: Acoustic influence of voicing on connected speech. In D. A. Robbin, K. M. Yorkston, & D. R. Beukelman (Eds.), *Disorders of motor speech: Assessment, treatment, and clinical characterization* (pp. 311–328). Baltimore: Paul H. Brookes.

Cannito, M. P., Murry, T., & Woodson, G. E. (1994). Attitudes toward communication in adductor spasmodic dysphonia before and after botulinum toxin injection. *Journal of Medical Speech-Language Pathology, 2,* 125–133.

Cannito, M. P., Woodson, G. E., Murry, T., & Newman, L. (1996, October). *Visual analog scaling of adductor spasmodic dysphonic speech before and after botulinum toxin injection.* Paper presented at First International Neurolaryngology Symposium, Bethesa, MD.

Carpenter, R. J., Snyder, G. G., & Henley-Cohn, J. L. (1981). Selective section of the recurrent laryngeal nerve for the treatment of spastic dysphonia: An experimental study and preliminary clinical report. *Otolaryngology Head and Neck Surgery, 89,* 986–991.

Chevrie-Muller, C., Arabia-Guidet, C., & Pfauwadel, M. (1987). Can one recover from spasmodic dysphonia? *British Journal of Disorders of Communication, 22,* 117–128.

Cohen, L. G., Ludlow, C. L., Warden, B. S., Estegui, M. Agostino, R. Sedory, S. E., Holloway, E., Dambrosia, J., & Hallett, M. (1989). Blink reflex excitability recovery curves in patients with spasmodic dsyphonia. *Neurology, 39,* 572–577.

Cooper, M. (1980). Recovery from spastic dyphonia by direct voice rehabilitation. *Proceedings of the 18th Congress of the International Association of Logopedics and Phoniatrics* (Vol. 1, pp. 579–584).

Darley, F. L., Aronson, A. E., & Brown, J. R. (1975). *Motor speech disorders*. Philadelphia: W.B. Saunders.

Davis, P. J., Boone, D. R., Carroll, R. L., Darveniza, P., & Harrison, G. A. (1988). Adductor spastic dysphonia: Heterogeneity of physiologic and phonatory characteristics. *Annals of Otology, Rhinology and Laryngology, 97,* 179–185.

Dedo, H. H. (1976) Recurrent laryngeal nerve section for spastic dysphonia. *Annals of Otolaryngology, 85,* 451–459.

Dedo, H. H. (1990). *Surgery of the larynx and the trachea* (p. 37). Philadelphia: B. C. Decker.

Dedo, H. H., & Izdebski, K. (1983). Problems with surgical (RLN section) treatment of spastic dysphonia. *Laryngoscope, 93,* 268–271.

Duffy, J. (1995). *Motor speech disorders: Substrates, differential diagnosis, and management.* St. Louis, MO: Mosby.

Finitzo, T., & Freeman, F. (1989). Spasmodic dysphonia, whether and where: Results of seven years of research. *Journal of Speech and Hearing Research, 32,* 541–555.

Ford, C. N., Bless, D. M., & Lowery, J. D. (1989). Treatment of spasmodic dysphonia with visually directed minimal injuctions of botulinum toxin. *Otolaryngology, Head and Neck Surgery, 101,* 151.

Ford, C. N., Bless, D. M., & Patel, N.Y. (1992). Botulinum toxin treatment of spasmodic dysphonia: Techniques, indications, efficacy. *Journal of Voice, 6,* 370–376.

Freeman, F., Cannito, M. P., & Finitzo-Hieber, T. (1985a). Classification of spasmodic dysphonia by perceptual-acoustic, visual means. In G. A. Gages (Ed.), *Spasmodic dysphonia: State of the art 1984* (pp. 5–13). New York: The Voice Foundation.

Freeman, F., Cannito, M. P., & Finitzo-Hieber, T. (1985b). Getting to know spasmodic dsyphonia patients. *Texas Journal of Speech Pathology, 10,* 14–19.

Friedman, M., Toriumi, D., Grybaukas, B. T., & Applebaum, E. L. (1989). Implantation of a recurrent laryngeal nerve stimulator for treatment of spasmodic dysphonia. *Annals of Otology, Rhinology and Laryngology, 98,* 130–134.

Genack, S. H., Woo, P., Colton, R. H., & Goyette, D. (1993). Partial thyroarytenoid myectomy: An animal study investigating a proposed new treatment for adductor spasmodic dysphonia. *Otolaryngology, Head and Neck Surgery, 108,* 256–264.

Ginsberg, B. I., Wallack, J. J., Srain, J. J., & Biller, H. F. (1988). Defining the psychiatric role in spastic dysphonia. *General Hospital Psychiatry, 10,* 132–137.

Greene, M., & Mathieson, L. (1989). *The voice and its disorders*. London: Whurr Publishers.

Hanson, D. G., Logemann, J. A., & Hain, T. (1992). Differential diagnosis of spasmodic dysphonia: A kinematic perspective. *Journal of Voice, 6,* 325–337.

Hartelius, L., Buder, E. H., & Strand, E. A. (1997). Long-term phonatory instability in individuals with multiple sclerosis. *Journal of Speech, Language, and Hearing Research, 40,* 1056–1072.

Hartman, D. E., & Aronson, A. E. (1981). Clinical investigations of intermittent breathy dysphonia. *Journal of Speech and Hearing Disorders, 46,* 428–432.

Hartman, D. E., Abbs, J. H., & Vishwanat, B. (1988). Clinical investigations of adductor spastic dysphonia. *Annals of Otology, Rhinology and Laryngology, 97,* 247–252.

Heaver, L. (1959). Spastic dysphonia: II. Psychiatric considerations. *Logos, 2,* 15–24.

Heuer, R. (1992). Behavioral therapy for spasmodic dysphonia. *Journal of Voice, 6,* 352–354.

Ingham, R. J., Fox, P. T., Ingham, J. C., Zamarripa, F., Martin, C., Jerabek, P., & Cotton, J. (1996). Functional-lesion investigation of developmental stuttering with positron emission tomography. *Journal of Speech and Hearing Research, 39,* 1208–1227.

Izdebski, K. (1992). Symptomatology of adductor spasmodic dysphonia: A physiologic model. *Journal of Voice, 6,* 306–319.

Jankovic, J., & Fahn, S. (1993). Dystonic disorders. In J. Jankovic & E. Tolosa (Eds.), *Parkinson's disease and movement disorders* (pp. 337–374). Baltimore: Williams & Wilkins.

Luchsinger, R., & Arnold, G.E. (1965). *Voice, speech, language, clinical communicology: Its physiology and pathology*. (G. E. Arnold, & E. R. Finkbeiner, Trans.). Belmont, CA: Wadsworth.

Ludlow, C. L., Bagley, J., Yin, S. G., & Koda, J. (1992). A comparison of injection techniques using botulinum toxin for treatment of the spasmodic dysphonias. *Journal of Voice, 6*, 380–386.

Ludlow, C. L., & Conner, N. P. (1987). Dynamic aspects of phonatory control in spasmodic dysphonia. *Journal of Speech and Hearing Research, 30*, 197–206.

Ludow, C. L., Hallet, M., Sedory, S. E., Fujita, M., & Naunton, R. F. (1990). The pathophysiology of spasmodic dysphonia and its modification by botulinum toxin. In A. Berardelli (Ed.), *Motor disturbances II: A selection of papers delivered at the 2nd Congress of the International Medical Society of Motor Disturbances held at Rome, Italy* (pp. 273–288). San Diego: Academic Press Limited.

Ludlow, C. L., Nauton, R. F., Sedory, S. E., Schulz, M. A., & Hallett, M. (1988). Effects of botulinum toxin injection on speech in adductor spasmodic dysphonia. *Neurology, 38*, 1220–1225.

Ludlow, C. L., Naunton, R. F., Terada, S., & Anderson, B. J. (1991). Successful treatment of selected cases of abductor spasmodic dysphonia using botulinum toxin injection. *Otolayngology, Head and Neck Surgery, 104*, 849–855.

Lundy, D. S., Casiano, R. R., Lu, F-L., & Xue, J. W. (1996). Abnormal soft palate posturing in patients with abnormal laryngeal movement disorders. *Journal of Voice, 10*, 348–353.

Maloney, A. P., & Morrison, M. D. (1994). A comparison of the efficacy of unilateral versus bilateral botulinum toxin injections in the treatment of spasmodic dysphonia. *Journal of Otolaryngology, 23*, 160–164.

Marsden, C. D. (1976). The problem of adult-onset ideopathic torsion dystonia and other isolated dyskinesias in adult life (including blepharospasm oromandubular dystonia, dystonic writer's cramp, and torticollis or axial dystonia.) In R. Eldridge & S. Fahn (Eds.), *Advances in neurology* (Vol. 14, pp. 259–275). New York: Raven Press.

McCall, G. N. (1974). Spasmodic dysphonia and the stuttering block: Commonalities or possible connections. In L. M. Webster & L. C. Furst (Eds.), *Vocal tract dynamics and dysfluency* (pp. 124–151). New York: Speech & Hearing Institute.

Merson, R., & Ginsberg, A. P. (1979). Spasmodic dysphonia: Abductor type. A clinical report of acoustic, aerodynamic, and perceptual characteristics. *Laryngoscope, 89*, 129–139.

Meyers, I., & Anderson, D. (1985). A stuttering therapy programme with spastic dysphonia. *South African Journal of Communication Disorders, 32*, 31–36.

Miller, R. H., Woodson, G. E., & Jankovic, J. (1987). Botulinum toxin injection of the vocal fold for spasmodic dysphonia: A preliminary report. *Archives of Otolaryngology, Head and Neck Surgery, 113*, 603–605.

Murry, T., Cannito, M. P., & Woodson, G. E., (1994). Spasmodic dysphonia: Emotional status and botulinum toxin treatment. *Archives of Otolaryngology—Head and Neck Surgery, 120*, 310–316.

Murry, T., & Woodson, G. E. (1995). Combined-modality treatment of adductor spasmodic dysphonia with botulinum toxin and voice therapy. *Journal of Voice, 9*, 460–465.

Netterville, J. L., Stone, R. E., Rainey, C., Zealear, D. L., & Ossoff, R. H. (1991). Recurrent laryngeal nerve avulsion for treatment of spastic dysphonia. *Annals of Otology, Rhinology and Laryngology, 100*, 10–14.

Pool, K. D., Freeman, F. J., Finitzo, T., Hagashi, M. M., Chapman, S. B., Devous, M. D., Sr., Close, L. G., Kondraske, G.V., Mendelsohn, D., Schaefer, S. D., & Watson, B. C. O. (1991). Heterogeneity in spasmodic dysphonia: Neurologic and voice findings. *Archives of Neurology, 48*, 305–309.

Rhew, K., Fiedler, D. A., & Ludlow, C. L. (1994). Technique for injection of botulinum toxin through the flexible nasolaryngoscope. *Oltolayngology, Head and Neck Surgery, 111*, 787–794.

Roark, R. M., Dowling, E. M., DeGroat, R. D., Watson, B. C., & Schaefer, S. D. (1995). Time-frequency analyses of thyroarytenoid myoelectric activity in normal and spasmodic dysphonia subjects. *Journal of Speech and Hearing Research, 38*, 289–303.

Rontal, M., Rontal, E., Rolnick, M., Merson, R., Silverman, B., & Truong, D. D. (1991). A method for the treatment of abductor spasmodic dsyphonia with botulinum toxin injections: A preliminary report. *Laryngoscope, 101*, 911–914.

Rosenfield, D. B. (1988). Spasmodic dysphonia. *Advances in Neurology, 49*, 317–327.

Rosenfield, D. B. (1991). Pharmacologic approaches to speech motor disorders. In D. Vogel & M. P. Cannito (Eds.), *Treating disordered speech motor control* (pp. 111–152). Austin, TX: Pro-Ed.

Rosenfield, D. B., Donovan, D. T., Sulek, M., Viswanath, N. S., Inbody, G. P., & Nudelman, H. B. (1990). Neurologic aspects of spasmodic dysphonia. *Journal of Otolaryngology, 19*, 231–236.

Sapienza, C. M., Cannito, M., & Erickson, M. (1996, November). *Temporal and volume indices associated with adductor spasmodic dysphonia*. Paper presented at the American Speech- Language-Hearing Association Convention, Seattle.

Sapir, S. (1993). Psychogenic spasmodic dysphonia: A case study with expert opinions. *Journal of Voice, 9*, 270–281.

Schaefer, S. D. (1983). Neuropathology of spasmodic dysphonia. *Laryngoscope, 93*, 1183–1204.

Schaefer, S., Freeman, F., Finitzo, T., Close, L., Cannito, M., Ross, E., Reisch, J., & Maravilla, K. (1985). Magnetic resonance imaging findings and correlations in spasmodic dysphonia patients. *Annals of Otology, Rhinology and Laryngology, 94*, 595–601.

Shipp, T., Izdebski, K., Reed, C., & Morrisey, P. (1985). Intrinsic laryngeal muscle activity in spastic dysphonia patient. *Journal of Speech and Hearing Disorders, 50*, 54–59.

Silverman, F. H., & Hummer, K. (1989). Spastic dysphonia: A fluency disorder? *Journal of Fluency Disorders, 14*, 285–291.

Simpson, L. L. (1992). Clinically relevant apects of the mechanism of action of botulinum neourotoxin. *Journal of Voice, 6*, 358–364.

Spielberger, C. D., Gorusch, R. L., Luschene, R., Vagg, P., & Jacobs, G. A. (1983). Manual for the State-Trait Anxiety Inventory (form Y): Self-Evaluation Questionnaire. Palo Alto, CA: Consulting Psychologists Press.

Stewart, C. F., Allen, E. L., Tureen, P., Diamond, B. E., Blitzer, A., & Brin, M. F. (1997). Adductor spasmodic dysphonia: Standard evaluation of symptoms and severity. *Journal of Voice, 11*, 95–103.

Swenson, M. R., Zwirner, P., Murry, T., & Woodson, G. E. (1992). Medical evaluation of patients with spasmodic dysphonia. *Journal of Voice, 6*, 320–324.

Tucker, H. (1989). Laryngeal framework surgery in the management of spasmodic dysphonia: Preliminary report. *Annals of Otology, Rhinology and Laryngology, 98*, 52–54.

Tucker, H. M. (1992). Combination surgical therapy for spasmodic dysphonia. *Journal of Voice, 6*, 355–357.

Watson, B. C., McIntire, D., Roark, R. M., & Schaefer, S. (1995). Statistical analyses of electromyographic activity in spasmodic dysphonic and normal control subjects. *Journal of Voice, 9*, 3–15.

Watson, B., Schaefer, S. D, Freeman, F. J., Dembowski, J., Kondraske, G., & Roark, R. (1991). Laryngeal electromyographic activity in adductor and abductor spasmodic dysphonia. *Journal of Speech and Hearing Research, 34*, 473–483.

Weed, D. T., Jewett, B. S., Rainey, C., Zealear, D. L., Stone, R. E., Ossoff, R. H., & Netterville, J. L. (1996). Long-term follow-up of recurrent laryngeal nerve avulsion for the treatment of spastic dysphonia. *Annals of Otology, Rhinology and Laryngology, 105*, 592–601.

Whurr, R., Lorch, M., Fontana, H., Brookes, G., Lees, A., & Marsden, C. D. (1993). The use of botulinum toxin in the treatment of adductor spasmodic dysphonia. *Journal of Neurology, Neurosurgery, and Psychiatry, 56*, 526–530.

Witsell, D. L., Weissler, M. C., Donovan, M. K., Howard, J. F., Jr., & Martinkosky, S. J. (1994). Measurement of laryngeal resistance in the evaluation of botulinum toxin injection for treatment of focal laryngeal dystonia. *Laryngoscope, 104*, 8–11.

Wolfe, V. I., Ratusnik, D. L., & Feldman, H. (1979). Acoustic and perceptual comparison of chronic and incipient spastic dysphonia. *Laryngoscope, 89*, 1478–1486.

Woo, P., Colton, R., Casper, J., & Brewer, D. (1992). Analysis of spasmodic dysphonia by aerodynamic and laryngostroboscopic measurements. *Journal of Voice, 6*, 344–351.

Woodson, G. E. (1994). Determining the optimal dose for botulinum toxin in spasmodic dysphonia. *Proceedings of the Third International symposium on Phonosurgery, June 1994* (pp. 155–157). Kyoto, Japan: International Association of Phonosurgeons.

Woodson, G. E., Zwirner, P., Murry, T., & Swenson, M. (1991). Use of flexible fiberoptic laryngoscopy to assess patients with spasmodic dysphonia. *Journal of Voice, 5*, 85–91.

Woodson, G. E, Zwirner, P., Murry, T., & Swenson, M. R. (1992). Functional assessment of patients with spasmodic dysphonia. *Journal of Voice, 6*, 338–343.

Zung, W. W. K. (1967). *The measurement of depression*. Milwaukee: Lakeside Laboratories.

Zwirner, P., Murry, T., Swenson, M., & Woodson, G. E. (1991). Acoustic changes in spasmodic dysphonia after botulinum toxin injection. *Journal of Voice, 5*, 78–84.

Zwirner, P., Murry, T., Swenson, M., & Woodson, G. E. (1992). Effects of botulinum toxin therapy in patients with adductor spasmodic dysphonia: Acoustic, aerodynamic and videoendoscopic findings. *Laryngoscope, 102*, 400–406.

Zwirner, P., Murry, T., & Woodson, G. E. (1993). A comparison of bilateral and unilateral botulinum toxin treatments for spasmodic dysphonia. *European Archives of Otorhinolaryngology, 250*, 271–276.

APPENDIX

VOCAL CHARACTERISTICS CHECKLIST FOR THE SPASMODIC DYSPHONIAS

Patient: ______________________ Examiner: ______________________

Date of Birth ______________________ Date of Evaluation ______________________

	Yes	No
1. Is voice quality persistently effortful?	______	______
2. Do you hear complete breaks in voicing?	______	______
3. Do you hear phonatory spasms?	______	______

4. If so: Abductor______ Adductor______ Mixed______

5. Nature of spasms:

Duration of spasms:

Long ______

Short ______

Frequency per breath group:

Less than one ________ One or more ________

Regularly ________ Irregularly ________

	Yes	No
6. Did you hear normal voice at all?	______	______
7. Was voice normal at least half the time?	______	______
8. Did speech/voice improve markedly when:		
Whispering	______	______
Phonating at high pitch	______	______

9. Nonspeech vocalizations:

	Relatively More	
	Normal	Abnormal
Singing	______	______

Chanting	______	______
Paralanguage	______	______
Laughing	______	______
Yawning	______	______
Coughing	______	______
Pushing "uh uh uh"	______	______

10. Voice/Speech qualities present while speaking:

	Reading	Spontaneous
Intermittent breathiness*	______	______
Strained-strangle quality*	______	______
Abnormal loudness*	______	______
Inspiratory voice*	______	______
Intermittent aphonia*	______	______
Hoarseness*	______	______
Glottal stops (catches)*	______	______
Vocal fry*	______	______
Audible voice tremor*	______	______
Pitch*		
Sudden pitch breaks	______	______
Habitual high pitch	______	______
Habitual low pitch	______	______
Monopitch	______	______
Respiratory grunting/gasping	______	______
Dysfluency	______	______
Dysprosody	______	______
Reduced intelligibility	______	______
Reduced speaking rate	______	______

*These features are also used to evaluate sustained vowels.

Note: Adapted with permission from *Extralaryngeal Functions in Spasmodic Dysphonia: Vocal Tract and Manual Control*, by M. Cannito (1986). Unpublished doctoral dissertation, The University of Texas at Dallas.

CHAPTER 21

Pediatric Voice Disorders

Kim Corbin-Lewis and Thomas S. Johnson

Pediatric clients are an important and frequently encountered patient group within the diagnosis and management of voice disorders. Conservative estimates of the voice disorder prevalence in children run between 4% and 9% of the population (Dobres, Lee, Stemple, Kummer, & Kretschmer, 1990; Herrington-Hall, Lee, Stemple, Niemi, & McHone, 1988; Hirschberg et al., 1995; Marge, 1991). Although some research indicates higher rates and considerable variability in prevalence at different age levels, the conclusion is that there are a substantial number of children with vocal disturbances or abnormalities (Lecoq & Drape, 1996; Senturia & Wilson, 1968; Silverman & Zimmer, 1975; Yairi, Currin, Bulian, & Yairi, 1974). This represents a potential number of voice patients with laryngeal structures that change over time, different patterns of voice use, and different vocal rehabilitative needs as compared to adults. Diagnostic methods currently in use with adult patients may require adaptation for use with a pediatric client. Moreover, the development of new and innovative methods is needed to meet the needs of this special group of voice patients.

The vocal characteristics that set children apart from adults include the childrens' anatomical immaturity and related unique physiological usage of immature laryngeal, respiratory, articulatory, and resonatory systems (Kent & Vorperian, 1995). Additional biomechanical constraints are placed on phonatory function by the layer differentiation of the vocal folds and the change in the ratio of the cartilaginous to membranous structures (Hirano, 1981b; Hirano, Kurita, & Nakashima, 1983; Kahane, 1982). The precise rate and schedule of anatomical and physiological change in children related to voice production remain unclear and largely unstudied. However, given the numerous documented anatomical and physiological differences between adult and pediatric laryngeal systems, most voice scientists agree that expectations about function cannot be based on study results of adult physiology. Recent data suggest that children not only differ from adults anatomically and physiologically but may show physiologic gender differences in the use of respiratory and laryngeal systems at prepubertal ages (Corbin-Lewis, 1996; Hoit, Hixon, Watson, & Morgan, 1990; Stathopoulos

& Sapienza, 1997). Clinical care and standards of practice for a pediatric patient with a voice disorder may depend, in part, on these identified functional differences between children and adults, as well as the consideration of gender differences among children.

1. THE UNIQUE NATURE OF PHONATORY FUNCTION IN CHILDREN

1.1. Differences in Structure and Function

Although our understanding of the pediatric larynx remains incomplete because of technical difficulties in documenting the maturational process in a noninvasive and longitudinal manner, we have a basic understanding of the pediatric laryngeal mechanism. In the larger context of pediatric voice measurement and management of disorders, our knowledge base must be founded on an understanding of the phonatory mechanism from the ultrastructural, or histochemical, level to the macroscopic, or voice production, level. A basis of comparison within these levels necessitates detailed information about normal laryngeal structure and function.

1.2. Histology

The ability to identify and measure the histological makeup of the vocal folds has increased significantly in the past 10 years (Gray, Hirano, & Sato, 1993; Gray, Pignatari, & Harding, 1994; Hammond, Zhou, Hammond, Pawlak, & Gray, 1997; Pawlak, Hammond, Hammond, & Gray, 1996). Information about the structure and function of the vocal folds furthers understanding of the results of trauma to this structure. Recent examination of the junction between the epithelial covering of the vocal fold and the superficial layer of the lamina propria with transmission electron microscopy has indicated significant variability in the number and location of anchoring fibers among individuals (Gray et al., 1994). These fibers are thought to be important in handling shearing and stress force during vibration and their population density and location may be one of the factors in predisposition or susceptibility to vocal injury.

Traditional microscopic examination of the vocal folds through staining techniques for cellular tissue has more recently been supplemented by staining methodologies that identify the predominant extracellular matrix constituents of the vocal folds. Electron microscopic imaging techniques that have allowed quantification of extracelluar constituents in recent morphologic studies have resulted in the preliminary identification of adult gender differences in the amount of hyaluronic acid, an interstitial protein found in the lamina propria. Hyaluronic acid is hypothesized to function, in part, as a buffer to vibrational stress (Hammond et al., 1997). Other protein constituents that may be equally important to the maintenance of vocal fold homeostasis or associated with trauma (use, abuse, and misuse) and repair are currently under investigation. Early results showing cellular level differences in protein constituents between adult males and females have led to speculation on the timing or emergence of this difference in structure. Increased sample sizes and inclusion of children in histological studies ultimately may assist understanding of the prevalence data that show age and gender differences for certain pathological states. For example, vocal fold nodules are most common in 8-year-old boys and middle-aged females (Silverman, 1975). Although mechanical trauma from vibratory friction, shearing forces, and impact in speakers with a high fundamental frequency may explain a manner of injury, it does not fully address the apparent gender differences at both pre- and postpubertal ages. The amount of extracellular level constituents may play a dominant role in the predisposition or susceptibility to damage as discussed by Johnson (1986, 1988, 1991) and Johnson and Child (1988). This new direction in research addressing cellular- and extracellular-level gender differences in children is just beginning.

1.3 Laryngeal Framework and Soft Tissues

Development of the laryngeal framework and soft tissues demonstrates significant anatomical and physiological differences between the immature and mature mechanisms across such parameters as size of the structures, position in the neck, consistency of tissues, and structure shape (Kent & Vorperian, 1995; Kirchner, 1970). These differences are not likely just differences of scale, but rather may reflect basic process differences in the systems and structures used in voice production (Titze, 1989). A limited number of specific examples can be found in Table 21–1. For a comprehensive examination of craniofacial-oral-laryngeal development see Kent and Vorperian (1995). For a thorough review of respiratory system development see Polgar and Weng (1979).

Morphological differences identified in Table 21–1 have physiological consequences. For example, the structural vocal fold edge shape difference has implications for the vibratory pattern, including a greater contact period per glottal cycle for adult males when compared to children and women. The inner structural changes and layer differentiation of the vocal folds are not complete until the end of puberty. The impact of the developmental process on the biomechanical performance of an immature and changing layered structure has not been fully addressed in research efforts to date, but it may be logical to assume that it needs to be considered a factor in the development of mechanically based vocal hyperfunction in children.

The respiratory system, which drives phonation, has been found to differ in both structure and function between adults and children. Children have demonstrated lower alternating glottal airflows and lower maximum flow declination rate than adults (Stathopoulos & Sapienza, 1993). The diameter of rib cage dimension (in the anterior-posterior plane) is far smaller in children, yet the rib cage movement during speech respiration is larger than in adults, and children use a higher percentage of their vital capacity to achieve speech production than do adults (Hoit et al., 1990; Stathopoulos & Sapienza, 1993, 1997). Tracheal pressure during speech has been found higher in children than in adults (Sapienza & Stathopoulos, 1994).

In summary, all of these functional differences between children and adults likely reflect children's phonation produced with a smaller mechanism across multiple physiologic systems and a primary vibratory structure with undifferentiated layers and differing membranous to cartilaginous ratios.

2. Phonatory Function Differences in Prepubertal Boys and Girls

Is phonatory function different between prepubertal boys and girls? The importance of determining if there are vocal differences among children is not simply an academic question and is far from resolved. If phonatory function differs between prepubescent boys and girls, the focus of prevention programs and therapeutic management decisions may be improved and more precisely accommodate the needs of all members of this special population. Continued inquiry into respiratory and laryngeal physiology in children will ultimately yield enough data to support or reject the need for reconsideration of management decisions and strategies.

The acoustic literature indicates that fundamental frequency decreases between birth and puberty and is a reflection of the growth of the laryngeal system. Gender differences in fundamental frequency, indicative of an increase in membranous vocal fold length, have begun to emerge by 8 years of age in some population samples. The exact age at which differences become evident is not agreed upon. Kent (1976) in his tutorial reported possible gender differences some time before 11 years of age. Hasek, Singh, and Murry (1980) in their examination of children from 5–10 years old reported gender differences in fundamental frequency by age 7. Corbin-Lewis (1996) found no statistically significant gender differences in fundamental fre-

Table 21–1. Differences in pediatric and adult laryngeal structures.

Structure	***Children***	***Adult***
Epithelium relative to total length of vocal fold	50% thicker epithelium to vocal fold length than in adults	10% epithelium to vocal fold length
Membranous to cartilaginous length	50% membranous: 50% cartilaginous	66% membranous: 33% cartilaginous
Vocal fold ligament	First observed near 4 years; matures through 16 years	Fully matured adding stiffness and mass to vocal folds
Vocal fold edge	Hypothesized to be thick and rectangular; no sexual dimorphism predicted until puberty	Males—medial edge bulging Females—linear convergent (wedge-shaped edge)
Vocal fold shape	Short, thick, circular	Long, thin, ovoid
Thyroid and cricoid than cartilages	Growth begins at prepubertal ages—unknown if linear or quantal	2–3 times larger in males females at maturity
Vocal fold length	Growth begins at prepubertal ages—unknown if linear or quantal	Twice as long in males than females at maturity

Note: Based on information from Hirano, 1981b; Hirano, Kurita, & Nakashima, 1983; Kahane, 1982; Kent & Vorperian, 1995; Titze, 1989.

quency at 9 years of age. It seems apparent that discrepancies are due, in part, to varying sample sizes, different speech samples used in protocols, and the use of cross-sectional, as opposed to longitudinal, data. Whether significant prepubertal gender differences exist in fundamental frequency (and by extension, laryngeal growth) is not known. A small sample size of cadaveric specimens examined by Kahane (1978) indicated no sexual dimorphism in anatomical structure until puberty. Whether physiologic (as opposed to anatomic) gender differences exist remains a question. Data on children are scarce but, at present, seem to indicate that there may be gender-based voice production differences in prepubescent children across specific speech production parameters. Vocal fold contact patterns differed between boys and girls in two studies that examined vocal fold contact patterns, electroglottographically (Corbin-Lewis, 1996; Robb & Simmons, 1990). Although interpretation of the data differed between the studies, the finding of boys having less contact per vibratory cycle when compared to girls was the same for both investigations.

In the literature examining speech respiration in prepubescent children, gender differences between boys and girls have been identified (Hoit et al., 1990; Stathopoulos & Sapienza, 1997). Girls produced syllable trains with higher lung volume initiations, lower volume terminations, and greater rib cage excursions than the boys. This pattern mimicked that of adult females to adult males. The statistically significant differences were attributed to more than just size differences between the genders (Stathopoulos & Sapienza, 1997) although not all researchers support the interpretation of prepubertal sexual dimorphism (Hoit et al., 1990).

3. Epidemiology

When looking at data on the prevalence (number of cases in the population) and incidence (new cases in a specified period) of voice disorders in children, it is evident that we have yet to adequately track these problems with any agreement or consistency. A number of difficulties, including the criteria and disorder definitions used, the disorders included, age ranges included, and the population from which subjects are drawn (biased as in an otolaryngologist's practice or not), have resulted in inconsistent data (Marge, 1991). Two recent studies have examined the distribution of laryngeal disorders in children and adults and have compared the data to earlier studies (Dobres et al., 1990; Herrington-Hall et al., 1988). The distribution of problem type indicated an increase in the number of cases attributed to vocal abuse from 50% in 1938 to 85% in the retrospective study of 1,262 records of adult otolaryngological patients completed in 1988. In a study that examined pediatric pathology, a similar finding emerged for a statistically significant increase in the prevalence of vocal abuse related pathology (Dobres et al., 1990). While data interpretation allows much speculation as to causal factors, what appears apparent is that we have more identified children in need of behavioral vocal rehabilitation.

Incidence and prevalence data are also important in helping resolve the age-old question of whether benign lesions in the pediatric population resolve without medical or behavioral therapeutic intervention. In an age of managed health care and accountability, this information is urgently needed. The debate about intervention has continued (see Kahane & Mayo, 1989; Sander, 1989), yet we still have little hard evidence from longitudinal studies. While the spontaneous resolution of vocal nodules and polyps during puberty remains a question, a study of 179 pediatric voice patients in Japan suggested that 15% of patients do not have an improvement in voice following puberty (Hirschberg et al., 1995). To date, this is one of the few longitudinal studies that has looked specifically at the number of documented benign lesions that did not resolve without intervention.

4. DIAGNOSIS: CURRENT STATE OF THE ART ON MEASUREMENT OF PEDIATRIC VOICE

The application of measures to clinically track vocal performance has been a long sought-after goal for use in the management of voice quality disorders (Hirano, 1981a; Johnson, 1986; Michel & Wendahl, 1971; Moore, 1977; Reed, 1980). In the past 10 years, the understanding of normal and abnormal pediatric phonatory function has increased significantly, with resulting improvement in diagnosis, management, and service delivery. This increase in the knowledge base has developed from both basic research efforts and an increased use of improved measurement and monitoring technology in clinical practice.

The current level of clinical practice takes into account the synergistic nature of the respiratory, phonatory, articulatory, and resonatory systems and stresses this integration as a consideration in development of assessment protocols. Simultaneous collection of aerodynamic, kinematic, and acoustic data is the developing standard of care in many voice clinics. Laryngeal visualization is frequently combined with collection of acoustic and electroglottographic data (Johnson, 1986). The Kay Elemetrics Computerized Stroboscopy System has this ability built into its instrumental array. In this way, the timing and coordination of multiple speech subsystems (such as the respiratory, laryngeal, articulatory, and resonatory systems) can be examined.

The use of instrumental measures has complemented perceptual data and assisted in the diagnosis and management of pediatric voice disorders. When repeated, appropriate measures collected under standard conditions provide excellent baseline and progress data. Perceptual judgments can be corroborated or called into question by the findings of instrumental measures. Instrumental methods are also used to provide biofeedback during voice therapy. In many instances, the use of computer technology has captured the interest and cooperation of young patients. Collection of acoustic data is quick and efficient when a child sees his or her voice "draw speech mountains" on the monitor. Although an assessment protocol is dictated by the signs and symptoms of a given child's voice difficulties, a basic pediatric assessment should include a detailed case history, aerodynamic, acoustic, and perceptual measures, along with visualization of the mechanism.

4.1. Case History

Perhaps the most critical component of a core assessment in pediatric voice disorders is a thorough case history. The essential components of a case history include demographic information, medical, educational, behavioral, and psychosocial history. In children, the focus is often centered on identifying the inappropriate behaviors that contribute to hyperfunctional use, abuse, or misuse of the vocal mechanism. It is often necessary to collect this information from more than one source and may include interviews with child-care workers, classroom teachers, and even coaches. Identifying inappropriate vocal behaviors and the situations in which they occur can assist a clinician in formulating specific behavioral objectives for a therapeutic program designed to meet a child's needs. There are numerous examples of effective case history forms in the literature (Andrews, 1995; Boone & McFarlane, 1994; Dworkin & Meleca, 1996; Johnson, 1985; Koschkee & Rammage, 1997).

4.2. Aerodynamic Measures

A number of measures have been used to infer the function of various aspects of respiratory support and drive. Currently, measures of glottal flow and estimated subglottal air pressure are most common in the research and clinical setting. Airflow data may be instrumentally collected with a circumferentially vented wire screen pneumotachograph mask (frequently referred to as a Rothenberg mask) connected to a flow transducer. Collected signals are frequently filtered using any number of computer software programs such as Cspeech (Milenkovic, 1989) or CASPER (Till, 1990). Dedicated devices, such as the Kay Elemetrics Aerophone, are also commercially available. Air pressure data may be simultaneously collected with flow data by connecting a pressure transducer to the Rothenberg mask. As with flow data, signal conditioning can be done with computer software. A number of measures can be gathered with these data including maximum flow declination rate; peak, alternating, and minimum glottal airflow rate; and estimated tracheal pressure (Sapienza & Stathopoulos, 1994; Smitheran & Hixon, 1981; Stathopoulos, 1986; Stathopoulos & Sapienza, 1993; Stathopoulos & Weismer, 1985).

Respirometric measures of vital capacity and phonation volume have been combined with maximum phonation time measures and used as the basis for mathematically derived measures of maximum predicted phonation time, phonation time ratio, mean flow rate, vocal velocity index, and the phonation volume/vital capacity ratio (Beckett, 1971; Johnson, 1988). Preliminary normative data were collected for college-aged adults and third-, fourth-, and sixth-graders. These measures were subsequently used to track progress during voice therapy using the Vocal Abuse Reduction Program (VARP) (Johnson, 1985). These measures were considered clinically useful for tracking individual performance but have not been validated against other measurement techniques to date.

Laryngeal resistance measurement has been suggested as an easily administered, noninvasive way of assessing the combined function of the respiratory and laryngeal systems in children (Smitheran & Hixon, 1981; Zajac, Farkas, Dindzans, & Stool, 1993).

Use of respiratory kinematic methods with children to examine how they use the chest wall and abdomen during speech breathing has been initiated in the research arena. To date, information on children with normal voice production and those with a limited number of disorders has been examined using kinematic methodologies (Hixon, 1987; Sapienza & Stathopoulos, 1994). Kinematic data allow examination of possible respiratory compensations for glottal inefficiencies. For example, in Sapienza & Stathopoulos (1994) children with bilateral nodules were observed to begin utterances at a higher lung volume level and terminate utterances at lower lung volumes than their counterparts with normal voice. As well, this relationship was correlated to peak glottal airflow. These techniques are presently used clinically with adults and will hopefully be extended to use with pediatric patients in the near future.

One simple, quick, and noninstrumental measure used historically has been the maximally sustained /s/ and /z/ phoneme and the ratio of the two durations. Its use was predicated on the undocumented assumption that phonation volume used to produce the two phonemes would be identical and that the airflow rate would be higher during the /z/ phoneme production if a mass lesion was located on the vibrating edge of the vocal folds, precluding complete glottal closure. The use of the s/z ratio, as either a screening tool to indicate vocal fold mass lesions or a measure designed to differentiate between respiratory support versus laryngeal efficiency, has come under close scrutiny and has been found lacking in validity (Hufnagle & Hufnagle, 1988; Trudeau & Forrest, 1997). Although the measure may be useful in documenting changes in phonatory function over time in individuals, it is important to realize that valid interpretation using this measure cannot address lesion size or separate respiratory from laryngeal function.

4.3. Acoustic Measures

Our basic understanding of the pediatric voice has long relied on noninvasive acoustic methodologies. There is a significant body of research on the acoustic properties of the pediatric voice and fundamental frequency, in particular, in the literature (Kent, 1976). In recent years, many technical problems with signal processing have been resolved and voices with high fundamental frequencies, such as found in women and children, have been closely examined (Glaze, Bless, Milenkovic, & Susser, 1988; Glaze, Bless, & Susser, 1990; Gilbert, Robb, & Chen, 1997; Klatt & Klatt, 1990). Kent (1993) addresses acoustic theory in relation to current voice measurement and laboratory methods.

A summary statement on current acoustic voice analysis methodologies and their applicability to normal and pathological voice is available from the National Center for Voice and Speech (Titze, 1995). This document provides recommendations for signal classification, basic analysis approach, fundamental frequency extraction and perturbation analysis methods, test utterances, signal acquisition, and data management. Following are highlights of the published recommendations. A type I acoustic signal is nearly periodic and use of perturbation analysis is considered reliable. In contrast, type II signals have periods of instability within stable productions resulting in unreliable perturbation analysis. In this case, a visual display method of analysis is suggested. Type III signals are random and aperiodic and are best analyzed perceptually. Recommended voice test utterances should include sustained high (/i/) and low (/a/) vowel productions for perturbation analysis, multiple tokens (approximately 10/task) for reliable analysis, and reporting of voice fundamental frequency, intensity, and quality, as these parameters can influence perturbation measures. High precision measurement of voice signals require acquisition with a condenser microphone with a minimum sensitivity of –60 dB; a constant mouth-to-microphone distance of 3–4 cm with off-axis positioning of 45°–90°; recordings made in a sound-treated room with limited reverberation and ambient noise and elimination of noise with 60 Hz hum; and DAT recording with amplifiers and filters with 85–95 dB signal-to-noise ratios, and data sampling frequencies of 20–100 kHz depending on the software analysis programs. The standard file format recommended for voice signals was SPHERE or the Microsoft RIFF format to encourage database sharing.

4.4. Perceptual Measures

Historically, auditory-perceptual measures in the evaluation of voice have often been the sole methodology used to categorize and classify disorders, most often across the parameters of pitch, quality, loudness, and resonance. As with all measures, auditory-perceptual evaluation of the voice has strengths and limitations. The limitations are frequently ignored, or worse, unrecognized. In a review of current thought on perceptual evaluation of voice and speech, Kent (1996) stated: "Auditory-perceptual methods carry strong advantages of convenience, economy, and robustness, but it is also clear that these judgments are susceptible to a variety of sources of error and biases" (p. 7). Some of the main problems Kent described include listeners' internal standards or differences in definitions of adjectives/traits used to describe voice, lack of agreement on the specific disordered characteristics/traits to be rated, ratings of dimensions that are not independent from each other, different traits are not rated with the same level of reliability across listeners, and differences between raters' judgments that are larger than levels needed to classify disorders or measure therapeutic change.

Because of the stated difficulties, perceptual voice evaluation is no longer restricted to equal-appearing interval scale measures that previously were commonly used in evaluating the pediatric voice (D. K. Wilson, 1987; F. B. Wilson, 1990). The difficulty with these types of measures has been in achieving acceptable reliability levels between and among trained listeners. A measure is not useful if individuals score the same voice differently across specific parameters or score the voice differently when listening to the same sample at a different point in time. Kreiman, Gerratt, Kempster, Erman, and Berke (1993) provided an extensive review and tutorial on the difficulties in selecting appropriate perceptual rating scales for assessing vocal quality. They discussed different types of scales, including equal-appearing interval scales, visual analog scales, direct magnitude estimation, and paired comparison tasks. One major problem in the field of voice disorder assessment is the lack of agreement between speech-language pathologists on disordered characteristics and terminology. Kreiman et al. (1993) suggested that one way to avoid the problem of internal standards held by individual listeners is to establish "reference voices" for specific vocal qualities. In this way, there would be a common reference or external standard among trained listeners. As Kent (1996) stated, for this type of a plan to succeed a national effort would be required to gather carefully selected samples, with systematic training based on appropriate criteria.

4.5. Endoscopic Imaging

It is intuitive that a direct view of the structure under assessment is preferable to indirect measures. The size discrepancy between the child and adult mechanism means that what is tolerable for an adult, such as use of a rigid oral endoscope for visualization, can be nearly impossible in the smaller oral cavity of a child. However, a number of centers report excellent results, with a success rate similar to that within the adult population, in using nasendoscopy with a flexible scope to examine children as young as 2 years of age (Chait & Lotz, 1991; Lotz, D'Antonio, Chait, & Netsell, 1993).

Studies addressing the efficacy of stroboscopic images in adults have shown increased diagnostic sensitivity and altered management decisions in 10–32% of voice disordered patients (Casiano, Zaveri, & Lundy, 1992; Sataloff, Spiegel, & Hawkshaw, 1991; Woo, Colton, Casper, & Brewer, 1991). The value of a video-recorded, magnified image of dynamic vibratory patterns of the vocal folds has become more recognized in the United States. in the past 10 years. Although nasendoscopic views have become common in the assessment of pediatric velopharyngeal function accompanied by a view of the larynx, endoscopy with stroboscopy specifically for assessment of laryngeal function has not been frequently reported. There is a need for efficacy research on use of laryngeal videostroboscopy in the pediatric population.

4.6. Electroglottography

Electroglottography (EGG) as a measurement technique is particularly well-suited for use with children, given its ease of use and noninvasiveness. The collected waveforms provide specific information about vocal fold kinematics on a cycle-by-cycle basis as measured by time-varying electrical impedance across the glottis, transmitted and recorded with surface electrodes. Validation studies on adult data have demonstrated that EGG is capable of examining fine details of each vibratory cycle (Childers, Smith, & Moore, 1984; Gilbert, Potter & Hoodin, 1984; Scherer, Druker, & Titze, 1988). However, to date, there is little published work in either EGG modeling of the pediatric vibratory cycle or examination of large pediatric datasets with children at various age levels. In a large study of pediatric vocal fold vibratory patterns, Corbin-Lewis (1996) found evidence of age and gender differences in 212 third- and sixth-grade children with perceptually normal voice. The shape of EGG waveforms, representing patterns of vocal fold contact, differed between boys and girls, and the amount of time the vocal folds were in contact was shorter for the boys. It is interesting to note that a shorter contact time for boys is in direct contrast to findings in the adult population, in which females have a shorter contact time. The examined age differences among subjects had less impact on parameters studied than did gender, even at the third-grade level. The beginning of a normative database has been established for comparison purposes to children with perceptually abnormal voices. In a recent study, sensitivity of EGG parameters were examined for voicing patterns in adults (Peterson, Verdolini-Marston, Barkmeier, & Hoffman, 1994). The closed quotient was sensitive in differentiating pressed, normal, and breathy voice patterns. This type of study needs to be replicated in the pediatric population.

The utility of EGG for diagnostic and therapeutic purposes will remain tentative until EGG data on large numbers of children with normal and disordered voice are collected and analyzed. However, the methodology holds promise as one tool in simultaneous measurement of speech production subsystems.

5. TREATMENT ISSUES IN THE PEDIATRIC POPULATION

The focus of this book is on current measurement techniques of voice. It is not within the scope of this chapter to outline specific treatment strategies for individual pediatric vocal disorders. However, the role of measurement in tracking progress or deterioration of vocal function specifically addressing pediatric problems is considered extremely important and is discussed next.

5.1. Management Principles

The management of childhood voice problems should be based on guiding principles that reflect current knowledge about vocal function and the physiological and structural processes that contribute to it. Although efficacy data validating these principles and techniques remain severely limited, the conceptual framework presented provides a reasonable rationale and starting point for inquiry.

Therapeutic intervention strategies for pediatric voice disorders have one primary goal—to change vocal behaviors to those that facilitate maximum glottal efficiency. This may be done surgically in the case of structural defects or behaviorally when symptoms suggest overuse, abuse, or misuse of the laryngeal system. Regardless of the framework used to classify voice disorders (functional versus organic or hypofunctional versus hyperfunctional), the speech-language pathologist's goal is to establish (or reestablish) behaviors resulting in the best possible voice the mechanism can maintain. To achieve that goal, a set of guiding principles may be postulated.

1. Voice disorders are not mysterious problems requiring unusual procedures for management. Fundamental clinical processes

are the same as those appropriate for other communication disorders.

2. Voice and its associated perceptual features are behaviors that can be modified in adults or children. The great majority of childhood voice problems spring from hyperfunctional action of the vocal mechanism and these behaviors can be modified. The utilization of careful behavioral inventory and identification of problems, stimulus control, and precise consequent management are as facilitative in voice therapy as in management of other communicative disorders.
3. Behavioral compensations or adjustments can often facilitate a maximally efficient voice, even in disorders with a primary structural or physiological basis.

Behrman and Orlikoff (1997) provided a conceptual approach that bases assessment and management of voice disorders on the scientific method of hypothesis construction and testing. They relied heavily on instrumental measures to provide data to support or reject a hypothesis under consideration. In their tutorial they describe the speech-language pathologist's role in diagnosing and managing disordered voice as consisting of (1) assessing, (2) determining severity, (3) determining etiology and maintaining factors, and (4) developing effective treatment. To accomplish these goals the speech-language pathologist must identify a symptom such as the perception of vocal hoarseness or roughness in the case of nodules and pose a hypothesis as to why and how the nodules developed and are being maintained in physiological terms. Advanced understanding of vocal physiology incorporating aerodynamic, phonatory, articulatory, and resonatory factors allows a clinician to speculate or hypothesize that a child is using increased vocal effort (increased vocal fold tension or glottal resistance and increased subglottal air pressure) to overcome the constraints presented by the mass-occupying lesions that inhibit total glottal closure. From that point the clinician needs to test the hypothesis by selecting measures that will either lend support to the hypothesis or provide data that may result in rejecting the hypothesis and formulating another. If measures of vocal intensity are higher than the appropriate normative data and glottal airflow values are lower than expected given assumed incomplete closure, the clinician might speculate that the hypothesis is supported and establish initial goals to decrease glottal tension and resistance, perhaps using a breathy onset or a confidential vocal pattern (Colton & Casper, 1996). Further use of instrumental measures can track progress and/or suggest to the clinician that the working hypothesis needs to be assessed. Although perceptual information provides one component used by the clinician to help develop and test hypotheses, it should not be the only component since it has the limitations outlined earlier in this chapter.

5.2. Management Strategies

5.2.1. Hyperfunctional Voice Disorders

Postinfancy, the single most common voice disorder in children is a hyperfunctional voice, with or without lesions (Johnson, 1988; Wilson, 1987).

Johnson (1985) recommends a basic three-step behavioral treatment strategy for children with persistent hoarseness resulting from overuse, misuse, or abuse resulting in vocal hyperfunction. The strategy includes first a systematic reduction of vocal misuse/abuse behavior detailed in the VARP; second the establishment of appropriate vocal quality with facilitative techniques (Boone & McFarlane, 1994); and third, the extension-generalization of appropriate vocal quality to all situations. The treatment model is summarized in Figure 21–1 and includes the targets for evaluation and assessment.

This treatment model is easily able to incorporate instrumental measures into evaluation and treatment goals. The VARP uses a self-control management strategy from applied behavior analysis with daily behavioral chart-

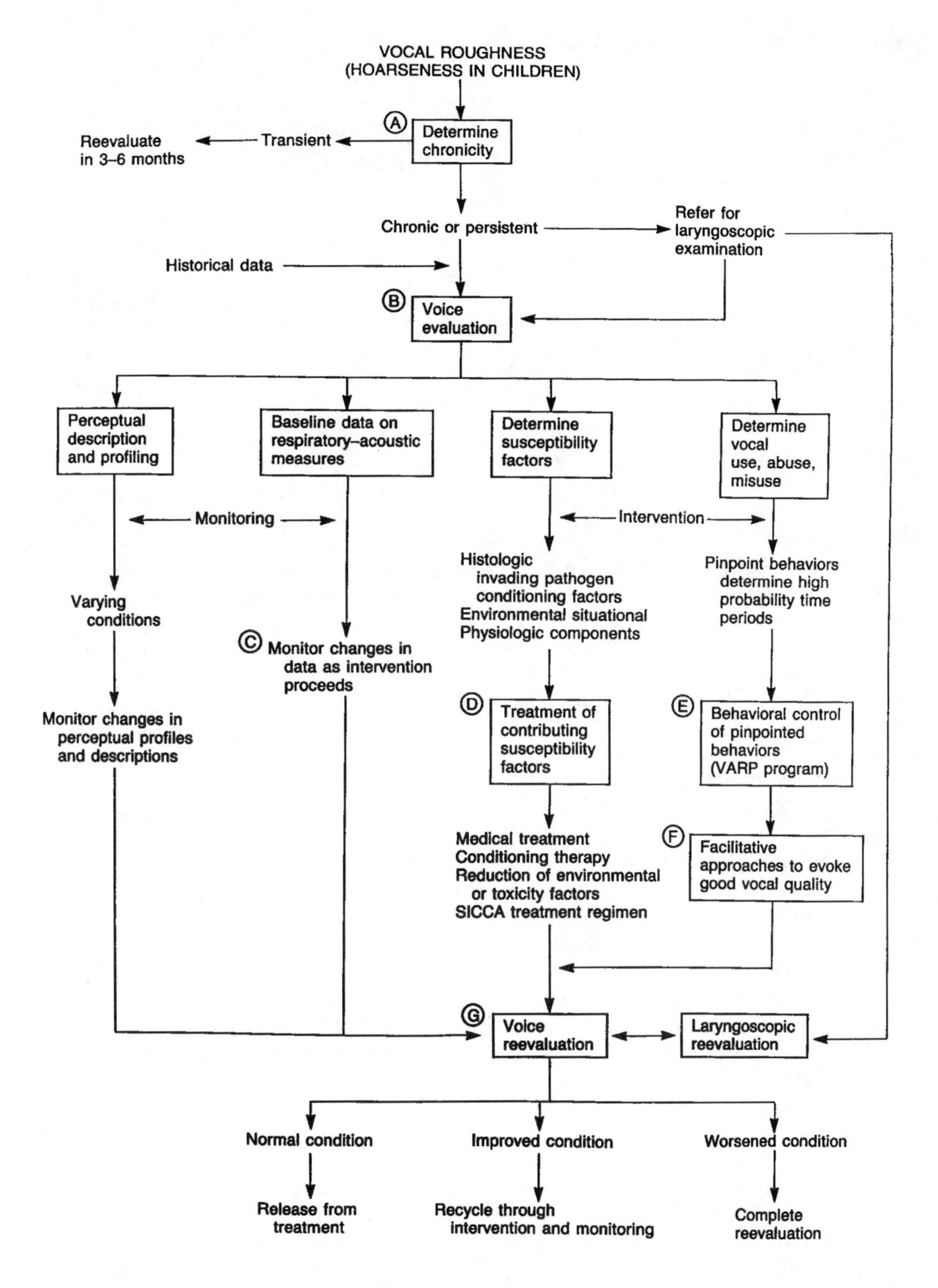

Figure 21–1. Treatment model for children with hoarseness. (From "Hoarseness in Children," by T. S. Johnson, 1988, p. 135 in *Decision Making in Speech-Language Pathology*, edited by D. E. Yoder and R. Kent, Philadelphia: B. C. Decker, Inc. Reprinted with permission.)

ing to effectively and efficiently reduce hyperfunctional voice behaviors. A clinician is able to monitor progress continuously over the course of therapy by viewing the daily behavior records of vocal abuse. The efficacy of the VARP (Johnson, 1985) is supported by 7 years of single-subject design research and multiple replication studies done at Utah State University (Johnson, unpublished data).

D. Kenneth Wilson has provided detailed management materials for modification of pediatric vocal function. His work (1987) suggested that the management of childhood voice problems proceed through a phased model including: (1) an introduction phase, (2) analyzing phase, (3) a change phase, and (4) a good voice establishment phase. Use of instrumental methodologies rather than sole reliance on perceptual scales is recommended.

Techniques to establish a maximally efficient voice are provided by Boone (1993) and Boone and McFarlane (1994). Although not specifically designed for pediatric voice problems, Boone and McFarlane's textbook integrates application of facilitative procedures into modes appropriate for both children and adults. *The Boone Voice Program for Children* (1993) similarly provides procedures and materials appropriately designed for implementation with pediatric clients. Again, these materials were well-designed and lend themselves to the incorporation of behavioral measurement and instrumental monitoring.

Moya Andrews' approach to pediatric phonatory disorders (1986, 1995) is likewise compatible with the previous methods. She suggests (1) symptomatic voice therapy; (2) a physiologic approach in which function of speech subsystems such as respiration, phonation, articulation, and resonation are examined to explain their role in the voice difficulty; (3) lifestyle and environment modification; and (4) the use of psychodynamic voice therapy techniques. Again, these methods can be best implemented with carefully chosen instrumental measures to establish baseline performance, differentiate between speech subsystem deficits, monitor progress, and provide direct feedback during therapy.

5.3. Medical-Surgical Considerations

There are times when surgical intervention may be considered for the elimination of laryngeal pathology secondary to vocal abuse in children. In the pediatric population, surgery should not usually be considered for the hyperfunctional group of disorders because of frequency of recurrence, the risk of vocal fold scarring, and because voice therapy, if properly applied, can effectively manage virtually all of them (Smith & Gray, 1995). The therapy of choice in children (and for that matter in adults) who have bilateral vocal pathology secondary to hyperfunction is vocal reeducation rather than surgical removal of the pathology. This conservative philosophy about management of childhood disorders currently prevails throughout the field of laryngology (Smith & Gray, 1995). The well-informed speech-language pathologist should be assertive in seeing that children be given appropriate behavioral treatment prior to any serious consideration of surgery. Such an advocacy position is both professionally appropriate and ethically sound when one has behavioral and/or valid instrumental data that support a diagnosis of a hyperfunctional voice disorder.

6. PREVALENT DISORDERS

6.1. Vocal Hoarseness and Gastroesophageal Reflux

Gastroesophageal reflux is defined as the backflow of gastric material through the lower esophageal sphincter (LES) into the esophagus and is most prevalent in children under 2 years of age and middle-aged adults (Arvedson, Bless, Ford, Robbins, & Singaram, 1997). Extraesophageal reflux or laryngopharyngeal reflux (LPR) occurs when material from the stomach refluxes above the upper esophageal sphincter (UES). The prevalence and incidence in school-aged children is not known now, but is thought to be implicated in three main pathological conditions presenting in older children—

asthma and cough, paradoxical vocal cord dysfunction, and voice disorders (Arvedson et al., 1997; Gumpert, Kalach, Dupont, & Contencin, 1998). Atypical presentation of GER/LPR may include hoarseness or chronic laryngitis, recurrent croup, chronic cough, chronic rhinosinusitis. The role of GER/LPR is currently under question in recurrent respiratory papillomas (Arvedson et al., 1997). The role of GER/LPR in the pathophysiology of benign vocal fold lesions warrants examination.

6.2. Vocal Fold Dysfunction

The disorder labeled paradoxical vocal cord dysfunction, vocal fold dysfunction, functional laryngeal stridor, chronic acute laryngospasms, Munchausen's stridor, and a host of other terms is a recently added disorder in the field of speech-language pathology. It is characterized by highly variable vocal fold closure patterns: one example being a closed pattern with a small posterior glottal chink during inspiration when the vocal folds should be abducted (hence, the term paradoxical), inhibiting air intake and resulting in severe air hunger. Pulmonary function studies or blood levels performed during an episode are suggestive of paradoxical vocal fold dysfunction. Paradoxical vocal fold dysfunction can be positively identified by visualizing the closure pattern during endoscopy. The disorder has often been misdiagnosed as bronchial asthma, exercise-induced asthma, or upper airway obstruction. The etiology and pathophysiology has not been identified to date but predisposing and precipitating factors hypothesized include neurologic (vagal reflex), gastrointestinal (microaspiration of acid), and psychogenic (somatization). The disorder has been identified in all age groups from infants to geriatric patients with a predominance of females to males (Bless & Swift, 1996; Martin, Blager, Gay, & Wood, 1987). Precise incidence and prevalence data are not yet available. It is estimated that approximately half of patients with paradoxical vocal fold dysfunction also have asthma (Arvedson et al., 1997). Data from the University of Wisconsin-Madison on 87 consecutive patients indicate different symptom profiles for a subset of adolescents compared to adults (Bless & Swift, 1996). Swift (personal communication) has found an increased prevalence in boys compared to girls in the 7- to 10-year-old age range. In her clinical practice, she has found that these children respond positively to counseling combined with behavioral treatment to gain control over the symptoms. In general, she has found that patients are intelligent, high-achieving individuals with extremely high self-expectations.

At present, treatment strategies for paradoxical vocal fold dysfunction are largely behavioral and address the symptoms, not the etiology of this disorder. Blager and colleagues, at the National Jewish Center for Immunology and Respiratory Medicine, developed one of the first behavioral treatment programs (Martin et al., 1987). Most programs are designed to focus the patient on the respiratory system to establish a controlled abdominal breathing pattern to be used during stridor or laryngeal tightness. This focus is initially intended as a distraction from the larynx and the vocal folds, enabling volitional relaxation of the neck region through controlled abdominal breathing. When volitional control over the breathing cycle is established and laryngeal abduction is under the patient's control, the panic sensation lessens and the cycle of the disorder is disrupted.

7. PREVENTION: THE FUTURE

Prevention of vocal abuse is a developing alternative to vocal abuse reduction therapy. It is believed that systematic approaches to vocal education can facilitate effective vocal use and reduce the number of hyperfunctional disorders of voice in children. Methods to improve vocal hygiene, such as increasing hydration levels have been shown empirically to effect vocal production (Hemler, Wieneke, & Dejonckere, 1997; Verdolini-Marston, Sandage, & Titze, 1994; Verdolini, Titze, & Fennell, 1994).

Nilson and Schneiderman (1983) developed an educational prevention program and used it with 155 second- and third-grade students.

Kaufmann and Johnson (1991) developed a program with a similar focus for adult educators. Educating students and educators in the prevention or control of vocally abusive behaviors may directly reduce the future need for specific voice therapy of this type. Prevention strategies are particularly appropriate for the hyperfunctional group of voice disorders since the basic causes of these problems are well known and amenable to behavioral change (Child & Johnson, 1991; Johnson, 1991; Kahane & Mayo, 1989; Marge, 1991; Stone, 1991). Certainly the future may reveal that the application of "best practices" in the care, health, and hygiene of the vocal mechanism will result in a reduction of the incidence of voice disorders.

REFERENCES

Andrews, M. L. (1986). *Voice therapy for children.* New York: Longman.

Andrews, M. L. (1995). *Manual of voice treatment: Pediatrics through geriatrics.* San Diego: Singular Publishing Group.

Arvedson, J., Bless, D., Ford, C., Robbins, J., & Singaram, C. (1997, November). *Reflux and airway protection across the age span: Clinical considerations.* Short course presented at the Convention of the American Speech-Language-Hearing Association, Boston.

Beckett, R. L. (1971). The respirometer as a diagnostic and clinical tool in the speech clinic. *Journal of Speech and Hearing Disorders, 36,* 235–241.

Behrman, A., & Orlikoff, R. F. (1997). Instrumentation in voice assessment and treatment: What's the use? *American Journal of Speech-Language Pathology, 6,* 9–16.

Bless, D. M., & Swift, E. (1996). *Vocal fold dysfunction (VFD): Diagnosis and management.* Presentation at the 4th Biennial Phonosurgery Symposium, Madison, WI.

Boone, D. R. (1993). *The Boone voice program for children* (2nd ed.). Austin, TX: Pro-Ed.

Boone, D. R., & McFarlane, S. C. (1994). *The voice and voice therapy* (5th ed.). Englewood Cliffs, NJ: Prentice-Hall, Inc.

Casiano, R. R., Zaveri, V., & Lundy, D. S. (1992). Efficacy of videostroboscopy in the diagnosis of voice disorders. *Otolaryngology—Head and Neck Surgery, 107,* 95–100.

Chait, D. H., & Lotz, W. K. (1991). Successful pediatric examinations using nasendoscopy. *Laryngoscope, 101,* 1016–1018.

Child, D. R., & Johnson, T. J. (1991). Preventable and nonpreventable causes of voice disorders. *Seminars in Speech and Language, 12*(1), 1–13.

Childers, D. G., Smith, A. M., & Moore, G. P. (1984). Relationships between electroglottograph, speech, and vocal cord contact. *Folia Phoniatrica, 36,* 105–118.

Colton, R. H., & Casper, J. K. (1996). *Understanding voice problems: A physiological perspective for diagnosis and treatment* (2nd ed.). Baltimore: William & Wilkins.

Corbin-Lewis, K. (1996). *Electroglottographic analysis of children with normal voice.* Unpublished doctoral dissertation, University of Wisconsin-Madison, Madison, WI.

Dobres, R., Lee, L., Stemple, J. C., Kummer, A. W., & Kretschmer, L. W. (1990). Description of laryngeal pathologies in children evaluated by otolaryngologists. *Journal of Speech and Hearing Disorders, 55,* 526–532.

Dworkin, J. P., & Meleca, R. J. (1996). *Vocal pathologies: Diagnosis, treatment, and case studies.* San Diego: Singular Publishing Group.

Gilbert, H. R., Potter, C. R., & Hoodin, R. (1984). Laryngograph as a measure of vocal fold contact area. *Journal of Speech and Hearing Research, 27,* 178–182.

Gilbert, H. R., Robb, M. P., & Chen, Y (1997). Formant frequency development: 15 to 36 months. *Journal of Voice, 11,* 260–266.

Glaze, L. E., Bless, D. M., Milenkovic, P., & Susser, R. D. (1988). Acoustic characteristics of children's voice. *Journal of Voice, 2,* 312–319.

Glaze, L. E., Bless, D. M., & Susser, R. D. (1990). Acoustic analysis of vowel and loudness differences in children's voice. *Journal of Voice, 4,* 37–44.

Gray, S. D., Hirano, M., & Sato, K. (1993). Molecular and cellular structure of vocal fold tissue. In I. R. Titze (Ed.), *Vocal fold physiology: Frontiers of basic science* (pp. 1–34). San Diego: Singular Publishing Group.

Gray, S. D., Pignatari, S. S., Harding, P. (1994). Morphologic ultrastructure of anchoring fibers in normal vocal fold basement membrane zone. *Journal of Voice, 8,* 48–52.

Gumpert, L., Kalach, N., Dupont, C., & Contencin, P. (1998). Hoarseness and gastroesophageal reflux in children. *Journal of Laryngology and Otology, 112,* 49–54.

Hammond, T. H., Zhou, R., Hammond, E. H., Pawlak, A., & Gray, S. D. (1997). The intermediate layer: A morphologic study of the elastin and hyaluronic acid constituents of normal, human vocal folds. *Journal of Voice*, 11, 59–66.

Hasek, C. S., Singh, S., & Murry, T. (1980). Acoustic attributes of preadolescent voices. *Journal of Acoustical Society of America, 68*, 1262–1265.

Hemler, R. J., Wieneke, G. H., & Dejonckere, P. H. (1997). The effect of relative humidity of inhaled air on acoustic parameters of voice in normal subjects. *Journal of Voice*, 11, 295–300.

Herrington-Hall, B. L., Lee, L., Stemple, J. C., Niemi, K. R., & McHone M. M. (1988). Description of laryngeal pathologies by age, sex, and occupation in a treatment-seeking sample. *Journal of Speech and Hearing Disorders, 53*, 57–64.

Hirano, M. (1981a). *Clinical examination of voice*. New York: Springer-Verlag.

Hirano, M. (1981b). Structure of the vocal fold in normal and disease states: Anatomical and physical studies. In C. L. Ludlow & M. O. Hart (Eds.), *Proceedings of the Conference on the Assessment of Vocal Pathology* (Vol. 11, pp. 11–30). Rockville, MD: American Speech and Hearing Association.

Hirano, M., Kurita, S., & Nakashima, T. (1983). Growth, development and aging of human vocal folds. In D. M. Bless & J. H. Abbs, (Eds.), *Vocal fold physiology* (pp. 22–44). San Diego: College-Hill Press.

Hirschberg, J., Dejonckere, P. H., Hirano, M., Mori, K., Schulz-Coulon,H.-J., & Vrticka, K. (1995). Voice disorders in children. *International Journal of Pediatric Oto-Rhino-Laryngology, 32*(Suppl.), S109–S125.

Hixon, T. J. (1987). *Respiratory function in speech and song*. Boston: College-Hill Press.

Hoit, J. D., Hixon, T. J., Watson, P. J., & Morgan, W. J. (1990). Speech breathing in children and adolescents. *Journal of Speech and Hearing Research, 33*, 51–69.

Hufnagle, J., & Hufnagle, K. K. (1988). S/Z ratio in dysphonic children with and without vocal cord nodules. *Language, Speech, and Hearing Services in the Schools, 19*, 418–422.

Johnson, T. S. (1985). *Vocal abuse reduction program*. San Diego: College-Hill Press.

Johnson, T. S. (1986). Vocal disorders: The measurement of clinical progress. In J. M. Costello & A. L. Holland (Eds.), *Handbook of speech and language disorders* (pp. 477–502). San Diego: College-Hill Press.

Johnson, T. S. (1988). Hoarseness in the child. In D. E. Yoder & R. D. Kent (Eds.), *Decision making in speech-language pathology* (pp. 134–135). Philadelphia: B. C. Decker, Inc.

Johnson, T. S. (1991). Principles and practices of prevention as applied to voice disorders. *Seminars in Speech and Language, 12*, 14–22.

Johnson, T. S., & Child, D. R. (1988). Voice disorders in the child. In N. J. Lass, L. V. McReynolds, J. L. Northern, & D. E. Yoder (Eds.), *Handbook of speech-language pathology and audiology* (pp. 787–808). Philadelphia: B. C. Decker, Inc.

Kahane, J. C. (1978). A morphological study of the human prepubertal and pubertal larynx. *American Journal of Anatomy, 151*, 11–20.

Kahane, J. C. (1982). Growth of the human prepubertal and pubertal larynx. *Journal of Speech and Hearing Research, 25*, 446–455.

Kahane, J., & Mayo, R. (1989). The need for aggressive pursuit of healthy childhood voices. *Language, Speech, and Hearing Services in Schools, 20*, 102–107.

Kaufmann, T. J., & Johnson, T. J. (1991). An exemplary preventative voice program for educators. *Seminars in Speech and Language, 12*, 40–48.

Kent, R. D. (1976). Anatomical and neuromuscular maturation of the speech mechanism: Evidence from acoustic studies. *Journal of Speech and Hearing Research, 19*, 421–447.

Kent, R. D. (1993). Vocal tract acoustics. *Journal of Voice, 7*, 97–117.

Kent, R. D. (1996). Hearing and believing: Some limits to the auditory-perceptual assessment of speech and voice disorders. *American Journal of Speech-Language Pathology, 5*, 7–23.

Kent, R. D., & Vorperian, H. (1995). Development of the craniofacial-oral-laryngeal anatomy: A review. *Journal of Medical Speech-Language Pathology, 3*, 145–190.

Kirchner, J. A. (1970). *Pressman & Kelemen's physiology of the larynx: Revised*. Washington, DC: American Academy of Otolaryngology-Head and Neck Surgery Foundation, Inc.

Klatt, D. H., & Klatt, L. C. (1990). Analysis, synthesis, and perception of voice quality variations among female and male talkers. *Journal of the Acoustical Society of America, 87*, 820–857.

Koschkee, D. L., & Rammage, L. (1997). *Voice care in the medical setting*. San Diego: Singular Publishing Group.

Kreiman, J., Gerratt B. R., Kempster, G. B., Erman, A., & Berke, G. S. (1993). Perceptual evaluation of voice quality: Review, tutorial, and a framework for future research. *Journal of Speech and Hearing Research, 36,* 21–40.

Lecoq, M., & Drape, F. (1996). An epidemiological survey of dysphonia in children at school entry. *Revue de Laryngologie, Otologie, Rhinologie, (Bordeaux), 117,* 323–325.

Lotz, W. K., D'Antonio, L. L., Chait, D. H., & Netsell, R. W. (1993). Successful nasendoscopic and aerodynamic examinations of children with speech/voice disorders. *International Journal of Pediatric Otorhinolaryngology, 26,* 165–172.

Marge, M. (1991). Introduction to the prevention and epidemiology of voice disorders. *Seminars in Speech and Language, 12,* 49–73.

Martin, R. J., Blager, F. B., Gay, M. L., & Wood, R. P. (1987). Paradoxic vocal cord motion in presumed asthmatics. *Seminars in Respiratory Medicine, 8,* 332–337.

Michel, J. F, & Wendahl, R. (1971). Correlates of voice production. In L. E. Travis (Ed.), *Handbook of speech pathology and audiology* (pp. 465–480). New York: Appleton-Century-Crofts.

Milenkovic, P. (1989). *Cspeech 3.0* [Computer software]. Madison: University of Wisconsin.

Moore, G. P. (1977). Have the major issues in voice disorders been answered by research in speech science? A 50-year retrospective. *Journal of Speech and Hearing Disorders, 42,* 152–160.

Nilson, H., & Schneiderman C. R. (1983). Classroom program for the prevention of vocal abuse in elementary school children. *Language, Speech, and Hearing Services in Schools, 14,* 172–178.

Pawlak, A., Hammond, T., Hammond, E., & Gray, S. (1996). Immunocytochemical study of proteoglycans in vocal folds. *Annals of Otology, Rhinology and Laryngology, 105,* 6–11.

Peterson, K. L., Verdolini-Marston, K., Barkmeier, J. M., & Hoffman, H. T. (1994). Comparison of aerodynamic and electroglottographic parameters in evaluating clinically relevant voicing patterns. *Annals of Otology, Rhinology and Laryngology, 103* (Pt. 1), 335–346.

Polgar, G., & Weng, T. R. (1979). The functional development of the respiratory system from the period of gestation to adulthood. *American Review of Respiratory Disease, 120,* 625–695.

Reed, C. G. (1980). Voice therapy: A need for research. *Journal of Speech and Hearing Disorders, 45,* 157–169.

Robb, M. P., & Simmons, J. O. (1990). Gender comparisons of children's vocal fold contact behavior. *Journal of the Acoustical Society of America, 88,* 1318–1322.

Sander, E. K. (1989). Arguments against the aggressive pursuit of voice therapy for children. *Language, Speech, and Hearing Services in Schools, 20,* 94–101.

Sapienza, C. M., & Stathopoulos, E. T. (1994). Respiratory and laryngeal measures of children and women with bilateral vocal fold nodules. *Journal of Speech and Hearing Research, 37,* 1229–1243.

Sataloff, R. T., Spiegel, J., & Hawkshaw, M. J. (1991). Strobovideolaryngoscopy: Results and clinical value. *Annals of Otology, Rhinology and Laryngology, 100,* 725–727.

Scherer, R. C., Druker, D., & Titze, I. (1988). Electroglottography and direct measurement of vocal fold contact area. In O. Fujimura (Ed.), *Vocal physiology* (Vol. 2, pp. 279–293). New York: Raven Press.

Senturia, B. H., & Wilson, F. B. (1968). Otorhinolaryngic findings in children with voice deviations. Preliminary report. *Annals of Otology, Rhinology and Laryngology, 77,* 1027–1042.

Silverman, E. M. (1975). Incidence of chronic hoarseness among school-age children. *Journal of Speech and Hearing Research, 40,* 211–215.

Smith, M. E., & Gray, S. D. (1995). Voice. In C. D. Bluestone, S. E. Stool, & M. A. Kenna (Eds.), *Pediatric otolaryngology* (3rd ed., pp. 1261–1274). Philadelphia: W. B. Saunders Company.

Smitheran, J. R., & Hixon, T. J. (1981). A clinical method for estimating laryngeal airway resistance during vowel production. *Journal of Speech and Hearing Disorders, 46,* 138–146.

Stathopoulos, E. T. (1986). Relationship between intraoral air pressure and vocal intensity in children and adults. *Journal of Speech and Hearing Research, 29,* 71–74.

Stathopoulos, E. T., & Sapienza, C. M. (1993). Respiratory and laryngeal measures of children during vocal intensity variation. *Journal of the Acoustical Society of America, 94,* 2531–2543.

Stathopoulos, E. T., & Sapienza, C. M. (1997). Developmental changes in laryngeal and respiratory function with variations in sound pressure level. *Journal of Speech, Language and Hearing Research, 40,* 595–614.

Stathopoulos, E. T., & Weismer, G. (1985). Oral airflow and air pressure during speech production. A comparative study of children, youths, and adults. *Folia Phoniatrica, 37,* 152–159.

Stone, R. E. (1991). Toward models for national issues in the prevention of voice disorders. *Seminars in Speech and Language, 12,* 23–39.

Till, J. A. (1990). *Computer assisted speech evaluation and rehabilitation.* Long Beach, CA: Speech Research

Laboratories, Long Beach Veterans Administration Medical Centers.

Titze, I. R. (1989). Physiologic and acoustic differences between male and female voices. *Journal of the Acoustical Society of America, 85,* 1699–1707.

Titze, I. R. (1995). *Workshop on acoustic voice analysis* (Summary statement). Iowa City, IA: National Center for Voice and Speech.

Trudeau, M. D., & Forrest, L. A. (1997). The contributions of phonatory volume and transglottal airflow to the s/z ratio. *American Journal of Speech-Language Pathology, 6,* 65–69.

Verdolini, K., Titze, I. R., & Fennell, A. (1994). Dependence of phonatory effort on hydration level. *Journal of Speech, Language and Hearing Research, 37,* 1001–1007.

Verdolini-Marston, K., Sandage, M., & Titze, I. R. (1994). Effect of hydration treatments on laryngeal nodules and polyps and related voice measures. *Journal of Voice, 8,* 30–47.

Wilson, D. K. (1987). *The voice problems of children* (3rd ed.). Baltimore: Williams & Wilkins.

Wilson, F. B. (1990). *A program of diagnosis and management for voice disorders.* Bellingham, WA: Voice Tapes, Inc.

Woo, P., Colton, R., Casper, J., & Brewer, D. (1991). Diagnostic value of stroboscopic examination in hoarse patients. *Journal of Voice, 5,* 231–238.

Yairi, E., Currin, L. H., Bulian, N., & Yairi, J. (1974). Incidence of hoarseness in school children over a 1-year period. *Journal of Communication Disorders, 7,* 321–328.

Zajac, D. J., Farkas, Z., Dindzans, L. J., & Stool, S. E. (1993). Aerodynamic and laryngographic assessment of pediatric vocal function. *Pediatric Pulmonology, 15,* 44–51.

CHAPTER 22

Voice Quality of Deaf Speakers

Evelyn Abberton

Nowhere is the relationship between speech perception and speech production more evident than in hearing impairment. Nevertheless, the relationship is far from straightforward. Not only is intelligibility often an issue, but social stereotyping and acceptability judgments made on the basis of their voices and other aspects of their spoken language can be causes of concern for deaf speakers. A major component of indexical information in speech is provided by voice quality.

Three interacting factors can be seen to influence the quality of the speech of deaf people:

- Degree and type of hearing loss and the age of the speaker at its onset
- Style of education and communication in the family: speech or sign
- Effect of hearing aids—including cochlear implants

Given the great variability in the intelligibility and acceptability of deaf people's speech—from essentially normal to unintelligible—it is not a simple question to ask what it is that characterizes "deaf" voice quality and how it might be described and measured. The fact that people claim to be able to recognize deaf speakers by simply hearing their voices—whatever language is being spoken—reinforces the essential starting point for a discussion of the definition or characterization and measurement of deaf voice quality: the nature of the voice must be sought not simply in descriptive perceptual or acoustic measures of phonetic and phonological patterns in speech output, but in relating these measures to the speech perceptual abilities and difficulties of the speaker. In other words, the qualities of the voice must be related to the role of auditory feedback in the control of speech production—a fact recognized in the last century by the auditory training pioneer, Urbantschitsch (1895). The easy recognition of a deaf voice also emphasizes the importance of the voice for conveying indexical information on personality and group identity (Scherer, 1995, and the many references included there); the social functioning of a voice and the social feedback it provides can be studied (Cowie & Douglas-Cowie, 1992) and measured as well as its acoustic and phonetic form and linguistic functioning.

1. RELATIONSHIP BETWEEN CHARACTERISTICS OF IMPAIRED HEARING AND SPEECH PRODUCTION

Conventional hearing aids are essentially amplifiers of the whole, or high frequency parts, of the speech signal. However, the deaf speaker's problem is not simply one of hearing acuity. Profoundly deaf speakers (with 5-frequency average pure tone losses greater than 95 dB) may have excellent spoken language and appropriate voices of better quality than those of less conventionally deaf speakers. Clearly, other aspects of speech perceptual processing must be taken into account in attempts to explain their speech quality. In recent years, there has been an increase of interest in this area of speech perception, particularly in the context of the design of signal processing hearing aids including cochlear implants (Walliker, Daley, Smith, Faulkner, & Fourcin, 1993). Fourcin, in an early account of this phonetic and psychoacoustically based approach, writes: "the objective is to show how an essentially auditory pattern approach towards an understanding of the important features of the mechanism of speech processing ability can lead to testable conclusions which are not otherwise obvious and which may have practical value" (Fourcin, 1979, p. 167). Speech production is regarded as being guided by essentially auditory pattern targets based on acoustic characteristics of laryngeal excitation patterns and formant structuring of the speech signal.

The psychoacoustic abilities beyond acuity that underlie speech perception are concerned with processing in the time and frequency domains. Detection thresholds, discomfort levels, dynamic range, intensity discrimination (static and dynamic), frequency selectivity, spectral shape discrimination, gap detection, tone/noise discrimination, frequency discrimination, and phase sensitivity may all contribute to speech perception ability (Rosen, Faulkner, & Smith, 1990) and, thus, to speech production. Features such as these are responsible for detection, discrimination, and identification of phonetic and phonological units in speech. They can also be related via auditory feedback to the characteristics of the voice and segmental organization of the spoken language of deaf speakers. In general, temporal resolving power is less impaired than frequency selectivity in even profoundly deaf(ened) speakers, who, given appropriate aids, should be able to develop or regain adequate phonation quality and pitch control. Tactile and kinesthetic feedback have a role in the interplay between perception and production of speech, as does speechreading. However, the striking characteristics of deaf voices and the improvements that can be achieved by enhancing auditory feedback in a principled way (Ball, Faulkner, & Fourcin, 1990; House, 1995; Oster, 1987; Toffin et al., 1995, for example) show that it is in auditory patterning that explanations can be most profitably sought.

2. DEFINITIONS OF VOICE QUALITY

The term voice quality is used in different ways. For some it refers to the laryngeal components in speech (Ní Chasaide & Gobl, 1997)—essentially phonation types. However, fundamental frequency variation in pitch and loudness patterning must also be considered in their phonetic and phonological contributions to perceived quality (Abberton, Fourcin, & Hazan, 1991; Parker, 1983). For others, voice quality is a continuous background effect to what is being said and encompasses not only phonation type but also aspects of resonance (such as nasality) and articulatory settings (Laver, 1980). Intermittent effects, particularly of phonation type, also contribute to a listener's overall perception of the auditory coloring of a voice.

Analytically, it is revealing to separate laryngeal excitation (the voice source) from its supraglottal modification (filtering) in the vocal tract. Although this may be considered artificial (as there is always larynx–vocal tract interaction in speech) there are also important practical as well as theoretical reasons for considering voice to be an essentially laryngeal phenomenon. This is evident in the design, use, and assessment of certain modern hearing aids and interactive visual feedback displays for speech perceptual and productive therapy. What is clear is that, without adequate input from the vibrating vocal folds, speech output cannot be adequate: The auditory and articulatory problems for deaf speakers in producing vowels and consonants must not be underestimated. But, without the essential framework provided by phonation type and pitch and loudness patterning, intelligibility and acceptability will suffer—sometimes drastically. In normal speech development, control of phonation and basic tone and intonation patterns precedes mastery of vowel and consonant systems (Fletcher & Garman, 1986; Fourcin, 1978); it is important to note that these skills are not simply a matter of reproducing the low frequency part of the speech signal, but are intimately bound up with pragmatic and syntactic development. The importance of allowing and encouraging laryngeal voice skills to develop (in family interaction and educational setting) as a prerequisite for later spoken language acquisitions has been emphasized by Clark (1989).

3. CHARACTERISTICS OF DEAF VOICE QUALITY

Quite elaborate systems of auditory perceptual assessment of voice quality are available; two well known systems are GRBAS (Grade, Roughness, Breathy, Asthenic, Strained) (Hirano, 1981) and the VPAS (Vocal Profile Analysis Scheme) (Wirz & Mackenzie Beck, 1995).

In much early descriptive work on deaf voice quality, there was no clear separation of source and vocal tract characteristics, phonetic and phonological patterns, or attempts to relate the perceived voice quality in any detailed or systematic way to the auditory abilities of the speaker. House (1995) gives a summary.

A major factor in the quality of the voices of speakers with hearing impairment is age of onset of hearing loss; prelingually deaf speakers tend to have less normal voices than people who become deaf after acquisition of spoken language. This is, of course, a generalization: As stated previously, even profoundly prelingually deaf speakers can have excellent voices if the hearing impairment is diagnosed early, appropriate hearing aids are used consistently from the time of diagnosis, and if the child is educated in a hearing–speaking environment. The effects of acquired deafness are variable. Some writers have claimed that there is little or no effect on speech in postlingual deafness. Ling (1976) considers that for adults with well established skills, feedforward and production mechanisms have become automatic and auditory feedback is therefore not essential. Espir and Rose (1976) assert that acquired deafness in adults does not usually interfere with ability to speak, but there is a tendency to shout. It is true that the speech quality of deafened adults may be preserved for many years in some people, but in others there is rapid deterioration, and it is interesting to note that Espir and Rose comment on an aspect of voice rather than articulation. Sooner or later, deficits in voice quality and intonation tend to appear and often also with imprecision in the production of sibilant fricative consonants (Lane & Webster, 1991; Zimmerman & Rettaliata, 1981).

The difficulty with keeping sibilant /s/ and /ʃ/ apart is of particular importance in a language like English in which there is a phonemic difference between them and where any merging of the qualities will be more noticeable (and contribute to the perception of "deaf" voice quality) than in a language that has only one sibilant fricative in the alveolar/palatal region. This demonstrates that the phonetic and phonological characteristics of a particular language may have a role to play in the perception and definition of a particular voice quality. A laryngeal example is provided by speakers of tone languages who will be especially handicapped if they lose control of fundamental frequency changes in profound acquired deafness. Laryngeal–vocal tract timing control may become less precise, with particular consequences for speakers of a language, like Thai, where there is a three-way contrast in Voice Onset Time (VOT) at bilabial and alveolar places of articulation (Carney et al., 1988). All of these features that contribute to perceived voice quality are even more problematic for the prelingually deaf child.

Despite wide individual variation, there are predictable tendencies in the voices of deaf speakers that are noted in studies of individuals or of groups of speakers. House (1995) gives a summary of findings from many authors, and Penn and Cowie and Douglas-Cowie describe group studies. Penn (1955) undertook a large-scale study of (moderately) war-deafened American veterans. Cowie and Douglas-Cowie (1983) describe their own group study of speakers in Belfast: of their 13 speakers, 12 were classed as profoundly deaf with no useful hearing, and the 13th as having some useful hearing, which was diminishing. Her speech was similar to the other 12. What Cowie and Douglas-Cowie, in a comparison of their data with that of Penn, refer to as "global errors" are aspects of laryngeal control and nasality. Speakers in both groups had problems in rate of speech, rhythm, volume, and pitch. In addition, some speakers had excessively nasalized speech and others denasalized. Voice quality is described as "retracted or hoarse, harsh or breathy." Pitch is described by Penn as being "monotonous" as is the speaking rate of a small number of speakers. The Belfast study refers to "little straightforward abnormality" of volume and pitch; Rahilly (1994) showed that a more fine-grained, linguistically based analysis revealed patterns of abnormality in the form and function of intonation in deaf Belfast speakers.

In a survey of work on "The Voice of the Deaf" Wirz (1986)—like Cowie, Sawey, and Douglas-Cowie (1995)—points out that most comments on deaf speakers' voices are adverse, and aims to disentangle different, confusing, uses of terminology and to separate laryngeal, supra-, and subglottal contributions to voice quality. For example, she points out that "over fortis" is frequently used to describe deaf speech, but with no indication as to whether this refers to loudness or articulation. Plant (1993) showed experimentally that listeners can easily identify speakers' hearing status and estimated the contributions of laryngeal and supraglottal features.

Jones (1967) lists the following as characteristics of deaf voice quality: tense, flat, breathy, harsh, throaty, monotone, lack of rhythm, and poor carrying power. Markides (1983) reports teachers' and lay people's ratings of the voice quality of deaf children and reports descriptions such as deep, throaty, hoarse or soft, fairly normal, and deep. The major difficulty with the use of such impressionistic terms is to know what they mean in articulatory or auditory terms or even whether, in the absence of knowledge of acoustic, articulatory or linguistic correlates, listeners can agree on the use of particular terms.

A particular example of this difficulty is seen in the common, undefined use of the term monotone. It could refer to loudness, average pitch level, narrow pitch range, or rhythm. However, it may also have a linguistic basis: For example, deaf children may be shown to have similar average fundamental frequencies to those of hearing children (Gilbert & Campbell, 1980) and similar fundamental frequency ranges (Abberton et al., 1991) but nevertheless may be said to sound "monotonous" and have perceptually narrow pitch ranges. Abberton et al. suggested that this is because of a restricted, stereotyped use of intonation patterns within the fundamental frequency range available to the child.

Conflicting appraisals of deaf voices appear in the literature: Deaf children are also sometimes found to have higher pitched voices and narrower pitch ranges than children with normal hearing (studies quoted in Wirz, 1986). As the Abberton et al. (1991) study suggests, it is essential to bear in mind the stage of linguistic development of the child, the type of material on which judgments are based, and to note that there can be developmental trends: Vocal fold vibration becomes more regular with use of speech and hearing, the fundamental frequency range widens, and a greater range of intonation patterns is used. The reverse is often seen in profound acquired deafness: The fundamental frequency range narrows, vocal fold vibration becomes irregular, and intonation may become stereotyped.

Quite elaborate perceptual descriptive systems have been devised in an attempt to get agreement among trained judges. One such is the Vocal Profiles Analysis Scheme (VPAS)

(Laver, Wirz, Mackenzie, & Miller, 1981; Wirz & Mackenzie Beck, 1995), which aims to produce a profile of deviations from the norm (neutral point) for a range of laryngeal and supralaryngeal parameters. For the larynx, as well as phonation type (harsh, whisper, creak, falsetto, or modal) tension is noted, as are prosodic features: pitch mean, range and variability; tremor; and loudness mean, range, and variability. Wirz (1986) describes the use of the VPAS in a comparison by three trained raters of the recorded voices of a group of severely deaf young adults and a group of normally hearing speakers. There was an interjudge reliability of 80%. The deaf speakers were judged to be markedly different from the hearing speakers in terms of the perceived range of articulatory movements. As far as larynx-related features are concerned, the deaf speakers, in comparison to the hearing speakers, were judged to have narrower pitch range, lower pitch variability, lower loudness mean, narrower loudness range, and lower loudness variability. Pitch mean judgments were not significicantly different. Nearly all the deaf speakers voices were judged to show harshness—probably related to laryngeal tension—and 20% showed falsetto. Wirz concludes that there is some justification for referring to such parameters as "typifying features" of deaf voice.

However one may choose to describe or measure deaf voice quality, the relationship of the features noted to paralinguistic (indexical) information and to phonetic and phonological organization provides other levels or layers of patterning to the description. The potential contribution of voice pitch patterning (not simply mean and range) to perceived voice quality has already been referred to, as have the linguistic consequences for different languages of an inadequate fricative system and of imperfect VOT control. Phonation type, similarly, can have phonetic or phonological implications: A continuously breathy voice may be characteristic of a given speaker, but may impede clear contrasts in languages in which breathy voice is phonemic. Thus, at the same time as a feature provides phonetic indexical information, it can also have implications for the speaker's phonology. A different sort of patterning is often seen in deaf speakers' use of falsetto voice; this may be continuous, but for some speakers, it only occurs with high vowels such as [i] and [u]. In these cases, there is no direct effect on contrastiveness, but it leads to a striking auditory effect occurring intermittently. A much richer account of deaf voice quality is potentially available if this kind of inter-relationship is investigated.

A simpler system, with clear physical and auditory underpinnings, could be based on the use of perceptually salient speech pattern elements (Fourcin, 1979) that may be affected by hearing impairment. At the laryngeal level, these elements would include phonation type (vocal register): modal, falsetto, or creaky and whether or not the phonation was breathy. Using electrolaryngography, these perceptually and potentially linguistically significant features can be analyzed and quantified and their relationship with fundamental frequency explored (see Chapter 13). Fundamental frequency in its physical aspects can be quantified in terms of range and measures of central tendency such as mean, mode, and median values. Such a quantitative approach allows correlations with perceptual descriptors such as wide/narrow pitch range or high/low voice, but, as Abberton et al. (1991) show, such relationships are not simple and involve consideration of the linguistic patterning of stress and intonation. Loudness is a useful descriptor of the element type, and its relationship with fundamental frequency can be explored by phonetograms. Supraglottal pattern elements such as frication and nasality are similarly accessible perceptually and can be measured and related to linguistic contrasts. Another advantage of this simpler but analytic approach is that it provides the basis for remediation: through speech and language therapy using interactive visual feedback to train perception as well as production and through novel hearing aids including cochlear implants (Abberton et al., 1985; Fourcin, Abberton, & Ball, 1993).

3.1. Quantitative Approaches

Different approaches to the measurement of characteristics of the voice quality of deaf speakers are described.

3.1.1. Global

The previous section referred to studies in which global features of deaf speech were noted by listeners. Cowie, Sawey et al. (1995) noted that traditional auditory segmental analysis may not capture the perceived abnormal qualities of deaf voices and were motivated to seek an acoustic measurement approach to find statistical properties in the speech signal characteristic of different groups of speakers. However, automatic analyses based on the signal as a whole would not produce such a rich description as approaches that incorporate preprocessing to extract key features and relationships whose properties could then be measured and summarized. The authors describe their ASSESS system: automatic statistical summary of elementary speech structures, which automatically segments the speech signal and provides "systematic statistical measures of the structures elicited" (p. 278). Statistical techniques seemed a helpful tool, because even simple observation of spectrograms of deaf speech showed gross differences, when compared with normal speech, such as, for example, intensity patterning.

Cowie, Douglas-Cowie, Sawey, and Mulhern (1995) used the ASSESS technique to study 75 postlingually deafened adult speakers who had received cochlear implants and 51 control speakers. "Pre-implant speech was abnormal in timing, intensity range, pitch height and change, frication and spectral balance. Implantation reduced some anomalies, left some unchanged, and aggravated others. Many effects were sex-related (p. 198)." The findings of this study are as follows:

Volume: Ratings on postimplant speakers showed a significant but small trend toward lowered volume. Twenty-four months post-implant the changes are appropriate for male speakers, but not for females, compared with the control speakers.

Timing: The deafened speakers spoke more slowly than the controls. Implantation had the effect, if any, of worsening this feature. The effect was not due to pausing, but the number of silences was high—significantly so after implant.

Features of intensity, timing, and fundamental frequency are, inevitably, entwined and some aspects of timing improve with implantation; the duration of rises and falls in intensity improved by becoming smaller, an improvement essentially complete 9 months after implantation.

For pitch changes, a similar trend was noted: Pitch falls decreased in duration postimplantation. Female speakers had pitch falls that were too rapid before being implanted, so, for them, the situation worsened postoperatively. Cowie et al. (1995) point out that these findings emphasize the need to be wary of global statements about timing.

Intensity: The clearest intensity effects involved spread measures, particularly interquartile range. Interquartile range was too high in preimplant speakers, but fell following implantation, an effect that sometimes continued after 9 months postimplantation. Implants narrow the intensity range by raising the lower limit. The changes are appropriate for men, but 24 months postimplantation, the women had shorter rises and falls in intensity than the control female speakers.

Pitch: No strong or straightforward fundamental frequency effects ("pitch" for the authors) are evident, but certain effects of hearing loss and implantation are reported. Although "pitch tunes" are referred to in the description, the approach is essentially statistical rather than linguistic. Extremes of F_0 range are measured, as are variability of initial and final "pitch movements in a tune (hertz/sec)," and "fitted mid-points of tunes" (p. 200). The findings are that female average pitch is not far from normal, but male pitch is high preimplant and remains so. As far as pitch change in rises and falls is concerned, implants reduce change, taking males toward control norms and females away from them. Pitch variability is strongly reduced 24 months after implantation both between and within individuals.

Frication and spectral effects: These measurements correlate with the well-known fact that deafened speakers lack energy in the higher part of the spectrum and fail to clearly distingish fricatives spectrally. Such measurements would correlate with auditory impressions of muffled speech quality and, especially, /s/–/S/ confusion.

The study described by Cowie et al. (1995) formed part of a large-scale investigation evaluating cochlear implantation in the UK, coordinated by the British Medical Research Council's Institute of Hearing Research. Results should be correlated with the signal processing provided by the implant used.

Another recent study (Kotby et al., 1996) shows results from a range of aerodynamic and acoustic analyses for deaf children's speech. The authors point to a possible breakdown in respiratory, phonatory, and articulatory coordination and suggest that the acoustic findings may represent a quantitative correlate to auditory perceptual assessment.

3.2. Analytic Approaches

In contrast to more global approaches taking stretches of the speech signal and their statistical properties as correlates/indicators of voice quality, another, analytic, acoustic approach is more phonetically (but not segmentally) motivated and explicitly linked with hearing aid and cochlear stimulation design and the residual auditory capabilities of the speaker (Fourcin, 1989, 1990). Particular speech pattern elements can be investigated separately or in combination and their predictable contribution to perceived voice quality described and quantified. Elements relevant to the present discussion are phonation type (including examination of regularity and open quotient measures, fundamental frequency patterning (range, measures of central tendency), related intensity and F_0 patterning (as in phonetograms), and frication. (See Fourcin, Chapter 13 in this volume, for examples of these measures.) Most of this work has been carried out for speakers who have become very profoundly deaf and whose auditory perceptual capabilities are extremely limited in the frequency domain and who have very small dynamic ranges, but whose temporal resolving abilities are relatively unimpaired. These auditory capabilities are well-matched to the voice pitch range of male speakers and thus vocal fold patterning (phonation type, tone, and intonation) is potentially available to them in the speech of others and in self-monitoring. The signal presented to these very auditorily impaired speakers via pattern processing hearing aids, such as SiVo (Faulkner et al., 1995) is derived algorithmically by neural networks trained on electrolaryn gograph signals—Lx waveforms (see Fourcin, Chapter 13 in this volume). Vocal fold patterning and auditory patterning are thus matched in a vary natural and linguistically relevant way. The signal can be transformed in terms of mean F_0 while preserving speaker- and language-specific variation. It is noteworthy that, if a female speaker hears her own voice lowered in this way (to bring it into her residual hearing range), she does not lower her own voice to match it—thus preserving its appropriate indexical characteristics. This is quite unlike the Lombard effect.

This approach also makes it possible to consider language-specific aids that would present features particularly important in a given language (Fourcin, 1990). Speakers of all languages benefit from a clear auditory sensation of voice pitch and phonation type.

Hearing aids of this type (explicitly designed to help speech production as well as perception) are intended for very profoundly deaf speakers who cannot benefit from conventional aids. The approach is also applicable to cochlear implants, and the first work was carried out with speakers receiving single-channel extra-cochlear stimulation (Fourcin et al., 1983). To help achieve the twin aims of perceptual and productive improvement, a rehabilitative program using interactive visual feedback of voice pitch and intensity and frication patterns has been developed (Abberton et al. 1985; Ball, 1991; Elbaz, Fresnel-Elbaz, & Legendre, 1988; Fourcin et al., 1993). Voice quality improvement, in vocal fold vibration regularity, voice pitch range, and intonation control are evident on auditory perceptual evaluation as well as in measurements.

A striking example of the effectiveness of reestablishing auditory self-monitoring for voice quality by profoundly deaf speakers is provided by Toffin et al. (1995) in the framework of a 5-nation European Union-funded project (STRIDE, 1995). The authors show how improvements in voice pitch range, loudness, and vocal fold vibration regularity, measured in F_0 histograms, and phonetograms, are produced as soon as a SiVo aid (whose output is a sinewave following the pich of the voice) is switched on, and how these improvements disappear when a familiar conventional hearing aid is used in the same recording session or when no auditory feedback is available. Oster (1987) and Svirsky, Lane, Perkell, and Wozniak, (1992) have demonstrated the same rapid effect of auditory feedback in speech production quality by switching implants off. The explanatory value of relating hearing ability to voice quality is also seen when breathy voice is considered. Many speakers with hearing impairment have breathy phonation because they do not have an adequate sensation of voice pitch and produce a noisy excitation spectrum that has proportionately more energy at the low end of the spectrum. As soon as adequate voice pitch monitoring is available, this aspect of voice quality improves.

3.3. Quantitative Assessment of Intonation

The contribution to perceived deaf voice quality of intonation has been referred to several times. Producing appropriate intonation patterns is not simply a matter of replicating a repertoire of low frequency pitch patterns, nor of expressing attitudes and emotions. Intonation is a language-specific system of rules relating pitch patterns to syntactic and pragmatic choices as well as playing an important role in the expression of affect.

House and Willstedt (1993) show how perceived emotion (anger versus happiness) in the voices of speakers with implants can be changed by altering F_0 mean values and ranges. Listeners could only identify happiness when the speakers were using their implants—demonstrating the use of auditory feedback in controlling fundamental frequency.

The linguistic dimensions of intonation patterning also lend themselves to quantitative appraisal, to complement physical F_0 measures. Phonological dimensions, such as the contrastiveness and sequencing of pitch rises and falls, and the contribution of the components of an intonation pattern to perceived (ab)normality can all be analytically studied and quantified (Cowie, Douglas-Cowie, & Rahilly, 1988); the phonetic implementation of these units may be abnormal even if a contrastive system is present (Abberton, Parker, & Fourcin, 1983; Parker, 1983; Rahilly, 1994; Waters, 1986).

4. CONCLUSION

An account such as the present chapter, although brief, at least serves several functions. At the simplest level it shows how, over the decades, many people have struggled to describe—and sometimes measure—the perceptually and physically elusive nature of deaf voice quality. Richer accounts are possible if different levels of representation of speech are considered: A degree of explanatory adequacy is achievable if observed characteristics of the speech of deaf people are related to the phonological patterning (segmental and nonsegmental) of the particular language being spoken. Recent work shows that further explanatory power can be achieved if speech output features are related to psychoacoustic abilities and to acoustic speech pattern elements. The advantage of such an analytic approach is that it provides the possibility of improving the quality of deaf speakers' voices through the provision of customized hearing aids and cochlear implants. The relationship between speech perceptual ability and the quality of speech production is thus exploited in a natural but principled way to the benefit of the deaf user whose speech becomes more acceptable and intelligible.

REFERENCES

Abberton, E., Parker, A., & Fourcin, A. (1983). Speech improvement in deaf adults using laryngograph displays. In J. M. Pickett (Ed.), *Papers from the re-*

displays. In J. M. Pickett (Ed.), *Papers from the research conference on speech-processing aids for the deaf, 1977* (pp. 172–188), Washington DC: Galaudet Research Institute.

Abberton, E., Fourcin, A., Rosen, S., Walliker, J., Howard, D., Moore, B., Douek, E., & Frampton, S. (1985). Speech perceptual and productive rehabilitation in electro-cochlear stimulation. In R. A. Schindler & M. M. Merzenich (Eds.), *Cochlear implants* (pp. 527–537). New York: Raven Press.

Abberton, E., Fourcin, A., & Hazan, V. (1991). Fundamental frequency range and the development of intonation in a group of profoundly deaf children. *Proceedings of the XIIth International Congress of Phonetic Sciences, 5,* 142–145.

Ball, V. (1991). Computer-based tools for assessment and remediation of speech. *British Journal of Disorders of Communication, 26,* 95–113.

Ball, V., Faulkner, A., & Fourcin, A. (1990). The effects of two different speech-coding strategies on voice fundamental frequency control in deafened adults. *British Journal of Audiology, 24,* 393–409.

Carney, A. E., Gandour, J., Petty, S., Robbins, A. Myres, W., & Miyamoto, R. (1988). The effect of adventitious deafness on the perception and production of voice onset time in Thai: A case study. *Language and Speech, 31,* 272–282.

Clark, M. (1989). *Language through living.* London: Hodder and Stoughton

Cowie, R., & Douglas-Cowie, E. (1983). Speech production in profound postlingual deafness. In M. E. Lutman & M. Haggard (Eds.), *Hearing science and hearing disorders* (pp. 183–230). London: Academic Press.

Cowie, R., & Douglas-Cowie, E. (1992). *Postlingually acquired deafness: Speech deterioration and the wider consequences.* Berlin: Mouton de Gruyter.

Cowie, R., Douglas-Cowie, E., & Rahilly, J. (1988). The intonation of adults with postlingually acquired deafness: Anomolous frequency and distribution of elements. In B. Ainsworth & J. Holmes (Eds.), *Proceedings SPEECH '88, 7th FASE Symposium, Edinburgh, 2,* 481–487.

Cowie, R., Douglas-Cowie, E., Sawey, M., & Mulhern, G. (1995). The effects of cochlear implants on speech production in postlingually acquired deafness. *Proceedings XIIIth International Congress of Phonetic Sciences, 3,* 198–201.

Cowie, R., Sawey, M., & Douglas-Cowie, E. (1995). A new speech analysis system: ASSESS (automatic statistical summary of elementary speech structures). *Proceedings XIIIth International Congress of Phonetic Sciences, 3,* 278–281.

Elbaz, P., Fresnel-Elbaz, E., & Legendre, M.-L. (1988). Testing et réeducation des candidats à la prothèse SIVO. *Annales d'Oto-Laryngologie (Paris), 105,* 623–627.

Espir, M., & Rose, F. C. (1976) *The basic neurology of speech.* Oxford: Blackwell.

Faulkner, A., Walliker, J., Coninx, F., Dahlqvist, M., Beijk, C., Fresnel-Elbaz, E., Smith, K. J., Wei, J., Bosman, A., Smoorenburg, G. F., & Fourcin, A. J. (1995). SIVO-II: A speech analysing hearing aid for profoundly hearing impaired people. *Proceedings XIIIth International Congress of Phonetic Sciences, 3,* 202–205.

Fletcher, P., & Garman, M. (1986). *Language acquisition.* Cambridge, UK: Cambridge University Press.

Fourcin, A. J. (1978). Acoustic patterns and speech acquisition. In N. Waterson & C. Snow, (Eds.), *The development of communication* (Sec. 3, Pt. 2, pp. 47–72). Chichester, UK: John Wiley.

Fourcin, A. J. (1979). Auditory patterning and vocal fold vibration. In B. Lindblom & S. Ohman (Eds), *Frontiers of speech communication research* (pp. 167–176). London: Academic Press.

Fourcin, A. J. (1989). Links between voice pattern perception and production. In B. A. G. Elsendoorn & H. Bouma (Eds.), *Working models of human perception* (pp. 67–91). London: Academic Press.

Fourcin, A. J. (1990). Prospects for speech pattern element aids. *Acta Otolaryngologica (Stockholm)* (Suppl.), *469,* 257–267.

Fourcin, A., & Abberton, E. (1995). Speech pattern elements in assessment, training and prosthetic provision. In G. Plant & K.-E. Spens (Eds.), *Profound deafness and speech communication* (pp. 492–509). London: Whurr.

Fourcin, A. J., Abberton, E., & Ball, V. (1993). Voice and intonation: Analysis, presentation and training. In B. A. G. Elsendoorn & F. Coninx (Eds.), *Interactive learning technology for the deaf* (pp. 137–150). NATO-ASI Series. New York: Springer Verlag.

Fourcin, A. J., Douek, E. E., Moore, B. C. J., Rosen, S., Walliker, J. R., Howard, D. M., Abberton, E., & Frampton, S. Speech perception with promontory stimulation. In C. Parkins & S. Anderson (Eds.), Cochlear prostheses: An international symposium. *Annals of the New York Academy of Sciences, 405,* 280–284.

Gilbert, H., & Campbell, M. (1980). Speaking fundamental frequency in three groups of hearing-impaired individuals. *Journal of Communication Disorders, 13,* 195–205.

House, D. (1995). Speech production by adults using cochlear implants. In G. Plant & K.-E. Spens (Eds.), *Profound deafness and speech communication* (pp. 285–296). London: Whurr.

House, D., & Willstedt, U. (1993). Changes in control of fundamental frequency and voice quality following cochlear implant activation and speech training. In A. Risberg, S. Felicetti, G. Plant, & K.-E. Spens (Eds.), *Proceedings 2nd International Conference on Tactile Aids, Hearing Aids and Cochlear Implants* (pp. 201–210). Stockholm: Department of Speech Communication and Music Acoustics, KTH.

Jones, C. (1967). "Deaf voice"—A description derived from a survey of the literature. *Volta Review, 69*, 507–508.

Kotby, M. N., Wafi, W. A., Rifaie, N. A., Abdel-Nasserr, N. H., Aref, E. E., & Elsharkawy, A. A. (1996). Multidimensional analysis of speech of hearing impaired children. *Scandinavian Audiology (Suppl.), 42*, 27–33.

Lane, H., & Webster, J. (1991). Speech deterioration in postlingually deafened adults. *Journal of the Acoustical Society of America, 89*, 859–866.

Laver, J. (1980). *A phonetic description of voice quality*. Cambridge, UK: Cambridge University Press.

Laver, J., Wirz, S., Mackenzie, J., & Miller, S. (1981). A perceptual protocol for the analysis of vocal profiles. University of Edinburgh Linguistics Dept. *Work in Progress, 14.*

Ling, D. (1976). *Speech and the hearing impaired child: Theory and practice.* Washington, DC: The Alexander Graham Bell Association for the Deaf Inc.

Markides, A. (1983). *The speech of hearing impaired children.* Manchester, UK: Manchester University Press.

Ní Chasaide, A., & Gobl, C. (1997). Voice source variation. In W. J. Hardcastle & J. Laver (Eds.), *The handbook of phonetic sciences* (pp. 427–461). Oxford, UK: Blackwell.

Oster, A.-M. (1987). Some effects of cochlear implantation on speech production. *STL-QPSR, 1*, 81–89, KTH, Stockholm.

Parker, A. (1983). Speech conservation. In W. J. Watts (Ed.), *Rehabilitation and acquired deafness* (pp. 234–250). London: Croom Helm.

Penn, J. P. (1955). Voice and speech patterns in the hard of hearing. *Acta Otolaryngologica (Suppl.), 124*. Quoted by Wirz, 1986.

Plant, G. (1993). The speech of adults with acquired profound hearing losses. I: A perceptual evaluation. *European Journal of Disorders of Communication 28*, 273–288.

Rahilly, J. (1994). *Intonation patterns in the postlingually deafened.* Amsterdam: John Benjamins.

Read, T. E. (1989). Improvement in speech production following the use of the UCH/RNID cochlear implant. *Journal of Laryngology and Otology Supplement, 18*, 45–49.

Rosen, S., Faulkner, A., & Smith, D. (1990). The psychoacoustics of profound hearing impairment. *Acta Otolaryngologica Supplement, 469*, 16–22.

Scherer, K. (1995). How emotion is expressed in speech and singing. *Proceedings XIIIth International Congress of Phonetic Sciences, 3*, 90–96.

STRIDE. (1995). Final report of TIDE project: TP 133/206 STRIDE. London: Department of Phonetics and Linguistics, University College, London.

Svirsky, M. A., Lane, H., Perkell, J. P., & Wozniak, J. (1992). Effects of short-term auditory deprivation on speech production in adult cochlear implant users. *Journal of the Acoustical Society of America, 92*(3), 1284–1300.

Toffin, C., Spens, K.-E., Smith, K., Powell, R., Lente, P., Fourcin, A., Faulkner, A., Dahlqvist. M. Fresnel-Elbaz, E., Coninx, F., Beijk, C., Agelfors, E., & Abberton, E. (1995). Voice production as a function of analytic perception with a speech element hearing aid. *Proceedings of the XIIIth International Congress of Phonetic Sciences, 3*, 206–209.

Urbantschitsch, V. (1895). *Horubugen bei Taubstummheit und bei Ertaubung im Spateren Lebensalter*, Wien: Urban und Schwarzenberg. [Translated by R. Silverman as *Auditory training for deaf mutism and acquired deafness*, (1981). Washington, DC: Alexander Graham Bell Association for the Deaf, Inc.]

Walliker, J., Daley, J., Smith, K., Faulkner, A., & Fourcin, A. (1993). Speech analytic hearing aids for the profoundly deaf: technical design aspects and user field trials results. In B. Granstrom, S. Hunnicutt, & K.-E. Spens (Eds.), *Speech and language technology for disabled persons*. Stockholm: ESCA/KTH.

Waters, T. (1986). Speech therapy with cochlear implant wearers. *British Journal of Audiology, 20*, 25–43.

Wirz, S. (1986), The voice of the deaf. In M. Fawcus (Ed.), *Voice disorders and their management* (pp. 240–259). London: Croom Helm.

Wirz, S., & Mackenzie Beck, J. (1995). Assessment of voice quality. The Vocal Profiles Analysis Scheme.

In S. L. Wirz (Ed.), *Perceptual approaches to communication disorders* (pp. 39–55). London: Whurr.
Zimmerman, G., & Rettaliata, P. (1981). Articulatory patterns of an adventitiously deaf speaker: Implications of the role of auditory information in speech production. *Journal of Speech and Hearing Research, 24,* 169–178.

CHAPTER

23

Toward a Theory of the Dispositional Bases of Functional Dysphonia and Vocal Nodules: Exploring the Role of Personality and Emotional Adjustment

Nelson Roy and Diane M. Bless

The human larynx is acutely responsive to sudden changes in affective states and as such it has been labeled a "barometer of emotions." Others have described the voice as one of the most characteristic expressions of the individual—"a mirror of personality" (Aronson, 1990; Diehl, 1960). Thus, when the voice becomes disordered, voice scientists and clinicians sometimes offer emotional or personality factors as likely causal explanations. However, considerable controversy surrounds when and whether such factors should be considered causal, concomitant, outcomes, or completely irrelevant. This debate is especially intense in the case of such disorders as functional dysphonia and vocal nodules. This chapter reviews some of the prevailing concepts, issues, controversies, and research literature on the role of psychological and personality processes in individuals with functional dysphonia and vocal nodules. Moreover, a theory is offered that identifies personality factors as important considerations in the development of these voice disorders.

The extant literature is replete with speculations linking functional dysphonia and vocal nodules to psychological precursors and personality variables. It has been suggested that personality and emotional maladjustment contribute to or are primary causes of these voice disorders, and that these voice disorders, in turn, create psychological problems or personality effects (Brodnitz, 1981). Unfortunately, dataless speculation and bias dominate both the anecdotal and scientific literature in this area. These biases usually reflect a clinician-researcher's general attitude of acceptance or willingness to consider psychological or emotional factors in voice disorders. Clinicians holding more global theories of psychosomatic causation seem more willing to connect patients' symptoms to psychosocial factors; any factors that correlate with the theory's explanatory constructs are often included as evidence for the psychogenic nature of symptoms. When the attitude toward these factors is one of skepticism, the attribution is made less often. On review of the literature, one must admit, as Goodstein (1958) did over 40 years ago, that much of this literature is unverifiable in a scientific sense. His comments remain germane today, as few advances have been made over the past several decades in our understanding of the relation between voice disorders, emotion, and personality. In the next few sections we review the available literature linking functional dysphonia and vocal nodules to psychological precursors.

1. FUNCTIONAL DYSPHONIA

1.1. Problems in Defining Functional Dysphonia

Most authors generally agree that functional dysphonia is a voice disturbance in the absence of visible neurological or structural pathology (Koufman & Blalock, 1982) or where the existing pathology is judged to be insufficient to account for the severity of the dysphonia. Functional dysphonia occurs predominantly in women and commonly follows upper respiratory infection symptoms (Aronson, Peterson, & Litin, 1966; Friedl, Friedrich, & Egger, 1990; Gerritsma, 1991; Kinzl, Biebl, & Rauchegger, 1988; Milutinovic, 1991). It is frequently transient and varies in its response to treatment (Bridger & Epstein, 1983; Fex, Fex, Shiromoto, & Hirano, 1994; Koufman & Blalock, 1982; Roy & Leeper, 1993). Because of imprecision in defining functional dysphonia, few reliable prevalence and incidence statistics exist.

Functional dysphonia and aphonia are sometimes regarded as disorders represented on a continuum of vocal severity and in some cases are believed to share a common etiology (Aronson, 1990; Aronson et al., 1966). In aphonia, patients lose their voice completely and articulate in a whisper, whereas dysphonia suggests phonation is preserved, but disturbed in quality, pitch, and/or loudness (Boone & McFarlane, 1988). Certain authors warn that distinctions must be made between aphonia and dysphonia to prevent overestimation of the role of psychological factors in dysphonia (Friedl, Friedrich, Egger, & Fitzek, 1993). Whether these vocal conditions simply represent quantitative differences along a single continuous dimension, for example laryngeal and extralaryngeal muscle tension, or are categorically and etiologically unique, is open for debate.

Some clinicians object to using the label of functional dysphonia because of its etiologic and symptomatologic ambiguity (Aronson, 1990; Morrison & Rammage, 1993; Pahn & Friemert, 1988). Functional implies a disturbance of physiological function rather than anatomical structure. In clinical circles, functional is usually contrasted with organic and often carries the added meaning of psychogenic. Stress and psychological conflict are frequently presumed to cause and/or exacerbate functional symptoms (Bass, 1990; Kirmayer & Robbins, 1991; Morrison, Nichol, & Rammage, 1986). Theorists' opinions differ, however, about the relative contribution of psychological factors to the formation of functional voice disorders.

The role of psychological or personality processes in functional dysphonia remains enigmatic partly because the term functional includes a range of medically unexplained voice disorders: psychogenic, conversion, hysterical, tension-fatigue syndrome, hyperkinetic, muscle misuse, or muscle tension dysphonia. It is therefore not understood whether functional dysphonia is one disorder or many. Although the previous diagnostic labels imply some degree of etiologic heterogeneity, whether these disorders are qualitatively different and etiologically distinct remains unclear. Voice disorder taxonomies have yet to be adequately operationalized; consequently, diagnostic categories often lack clear thresholds or discrete boundaries for determining patient inclusion or exclusion. At the purely phenomenological level, there may be little difference between these disorders. This nosological imprecision may account for differences found in the literature regarding the voice-psychology relationship.

1.2. Causal Models of Functional Dysphonia

The search for the link between functional voice symptoms and psychosocial factors is guided by theories of causality. Authors have described assorted psychopathological processes that may be active in voice symptom formation.

The dominant psychological explanation for medically unexplained voice loss is the concept of conversion disorder introduced by Freud (Aronson, 1990; Butcher, 1995; Greene & Mathieson, 1989; Stemple, 1984, 1993). Conversion disorder involves unexplained symptoms or deficits influencing voluntary motor or sensory function that suggest a neurological or other general medical condition (American Psychiatric Association [APA], DSM-IV, 1994). When the laryngeal system is involved, voice loss is called conversion dysphonia or aphonia. The voice loss, whether partial or complete, is often interpreted to have symbolic meaning. In short, it is posited that patients convert intrapsychic distress into a voice symptom.

Psychological factors are judged to be associated with the voice symptoms because conflicts or other stressors precede the onset or exacerbation of the dysphonia. Primary or secondary gains are thought to play an important role in maintaining and reinforcing the conversion voice disorder. Primary gain is anxiety alleviation through prevention of the psychological conflict from entering conscious awareness. Secondary gain is the avoidance of an undesirable activity/responsibility and the extra attention or support conferred to the patient.

Conversion disorder has historically been associated with histrionic-hysterical (superficial, melodramatic) personality features. In some cases, individuals with conversion symptoms seem to possess a complacent or serene attitude toward their voice symptoms. This relative lack of emotional concern, which is incongruous with their loss of voice function, has been referred to as "la belle indifference." More recent descriptions of conversion disorder minimize the significance of the symbolic nature of symptoms, hysterical personality traits, and la belle indifference (APA, 1994; Kirmayer & Robbins, 1991).

Butcher and colleagues (Butcher, 1995; Butcher, Elias, & Raven, 1993; Butcher, Elias, Raven, Yeatman, & Littlejohns, 1987) argue that there is little research evidence that hysterical conversion disorder, as defined by Freud, is the most common cause of voice loss unaccounted for by pathological findings. P. Butcher advises that the conversion label should be reserved for cases of aphonia, in which la belle indifference and lack of motivation to improve the voice coexist with clear evidence of a temporally linked psychosocial stressor. In the place of conversion, Butcher (1995) offers two alternative models to account for psychogenic voice loss. Both models minimize the role of primary and secondary gain in maintaining the voice disorder. The first is a slightly reformulated psychoanalytic model that states: "if predisposed by social and cultural bias as well as early learning experiences, and then exposed to interpersonal difficulties that stimulate internal conflict, particularly in situations involving conflict over self-expression or voicing feelings, intrapsychic conflict or stress becomes channeled into musculoskeletal tension, which physically inhibits voice production" (p. 472). The second model, based on cognitive-behavioral principles, states that: "life stresses and interpersonal problems in an individual predisposed to having difficulties expressing feelings or views would produce involuntary anxiety symptoms and musculoskeletal tension, which would center on and inhibit voice production" (p. 473). Both models clearly emphasize the inhibitory effects of excess laryngeal muscle tension on voice production, although through slightly different causal mechanisms.

The subject of poorly regulated laryngeal muscle tension is also a topic in the writings of Rammage and colleagues (Morrison & Rammage, 1993; Nichol, Morrison, & Rammage, 1993; Rammage, Nichol, & Morrison, 1987) and Aronson (1990) among others (Colton & Casper, 1996; Greene & Mathieson, 1989). In addition to acknowledging the conversion explanation for functional dysphonia, Nichol and associates (1993) proposed that "tensional symptoms arise from the overactivity of autonomic and voluntary nervous systems in individuals who are unduly aroused and anxious" (p. 644). They added that such overactivity leads to hypertonicity of the intrinsic and extrinsic laryngeal muscles, resulting in muscle tension dysphonias sometimes associated with adjustment or anxiety disorders or with certain personality trait disturbances.

Another possible explanation for functional dysphonia is the interaction between organic and psychogenic mechanisms. One example of this interaction is the specificity hypothesis advanced by Alexander (Alexander, 1950; Alexander, French, & Pollock, 1968). This theory suggests that a specific stimulus (e.g., emotional conflict) elicits a distinctive response, or illness, and the organ affected (larynx) is determined by a genetic weakness or vulnerability. Milutinovic (1991) recognized the extensive etiologic overlapping of organic and functional voice disturbances and stated that "genetic factors, the state of the endocrine and neurovegetative systems, and psychological factors are significant in the development of functional dysphonia" (p. 179). He suggested that psychogenic aphonia and dysphonia should be considered "phononeuroses." As more than half of his "phononeurotic" patients had documented infection of the upper respiratory airways preceding the voice disturbance, he concluded that there was a direct connection between the pathological state of the mucosa and development of functional dysphonia. Milutinovic speculated that organic changes in the larynx, pharynx, and nose facilitate the appearance of a functional voice problem; that is, the change directs the somatization of psychodynamic conflict.

Similarly, Schalen and Andersson (1992) noted that their "psychogenic dysphonia and aphonia" patients had an abnormally high number of reported allergy/asthma symptoms (37.5%). This suggested the need for a more detailed examination of the interrelationship between psychological factors and respiratory and phonatory disorders. Likewise, Rammage et al. (1987) proposed that a relatively minor organic change such as edema, infection, or reflux laryngitis may trigger functional misuse, particularly if an individual is exceedingly anxious about his or her voice or health. In a similar vein, the same authors felt that anticipation of poor voice production in hypochondriacal, dependent, or obsessive-compulsive individuals leads to excessive vigilance about sensations arising from the throat (larynx) and respiratory system that may lead to altered voice production.

Finally, although most authors have viewed psychological factors as strongly influential in the development of functional dysphonia, they have virtually ignored the possibility that such processes could be the consequence of coping with an incapacitating voice disorder (i.e., the scar hypothesis). Because voice problems can be associated with a number of adverse consequences including laryngeal discomfort, fatigue, and impairment of social and/or occupational functioning (with a concomitant loss of self-esteem and social support), it is not unreasonable to posit that chronic voice problems might lead to general personality or psychological changes, such as heightened feelings of distress and social withdrawal/introversion. Depression, anxiety, and tension are frequent psychological concomitants of chronic illness (Dembo, Levitan, & Wright, 1975; Dubovsky & Weissberg, 1982; Reiser, 1980). To our knowledge, the notion that such sequelae could be considered outcomes of a severe voice disturbance, rather than causal agents, has been investigated only once. Murry, Cannito, and Woodson (1994) evaluated changes in measures of depression and anxiety in patients with spasmodic dysphonia following Botox injections. Reduced levels of depression and anxiety were observed 1 week after injection, and these reduced levels were maintained during the ensuing 2-month postinjection period. In voice disorders such as functional dysphonia, it is therefore unknown whether elevated depression and anxiety might be more accurately regarded as state-dependent characteristics, more suitably viewed as concomitant than as causal.

1.3. Psychological Factors as Causal or Concomitant?

Most research studies investigating personality and/or psychological processes group both functional aphonia and dysphonia under the presumptive designation "psychogenic voice disorder," reflecting the etiological supposition. This causal inference is, in fact, often difficult to verify in either research or clinical practice. Sapir (1995) suggests that three criteria should be met to warrant the diagnosis of psychogenic voice disorder: symptom incongruity, symptom reversibility, and symptom psychogenicity.

Symptom incongruity is the observation that vocal symptoms are physiologically incompatible with existing or suspected disease, are internally inconsistent, and are incongruent with other speech and language characteristics. Often-cited examples of symptom incongruity are (1) complete aphonia in the context of minor vocal fold mucosal changes deemed insufficient to explain the severity of vocal dysfunction, or (2) aphonia in a patient who demonstrates a normal throat clear, cough, laugh, or hum, whereby the presence of such normal nonspeech vocalization is at odds with assumptions regarding neural integrity and function of the laryngeal system.

Symptom reversibility is the complete, sustained amelioration of the voice disorder with short-term voice therapy (usually one or two sessions) and/or through psychological abreaction. Furthermore, maintenance of voice improvement requires no compensatory effort on the part of a patient. Sapir (1995) advises that symptom reversibility must be distinguished from spontaneous recovery, the latter being the eventual resolution of symptoms as the underlying disease process abates.

Finally, symptom psychogenicity is the finding that the voice disorder is logically linked in time of onset, course, and severity to an identifiable psychological antecedent, such as a stressful life event or interpersonal conflict. In general, Sapir (1995) adds that "psychogenic dysphonia should be suspected when there is strong evidence for symptom incongruity and symptom psychogenicity, but confirmed only when there is unambiguous evidence of symptom reversibility" (p. 275).

Although this attempt to delineate criteria for establishing psychogenicity is commendable, some critics suggest that, in reality, there is rarely a clear demonstration that a symptom is psychogenic. Occasionally, symptoms will come and go in strict association with a salient psychological event or state, and this will allow a degree of confidence that the psychological factor is contributory. More commonly, potential psychosocial contributors are identified, but it cannot be precisely ascertained whether they antedated the voice problem or arose in conjunction with it. Once the voice symptom has developed, the recollection of recent life events may be biased by the tendency of both clinician and client to search for explanations and reassess the salience and negativity of events or mood states. In many cases, the dysphonia has been present for a long time. This leads to difficulty in determining the precise etiological factors. Not only do patients forget important historical information, but also some of the precipitating factors may have been resolved with passage of time. At the time of assessment, the patient may seem relatively free of psychological distress.

When linking a voice symptom and a psychosocial cause or context, it would seem that there is an underlying assumption that the antecedent conflict or ongoing stressors are of sufficient *intensity* and/or *duration* to account for the voice symptomatology. It is therefore not only the presence, but also the severity of stressors that makes them plausible causes of a voice disorder. An emotional event or interpersonal conflict must be viewed as sufficient to account for comparably severe somatic distress or tension. The problem here is that there are few reliable measures of the severity of a stressor. Severity of the antecedent event/conflict seems to depend on the personal meaning of events and an individual's idiosyncratic judgment of his or her ability to cope adequately with the challenge. Estimates of the intensity of social stress are thus confused with the symptomatic distress that they are intended to explain.

The identification of psychological factors that accompany or even exacerbate a symptom is customarily offered as evidence that the symptom itself is psychogenic. Skeptics suggest that such covariation still does not establish anything beyond concomitance. The covariation of symptom severity with psychological distress establishes a link but does not distinguish functional symptoms from those with obvious organic causes. Such correspondence, even if perfect, does not permit one to infer that a maladjustment caused a voice problem, or the voice problem caused the maladjustment, or that the two caused each other, or that both stem from a single common cause (Irwin, 1960). Spasmodic dysphonia for instance, once was regarded as solely psychogenic (Brodnitz, 1962; Heaver, 1960). But, recent investigations have suggested that spasmodic dysphonia appears to be an action-induced focal dystonia, whose onset of symptoms is often related to emotional upset or environmental stresses (Cannito, 1991). Patients with spasmodic dysphonia report condition worsening in conjunction with stressful events and improvement when the emotional and social conditions change for the better. Therefore in actual practice, the criterion of recent stressor does not distinguish functional symptoms from those of organic disease that may be aggravated by stress. In many cases, some ambiguity regarding psychogenicity remains, especially in cases in which functional dysphonia masquerades as spasmodic dysphonia.

The mere presence of symptom psychogenicity and incongruity raises the index of suspicion regarding the contribution of psychological factors, but as Sapir suggests, confirmation requires symptom reversibility. A clinician may have a strong suspicion that a voice disorder has psychological underpinnings; however, confirmation depends on complete sustained symptom reversal without compensatory effort. In this regard, numerous voice-facilitating techniques are available to practicing voice clinicians. However, documentation about which therapies are the most effective is scant. If symptoms do not remit with brief therapy, one is left to wonder whether therapy failure is related to differences in disorder or inappropriately selected or applied techniques by clinicians that vary in levels of confidence, experience, and expectation.

To complicate matters, the same clinician who suspects a psychogenic etiology may ascribe voice therapy failure to psychological causes, such as secondary gain, or incomplete resolution of the interpersonal conflict (or persistent personality characteristics that interfere with resolution). If patients deny psychological precursors or antecedent events, the clinician may also conclude that the patient is psychologically defended and resistant to psychological insight. Thus, the same assumptions used to explain causation are then invoked to explain voice therapy failure. The circularity of this logic becomes apparent. As Irwin observed, "grant the assumptions, and the evidence is good; doubt the assumptions and there is no evidence" (Irwin, 1960, p. 311).

It is apparent from the previous discussion that, in the clinical domain at least, the evidence pointing to a psychological basis for functional dysphonia is often inferential and circumstantial. In the scientific realm then, what objective data do we have documenting the presence of predisposing psychological and personality factors in functional dysphonia? The major results of the relevant research to date are reviewed in the next section.

1.4. Standardized Assessment of Psychological Processes in Functional Dysphonia

Although the previous review of potential psychological mechanisms contributing to functional dysphonia represents engaging speculation, empirical evidence to support these explanations is lacking. There are only a handful of studies that have used standardized instruments to assess the personality or psychological characteristics of patients with functional dysphonia. The existing research is generally disappointing for a variety of reasons:

1. Most data have been collected using test instruments of unknown psychometric properties.
2. The terminology used to classify voice disorders is often ambiguous and imprecise. Thus, it is not clear whether patients with structural pathology have been included or excluded. This is especially true in the case of so-called "functional" voice disorders, where some studies included subjects with vocal nodules and others did not (Deary et al., 1997). The inclusion of both sexes and the failure of the investigators to distinguish aphonic from dysphonic subjects complicate these problems. Mixing voice disorder types and sexes into a single study group renders interpretation difficult, if not impossible. Furthermore, recent technical advancements in observing and evaluating the larynx have improved diagnostic precision. Consequently, subjects with sulcus vocalis, vocal fold scarring, or cysts may have been previously mislabeled as having functional dysphonia or vocal nodules, thereby obscuring potential differences between and within groups.
3. Most studies neglect to compare their findings with other voice disorder groups. This hinders interpretations of commonality versus specificity.
4. The use of non-voice-disordered controls or normative data has been largely neglected, or researchers have selected dis-proportionately large comparison groups with unmatched or unspecified characteristics (Green, 1988).
5. There are few data that have been satisfactorily analyzed using suitable statistical methods.
6. Most investigators do not describe whether subjects were vocally asymptomatic at the time of testing. It is therefore difficult to judge whether psychological attributes reflect long-term "trait-like" characteristics, or merely represent transient reaction to the voice disorder (i.e., "state" or "scar" attributes). Information is not provided regarding the severity of vocal handicap or duration of the vocal symptoms; therefore, it is not known whether positive psychological findings represent the effects of attempting to cope with the voice disorder.

These deficits notwithstanding, a review of the major findings and interpretations of the empirical research is provided in Table 23–1. Direct comparison and generalization of the results is difficult because of significant methodological variance. This might partly explain the diverse results about the frequency and degree of hysterical personality traits (Aronson et al., 1966; Gerritsma, 1991; Kinzl et al., 1988), conversion reaction (House & Andrews, 1987; Pfau, 1975) and psychopathological symptoms (Aronson et al., 1966; Gerritsma, 1991; House & Andrews, 1987; Kinzl et al., 1988; Pfau, 1975). Despite their shortcomings, these studies have identified a general pattern of results consistent with elevated levels of anxiety, somatic complaints, and introversion in the functional dysphonia population. Patients have been described as socially anxious and nonassertive, with a tendency toward restraint (Friedl et al., 1990; Gerritsma, 1991). None of these researchers have attempted to explicitly integrate their findings into a coherent theory of personality structure as a vulnerability for functional dysphonia. As Green (1988, p. 34) states, "until more adequate research is conducted, psycho-

Table 23-1. Literature review: Description of subjects, test instrument(s), and major findings of the FD-psychology-personality relationship (reported in chronological order).

Authors	*Subjects*	*Test Instrument(s)*	*Major Findings and Interpretations*
Aronson et al. (1966)	■ psychogenic aphonia/ dysphonia ■ $n = 24$ F; 3 M 1 mute, 11 continuous whisper, 7 intermittent whisper/phonation, 8 continuous phonation	■ Minnesota Multiphasic Personality Inventory (MMPI) ■ Clinical psychiatric interview	■ A period of acute/chronic stress antedated the onset of dysphonia in 74% of the patients. ■ 93% were judged to have difficulty dealing with anger. ■ 26% reported excessive somatic complaints. ■ No patient in acute psychiatric distress. ■ A clinical impression of hysteria was observed in less than half and 30% exhibited a conversion "V" profile. ■ The authors suggested that the entire group had a "hysterical flavor."
Pfau (1975)	■ psychogenic aphonia/ dysphonia ■ $n = 46$ F; 8 M	■ German equivalent of MMPI	■ Results suggested neurosis in 35% of females patients, 20% of whom were considered a hysterical reaction type. ■ The majority of individual profiles were either uninterpretable (37%), or considered within normal limits (28%).
House & Andrews (1987)	■ functional dysphonia/ aphonia ■ dysphonia (65) ■ aphonia (4) ■ spastic (2)	■ Present State Examination (PSE) ■ Bedford College Life Events & Difficulties Interview (BCLEDI)	■ Authors failed to find an association between voice type and PSE score or psychiatric diagnosis. ■ "The majority of patients were remarkable for the apparent normality of their premorbid psychological and social functioning. Major mental illness was infrequently diagnosed and minor states of tension and anxiety predominated (33%)" (p. 488). ■ FD is not usually found in markedly abnormal personalities and previous episodes of conversion disorder are rare.
Kinzl et al. (1988)	■ "hyperfunctional" and "hypo-functional" aphonia ■ $n = 22$ F	■ Psychiatric evaluations ■ Social support network assessments	■ Patients did not have particular personality traits in common, nor exposed to comparable conflict situations.

Authors	Subjects	Test Instrument(s)	Major Findings and Interpretations
		■ Life event histories	■ "Personality structures and psychopathological symptoms. . . ranged from mild impairment to severe neurosis" (p.134). ■ Hysterical personality traits were frequent, but not always. . . pre-
sent.			
			■ 75% of patients have other psychosomatic functional disturbances in their histories. ■ Authors suggest that aphonia is a homogeneous clinical syndrome with heterogeneous personality structures and psychopathologies underlying its development.
Friedl et al. (1990)	■ functional dysphonia/ aphonia (20) ■ organic dysphonia (14) ■ normal control (20)	■ Multiple measures of personality and anxiety	■ FD patients show a tendency toward restraint, and in stressful situations, the result is an intensified anxiety state. ■ Life events may influence the pathogenesis of FD.
Gerritsma (1991)	■ psychogenic dysphonia/ aphonia ■ *n* = 75 F; 7 M	■ Wilde's Amsterdam Biographical Questionnaire ■ Social Anxiety Scale (SAS) ■ Wolpe-Lazarus Assertiveness Scale (WLAS)	■ 42% of patients scored high on neuroticism (N) and neurotic somatization (NS) scales, a pattern consistent with conversion symptoms; and, 40% scored low on the extraversion (E) scale, suggesting a tendency toward introversion. ■ 4% met DSM (III) criteria for hysterical personality. ■ 65% of subjects were socially anxious, nonassertive or both. ■ Author suggests dropping the term hysterical dysphonia in favor of one of "conversion, psychogenic, or functional" aphonia
Friedl et al. (1993)	■ functional dysphonia/ aphonia	■ "Empirical-psychological procedure"	■ Psychological conditions were major etiologic factors in aphonia, but only partially relevant in
patients			

logical-personality variables must be considered possible etiological, consequential and therapeutic factors."

In a recent work, Roy and coworkers (Roy et al., 1997) attempted to shed further light on the voice–personality relationship. They described the personality/psychological characteristics of 25 female subjects who had received the diagnosis of functional dysphonia. All subjects experienced symptom resolution following voice therapy. While vocally asymptomatic, these remitted functional dysphonia subjects completed the Minnesota Multiphasic Personality Inventory (MMPI), an objective personality questionnaire (Hathaway & McKinley, 1972). When compared to a medical outpatient control group, the results showed that functional dysphonia subjects scored significantly higher on 7 of 10 clinical scales, suggesting an elevated degree of emotional maladjustment. A stepwise discriminant analysis identified two clinical scales that provided valuable discriminatory information. Scale 1 (Hs-Hypochondriasis), which measures number and type of reported somatic complaints, and scale 7 (Pt-Psychaesthenia), a measure of diffuse anxiety, discriminated the groups with 88% sensitivity and 89% specificity. The results suggested that in spite of symptom improvement after voice therapy, the subjects with functional dysphonia continued to exhibit poor levels of adaptive functioning, which may represent trait-like stability. Figure 23–1 illustrates the differences between the functional dysphonia group and the medical controls. The elevations on scales 1, 2, and 3 have come to be known as the neurotic triad and are highly related to the personality dimension of neuroticism, to be discussed later. Furthermore, elevation on scale 7 measures not only diffuse anxiety, but also self-doubt about adequacy in interpersonal situations. When combined with elevation on Scale 0-Social Introversion (Si) (an index of a person's preference for being alone (high 0) or being with others (low 0), a strong case can be made for a tendency toward introversion. High scorers tend to be withdrawn, socially insecure, and anxious when in contact with people. With the exception of Scale 2 (Depression), all clinical scales are viewed as assessments of character, not mood (Butcher, Dahlstrom, Graham, Tellegen & Kaemmer, 1989; Duckworth & Anderson, 1995; Graham, 1987; Graham, 1990; Greene, 1989; Marks et al., 1974; Newmark, 1979). The scatterplot of the distribution of scores for the functional dysphonia subjects versus the controls (Figure 23–2) clearly illustrates the discriminatory value of the two clinical scale variables (i.e., Scales 1 and 7). These data seem to support a dispositional vulnerability for the development of functional symptoms, including laryngeal problems.

2. VOCAL NODULES

Vocal nodules are another voice disorder that potentially illustrates a link between vocal pathology and personality–psychological factors, but much less has been reported on this topic. Vocal nodules are benign callous-like lesions of the vocal folds often attributed to chronic, repetitive phonotrauma creating excessive mechanical tissue stresses and reactive histological changes. They are considered to be one of the most common manifestations of vocal hyperfunction—that is, abuse and/or misuse of the vocal mechanism due to excessive and/or "imbalanced" muscular forces (Hillman, Holmberg, Perkell, Walsh, & Vaughan, 1989), and may account for almost 4% of an otolaryngologic caseload (Nagata et al., 1983). Vocal nodules tend to occur in prepubescent males and postpubescent/premenopausal females. In adults, at least two-thirds of patients with nodules are female (Herrington-Hall, Lee, Stemple, Niemi, & McHone, 1988; Nagata et al., 1983). Surgical removal is one method of treatment; however, a more conservative approach is behavioral voice therapy that attempts to eliminate the putative cause(s) of the vocal nodule rather than the nodule itself. The short-term results of behavioral therapy or surgical excision are generally favorable (Bouchayer & Cornut, 1988; Lancer, Syder, & Jones, 1988; Murry & Woodson, 1992). But few studies have *objectively* evaluated long-term clinical outcomes. At least anecdotally, it appears that despite the efforts of surgeons and voice therapists, the lesions in some adults are resistant to therapy and/or tend to recur (Arnold, 1962; Bridger & Epstein, 1983).

For the most part, authors have attempted to distinguish vocal nodules from other voice disorders, such as functional dysphonia. However, some authors have classified vocal nodules as a functional disorder and have emphasized the role of psychological precursors and predisposing personality factors (Arnold, 1962; Aronson,

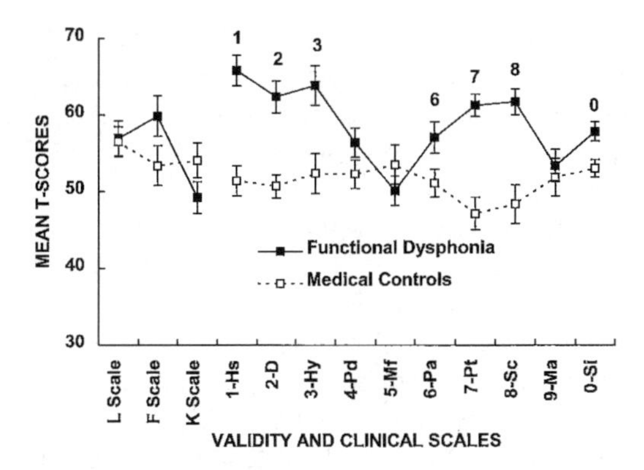

Figure 23–1. Composite MMPI Profiles for Functional Dysphonia and Medical Control Groups using mean T-Scores (± standard error). Numbers placed above select scales indicate significant differences between groups.

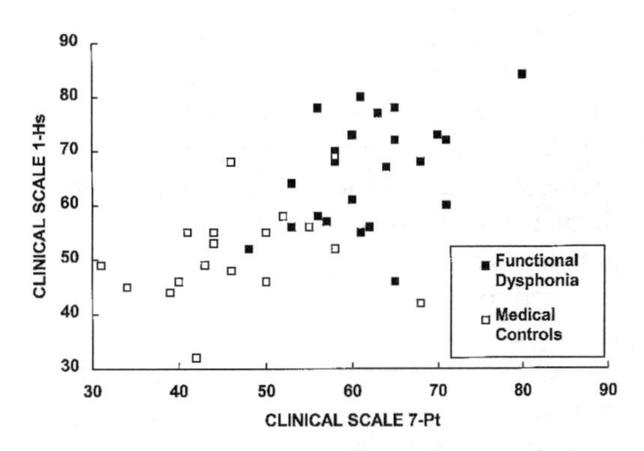

Figure 23–2. Scatterplot of T-Scores obtained for Clinical Scale 1-Hs (ordinate) and Clinical Scale 7-Pt (abscissa) from individual Functional Dysphonia and Medical Control Subjects.

1990; Wilson, 1987). One common assertion is that people with vocal nodules are talkative and have aggressive tendencies (Arnold, 1962; Green, 1989; Mosby, 1970; Nemec, 1961; Toohill, 1975; Wilson, 1971; Wilson & Lamb, 1974; Withers & Dawson, 1960). Elevated levels of anxiety, reduced self-concept, emotional maladjustment, and high levels of extraversion have also been found in patients with vocal nodules (Mosby, 1970; Peter & Brandell, 1980; Toohill, 1975; Yano, Ichimura, Hoshino, & Nozue, 1982).

In a recent study using the MMPI, we identified elevated levels of psychological distress and somatic complaints in a group of adult female vocal nodule patients when compared to a medical out-patient control group (Roy, McGrory, & Bless, 1995). Goldman, Hargrave, Hillman, Holmberg, and Gress (1996) confirmed these findings when they also identified elevated levels of anxiety, somatic complaints, and voice use when compared to non-voice-disordered controls. No differences, however, were identified between the subjects with vocal nodules and a nonpathological-voice disordered control group.

Recently, White, Deary, and Wilson (1997) using the General Health Questionnaire (GHQ), a measure of an individual's number and variety of health complaints, and the Eysenck Personality Questionnaire (EPQ) found no significant differences in personality traits when comparing dysphonic patients (both functional and organic) with ENT outpatient controls. They did, however, identify elevated levels of psychological distress in both voice-disordered groups and concluded that the mere presence or absence of laryngeal pathology was insufficient to identify those dysphonia patients with a major underlying psychological upset. Thus the pattern of results, although by no means definitive, suggests a trend toward elevated levels of extraversion and anxiety among subjects with vocal nodules.

3. TOWARD A THEORY OF THE DISPOSITIONAL BASES OF FUNCTIONAL DYSPHONIA AND VOCAL NODULES

From the previous literature review, it is apparent that the origin of common voice problems such as functional dysphonia and vocal nodules is poorly understood and likely involves the convergence of multiple factors including organic, psychological, and social features. A major obstacle limiting progress in the field of voice pathology is the difficulty in conceptualizing personality–psychological processes that might contribute to the development and maintenance of these voice disorders. An effective theoretical perspective is needed to promote intuitive understanding of these disorders, reconcile divergent research findings, arouse interest in the etiology and treatment of such voice problems, and generate research designed to contrast alternative hypotheses.

Toward this end, we speculate that personality composition, and consequent cognitive processing and behavioral patterns, provides an important footing for the development of both functional dysphonia and vocal nodules. A theory is proposed that couples aspects of a biological theory of personality (Eysenck, 1967; Eysenck & Eysenck, 1985) with a neuropsychological model of the conceptual nervous system (Gray, 1975). Based on differences in personality, this theory predicts *unique* and *contrasting* signal sensitivities and behavioral response biases for individuals with functional dysphonia and vocal nodules. It is proposed that specific personality traits predispose one to develop these disorders, and moderate the symptomatology and course of the voice pathology. Moreover, by virtue of its enduring nature, personality serves as a persistent vulnerability, rendering an individual susceptible for recurrence of symptoms. The following sections describe the theory's foundations and its predictions.

3.1. Defining Personality, Personality Traits, and Trait Structure

Most definitions of personality indicate that it is internal, organized, enduring—characteristic of an individual over time and situations and related to how an individual functions in the world. The term personality implies a complex organization of systematically interrelated trait dispositions (Watson, Clark & Harkness, 1994). It is widely acknowledged that personality traits are hierarchically arranged, with specific but narrow traits at lower levels in the hierarchy and global but broad trait dimensions or domains at the top (Goldberg, 1993; John, 1990). At the highest level of the trait hierarchy are three stable, heritable, general personality dimensions, or "superfactors." These relatively orthogonal superfactors provide for the global classification of personality traits (Costa & McCrae, 1995; Digman & Takemoto-Chock, 1981). The so-called "big three" dimensions have been identified in a wide range of data sources, instruments, samples, and languages (John, 1990) and are commonly known as (1) extraversion versus introversion, (2) neuroticism versus stability, and (3) constraint versus disinhibition.[1] These personality dimensions are typically derived using factor analytic techniques and thus, are not necessarily tied to actual psychobiological processes. However, some investigators such as Hans Eysenck (1967; Eysenck & Eysenck, 1985) and Jeffrey Gray (1982, 1987) have linked the superfactors to specific psychophysiological processes. These associations provide the foundation for a theory linking personality and voice pathology. Extraversion (E) and neuroticism (N) play a vital role in our theory, which synthesizes Eysenck's and Gray's biological theories of personality to account for the development of functional dysphonia and vocal nodules.

3.2. Eysenck's Personality System

Eysenck (1967) developed an integrated biopsychosocial theory of personality that is based primarily on the dimensions of personality, extraversion (E) and neuroticism (N). Extraversion is related to sociable, lively, active, assertive, sensation-seeking, carefree, dominant,

[1]Constraint versus disinhibition is centered on the basic issue of impulse control. High constraint individuals are cautious, restrained, as refraining from risky adventures, and as accepting the conventions of society. These individuals plan carefully before acting and avoid situations involving risk or danger. Low constraint persons are relatively impulsive, adventurous, and inclined to reject conventional restrictions (Clark, Watson, & Mineka, 1994).

and venturesome characteristics. Extraversion involves the willingness to engage and confront the environment, including the social environment. Extraverts (i.e., high E) tend to be dominant, sociable, and active; whereas introverts (i.e., low E) tend to be quiet, unsociable, passive, and careful. Eysenck views E as reflecting stable differences in the tonic activity level of the ascending reticular activating system and, thus, cortical arousal. Introverts are thought to exhibit higher tonic levels of cortical arousal than extraverts. Extraverts are therefore expected to seek stimulation to raise their arousal to more optimal levels. On the other hand, introverts' high level of arousal is associated with the avoidance of excessive stimulation.

N, the second personality dimension, can be likened to emotionality and is related to anxious, depressed, tense, shy, moody, and emotional characteristics, as well as guilt feelings and low self-esteem. High N individuals tend to be emotionally unstable, worried, anxious, or highly reactive to environmental stimuli. Eysenck proposed the visceral brain, consisting of the septum, hippocampus, cingulum, amygdala, and hypothalamus as the neurological substrate (Eysenck & Eysenck, 1985). Neuroticism magnifies response tendencies derived from E (Eysenck & Eysenck, 1975a). Therefore, neurotic introverts tend to be more introverted, and neurotic extraverts tend to be more extraverted, when compared to their stable counterparts.[2]

3.3. Gray's Theory of Personality and Nervous System Function

Gray (1975, 1982, 1985, 1987) has integrated findings from learning, psychometry, pharmacology, neurophysiology, and other areas of research into a general model of personality and functional neuropsychology. He proposed a neuropsychological model of the conceptual nervous system that consists of a set of three interacting components (Figure 23–3): a behavioral activation system (BAS), a behavioral inhibition system (BIS), and a nonspecific arousal system (NAS). The BAS, which is the reward system, is responsive to signals of conditioned reward and nonpunishment; activity increases in the presence of such stimuli. Hence, the BAS—as a functional system—can be conceived as associated with the attainment of motivationally significant goals (i.e., approach behavior). The BAS is considered the "go" system, and promotes the initiation of goal-directed motor behavior including approach, escape, and active avoidance. The BIS, on the other hand, is responsible for organizing reactions to conditioned signals of punishment; signals of frustrative nonreward, novel, or threat stimuli; and a class of innate fear stimuli. Nonreward refers to a context in which a reward is omitted following a response in a situation in which the response had previously been rewarded or in which a reward for the response was anticipated. The psychological state instantiated by the occurrence of such nonrewards is called frustration.

Each of these types of input stimuli is presumed to influence common neural structures located in the septohippocampal system, with connections to the prefrontal cortex. Because the inputs of punishment and frustrative nonreward act on the same neural structures, the effects of nonreward and punishment are considered functionally equivalent. These input signals increase BIS activity, resulting in increased arousal, inhibition of ongoing behavior, and increased attention to the environment. The BIS inhibits or decelerates responses that may lead to punishment or nonreward, producing passive avoidance or extinction. In passive avoidance, an organism can avoid

[2]Eysenck also proposed a third personality dimension known as psychoticism (P) or "tough-mindedness" (Eysenck & Eysenck, 1975b). This broad personality factor shares many of the impulsive features of the constraint dimension (reversed), but also includes a predilection for antisocial and aggressive behavior. The biological substrate of P has been more problematic for Eysenck, and he has suggested that it may be related to individual differences in serotonergic systems (McBurnett, 1992).

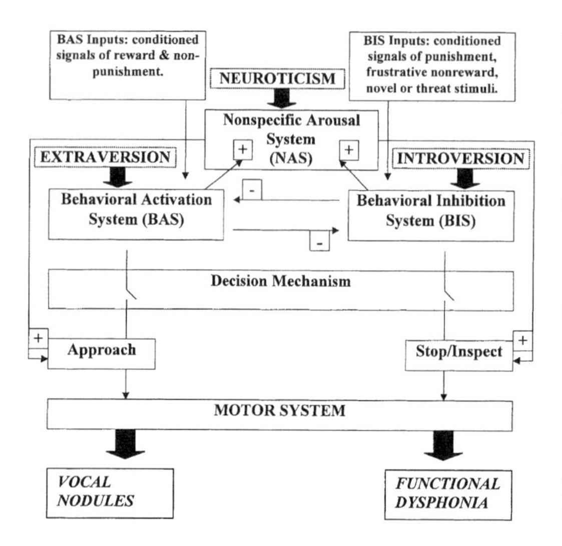

Figure 23–3. A Theory of the Dispositional Bases of Vocal Nodules and Functional Dysphonia. (Adapted from Newman and colleagues, synthesis of Eysenck's [1967] and Gray's [1975] biological theories of personality.) E and N are mapped onto the three systems within Gray's conceptual nervous system model. Functional dysphonia and vocal nodules are seen as behavioral consequences of the signal sensitivities and response biases of BIS dominant neurotic introverts and BAS dominant neurotic extraverts respectively.

receiving punishment or nonreward by not performing a given action (i.e., response suppression). Gray distinguishes this type of avoidance from active avoidance, in which punishment can be avoided if an organism performs a given action.

The third component of Gray's model—the nonspecific arousal system (NAS)—serves to prepare or make ready the organism to respond to BAS or BIS inputs that have motivational or emotional significance. This NAS has been linked to major changes in the functioning of the autonomic nervous system similar to the fight/flight response.

Several general points regarding Gray's theory should be recognized: (1) Reciprocal inhibitory inputs connect the two behavioral systems, such that an increase in the activity of one results in a decrease in the activity of the other. (2) An increase in the activity of either behavioral system results in heightened NAS activity via excitatory outputs from the BAS and BIS. (3) The NAS has excitatory connections affecting responses mediated by the behavioral systems, so that as NAS activity increases, the speed and strength of behavioral responses increase proportionately.

3.4. Dispositional Vulnerability in Functional Dysphonia and Vocal Nodules: The Importance of Extraversion and Neuroticism

Newman and colleagues (Newman & Wallace, 1993a, 1993b; Patterson & Newman, 1993; Wallace & Newman, 1991) proposed a synthesis of Eysenck's and Gray's theoretical formulations to account for breakdowns in self-regulatory behavior observed in disinhibited adults and children. It is this synthesis that provides the foundation for our theory of the dispositional bases of functional dysphonia and vocal nodules (Figure 23–3).

Briefly, the three components of Gray's model are mapped onto Eysenck's personality dimensions of extraversion (E) and neuroticism (N). An individual's position on E reflects the relative strengths of the behavioral systems. For example, in extraverts the BAS is stronger than the BIS, and for introverts the BIS is the stronger of the two systems. Thus, extraverts = BAS dominance = reward sensitive = approach behavior; introverts = BIS dominance = punishment, threat sensitive = stop/reflect behavior. Neuroticism directly reflects the reactivity or lability of the NAS: an individual is neurotic by reason of possessing a more reactive NAS than a stable individual. Neuroticism (N) amplifies response tendencies associated with the two behavioral systems; therefore, as N increases, extraverts tend to act in a more extraverted manner and introverts tend to behave in a more introverted manner. In this model, the combination of neuroticism and extraversion leads to impulsivity (disinhibition), whereas the combination of neuroticism and introversion leads to anxiety/distress (inhibition). Neurotic extraverts are highly reactive, especially to potential rewards, and initiate goal-directed behavior (e.g., approach). On the other hand, neurotic introverts are highly reactive to threatening and unexpected stimuli and are prone to engage in BIS-mediated activities (e.g., motor inhibition, inspecting the environment for potential threats, and passive avoidance).[3]

An important feature of this model is that BAS-dominated neurotic extraverts do not engage in BIS-mediated processes that underlie response modulation (i.e., response interruption, initiation of information gathering and processing) and therefore do not adjust dominant or ongoing responses. This ultimately manifests in forms of perseverative behavior; for example, persistent approach behavior in spite of unfavorable effects. By virtue of heightened NAS activity, impulsive (neurotic extraverts) and anxious individuals (neurotic introverts) are inclined to focus selectively on stimuli of direct relevance to the attainment of their goal, to the exclusion of information that is of peripheral relevance to the current response set. BIS-dominated neurotic introverts are unable to alter dominant response sets such as motor inhibition–passive avoidance, by attending to other information. This model and its presumed signal sensitivities and response biases have implications for both types of voice disorders—functional dysphonia and vocal nodules—which are described in the section that follows.

3.5. Applying the Theory to Individuals With Functional Dysphonia and Vocal Nodules

This theoretical synthesis serves as the foundation for a theory describing the dispositional bases of functional dysphonia and vocal nodules. Functional dysphonia is a voice disorder in the absence of visible structural or neurological pathology. As mentioned previously, psychological processes have been identified as pathogenic; however the underlying mechanism has not been fully elucidated. Earlier we identified that elevated scores on measures of anxiety, somatic complaints, and introversion (see literature review) characterized diagnosed individuals. Excessive voice use has not been confirmed as a causative agent in this form of dysphonia. We contend that functional voice loss is related to anxiety, motor inhibition, and elevated tension states. By virtue of BIS dominance and elevated NAS, *neurotic introverts* tend to have difficulty in evaluating and, if necessary, appropriately altering ongoing responses or response sets in the presence of BIS inputs such as uncertainty, frustrative nonreward, punishment, or potential threats. We speculate that these input signals ultimately contribute to inhibitory laryngeal motor behavior in at least two possible ways. These mechanisms are not independent or mutually exclusive and, therefore, could be operating in combination within a single individual.

First, individuals who are BIS-dominant will exhibit hypervigilance concerning their environment, including their internal body environment. A chief function of the BIS is to compare actual with expected stimuli. The system exercises selective control over the sensory information that reaches it, and tags it as important or filters it out as unimportant. Once activated, the system is assumed to heighten attentional awareness and focus on potential threats. Ambiguous sensory changes accompanying minor alterations in laryngeal function as a result of infection, edema, reflux laryngitis, or emotional states are tagged by the BIS as a mismatch: novel and perhaps threatening. In combination with increased

[3] **"Neurotic" as it is used in the context of this chapter should not be misinterpreted as synonymous with the Freudian notion of the neurotic (i.e., an individual manifesting a clinical neurosis). Rather, neurotic is used here to describe individuals who score above the median on N- sensitive measures, such as the Eysenck Personality Questionnaire (Eysenck & Eysenck, 1975). It is essential to recognize that individuals who are high scorers on N are not necessarily clinically disturbed or even dysfunctional.**

arousal, further attentional resources are directed to the circumlaryngeal area combined with interruption of ongoing motor programs, that is, laryngeal motor inhibition. In this control mode, the inputs of uncertainty persist, the problem is intensified, and the patient is unable to interrupt this inhibitory response pattern. The neocortical control of speech and language is unaffected, but inhibitory control by the septohippocampal system dominates, preventing normal phonation. Sustained motor inhibition without appropriate release leads to unnecessarily high muscular tonus. Partial or complete voice loss reflects the cumulative effects of heightened NAS and BIS, with resultant motor inhibition and elevated tension states.

The second pathway to vocal dysregulation emphasizes frustrative nonreward and punishment as important inputs for BIS activation. Recall that frustrative nonreward occurs in circumstances in which a reward is omitted following a response in a situation in which the response had been previously rewarded or in which a reward for the response was anticipated. The effects of nonreward where it had been anticipated are functionally equivalent to punishment. Thus, the BIS inhibits responses that may lead to frustration. The inhibition system is activated only when the individual anticipates the omission of a reward or punishment following a response. The BIS system takes active control over vocal behavior on receipt of stimuli, which have preceded (on a previous occasion), the disruptive event (frustrative nonreward or punishment). If vocalization (speaking out) has resulted in frustrative nonreward or punishment in the past, such vocalization will be inhibited (i.e., passive avoidance). Recall that in passive avoidance an organism can avoid receiving punishment by not performing a given action. The failure to respond removes the potential for punishment. The BIS is assumed to increase passive avoidance and inhibits actions that might result in punishment.

A common theme in most writings about antecedents to psychogenic voice loss involves (1) a conflict over speaking out or expressing an unfavorable opinion and/or (2) chronic stress involving job and family responsibilities, marital dissatisfaction, or long-standing communication breakdowns (Aronson, 1990; Butcher, 1995; House & Andrews, 1988). When the subject has experienced undesirable punishing or frustrating outcomes paired with previous attempts to speak out, these become conditioned inputs for the BIS. The BIS outputs remain the same regardless of the inputs. In the case of human voice production, the newer phylogenetic system (neocortex) competes with inputs from the older phylogenetic system (septohippocampal system). By way of the BIS, this older brain region may stimulate inhibition of vocalization (i.e., laryngeal "freezing" behavior); whereas the neocortex carries out its communicative intent/goal. This conflict between inhibition and activation may give rise to incomplete or disordered vocalization in a structurally and neurologically intact larynx.

As mentioned earlier, vocal nodules are benign lesions of the vocal folds thought to be caused by repetitive mucosal injury leading to histological changes and concomitant voice mutation. Excessive voice use and abuse have been implicated as causative agents. Although treatment (surgical and/or voice therapy) may improve the voice in the short term, less is known regarding long-term outcomes. Recurrence of dysphonia seems common, rather than the exception. We allege that vocal nodule development is in part a result of an information processing pattern related to the *impulsive behavior of neurotic extraverts* (i.e., BAS dominance with elevated NAS activity). In spite of the obvious harmful effects (voice change, laryngeal discomfort) of this perseverative behavior, patients with vocal nodules often appear unable to engage in appropriate response modulation (i.e., to stop vocal overuse and abuse) in the presence of salient "social" reward cues. Consequently, we reason that vocal nodule patients should score high on indices of extraversion (dominance, sociability) and neuroticism (emotional reactivity) and low on measures of constraint (i.e., reflecting impulsivity). Neuroticism serves to potentiate the signal sensitivities and response biases of extraversion leading to impulsivity.

The role of impulsivity in the development and maintenance of vocal nodules has not received much attention in the voice literature. Impulsivity is admittedly a complicated construct, but most current descriptions of impulsivity include some form of behavioral excess, in the sense of doing something that potentially leads to trouble. The behavior is viewed as impulsive, because good judgment would suggest that it be inhibited (Fowles, 1987). Vocal nodules are presumed to be related to forms of behavioral excess, for instance excessive voice use and abuse. The theory espoused here holds that when anticipating social rewards, individuals with vocal nodules will fail to inhibit vocal overuse and abuse in spite of obvious signs of trouble, such as audible voice deterioration and laryngeal discomfort. Engaging in persistent vocal behavior in spite of its untoward effects is viewed as impulsive, because good judgment would suggest that it be inhibited.

To summarize, we connect the development of functional dysphonia and vocal nodules to personality differences related to dissimilar signal sensitivities and response biases of neurotic introverts and neurotic extraverts, respectively. We credit hyperreactivity of the BIS as a prime constituent in the pathogenesis of functional dysphonia, whereas hyperreactivity of the BAS is pathogenic in vocal nodule development. Both behavioral systems are potentiated by the NAS. This synthesis of two biological theories of personality as an explanatory model serves as a heuristic for future research. If a theory is to have scientific value, it must be open to test. One must be able to derive hypotheses from it that allow new evidence to be gathered that either refutes the theory or fails to do so, thus adding to its credibility. From this perspective, we believe that this theory and its derivations presents a decided advantage over other psychoanalytically-based formulations of being open to test by a variety of approaches. We look forward to such scientific inquiry.

Assessment of these broad personality dimensions, and the traits subsumed within, is needed to help clinicians better appreciate the relation between personality, psychological factors, and voice pathology. Until the role of personality in the pathogenesis of voice disorders is better understood, *long-term* clinical outcomes for these populations may remain unsatisfactory (Bridger & Epstein, 1983; Roy, Bless, Heisey, & Ford, 1997). Improved understanding of its influence could help to explain voice therapy failure and refine treatment strategies in some cases. If personality represents a persistent predisposition for the development, maintenance, and recurrence of certain voice pathologies, then assessment and management practices may need to be revised.

REFERENCES

American Psychiatric Association (APA), (1994). *Diagnostic and statistical manual of mental disorders* (DSM-IV) (4th ed.).Washington, DC: Author.

Alexander, F. (1950). *Psychosomatic medicine: Its principles and applications.* New York: W. W. Norton and Company.

Alexander, F., French, T. M., & Pollock, G. H. (Eds.). (1968). *Psychosomatic specificity. Vol. 1: Experimental study and results.* Chicago: University of Chicago Press.

Aronson, A. E. (1990). *Clinical voice disorders: An interdisciplinary approach* (3rd ed.). New York: Thieme.

Aronson, A. E., Peterson, H. W., & Litin, E. M. (1966). Psychiatric symptomatology in functional dysphonia and aphonia. *Journal of Speech and Hearing Disorders, 31,* 115–127.

Arnold, G. A. (1962). Vocal nodules and polyps: Laryngeal tissue reaction to hyperkinetic dysphonia. *Journal of Speech and Hearing Disorders, 27,* 205–217.

Bass, C. M. (Ed.). (1990). *Somatization: Physical symptoms and psychological illness.* London: Blackwell Scientific Publications.

Boone, D. R., McFarlane, S.C. (1988). *The voice and voice therapy* (4th ed.). Englewood Cliffs, NJ: Prentice-Hall.

Bouchayer, M., & Cornut, G. (1988). Microsurgery for benign lesions of the vocal folds. *Ear, Nose, and Throat Journal, 67,* 446–466.

Bridger, M. W., & Epstein, R. (1983). Functional voice disorders: A review of 109 patients. *Journal of Laryngology and Otology, 97,* 1145–1148.

Brodnitz, F. S. (1962). Functional disorders of the voice. In N. M. Levin (Ed.), *Voice and speech disor-*

ders: Medical aspects (pp. 453–481). Springfield, IL: Charles C. Thomas.

Brodnitz, F. S. (1981). Psychological considerations in vocal rehabilitation. *Journal of Speech and Hearing Disorders, 42,* 21–26.

Butcher, J. N., Dahlstrom, W. G., Graham, J. R., Tellegen, A., & Kaemmer, B. (1989). *MMPI-2 (Minnesota Multiphasic Personality Inventory—2): Manual of administration and scoring.* Minneapolis: University of Minnesota Press.

Butcher, P. (1995). Psychological processes in psychogenic voice disorder. *European Journal of Disorders of Communication, 30,* 467–474.

Butcher, P., Elias, A., & Raven, R. (1993). *Psychogenic voice disorders and cognitive behaviour therapy.* San Diego: Singular Publishing Group.

Butcher, P., Elias, A., Raven, R., Yeatman, J., & Littlejohns, D. (1987). Psychogenic voice disorder unresponsive to speech therapy: Psychological characteristics and cognitive-behaviour therapy. *British Journal of Disorders of Communication, 22,* 81–92.

Cannito, M. P. (1991). Emotional considerations in spasmodic dysphonia: Psychometric Quantification. *Journal of Communicative Disorders, 24,* 313–329

Clark, L. A., Watson, D., & Mineka, S. (1994). Temperament, personality, and the mood and anxiety disorders. *Journal of Abnormal Psychology, 103,* 103–116.

Colton, R., & Casper, J. K. (1996). *Understanding voice problems: A physiological perspective for diagnosis and treatment.* Baltimore: Williams & Wilkins.

Costa, P. T., Jr., & McCrae, R. R. (1995). Domains and facets: Hierarchical personality assessment using the Revised NEO Personality Inventory. *Journal of Personality Assessment, 64,* 21–50.

Deary, I. J., Scott, S., Wilson, I. M., White, A., MacKenzie, K., & Wilson, J. A. (1997). Personality and psychological distress in dysphonia. *British Journal of Health Psychology, 2,* 333–341.

Dembo, T., Levitan, G., & Wright, B. (1975). Adjustment to misfortune: A problem of social psychology rehabilitation. *Rehabilitation Psychology, 22,* 1–100.

Diehl, C. F. (1960). Voice and personality: An evaluation. In D. A. Barbara (Ed.), *Psychological and psychiatric aspects of speech and hearing* (pp. 171–203). Springfield, IL: Charles C. Thomas

Digman, J. M., & Takemoto-Chock, N. K. (1981). Factors in the natural language of personality: Re-analysis and comparison of six major studies. *Multivariate Behavioral Research, 16,* 149–170.

Dubovsky, S. L., & Weissberg, M. P. (1982). *Reactions to illness: In clinical psychiatry in primary care* (2nd ed.). Baltimore: Williams & Wilkins.

Duckworth, J. C., & Anderson, W. P. (1995). *MMPI and MMPI—2: Interpretation manual for counselors and clinicians.* Philadelphia: Taylor and Francis Group.

Epstein. S. (1979). The stability of behavior: I. On predicting most of the people much of the time. *Journal of Personality and Social Psychology, 37,* 1097–1126.

Eysenck, H .J. (1967). *The biological basis of personality.* Springfield, IL: Thomas.

Eysenck, H. J., & Eysenck, S. B. (1975a). *Manual of the Eysenck Personality Questionnaire.* San Diego, CA: Educational and Industrial Testing Service.

Eysenck, H. J., & Eysenck, S. B. (1975b). *Psychoticism as a dimension of personality.* London: Hodder & Stoughton.

Eysenck, H. J., & Eysenck, M. W. (1987). *Personality and individual differences: A natural science approach.* New York/London: Plenum Press.

Fex, B.F., Fex, S., Shiromoto, O., & Hirano, M. (1994). Acoustic analysis of functional dysphonia: Before and after voice therapy (Accent Method). *Journal of Voice, 8,* 163–167.

Fowles, D. C. (1987). Application of a behavioral theory of motivation to the concepts of anxiety and impulsivity. *Journal of Research in Personality,* 21, 417–435.

Friedl, W., Friedrich, G., & Egger, J. (1990). Personality and coping with stress in patients suffering from functional dysphonia. *Folia Phoniatrica, 42,* 144–149.

Friedl, W., Friedrich, G, Egger, J., & Fitzek, I. (1993). Psychogenic aspects of functional dysphonia. *Folia Phoniatrica, 45,* 10–13.

Gerritsma, E. J. (1991). An investigation into some personality characteristics of patients with psychogenic aphonia and dysphonia. *Folia Phoniatrica, 43,* 13–20.

Goldberg, L. R. (1993). The structure of phenotypic personality traits. *American Psychologist, 48,* 26–34.

Goldman, S. L., Hargrave, J., Hillman, R. E., Holmberg, E., & Gress, C. (1996). Stress, anxiety, somatic complaints, and voice use in women with vocal nodules: Preliminary findings. *American Journal of Speech-Language Pathology: A Journal of Clinical Practice, 5,* 44–54.

Goodstein, L. D. (1958). Functional speech disorders and personality: A survey of the research. *Journal of Speech and Hearing Research, 1,* 359–376.

Graham, J. R. (1987). *The MMPI: A practical guide* (2nd ed.). New York: Oxford University Press.

Graham, J. R. (1990). *MMPI—2: Assessing personality and psychopathology*. New York: Oxford University Press.

Gray, J. A. (1975). *Elements of a two-process theory of learning*. London: Academic Press.

Gray, J. A. (1981). A critique of Eysenck's theory of personality. In H. J. Eysenck (Ed.), *A model for personality* (pp. 246–276). New York: Springer-Verlag.

Gray, J. A. (1982). *The neuropsychology of anxiety*. New York: Oxford University Press.

Gray, J. A. (1985). Issues in the neuro-psychology of anxiety. In A. H. Tuma & J. D. Maser (Eds.), *Anxiety and the anxiety disorders* (pp. 5–25). Hillsdale, NJ: Erlbaum.

Gray, J. A. (1987). *The psychology of fear and stress* (2nd ed.). New York: Cambridge University Press.

Green, G. (1988). The inter-relationship between vocal and psychological characteristics: A literature review. *Australian Journal of Human Communication Disorders, 16*, 31–43.

Green, G. (1989). Psycho-behavioral characteristics of children with vocal nodules: WPBIC ratings. *Journal of Speech and Hearing Disorders, 54*, 306–312.

Greene, M. C., & Mathieson, L. (1989). *The voice and its disorders* (5th ed). London: Whurr Publishers.

Greene, R. L. (1989). *The MMPI: An interpretive manual* (2nd ed.). New York: Grune & Stratton.

Hathaway, S. R., & McKinley, J. C. (1972). *The Minnesota Multiphasic Personality Inventory*. New York: Psychological Corporation.

Heaver, L (1960). Spastic dysphonia: A psychosomatic voice disorder. In D. A. Barbara (Ed.), *Psychological and psychiatric aspects of speech and hearing* (pp. 250–263). Springfield, IL: Charles C. Thomas.

Herrington-Hall, B. L., Lee, L., Stemple, J. C., Niemi, K. R., & McHone, M. M. (1988). Description of laryngeal pathologies by age, sex, and occupation in a treatment-seeking sample. *Journal of Speech and Hearing Disorders, 53*, 57–64.

Hillman, R. E., Holmberg, E. B., Perkell, J. S., Walsh, M., & Vaughan, C. (1989). Objective assessment of vocal hyperfunction: An experimental framework and initial results. *Journal of Speech and Hearing Research, 32*, 373–392.

House, A. O., & Andrews, H. B. (1987). The psychiatric and social characteristics of patients with functional dysphonia. *Journal of Psychosomatic Research, 3*, 483–490.

House, A. O., & Andrews, H. B. (1988). Life events and difficulties preceding the onset of functional dysphonia. *Journal of Psychosomatic Research, 31*, 311–319.

Irwin, J. V. (1960). Psychological implications of voice and articulation disturbances. In D. A. Barbara (Ed.). *Psychological and psychiatric aspects of speech and hearing* (pp. 288–317). Springfield, IL: Charles C. Thomas.

John, O. P. (1990). The "Big Five" factor taxonomy: Dimension of personality in the natural language and in questionnaires. In L. A. Pervin (Ed.), *Handbook of personality: Theory and research* (pp. 66–100). New York: Guilford Press.

Kirmayer, L. J., & Robbins, J. M. (Eds.). (1991). *Current concepts of somatization: Research and clinical perspectives*. Washington, DC: American Psychiatric Press, Inc.

Kinzl, J., Biebl, W., & Rauchegger, H. (1988). Functional aphonia: Psychosomatic aspects of diagnosis and therapy. *Folia Phoniatrica, 40*, 131–137.

Koufman, J. A., & Blalock, P. D. (1982). Classification and approach to patients with functional voice disorders. *Annals of Otology, Rhinology and Laryngology, 91*, 372–377.

Lancer, J. M., Syder D., Jones A. S., & Boutillier, A. L. (1988). The outcome of different management patterns for vocal cord nodules. *Journal of Laryngology and Otology, 102*, 423–427.

Mans, E. J. (1994). Psychotherapeutic treatment of patients with functional voice disorders. *Folia Phoniatrica, 46*, 1–8.

Marks, P. A., Seeman, W., & Haller, D. L. (1974). *The actuarial use of the MMPI with adolescents and adults*. Baltimore: Williams & Wilkins Company.

McBurnett, K. (1992). Psychobiological approaches to personality and their applications to child psychopathology. In B. B. Lahey & A. E. Kazdin (Eds.), *Advances in Clinical Child Psychology* (Vol. 14). New York: Plenum Press.

Milutinovic, Z. (1991). Inflammatory changes as a risk factor in the development of phononeurosis. *Folia Phoniatrica, 43*, 177–180.

Morrison, M. D., Nichol, H., & Rammage, L. A. (1986). Diagnostic criteria in functional dysphonia. *Laryngoscope, 96*, 1–8.

Morrison, M. D., & Rammage, L.A. (1993). Muscle misuse voice disorders: Description and classification. *Acta Otolaryngologica (Stockholm), 113*, 428–434.

Mosby, D. P. (1970). Psychotherapy versus voice therapy for a child with a deviant voice. A case study. *Perceptual Motor Skills, 30*, 887–891.

Murry, T., & Woodson, G., (1992). Comparison of three methods for the management of vocal fold nodules. *Journal of Voice, 6*, 271–276.

Murry, T., Cannito, M. P., & Woodson, G. E. (1994). Spasmodic dysphonia: Emotional status and botulinum toxin treatment. *Archives of Otolaryngology, Head and Neck Surgery, 120,* 310–316.

Nagata, K., Kurita, S., Yasumoto, S., Maeda, T., Kawasaki, H., & Hirano, M. (1983). Vocal fold polyps and nodules: A 10 year review of 1,156 patients. *Auris, Nasus, Larynx, 10* (Suppl.), S27–S35.

Nemec, J. (1961). The motivation background of hyperkinetic dysphonia in children: A contribution to psychologic research in phoniatry. *LOGOS, 4,* 28–31.

Newman, J. P., & Wallace, J. F. (1993a). Cognition and Psychopathy. In K. S. Dobson & P. C. Kendall (Eds.), *Psychopathology and cognition.* New York: Academic Press.

Newman, J. P., & Wallace, J. F. (1993b). Diverse pathways to deficient self-regulation: Implications for disinhibitory psychopathology in children. *Clinical Psychology Review, 13,* 699–720.

Newmark, C. S. (1979). *MMPI clinical and research trends.* New York: Praeger.

Nichol, H., Morrison, M. D., & Rammage, L. A. (1993). Interdisciplinary approach to functional voice disorders: The psychiatrist's role. *Otolaryngology Head and Neck Surgery, 108,* 643–647.

Pahn, J., & Friemart, K. (1988). Differential Diagnostische und terminologische Erwagungen bei sogenannten; funktionellen Störungen im neuropsychiatrischen und Phoniatrischen. Fachgebiet. 2. Phoniatrischer Aspeckt. *Folia Phoniatrica, 40,* 168–174.

Patterson, C. M., & Newman, J. P. (1993). Reflectivity and learning from aversive events: Toward a psychological mechanism for the syndromes of disinhibition. *Psychological Review, 4,* 716–736.

Peter, F., & Brandell, M. E. (1980 November), *A study on the self-concept of children with vocal nodules.* Paper presented at the American Speech-Language-Hearing Association, Boston, MA.

Pfau, E. M. (1975). Psychologische Untersuchungsergegnisse sur atiologie der psychogenen Dysphonien. *Folia Phoniatrica, 27,* 298–306.

Rammage, L. A., Nichol, H., & Morrison, M. D. (1987). The psychopathology of voice disorders. *Human Communications Canada, 11,* 21–25.

Reiser, D.E. (1980). Reactions to illness. In D.E. Reiser & A.K. Schroder, (Eds.). *Patient interviewing: The human dimension.* Baltimore: Williams & Wilkins.

Roy, N., & Leeper, H. A. (1993). Effects of the manual laryngeal musculoskeletal tension reduction technique as a treatment for functional voice disorders: Perceptual and acoustic measures. *Journal of Voice, 7,* 242–249.

Roy, N., McGrory, J. J., & Bless, D. M. (1995). *Psychological correlates of patients with vocal nodules.* Paper presented at the American Speech and Hearing Association convention, New Orleans, LA.

Roy, N., McGrory, J .J., Tasko, S. M., Bless, D. M., Heisey, D., & Ford, C. N. (1997). Psychological correlates of functional dysphonia: An investigation using the Minnesota Multiphasic Personality Inventory. *Journal of Voice, 11,* 443–451.

Roy, N., Bless, D. M., Heisey, D., & Ford, C. N. (1997). Manual circumlaryngeal therapy for functional dysphonia: An evaluation of short- and long-term treatment outcomes. *Journal of Voice, 11,* 321–331.

Sapir, S. (1995). Psychogenic spasmodic dysphonia: A case study with expert opinions. *Journal of Voice, 9,* 270–281.

Schalen, L., & Andersson, K. (1992). Differential diagnosis and treatment of psychogenic voice disorder. *Clinical Otolaryngology, 17,* 225–230.

Stemple, J. C. (1984). *Clinical voice pathology: Theory and management.* Columbus, OH: Charles E. Merrill.

Stemple, J. C. (1993). *Voice therapy: Clinical studies.* St. Louis: Mosby-Year Book.

Toohill, R. J. (1975). The psychosomatic aspects of children with vocal nodules. *Archives of Otolaryngology, 101,* 591–595.

Wallace, J. F., & Newman, J. P. (1991). Failures of response modulation: Impulsive behavior in anxious and impulsive individuals. *Journal of Research in Personality, 25,* 23–44.

Watson, D., Clark, L. A., & Harkness, A. R. (1994). Structures of personality and their relevance to psychopathology. *Journal of Abnormal Psychology, 103,* 18–31.

White, A., Deary, I. J., & Wilson, J. A. (1997). Psychiatric disturbance and personality traits in dysphonic patients. *European Journal of Disorders in Communication, 32,* 307–314.

Wilson, F. B. (1971). Emotional stress may cause voice anomalies in kids. *Journal of the American Medical Association, 216,* 2085.

Wilson, F. B., & Lamb, M. (1974) Comparison of personality characteristics of children with and without vocal nodules based on Rorschach protocol interpretation. *Acta Symbolica,* 43–55.

Wilson, D. K. (1987). *Voice problems of children* (3rd ed.). Baltimore, MD: Williams & Wilkins.

Withers, B. T., & Dawson, M. H. (1960). Psychological aspects: Treatment of vocal nodule cases. *Texas State Journal of Medicine, 56,* 43–46.

Yano, J., Ichimura, K., Hoshino, T., & Nozue, M. (1982). Personality factors in pathogenesis of polyps and nodules of vocal cords. *Auris, Nasus, Larynx, 9,* 105–110.

INDEX

E

F

N

O

P

Q

R

S

T

U

V

W